Essentials of
GYNECOLOGY

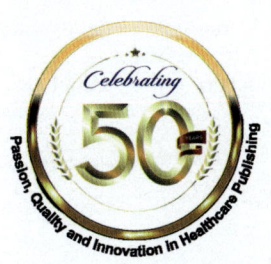

Essentials of GYNECOLOGY

Third Edition

Editors

Sabaratnam Arulkumaran
DCH FRCS FRCOG FAMS MD PhD Hon FACOG FSLCOG FSOGC
Emeritus Professor, Department of Obstetrics and Gynecology
St George's University of London, London, United Kingdom

V Sivanesaratnam
MBBS (S'pore) FRCOG FICS FACS FAMM FAOFOG
Consultant Gynecologist/Gynecologic Oncologist
University of Malaya Specialist Centre, Kuala Lumpur, Malaysia
Emeritus Professor, Department of Obstetrics and Gynecology
University of Malaya, Kuala Lumpur

Formerly, Professor, Head and Senior Consultant
Department of Obstetrics and Gynecology
University of Malaya, Kuala Lumpur, Malaysia

Alokendu Chatterjee
FRCOG FICS
Formerly, Head, Department of Obstetrics and Gynecology
NRS Medical College and Hospital
Kolkata, West Bengal, India

Pratap Kumar
MD DNB
Professor, Department of Obstetrics and Gynecology
Kasturba Medical College, Manipal University
Manipal, Karnataka, India

Foreword
Shirish S Sheth

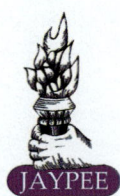

JAYPEE BROTHERS MEDICAL PUBLISHERS
The Health Sciences Publisher
New Delhi | London | Panama

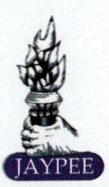

Jaypee Brothers Medical Publishers (P) Ltd

Headquarters
Jaypee Brothers Medical Publishers (P) Ltd
4838/24, Ansari Road, Daryaganj
New Delhi 110 002, India
Phone: +91-11-43574357
Fax: +91-11-43574314
Email: jaypee@jaypeebrothers.com

Overseas Offices

J.P. Medical Ltd
83 Victoria Street, London
SW1H 0HW (UK)
Phone: +44 20 3170 8910
Fax: +44 (0)20 3008 6180
Email: info@jpmedpub.com

Jaypee-Highlights Medical Publishers Inc
City of Knowledge, Bld. 235, 2nd Floor
Clayton, Panama City, Panama
Phone: +1 507-301-0496
Fax: +1 507-301-0499
Email: cservice@jphmedical.com

Jaypee Brothers Medical Publishers (P) Ltd
Bhotahity, Kathmandu, Nepal
Phone: +977-9741283608
Email: kathmandu@jaypeebrothers.com

Website: www.jaypeebrothers.com
Website: www.jaypeedigital.com

© 2019, Jaypee Brothers Medical Publishers

The views and opinions expressed in this book are solely those of the original contributor(s)/author(s) and do not necessarily represent those of editor(s) of the book.

All rights reserved. No part of this publication may be reproduced, stored or transmitted in any form or by any means, electronic, mechanical, photocopying, recording or otherwise, without the prior permission in writing of the publishers.

All brand names and product names used in this book are trade names, service marks, trademarks or registered trademarks of their respective owners. The publisher is not associated with any product or vendor mentioned in this book.

Medical knowledge and practice change constantly. This book is designed to provide accurate, authoritative information about the subject matter in question. However, readers are advised to check the most current information available on procedures included and check information from the manufacturer of each product to be administered, to verify the recommended dose, formula, method and duration of administration, adverse effects and contraindications. It is the responsibility of the practitioner to take all appropriate safety precautions. Neither the publisher nor the author(s)/editor(s) assume any liability for any injury and/or damage to persons or property arising from or related to use of material in this book.

This book is sold on the understanding that the publisher is not engaged in providing professional medical services. If such advice or services are required, the services of a competent medical professional should be sought.

Every effort has been made where necessary to contact holders of copyright to obtain permission to reproduce copyright material. If any have been inadvertently overlooked, the publisher will be pleased to make the necessary arrangements at the first opportunity. The **CD/DVD-ROM** (if any) provided in the sealed envelope with this book is complimentary and free of cost. **Not meant for sale.**

Inquiries for bulk sales may be solicited at: jaypee@jaypeebrothers.com

Essentials of Gynecology

First Edition: 1996
Second Edition: 2011
Third Edition: **2019**

ISBN 978-93-86261-69-4

Printed at: Samrat Offset Pvt. Ltd.

Contributors

Akhila Vasudeva MD DGO
Associate Professor
Department of Obstetrics and Gynecology
Kasturba Medical College and Hospital
Manipal, Karnataka, India
Chapter: 26

Alok Sharma MD
Registrar
Kamla Nehru State Hospital for Mother and Child
Indira Gandhi Medical College
Shimla, Himachal Pradesh, India
Chapter: 30

Anna Gracia Perez-Bonfils MD
Consultant Gynecologist
Institut Marquès
Paseo Manuel Girona, Barcelona, Spain
Chapter: 4

AP Manjunath MD
Ex-Assistant Professor
Department of Obstetrics and Gynecology
Kasturba Medical College and Hospital
Manipal, Karnataka, India
Chapters: 3 and 23

Arun Nagrath MS FICOG FICMCH FICMU MIAC
Professor
Department of Obstetrics and Gynecology
SN Medical College
Agra, Uttar Pradesh, India
Chapter: 5

B Kanchana Devi MD
Assistant Professor
Chettinad Hospital and Research Institute
Chennai, Tamil Nadu, India
Chapter: 9

Christina Portelli MD MRCOG
Post CCT Fellow
Department of Obstetrics and Gynecology
Norfolk and Norwich University Hospital
Norwich, United Kingdom
Chapter: 38

Claire Stewart MD
Research Fellow
Department of Gynae-oncology and Palliative Care
Royal Derby Hospital
Derby, United Kingdom
Chapter: 42

Claudine Domoney FRCOG
Consultant
Department of Obstetrics and Gynecology
Chelsea & Westminster Hospital NHS Trust
London, United Kingdom
Chapter: 17

Deeksha Pandey MD
Associate Professor
Department of Obstetrics and Gynecology
Kasturba Medical College, Manipal University
Manipal, Karnataka, India
Chapter: 19

Edwin Chandraharan FRCOG
Labour Ward Lead/Clinical Director for Women's Services
Department of Obstetrics and Gynecology
St George's University Hospitals NHS Foundation Trust
London, United Kingdom
Chapter: 4

Jaideep Malhotra MD FICOG FICMCH FICS FRCOG FMAS
Director, Malhotra Nursing and Maternity Home (P) Ltd.
Consultant, Apollo Pankaj Hospital
Agra, Uttar Pradesh, India
Vice-President
Elect FOGSI 2010
Chapter: 22

Jayaraman Nambiar MD DGO
Associate Professor
Department of Obstetrics and Gynecology
Kasturba Medical College
Manipal University
Manipal, Karnataka, India
Chapters: 3 and 23

K Jayakrishnan MD DGO DIPNB
Director
KJK Hospital
Thiruvananthapuram, Kerala, India
Chapters: 15 and 16

Keshav Pai MD
Consultant Obstetrician and Gynecologist
Seth GS Medical College and KEM Hospital
Mumbai, Maharashtra, India
Chapter: 7

Krishnendu Mukherjee MS FRCS FRCS (Ed)
Chairman, Dillons Kidney Foundation
Consultant, General and Vascular Surgeon, AMRI Hospitals
Consultant and Surgeon, Belle Vue Clinic
Kolkata, West Bengal, India
Examiner, Royal College of Surgeons of Edinburgh
Edinburgh, Scotland
Chapter: 24

Lim Boon Kiong MBBS (UM), MRCOG
Associate Professor and Consultant
Department of Obstetrics and Gynecology
University of Malaya
Kuala Lumpur, Malaysia
Chapter: 37

Muralidhar V Pai MD
Professor
Department of Obstetrics and Gynecology
Kasturba Medical College and Hospital
Manipal, Karnataka, India
Chapters: 31 and 32

N Pandiyan MBBS MD
Chief Consultant and Head
Department of Andrology and Reproductive Medicine
Chettinad Hospital and Research Institute
Director, Chettinad Hospital and Research Institute
Chennai, Tamil Nadu, India
Chapter: 9

Narendra Malhotra MD FICOG FICMCH FRCOG FICS FMAS FIAP
Professor and Head
Malhotra Nursing and Maternity Home (P) Ltd.
Agra, Uttar Pradesh, India
Chapter: 22

Neharika Malhotra Bora MD FICMCH FMAS MS
Consultant Obstetrician and Gynecologist
Malhotra Nursing and Maternity Home (P) Ltd.
Agra, Uttar Pradesh, India
Chapter: 22

Nozer Sheriar MD DNBE FCPS FICOG DGO
Consultant Obstetrician and Gynecologist
BD Petit Parsee General Hospital
Mumbai, Maharashtra, India
Chapter: 1

Nuguelis Razali MBBS (UM) Master O&G(UM)
Senior Lecturer
Department of Obstetrics and Gynecology
University of Malaya
Kuala Lumpur, Malaysia
Chapter: 29

Onnig Tamizian FRCOG LLM (Medical Law)
Consultant Obstetrician and Gynecologist
Lead Colposcopy
Royal Derby Hospital
United Kingdom
Chapter: 42

P Manjula MBBS MD
Consultant
Department of Obstetrics and Gynecology
Fernandez Hospital
Hyderabad, Telangana, India
Chapters: 15 and 16

PK Sekharan MD
Former Professor and Head
Department of Obstetrics and Gynecology
Institute of Maternal and Child Health Medical College,
Calicut, Kerala, India
Chapter: 8

PK Shah MD FICOG FCPS FICMU FICM CH DGO DFP
Professor and Unit Head
Department of Obstetrics and Gynecology
Seth GS Medical College and KEM Hospital
Mumbai, Maharashtra, India
Chapter: 7

Contributors

Pralhad Kushtagi MD DNB FICOG
Professor
Department of Obstetrics and Gynecology
Kasturba Medical College
Mangaluru, Karnataka, India
Chapter: 18

Prashant Nadkarni MBBS (UM) FRCOG
Consultant Gynecologist
Kuala Lumpur Fertility and Gynaecology Centre
Kuala Lumpur, Malaysia
Chapter: 33

Prashanth K Adiga MD
Professor and Head
Department of Obstetrics and Gynecology
Gadag Institute of Medical Sciences
Gadag, Karnataka, India
Chapter: 25

Pratap Kumar MD DGO FICS FICOG FICMCH
Professor, Department of Obstetrics and Gynecology
Kasturba Medical College
Manipal University
Manipal, Karnataka, India
Chapters: 2, 3, 5, 12, 13, 14, 25, 26 and 30

Premitha Damodaran MBBS Master O&G (UM)
Consultant Obstetrican and Gynaecologist
Pantai Medical Centre
Formerly Lecturer
Department of Obstetrics and Gynecology
University of Malaya
Kuala Lumpur, Malaysia
Chapter: 34

Rajesh Bhakta MD
Consultant
Department of Obstetrics and Gynecology
Roshni Laparoscopy and Infertility Centre
Kamath Nursing Home
Bengaluru, Karnataka, India
Chapters: 21, 27

Rishabh Bora MD MS Radio Diagnosis
Consultant Obstetrican and Gynaecologist
Malhotra Nursing and Maternity Home
Agra, Uttar Pradesh, India
Chapter: 22

Robert Wade MRCOG
Consultant Clinical Oncologist
Department of Obstetrics and Gynecology
Norfolk and Norwich University Hospitals
NHS Foundation Trust
Norwich, Norfolk, United Kingdom
Chapter: 41

Rupinder Kaur Ruprai MD
Consultant Obstetrician and Gynecologist
Medstar Day Surgery Center
Dubai, UAE
Chapters: 5 and 6

Sambit Mukhopadhyay MS MD FRCOG
Consultant Gynecologist
Department of Obstetrics and Gynecology
Norfolk and Norwich University Hospital
NHS Foundation Trust
Norwich, United Kingdom
Chapters: 10

Sapna Vinit Amin (Goni) MD DNB
Associate Professor
Department of Obstetrics and Gynecology
Kasturba Medical College
Manipal University
Manipal, Karnataka, India
Chapter: 2

Shyamala Guruvare MD
Associate Professor
Department of Obstetrics and Gynecology
Kasturba Medical College
Manipal University
Manipal, Karnataka, India
Chapter: 5

Siti Zawiah Omar MBBS (UM) Master O&G (UM)
Professor and Senior Consultant
Department of Obstetrics and Gynecology
University of Malaya
Kuala Lumpur, Malaysia
Chapter: 11

Siya Sharan Sharma MRCOG MD DNB DGO MBBS
Consultant Gynecologist and Obstetrician
Department of Reproductive Medicine
The Queen Elizabeth Hospital, King's Lynn
NHS Foundation Trust
United Kingdom
Chapters: 12, 13 and 14

Sonal Panchal MD
Consultant Radiologist
Dr Nagori Hospital
Ahmedabad, Gujarat, India
Chapter: 22

Sucheta Jindal MD MRCOG
Consultant
Department of Obstetrics and Gynecology
Calderdale and Huddersfield NHS Foundation Trust
West Yorkshire, England
Chapters: 12, 13 and 14

SS Prasad MD
Professor
Department of Surgery
Kasturba Medical College
Manipal University
Manipal, Karnataka, India
Chapter: 20

Tim Duncan FRCOG
Consultant Gynecologist
Department of Obstetrics and Gynecology
Norfolk and Norwich University Hospital
Norwich, United Kingdom
Chapter: 38

V Sivanesaratnam MBBS FRCOG FICS FACS FAMM FAOFOG
Consultant
Department of Gynecology and Oncology
University of Malaya Specialist Centre
Kuala Lumpur, Malaysia
Emeritus Professor (Formerly: Professor(Chair), Head and Senior Consultant, Department of Obstetrics and Gynecology, University of Malaya, Kuala Lumpur Malaysia)
Chapters: 35, 36, 37, 39 and 40

Vani Ramkumar MD
Professor
Department of Obstetrics and Gynecology
St. Johns Medical College
Bengaluru, Karnataka, India
Chapter: 28

WC Maina MRCOG
Speciality Doctor
Department of Obstetrics and Gynecology
Norfolk and Norwich University Hospital NHS Foundation Trust
Norwich, United Kingdom
Chapter: 10

Foreword

We are fortunate to have lived through a period of historic milestones, and the turn of the millennium. The last millennium saw dramatic technical advances in the field of medicine. The greatest single difference between women in rich countries and women in developing ones is in their reproductive health status, particularly the availability, affordability and access to the same.

The book *Essentials of Gynecology* is the work of leading experts in the field, detailing the methodology for clinical practice and modus operandi for appropriate treatment for the disease. The contributors are experienced professionals, who have distilled their wealth of expertise to provide invaluable guide for the problems faced in day-to-day practice and emphasize practical aspects. Utmost care has been taken to include essentials ranging from embryology to cancer detection, suited to all different geographical regions.

The substance as presented, invites readers to appreciate and engage themselves in a rational and logical approach to problems. The contents of this treatise will reiterate the importance of the art of clinical practice and the principles involved in scientific management. I hope it would become a springboard for some to rise to great heights in managing the selected subjects.

Shirish S Sheth
MD FRCOG FICS
Consultant Gynecologist
Department of Obstetrics and Gynecology
Breach Candy Hospital
Mumbai, Maharashtra, India

Past President, FIGO

Preface to the Third Edition

The third edition of this popular book has 42 chapters. Chapter 1 sets the scene with the basic embryological development of the genital tract and this is immediately followed by developmental abnormalities of the genital tract. This leads to functional aspects of ovulation and menstruation in chapter 3 followed by basic clinical history taking and gynecological examination in chapter 4. The next two chapters cover pediatric and adolescent gynecology followed by the chapters on dysmenorrhea, abnormal uterine bleeding and amenorrhea and oligomenorrhea.

After the anatomical and functional disorders are described the next several chapters deal with benign gynecology of endometriosis, adenomyosis and benign lesions of the reproductive tract. Operative procedures, contraception, breast diseases are other important areas that are well described. Special attention is paid to pelvic floor disorders and endoscopic surgery whilst not missing out on rare problems such as tuberculosis of the genital tract. Subfertility affects 80 million couples globally and 10 to 20% of clinic attendance is due to subfertility. Management of this important problem is covered in detail. Globally 3 to 4 hundred thousand women die of reproductive tract cancers. Hence, the final few chapters are devoted for dealing with the clinical screening, diagnosis and management of gynecological malignancies.

The authors who have contributed chapters to this book are teachers for undergraduates and postgraduates and are well recognized nationally and internationally. They have published original research articles in indexed journals and chapters in popular books. Each chapter is well illustrated and easy to read. The entire spectrum of gynecology is covered in this book. Hence, little additional reading is required by the students. We are hopeful that this book would enjoy the same popularity as the previous editions. As authors and editors we would greatly appreciate your comments and criticisms. If any errors are observed—our apologies but please write to us, so that we can rectify these in the next reprint or edition of the book.

Sabaratnam Arulkumaran
V Sivanesaratnam
Alokendu Chatterjee
Pratap Kumar

Preface to the First Edition

Gynecology has always been a fascinating subject looking at the health issues of a female from birth to the menopause. This book takes the life cycle approach starting in sex differentiation, abnormal development of reproductive organs to pediatric and adolescent health. This is followed by menarche, menstruation and menstrual problems. The issues related to contraception and subfertility are dealt with in detail. Sexually transmitted diseases and pelvic inflammatory diseases are described followed by benign and malignant neoplasms of the reproductive tract. Menopause and cancer screening is discussed based on the current data and available evidence. There is little doubt that gynecological problems are increasingly managed medically and by minimally invasive surgery and where possible by out-patient procedures. Detailed descriptions of these are provided including the latest in technology.

The contributors for each chapter have specially been selected based on their expertise and experience. A large number of figures have been included to make the subject easy to understand and to make an "imprint" in the reader's mind, so that the subject matter will remain for years to come. We have no doubt that this book will be of great value to those interested in the subject.

There are bound to be some overlap of subject matter due to the contributory nature of the book and the need to repeat certain basic facts to provide a continuous flow of the subject matter. No book is perfect and ageless. With progress of time, there will be changes in practice and the editors would provide this in the next edition. The readers are kindly requested to communicate any mistakes and omissions to the publishers or the editors, so that they can be incorporated in the next/reprint edition.

Sabaratnam Arulkumaran
V Sivanesaratnam
Alokendu Chatterjee
Pratap Kumar

Contents

SECTION 1: GENERAL GYNECOLOGY

1. **Embryology and Development of the Female Genital Tract** — 3
   Nozer Sheriar
   Indifferent Embryo   3
   Female Gonadal Differentiation   4
   Female Genital Duct Differentiation   5

2. **Disorders of the Development of Müllerian System** — 7
   Pratap Kumar, Sapna Vinit Amin
   Anomalies of the Female Reproductive Tract   7

3. **Ovulation and Menstruation** — 13
   AP Manjunath, Pratap Kumar, Jayaraman Nambiar
   Ovulation and Menstruation   13
   Feedback Oscillation of the Hypothalamo-pituitary Ovarian System   17

4. **Gynecological History and Examination** — 19
   Anna Gracia Perez-Bonfils, Edwin Chandraharan
   History-Taking   20
   Menstrual History   21
   Contraceptive History   22
   Past Obstetric History   22
   Past Gynecological History   22
   Past Medical/Surgical History   22
   Drug History/Allergies   22
   Sexual History   22
   Social History   23
   Family History   23
   General Examination   23
   Abdominal Examination   23
   Gynecological Examination   24
   Position   24
   Technique of Bimanual Examination   24
   Bimanual Examination of the Uterus and the Adnexae   26
   Rectal Examination   26
   Rectovaginal Examination   27

Essentials of Gynecology

5. Pediatric Gynecology — 28
Pratap Kumar, Shyamala Guruvare, Arun Nagrath, Rupinder Kaur Ruprai

- Normal Anatomy and Physiology 28
- Disorders of Sexual Differentiation and Sexual Ambiguity 30
- Vulvovaginal Disorders 33
- Vaginal Discharge 35
- Viral Infections 35
- Urethral Prolapse 36
- Foreign Bodies 36
- Imperforate Hymen 36
- Precocious Puberty 36
- Ovarian Cysts 39

6. Adolescent Gynecology — 42
Rupinder Kaur Ruprai

- Puberty 42
- Clinical Evaluation of the Adolescent Girl 44
- Conditions Affecting the Adolescent Girl 46
- Delayed Sexual Development 46
- Turner's Syndrome 47
- Congenital Adrenal Hyperplasia 47
- Cystic Fibrosis 51
- Menstrual Disorders 52
- Amenorrhea 56
- Hyperandrogenism in Adolescent Girls 58
- Functional Ovarian Hyperandrogenism 61
- Premenstrual Syndrome 62
- Pelvic Pain and Recurrent Abdominal Pain 63
- Dysmenorrhea 63
- Endometriosis 65
- Ovarian Enlargements in Adolescent Girl 68
- Vulvovaginal Complaints 70
- Cervical Cytology, Histology, and Human Papillomavirus 70
- Müllerian Abnormalities 71
- Eating Disorders 71
- Athletic Adolescents 72
- Epilepsy 72
- Childhood Cancer Survivors 72
- Adolescent Pregnancy 72
- Termination of Pregnancy 72
- Sexual Abuse 73
- Female Cosmetic Genital Surgery 73

7. Dysmenorrhea — 77
PK Shah, Keshav Pai

- Definition 77
- Incidence 77

Risk Factors for Dysmenorrhea 77
Classification or Types 78
Recent Advances 82

8. Abnormal Uterine Bleeding 84
PK Sekharan

Normal Menstrual Bleeding 84
The New Classification of AUB 84
Salient Features of PALM-COEIN Classification 86
Evaluation of Abnormal Uterine Bleeding 86
Management 88
Danazol and Gestrinone 90

9. Amenorrhea and Oligomenorrhea 93
B Kanchana Devi, N Pandiyan

Physiology of Menstruation 93

10. Reproductive Health 101
WC Maina, Sambit Mukhopadhyay

Adolescent Health 101
Female Genital Mutilation 102
Overweight and Obesity 103
Unsafe Abortion 105
Pelvic Inflammatory Disease and Sexually Transmitted Infections 106
Childbirth and Maternal Mortality 107

11. Endometriosis and Adenomyosis 109
Siti Zawiah Omar

Occurrence 109
Etiology 109
Clinical Manifestations 110
Investigations 110
Staging 111
Management 111
Other Options 113
Surgical Treatment 113
Endometriosis and Infertility 114
Adenomyosis 114

12. Pelvic Inflammatory Disease 117
Siya Sharan Sharma, Sucheta Jindal

Natural Barriers to PID 117
Vulnerability to PID 117
Etiological Factors of PID 117
Clinical Features of PID 119
Treatment 121

13. Sexually Transmitted Infections (Formerly Known as Sexually Transmitted Diseases) ... 125
Siya Sharan Sharma, Sucheta Jindal

Defense Mechanism of Female Genital Tract 125
Sexually Transmitted Infections 126
Chlamydial Infection 127
Gonorrhea 128
Acute Gonorrhea 129
Trichomonas Vaginitis 130
Vulvovaginal Candidiasis (Moniliasis) 131
Chronic Vulvovaginal Candidiasis 132
Genital Ulcerative Diseases 133
Herpes in Pregnancy 134
Syphilis 135
Chancroid 139
Lymphogranuloma Venereum 139
Granuloma Inguinale 140
Genital Warts (Condyloma Acuminata) 141

14. Human Immunodeficiency Virus in Women (Including in Pregnancy) ... 144
Siya Sharan Sharma, Sucheta Jindal

Epidemiology 144
Pathophysiology 144
Clinical Progression of HIV 145
Diagnosis 145
Prevention of Spread 146
Gynecological Problems due to HIV 146
Clinical Assessment after Initial Diagnosis 147
Prevention of Mother-to-Child Transmission 148

15. Benign Lesions of the Genital Tract ... 150
K Jayakrishnan, P Manjula

Benign Lesions of Vulva 150
Benign Tumors of Vulva 151
Benign lesions of the Vagina 152
Benign Lesions of the Cervix 152
Benign Tumors of Uterus 152
Uterine Polyps 156
Benign Tumors of Ovary 156

16. Contraception and Sterilization ... 162
K Jayakrishnan, P Manjula

Definition 162
Classification of Contraceptive Agents 163
Traditional Methods 163
Barrier Methods 165
Hormonal Contraceptives 166
Progesterone only Pills (Mini Pills) 169

Transdermal Patch 169
Vaginal Ring 169
Injectable Contraception 169
Contraceptive Implants 170
Emergency Contraception (Postcoital Contraception) 171
Intrauterine Devices 171
Surgical Sterilization 175
Newer Methods 179

17. Psychosexual Problems and Sexual Dysfunction 181
Claudine Domoney

Presentation of Sexual Difficulties 182
Definitions of Sexual Disorders in Women 183
Management 184
Investigations 185
Treatment 185
Partners 189
Phases of Life 189

18. Pelvic Organ Prolapse 193
Pralhad Kushtagi

Definition and Incidence 193
Classification 193
Etiology 194
Anatomy of the Pelvic Floor 196
Secondary Anatomical Changes 197
Symptoms 198
Clinical Evaluation 199
Differential Diagnosis 200
Treatment of Pelvic Organ Prolapse 200
Conservative Management 204

19. Urinary and Fecal Incontinence (Including Fistulae) 206
Deeksha Pandey

Background 206
Etiology and Risk Factors 207
Urinary Incontinence 207
Fecal Incontinence 212
Genital Fistulae 213

20. A Simplified Approach to Breast Diseases for Obstetricians and Gynecologists 216
SS Prasad

Relevant Anatomy and Physiology 216
Common Breast-related Symptoms 216
Investigations for Breast Diseases 217
Common Benign Breast Diseases 218
Breast Cancer 219
Breast Problems in Pregnancy and Lactation 220

Essentials of Gynecology

21. **Instruments Used in Obstetrics and Gynecology**   221
    Rajesh Bhakta
    Sim's Vaginal Speculum   221
    Cusco's Vaginal Speculum   221
    Sim's Anterior Vaginal Wall Retractor   222
    Uterine Sound   222
    Vulsellum Forceps   222
    Tenaculum   222
    Cervical Dilators   223
    Uterine Curette   223
    Suction Cannula   224
    Manual Vacuum Aspirator   224
    Ayer's Spatula   224
    Punch Biopsy Forceps   225
    Endometrial Biopsy Curette   225
    Red Rubber Catheter   225
    Foley's Catheter   225
    Leech Wilkinson's Cannula   226
    Shirodkar's Hook   226
    Pessary (Hodge, Smith or Ring Pessary)   226
    Doyen's Retractor   227
    Richardson's Tetractor   227
    Episiotomy Scissors   227
    Umbilical Cord Cutting Scissor   227
    Kocher's Artery Forceps   227
    Green-armytage's Forceps   228
    Babcock's Forceps   228
    Forceps   228
    Vacuum Delivery (Ventouse)   229
    Malmstrom Cup   229
    Vacuum Extractor   229
    Sponge Holding Forceps   229
    Pinard's Fetal Stethoscope   230
    Lamineria Tent   230

22. **Ultrasound and Color Doppler in Gynecology**   231
    Neharika Malhotra Bora, Rishabh Bora, Narendra Malhotra, Jaideep Malhotra, Sonal Panchal

    Ultrasonography in Gynecology   231
    Normal Female Pelvis   232
    Uterus   232
    Ovaries   232
    Folliculogenesis   232
    Fallopian Tubes   233
    Pouch of Douglas   233
    Ultrasound of the Uterus   234
    Diseases of the Myometrium   234

Diseases of the Endometrium 236
Diseases of the Uterine Cavity 236
Sonohysterography 240
Ultrasound and Puerperium 240
Diseases of Cervix 241
Vagina 242
Ovarian Sonography 242
Evaluation of an Ovarian Mass 248
Gestational Trophoblastic Disorders 248
Pelvic Kidney 249

3D Ultrasound in Gynecology 251
Uterine Lesions 252
3D of Endometrium 252
Endometrial Volume 252
Endometrial Perfusion 252
Ovarian Lesions 254
Other Adnexal Lesions 256
Endometriosis 258
Paraovarian Cysts 258
Ovarian Dermoid Cysts 258
Other Ovarian Masses 258

23. **Gynecological Operations** 261
    AP Manjunath, Jayaraman Nambiar
    Abdominal Hysterectomy 261
    Laparoscopy 273
    Hysteroscopy 276

24. **General Surgical Problems in Gynecology** 279
    Krishnendu Mukherjee
    Categories of General Surgical Problems in Gynecology 279

25. **Genital Tuberculosis** 285
    Prashanth K Adiga, Pratap Kumar
    Incidence 285
    Pathology 285
    Clinical features 286

26. **Uterine Displacements including Retroversion and Uterine Inversion** 290
    Akhila Vasudeva, Pratap Kumar
    Upward Displacement of the Uterus 290
    Lateral Displacement of the Uterus 291
    Retroversion 291
    Symptoms of Retroversion 291
    Diagnosis 292
    Management 292
    Retroverted Gravid Uterus 293

Uterine Inversion 293
Acute Inversion 293
Prevention of Puerperal Inversion 294
Management 294
Chronic Inversion 295

27. Endoscopy in Gynecology — 298
Rajesh Bhakta

Indications of Laparoscopic Surgery 298
Contraindications 298
Technique of Laparoscopy 301
Complications of Laparoscopy 302
Hysteroscopy 302

SECTION 2: REPRODUCTIVE ENDOCRINOLOGY AND ASSISTED CONCEPTION

28. Puberty — 307
Vani Ramkumar

Physiology of Puberty 307
Factors Influencing Puberty 308
Definitions 308
Physical Changes of Puberty 309
Puberty in Boys 310
Psychologic Changes of Puberty 310
Problems Associated with Adolescence 310
Recent Trends 311

29. Disorders of Ovulation — 312
Nuguelis Razali

Classification 312
History 314
Investigations 314
Management 315
Ovulation Induction 315

30. Polycystic Ovarian Syndrome — 318
Pratap Kumar, Alok Sharma

Pathophysiology 318
Puberty and PCOS 319
Diagnosis 319
Approach to Infertility in a Patient with PCOS 320

31. Hirsutism — 323
Muralidhar V Pai

Definition 323
Hypertrichosis 323
Pathophysiology 323

Etiology   324
Diagnosis   324
Treatment   325

32. Disorders of Sexual Differentiation and Development (Intersex) — 328
Muralidhar V Pai

Sexual Differentiation of the Fetus   328
Other Intersex Syndromes   334
Diagnosis of Intersex (Disorders of Sexual Development)   335
Management of Intersex   335
Gender Assignment   336

33. Infertility — 337
Prashant Nadkarni

Causes of Infertility   337
Assessment of the Infertile Couple   338
Investigation of the Infertile Couple   339
Treatment Options   340
Future Directions   341

34. Menopause and Hormone Therapy — 343
Premitha Damodaran

Endocrinology   345
Signs and Symptoms of Menopause   345
Early Menopausal Problems   345
Medium-Term problems   346
Late Menopausal Problems   347
Hormone Therapy Delivery Systems   351
Action of Estrogen   351
Prescribing Hormone Therapy   351
Hormone Therapy and Cancers   352
Ovarian Cancer   353
Colorectal Cancer   354
Lung Cancer   354
Hormone Therapy and Diabetes   354
Hormone Therapy and Gallbladder Disease   354
Other Effects of Hormone Replacement Therapy   355
Duration of Use   355
Recommendations   356

SECTION 3: GYNECOLOGIC ONCOLOGY

35. Gynecological Cancer Screening — 363
V Sivanesaratnam

Cervical Cancer   364
Ovarian Cancer   368
Endometrial Cancer   369

Essentials of Gynecology

36. Preinvasive and Invasive Cancer of the Cervix — 372
V Sivanesaratnam

Preinvasive Lesions of the Cervix 373
Adenocarcinoma in situ 377
Invasive Carcinoma of the Cervix 377

37. Ovarian Cancer — 383
V Sivanesaratnam, Lim Boon Kiong

Epidemiology 383
Anatomy 384
Etiological Factors 384
Screening for Ovarian Cancer 385
Prevention of Ovarian Cancer 385
Classification of Ovarian Neoplasms 385
Diagnosis 386
Examination 387
Preoperative Evaluation 387
Stages of Ovarian Cancer 387
Treatment of Ovarian Carcinoma 388

38. Uterine Malignancy — 393
Christina Portelli, Tim Duncan

Epidemiology and Risk Factors 394
Histopathology 394
Leiomyosarcoma 395
Patterns of Spread 396
Risk Factors 396
Clinical Features 396
Diagnosis and Investigations 397
Revised FIGO Staging 2009 397
Prognostic Factors 398
Management 398

39. Vulvar Cancer — 401
V Sivanesaratnam

Etiology 401
Squamous Cell Carcinoma 402
Diagnosis 403
Pattern of Spread 403
Management 404
Special Situations 405
Lymphatic Mapping 407
Other Vulvar Malignancies 407

40. Gestational Trophoblastic Neoplasia — 411
V Sivanesaratnam

Hydatidiform Mole 412
Prophylaxis Against Choriocarcinoma 414

Placental Site Trophoblastic Tumor 415
Epithelioid Trophoblastic Tumor 415
Choriocarcinoma 415

41. Radiotherapy and Systemic Anticancer Therapy in Gynecological Malignancy   421
Robert Wade

Radiotherapy 421
Systemic Anticancer Cancer Therapy 422
Oncological Treatment of Specific Cancers 423
Cervical Cancer 423
Endometrial Cancer 424
Ovarian Cancer 424
Vulval Cancer 425
Vaginal Cancer 425
Trophoblastic Tumors 425

42. Palliative Care   426
Claire Stewart, Onnig Tamizian

Symptom Management 426

Index   437

SECTION 1

General Gynecology

1. Embryology and Development of the Female Genital Tract
2. Disorders of the Development of Müllerian System
3. Ovulation and Menstruation
4. Gynecological History and Examination
5. Pediatric Gynecology
6. Adolescent Gynecology
7. Dysmenorrhea
8. Abnormal Uterine Bleeding
9. Amenorrhea and Oligomenorrhea
10. Reproductive Health
11. Endometriosis and Adenomyosis
12. Pelvic Inflammatory Disease
13. Sexually Transmitted Infections
14. Human Immunodeficiency Virus in Women (Including in Pregnancy)
15. Benign Lesions of the Genital Tract
16. Contraception and Sterilization
17. Psychosexual Problems and Sexual Dysfunction
18. Pelvic Organ Prolapse
19. Urinary and Fecal Incontinence (Including Fistulae)
20. A Simplified Approach to Breast Diseases for Obstetricians and Gynecologists
21. Instruments Used in Obstetrics and Gynecology
22. Ultrasound and Color Doppler in Gynecology
23. Gynecological Operations
24. General Surgical Problems in Gynecology
25. Genital Tuberculosis
26. Uterine Displacements including Retroversion and Uterine Inversion
27. Endoscopy in Gynecology

CHAPTER 1

Embryology and Development of the Female Genital Tract

Nozer Sheriar

Overview

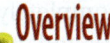

- Wolffian ducts (mesonephric) are the male reproductive system and the Müllerian ducts (paramesonephric) are the female system.
- The Leydig cells in the testes produce *testosterone*, while the Sertoli cells synthesize the *anti-Müllerian hormone* which inhibits the female development.
- The paired müllerian ducts meet in the midline, fusing within the urorectal septum at the end of the embryonic period and forms the fallopian tubes, uterus and the upper part of vagina. The lower part of vagina is by the urogenital sinus.

The reproductive organs in the female (as also in the male) consist of gonads, external genitalia and an internal duct system between the two. Since, these three components originate from different primordia in close association with the urinary system and the hindgut, the embryological development is complex and developmental abnormalities are often inter-related.[1]

INDIFFERENT EMBRYO

The hindgut appears about the twentieth postovulatory day. The intermediate mesoderm develops adjacent to the midline dorsal mesentery of the gut, extending through the length of the body cavity (celom). A part of this intermediate cell mass medial to the mesonephros (primitive kidney), proliferates to form the gonadal ridges. These bilateral thickenings being recognizable in the 4 to 5 mm embryo (Fig. 1.1).

Indifferent Gonad

Primordial germ cells that are subsequently capable of meiosis, separate out from the pool of somatic cells that are capable only of mitosis. These germ cells are present in the allantoic diverticulum and the adjacent parts of the yolk sac in 17 to 20 day embryos. From here they migrate through the dorsal mesentery of the hindgut, reaching the gonadal

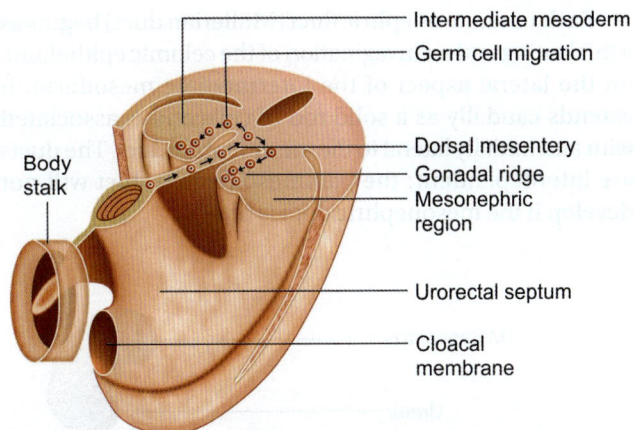

Fig. 1.1: The caudal half of the embryo (30-35 days).

ridge in the human embryo at 35 days (Fig. 1.1). The cause of this migration of the germ cells is yet unknown.

The area to which the germ cells migrate is referred to as the indifferent gonad until gonadal sex is established. At 35 days the indifferent gonad is formed by the primordial germ cells, cells from the overlying celomic epithelium and the cells of the adjacent mesonephros. The germ cells now undergo rapid mitotic proliferation and are enclosed by extensions of the celomic epithelium (sex cords) and the mesonephric ducts.

Mesonephric (Wolffian) Ducts

In 1759, Caspar Wolff studying the embryology of the chick described a symmetrical pair of paravertebral swellings as the precursors of the kidneys. The term Wolffian has been subsequently used to describe the mesonephric ducts and vesicles.

The first indication of the urinary system appears at 21 days when the mesonephric vesicles develop. These are associated with a solid cord of cells in the intermediate mesoderm, that acquire a lumen at 26 days, forming the mesonephric ducts. Skirting the hindgut the bilateral mesonephric ducts open into the urogenital sinus at 28 days (Fig. 1.2). At 32 days, the caudal end of each mesonephric duct gives rise to the ureteric bud and is incorporated into the posterior wall of the urogenital sinus, subsequently forming the trigone of the bladder and the posterior wall of the urethra. The mesonephros attains maximum size and function at 42 days, the metanephros taking over excretory function after 50 days.

Paramesonephric (Müllerian) Ducts

In 1830, Johannes Müller described a cord on the outer aspect of the Wolffian body, but thinner than the Wolffian cord. These Müllerian cords now referred to as the paramesonephric ducts, appear at about 40 days.

Each paramesonephric duct (Müllerian duct) begins as a thickening and an invagination of the celomic epithelium, on the lateral aspect of the intermediate mesoderm. It extends caudally as a solid rod of cells and is associated with and initially lateral to the mesonephric duct. The ducts are interdependent; the paramesonephric duct will not develop if the mesonephric duct is absent.[2]

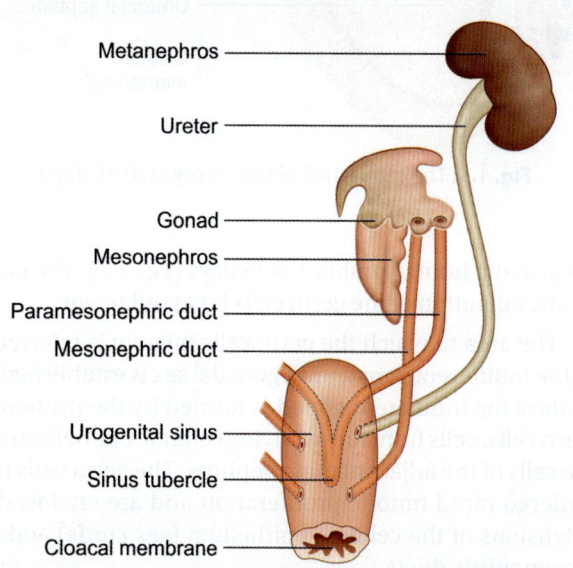

Fig. 1.2: The embryo with urogenital ducts (after 40 days).

As the paramesonephric cord of cells continues its descent, a lumen appears in its cranial portion in continuity with the intraembryonic body cavity. The lumen extends caudally, as the ducts pass ventral to the mesonephric ducts, come in close association with each other and reach the posterior aspect of the urogenital sinus (Fig. 1.2).

Urogenital Sinus

The hindgut and the cloaca are established by a process of flexion, as that part of the yolk sac enclosed within the tail fold of the embryo. At an early stage the hindgut and the urogenital ducts open into a common cloaca (Fig. 1.3A). The mesoderm between the allantoic diverticulum and the hindgut then extends caudally in line with the curvature of the tail fold as the urorectal septum. The urorectal septum fuses with the cloacal membrane at 30–32 days, completely dividing the cloaca into the ventral urogenital sinus and the dorsal rectum (Fig. 1.3B).

The functioning mesonephros now produces an increase in the pressure in the closed urogenital sinus, rupturing the ventral part of the cloacal membrane and allowing the urogenital sinus to communicate with the amniotic cavity.

FEMALE GONADAL DIFFERENTIATION

Male and female embryos are morphologically indistinguishable till 42 days when the transformation of the indifferent gonad into an embryonic testis begins to occur. The Leydig cells in the testes produce testosterone from 56 days onwards, while the Sertoli cells synthesize the anti-Müllerian hormone. The secretion of the anti-Müllerian hormone begins soon after testicular differentiation and continues into the prenatal period, though, it is functional only for a short period during early gestation.

The transformation of the indifferent gonad into an embryonic ovary occurs gradually between 45 and 55 days.

Development of the Ovary

A gonad with the germ cells in meiosis is always an ovary since meiotic division does not occur in the testes until puberty. Meiosis I begins in the ovary in intrauterine life, only to be completed at ovulation some 15–45 years later. Meiosis II occurs at fertilization. During the early fetal stage, the ovaries contain five million germ cells, that along with the sex cords from the celomic epithelium, remain in the superficial part of the ovary, the future cortex. The cords lose contact with the surface, forming small groups of cells each with a germ cell, a primitive follicle.

Meanwhile, the ovary descends extraperitoneally, its descent controlled by the suspensory ligament that connects it to its site of origin on the genital ridge, and the

CHAPTER 1 Embryology and Development of the Female Genital Tract

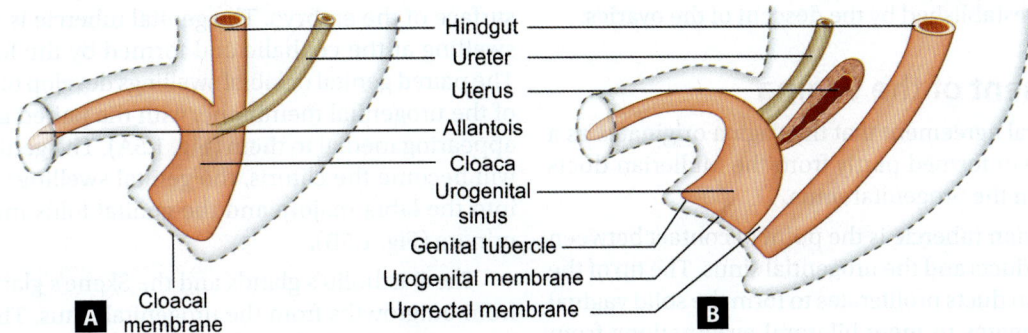

Figs. 1.3A and B: (A) The hindgut and urogenital ducts opening into the cloaca; (B) Fusion of the urorectal septum with the cloacal membrane.

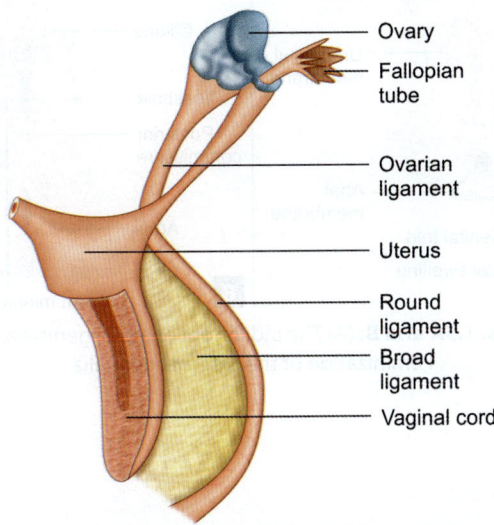

Fig. 1.4: Descent of the ovary into the pelvis.

gubernaculum. The gubernaculum is the inferior continuation of the genital mesentery, that becomes attached to the uterine cornu forming the proximal ovarian ligament and continues as the distal round ligament passing through the inguinal canal and ending in the labium majus[3] (Fig. 1.4).

The total number of germ cells in the ovary decline to about two million at birth and only 4,00,000 oocytes at the onset of puberty. Of these 400 will be ovulated during reproductive life, the remaining 99.9% undergoing atresia.

FEMALE GENITAL DUCT DIFFERENTIATION

At the end of the embryonic period the fetus has gonads recognizable as either testes or ovaries, but possesses both the mesonephric ducts and the paramesonephric ducts. The subsequent differentiation of the ducts is governed by fetal testicular hormones. In the male fetus, Müllerian duct regression begins under the influence of the anti-Müllerian hormone at 50–60 days,[4] while the mesonephric ducts are stabilized under the influence of testosterone between 56 and 70 days. In contrast, the absence of testicular hormones in the female fetus allows the stabilization of the Müllerian ducts and a regression of the mesonephric ducts to take place.

The basic sequence of change from the bipotential state is directed by chromosomal sex determined gonad formation, which then favors the development of male or female duct systems and external genitalia. In final analysis, this depends on endocrine effects and not chromosomal sex.[5]

The development of the female genitourinary tract is nearly complete at the end of the first trimester, with some changes such as the final canalization of the vagina and repositioning of the gonads taking place later.

Development of the Uterus

The paired Müllerian ducts meet in the midline, fusing within the urorectal septum at the end of the embryonic period. The Müllerian ducts fuse, forming the uterus around 63 days, the median septum being completely reabsorbed by 80 days, forming a single uterovaginal canal. While, the complete failure of fusion between the ducts results in a didelphic uterus, a partial failure results in an arcuate or a bicornuate uterus, and a failure of septal resorption results in variants ranging from a subseptate to a septate uterus.[5,6]

In the fetus, the cervix forms two-thirds of the uterus. The corpus differentiates into the serosal, muscular and mucosal layers at 19 weeks, the endometrial glands forming a week later. The uterus at birth and during childhood is devoid of flexion and version, these characteristics develop at puberty.

Development of the Fallopian Tubes

The separated upper part of each Müllerian duct retains its identity to form the fallopian tube, the open cranial segment of the duct develops fimbriae. The transverse lie of the tubes is established by the descent of the ovaries.

Development of the Vagina

There is general agreement that the vagina originates as a composite organ formed partly from the Müllerian ducts and partly from the urogenital sinus.

The Müllerian tubercle is the point of contact between the Müllerian ducts and the urogenital sinus. The tip of the fused Müllerian ducts proliferates to form the solid vaginal cord that elongates to meet bilateral evaginations from the urogenital sinus (sinovaginal bulbs). The sinovaginal bulbs fuse with the vaginal cord to form the vaginal plate. Canalization of the vaginal cord occurs, followed by epithelialization, mostly with cells from the urogenital sinus.

According to current hypothesis, only the upper third of the vagina is formed from the Müllerian ducts, with the lower vagina developing from the vaginal plate of the urogenital sinus below.

Development of the External Genitalia

The external genitalia develop in the area bound by the body stalk above and the tail below, the sex of the external genitalia being unrecognizable till the twelfth week.

Five swellings appear around the urogenital sinus on the surface of the embryo. The genital tubercle is the midline swelling at the cephalic end formed by the fourth week. The paired genital or labial swellings develop on either side of the urogenital membrane, with the paired genital folds appearing medial to them (Fig. 1.5A). The genital tubercle will become the clitoris, the genital swellings developing into the labia majora and the genital folds into the labia minora (Fig. 1.5B).

The Bartholin's glands and the Skene's glands develop from outgrowths from the urogenital sinus. The urorectal septum will finally form the perineal body.

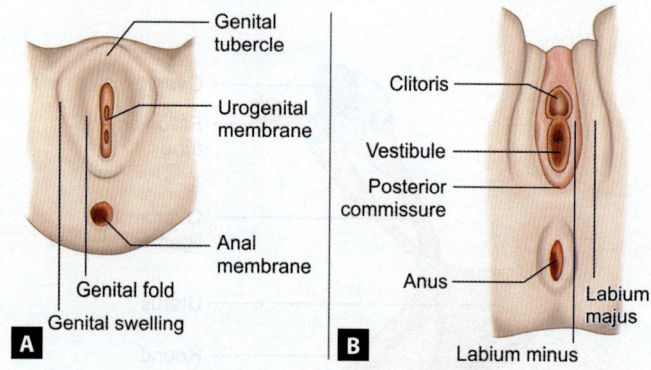

Figs. 1.5A and B: (A) The indifferent external genitalia; (B) Feminization of the external genitalia.

REFERENCES

1. Boyd ME, Daniels E. Development of the female genital tract and external genitalia. In: Gidwani G, Falcone T (Eds). Congenital malformations of the female genital tract. Philadelphia: Lippincott Williams & Wilkins; 1999;1-20.
2. Lytle W. The deep inguinal ring: development, function and repair. Br J Surg. 1970;57:531-7.
3. Terruhn V. A study of impression moulds of the genital tract of female fetuses. Arch Gynecol. 1980;229:207-17.
4. Josso N, Picard JY, Tran D. The antimüllerian hormone. Recent Prog Horm Res. 1977;37:117-20.
5. Duncan S. Embryology of the female genital tract: its genetic defects and congenital anomalies. In: Shaw R, Soutter W, Stanton S (Eds). Gynecology. New York: Churchill Livingstone; 1997;1-22.
6. Rock J, Schlaff W. The obstetric consequences of uterovaginal anomalies. Fertil Steril. 1985;43:681-92.

CHAPTER 2

Disorders of the Development of Müllerian System

Pratap Kumar, Sapna Vinit Amin

Overview

- Development of genital system is interesting and intricating.
- The etiology of this developmental abnormality, though not very clear, is controlled by genetic, hormonal and environmental factors.
- Müllerian duct fusion defect causes different kinds of uterus like the bicornuate uterus, unicornuate uterus, etc. The defective resorption may lead to septae.
- Absence of vagina or complete septa in the vagina can lead to collection of blood beyond causing hematocolpos. Uterus also may be totally absent.
- Surgical correction may be as simple as cruciate incision for hematocolpos to complex one done for vaginoplasty and corrective surgery for obstetric indications, is rarely required.
- Müllerian anomalies are second most common cause for primary amenorrhea, next only to Turner's syndrome.
- Functionally urogenital systems are two different components, however embryologically and anatomically they are intimately interconnected. Hence may be associated with renal anomalies in 20–30% of cases or vice versa.
- Various surgical and nonsurgical procedures are available to reconstruct vagina when there is absence of the same.

ANOMALIES OF THE FEMALE REPRODUCTIVE TRACT

Female genital tract anomalies incidence: 1–3% of the female population, and 5% of infertile women.

Anomalies of the female reproductive tract can result from agenesis or hypoplasia, fusion and/or canalization defects, duplication abnormalities, or failure of resorption, resulting in septa.

Arrest in the normal development of the Müllerian ducts can cause several anomalies:

1. Aplasia— in which the organs fail to develop.
2. Hypoplasia—in which the organs are rudimentary.
3. Atresia—in which there is partial or complete failure of canalization of these ducts leading to varying degrees of gynatresia.
4. Müllerian duct anomalies like:
   - Unicornuate uterus (asymmetrical development) (Fig. 2.1) with or without rudimentary horn.

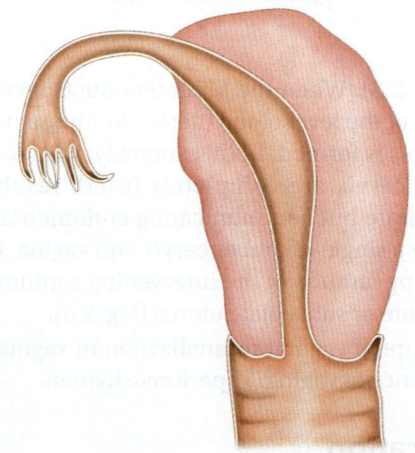

Fig. 2.1: Unicornuate uterus.

- Failure of fusion in part or whole may lead to duplication of the genital tract uterus didelphys (two separate uterus, two cervix; or a bicornuate uterus

SECTION 1 *General Gynecology*

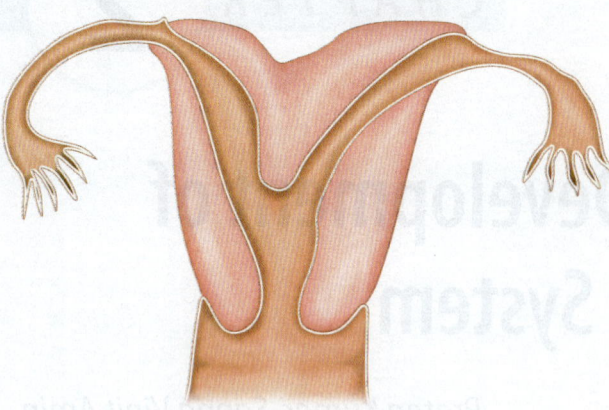

Fig. 2.2: Bicornuate uterus.

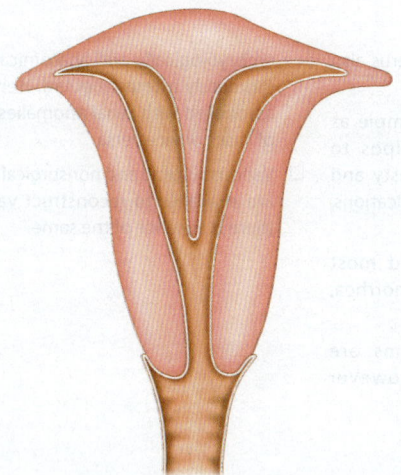

Fig. 2.3: Uterus subseptus.

(Fig. 2.2). When the Müllerian ducts incompletely fuse at the level of the uterine fundus, a bicornuate uterus is formed. In this anomaly, the lower uterus and cervix are completely fused, resulting in 2 separate but communicating endometrial cavities with a single-chamber cervix and vagina. Failure of disappearance of the intervening septum leads to septate or subseptate uterus (Fig. 2.3).
- Failure of vaginal recanalization of vagina leads to absence of vagina/imperforate hymen.

Classification

Mullerian anomalies have been classified in various ways.
- Jones classification
  - Agenesis/Aplasia: Agenesis of vagina, cervix, uterus, or of the complete reproductive tract
- Fusion, canalization and resorption of septum abnormalities (vertical and lateral fusion defects)

Table 2.1: Classification of Müllerian anomalies according to American Society for Reproductive Medicine (American Fertility Society, 1988).

I. Segmental Müllerian hypoplasia or agenesis
  a. Vaginal
  b. Cervical
  c. Uterine
  d. Tubal
  e. Combined

II. Unicornuate uterus
  a. Rudimentary horn with cavity, communicating to unicornuate uterus
  b. Rudimentary horn with cavity, not communicating to unicornuate uterus
  c. Rudimentary horn with no cavity
  d. Unicornuate uterus without a rudimentary horn

III. Uterine didelphys

IV. Bicornuate uterus
  a. Complete bifurcation (bicollis)
  b. Partial bifurcation (unicollis)

V. Septate uterus
  a. Complete septation
  b. Partial septation

VI. Arcuate uterus
VII. Diethylstilbestrol- related anomalies (1938–1975)

Clinical Problems (General)

- Gynecological
  - Primary amenorrhea
  - Out-flow tract obstruction
  - Dysmenorrhea
  - Infertility
  - Endometriosis.
- Obstetric: 5–10% in women with recurrent miscarriages
  - Recurrent pregnancy loss (mid trimester)
  - Rupture of rudimentary horn
  - Preterm labor.
- Malpresentations (breech, transverse lie)
- Fetal growth restriction
- Dystocia
- Ruptured uterus
- Operative delivery
- Retained placenta
- Postpartum hemorrhage
- Subinvolution of the uterus.

Problems connected to each of the anomalies can be as follows:

1. **Ovary:** Ovarian absence is called as ovarian agenesis/dysgenesis and this leads to Turner's syndrome (chromosomes will be 45XO) and this will present a primary amenorrhea, and has special characters like short stature web neck.

CHAPTER 2 Disorders of the Development of Müllerian System

2. **Uterus:** Uterine anomalies described above usually does not cause problems. However, in obstetrics, it may cause increased incidence of abortions, preterm labors, malpresentations.
3. **Vagina:** Noncanalization of vagina leads to crypto menorrhea (hidden menses) and may present during adolescent age as primary amenorrhea. There will be cyclical pain (because of menses which is collected above the noncanalized vagina). If there is only imperforate hymen then the bulge is at the exterior. At this stage, there can be retention of urine also along with primary amenorrhea.

Diagnosis in Infancy or Childhood

Occasionally, diagnosis is possible in infancy. The infant may present with a bulging yellow-gray mass at or beyond the introitus. The presence of an abdominal mass can occur in association with urinary obstruction.

Diagnosis in utero can be done with obstetric ultrasonography. Ultrasonography is an essential first step in diagnosis.

Hymenal Obstruction

Usually, the problems are seen only at puberty when they present with primary amenorrhea. Unfortunately, the typical findings at diagnosis include a large collection of blood within the uterus (hematometra) and an even larger collection of blood within the distensible vagina (hematocolpos) (Fig. 2.4). Additional findings may include blood-filled fallopian tubes (hematosalpinges) and signs of retrograde menses, occasionally to the point of the development of intra-abdominal endometriosis and severe adhesions. An imperforate hymen must be corrected surgically. Surgical decision-making should focus on appropriate diagnosis and timing of surgical repair.

- Pelvic and abdominal ultrasound/MRI
  - A pelvic ultrasound is the essential initial diagnostic test to confirm, and a transabdominal route is needed. Renal anomalies should be ruled out when other Müllerian defects of the uterus and vagina are suspected
  - Pelvic and abdominal MRI: If the diagnosis of imperforate hymen is not absolutely certain based on physical examination or pelvic ultrasound findings, MRI is indicated to clearly define the anatomy prior to any planned surgical procedure.

Surgical Procedure for Imperforate Hymen

A cruciate incision along the diagonal diameters of the hymen, rather than anterior to posterior, avoids injury to the urethra directly anteriorly and can be enlarged by removal of excess hymenal tissue. In either approach, the vaginal epithelium then is sutured to the hymenal ring using interrupted stitches with fine absorbable suture (e.g. 4-0 polyglycolic acid suture). The application of 2% lidocaine jelly to the suture line to provide postoperative analgesia is suggested.

Aspiration or puncture of the mucocolpos or hematocolpos without definitive enlargement of the vaginal orifice should be avoided because a pyocolpos or ascending infection may develop. Pelvic examination should not be done since it will cause ascending infection.

Surgical Management of Vaginal Agenesis

Surgical and nonsurgical methods of treatment have been utilized. The nonsurgical approach relies on the use of graduated dilators (Frank's dilation) and may take several months or a few years before a functional vagina is formed. Surgery remains the most effective method of treatment for vaginal agenesis.

Choosing the proper time to perform a vaginoplasty is of paramount importance. Surgical treatment should be considered only when the patient wishes to become sexually active and is highly motivated to use a vaginal prosthesis for several months postoperatively.[1]

Preoperative Evaluation

Routine preoperative evaluation should include an intravenous pyelogram (IVP) and renal ultrasound to exclude urinary tract anomalies. Discovery of a pelvic kidney is important in planning corrective surgery since its presence may limit the amount of potential space.

Surgical Techniques for Vaginal Agenesis

McIndoe operation: The aim of surgical treatment is to create a neovagina. The modified McIndoe's procedure remains the most common surgical approach to vaginoplasty for vaginal agenesis. Obtaining a satisfactory

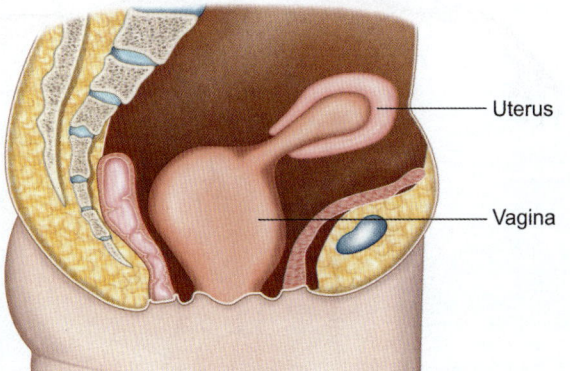

Fig. 2.4: Hematocolpos (distended vagina filled with blood).

split-thickness graft is one of the most important steps in performing the modified McIndoe's procedure. A space is created between the bladder and the rectum.

- **Prosthesis assembly:** The stent should be made from material that can maintain patency of the vaginal cavity. A foam rubber form measuring 10 cm by 2 cm works well. The prosthetic device is sterilized, and the size is customized to fit the patient's vagina. The prosthetic material is cut to twice the desired size of the vagina, folded in half, and compressed by the placement of 2 condoms over the surface. The condoms are tied at the open end.
- **Graft attachment to prosthesis:** The skin graft is placed over the stent, dermal aspect out, and sutured over the form using 5-0 synthetic absorbable sutures. The graft-covered prosthesis is carefully inserted into the vaginal canal. The edges of the graft are sutured to the previously cut edges of the mucosal margins of the vaginal introitus. This contact is often adequate, rendering sutures unnecessary. If the contact between the graft and the vaginal space is too tight, serum may collect and compromise the engraftment. The labia minora are sutured around the stent using nonreactive sutures.

Patient education regarding the importance of continuous, prolonged dilatation as well as stent care during the healing phase is essential. The foam is worn continuously for 6 weeks and is removed only for urination and defecation. Low-pressure douches with warm water are performed daily. At the same time, the form is cleaned with a povidone-iodine solution, covered with a fresh condom, lubricated, and reintroduced into the neovagina. After 6 weeks, a silicone form that is inserted nightly for the next 12 months replaces the original stent. In most cases, the vagina is functional 6–10 weeks postoperatively.[2,3]

Williams vulvovaginoplasty is an alternative to the McIndoe procedure. This procedure is particularly useful for patients with previously failed vaginoplasty. It utilizes full-thickness skin flaps from the labia majora to create a vaginal pouch. Unlike the McIndoe procedure, vaginal dilation is required for only 3–4 weeks. The vagina created by this approach is not anatomically similar to a normal vagina or the neovagina created by the McIndoe procedure. Instead, the vaginal pouch axis is directly posterior and horizontal to the perineum; however, the vagina is functional and well-received by patients. Fistula formation, which can occur with the McIndoe procedure, is rare.[4]

Sigmoid vaginoplasty in which sigmoid colon is used to create neovagina, is another operative option. It provides good vaginal length, adequate secretion allowing lubrication, less incidence of vaginal stenosis, also does not need prolonged neovaginal dilatation. More importantly has short recovery time with good patient satisfaction.

In the recent decades, novel vaginoplasty techniques like Vecchietti and Davydov procedures are becoming popular (both open and laparoscopic techniques).[5]

Uterus Didelphys, Nonobstructed (Fig. 2.5)

Women with nonobstructed didelphys uterus usually are not candidates for surgical unification. The decision to perform metroplasty should be individualized, and only selected patients may benefit from surgical reconstruction. Metroplasty using the Strassman procedure[6] deals with the method of unification of the uterine cavities at the fundus while the cervices are left intact. This is not done in modern gynecology, since unification was causing higher incidence of rupture of uterus during subsequent pregnancy. Rarely, they can present with double uterus and double vagina (Fig. 2.6).

Bicornuate Uterus

Bicornuate uterus is considered an incidental finding. Patients usually have no difficulty becoming pregnant and usually do not have much of obstetrical problem except rarely it may be the cause of preterm labor. At times they have one rudimentary horn (Fig. 2.7).

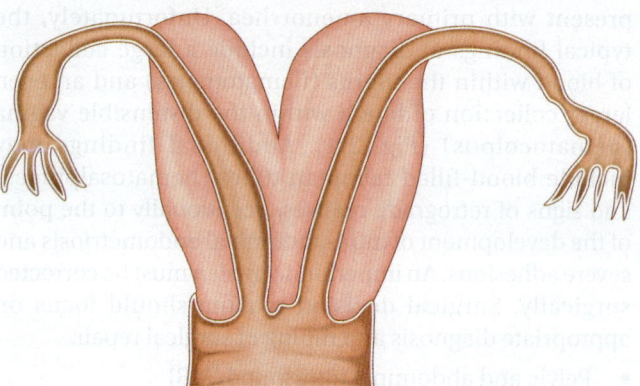

Fig. 2.5: Double uterus with single vagina.

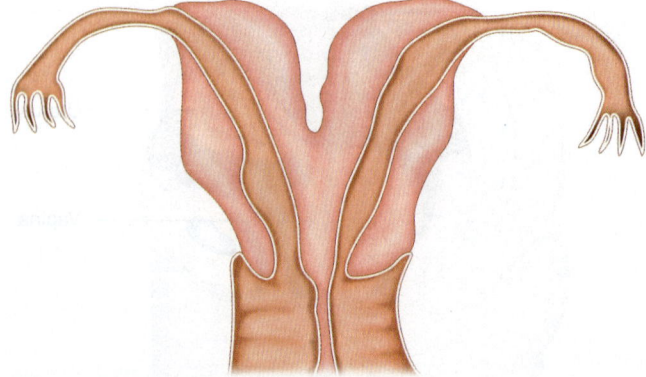

Fig. 2.6: Double uterus with double vagina.

CHAPTER 2   Disorders of the Development of Müllerian System

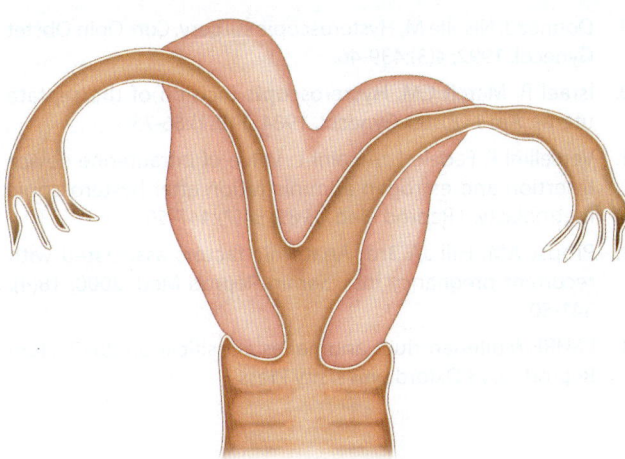

Fig. 2.7: Bicornuate uterus with rudimentary left horn.

Surgical Techniques for Bicornuate Uterus

Although, a number of metroplasty procedures are available, the Strassman procedure was the surgical treatment of choice for bicornuate uterus and didelphys uterus. This approach involves the removal of the septum by wedge resection with subsequent unification of the 2 cavities. Since, it causes a weak uterus, this procedure is not recommended in recent times.

Septate Uterus (Fig. 2.3)

The septum is considered complete if it extends to the internal os, thus dividing the endometrial cavity, and partial if it does not. In addition, septa may be segmental, which results in partial communication between the endometrial cavities. Although, fertility does not appear to be significantly compromised its presence alone is not an indication for surgery.

Transvaginal ultrasound is a useful aid in diagnosing septate uterus, with one study demonstrating a sensitivity of 100% and a specificity of 80%.[7]

Surgical Management of Septate Uterus

Surgical techniques: As the surgical procedure of choice, transabdominal Tompkin's metroplasty has been replaced by operative hysteroscopy. Currently, surgical correction of septate uterus is rendered through hysteroscopic division of the septum.[8–10] The surgical approach utilizes concurrent laparoscopy and hysteroscopy. Laparoscopy is essential to the success of the surgery; it helps confirm the diagnosis of septate uterus as opposed to bicornuate uterus, and it helps reduce the risk of uterine perforation during septal incision.[9,10]

Postoperative Management

Postoperative placement of a Lippes Loop intrauterine device for a month is controversial.[9] Some think that it may prevent intrauterine adhesion formation, while others maintain that this procedure is unnecessary and may provoke local inflammation with subsequent synechiae.[11] Currently, no unanimity exists for this practice.

Conjugated estrogens (1.25 mg/d for 25 days) and progesterone (10 mg/d added on days 21–25) are frequently prescribed postoperatively to assist epithelialization. At present, there is no consensus on this practice. Some experts believe that hormonal therapy has not been proven necessary and can often be withheld.[12]

A 1 month postoperative follow-up examination is recommended. Either hysteroscopy or hysterosalpingography can be performed to assess the uterine cavity. Ultrasound can also be performed.

The risk of pelvic adhesions is limited, and recovery is rapid with no prolonged postoperative delay in conception. Hysteroscopic metroplasty allows vaginal delivery, obviating the need for subsequent cesarean section as was recommended using the transabdominal approach.

CONCLUSION

Müllerian duct anomalies are a morphologically diverse group of congenital disorders involving the female reproductive tract.[13] Establishing an accurate diagnosis is essential for patient management and planning treatment strategies. Uterine shape or anomalies do not require active measures of surgery most often, except for the wide uterine septum. Vaginal reconstruction operations have a place in those whose vagina is absent.

REFERENCES

1. Coney P. Effect of vaginal agenesis on the adolescent: prognosis for normal sexual and psychological adjustment. Adolesc Pediatr Gynecol. 1992; 5:8.
2. Rock JA. Surgery for anomalies of the müllerian ducts. In: Thompson JD, Rock JA (Eds). Telinde's Operative Gynecology, 7th ed. Philadelphia: JB Lippincott; 1992:603-46.
3. Mc Indoe. The treatment of congenital absence and obliterative condition of the vagina. Br J Plast Surg. 1950; 2:254-67.
4. Williams EA. Congenital absence of the vagina: a simple operation for its relief. J Obstet Gynecol Br Commonwealth. 1964; 71:511.

5. Ismail IS, Cutner AS, Creighton SM. Laparoscopic vaginoplasty: alternative techniques in vaginal reconstruction. BJOG. 2006; 113:340-3.
6. Strassman EO. Fertility and unification of the pregnant uterus. Fertil Steril. 1966; 17:165.
7. Pellerito JS, McCarthy SM, Doyle MB. Diagnosis of uterine anomalies: relative accuracy of MR imaging, endovaginal sonography, and hysterosalpingography. Radiology. 1992; 183(3): 795-800.
8. DeCherney AH, Russell JB, Graebe RA. Resectoscopic management of mullerian fusion defects. Fertil Steril. 1986; 45(5):726-28.
9. Donnez J, Nisolle M. Hysteroscopic surgery. Curr Opin Obstet Gynecol. 1992; 4(3):439-46.
10. Israel R, March CM. Hysteroscopic incision of the septate uterus. Am J Obstet Gynecol. 1984; 149(1):66-73.
11. Vercellini P, Fedele L, Arcaini L. Value of intrauterine device insertion and estrogen administration after hysteroscopic metroplasty. J Reprod Med. 1989; 34(7):447-50.
12. Propst AM, Hill JA 3rd. Anatomic factors associated with recurrent pregnancy loss. Semin Reprod Med. 2000; 18(4): 341-50.
13. ESHRE Mullerian duct anomalies classification 2013, Hum Reprod. 2013 Oxford university Press.

CHAPTER 3

Ovulation and Menstruation

AP Manjunath, Pratap Kumar, Jayaraman Nambiar

Overview

- Menstruation is initiated in response to changes in the hormonal production by the ovaries which themselves are controlled by the pituitary and hypothalamus.
- The ovary has two functional roles. First gametogenesis and second hormonogenesis.
- Less than 500 of the original 6 million ovarian follicles will be selected to ovulate in the reproductive years.
- The hormonogenesis is functionally compartmentalized within the follicle as "two cell two gonadotropin system". LH receptors are present only on the theca cells and FSH receptors only on granulosa cells. In response to LH, the thecal cells are stimulated to produce androgens. The FSH induces aromatization in the granulosa cells, which converts the thecally-derived androgens into estrogen.
- During the follicular phase, an orderly sequence of events takes place, the end results of which is one surviving mature follicle. Recruitment, selection, dominance and ovulation are the processes.
- After ovulation the corpus luteum is formed. The lifespan of corpus luteum is fixed being around 14 days. At the end of the luteal phase the corpus luteum regresses unless rescued by human chorionic gonadotropin (hCG) from the implanting embryo.
- The endometrial events can be divided into three phases: Menstrual phase, proliferative phase and the secretory phase.

INTRODUCTION

Menstrual problems are one of the commonest presentations to the physicians. The understanding of the physiological spectrum of menstruation is essential to tackle such problems. We hope to provide a fundamental basis for better understanding of normal ovarian physiologic process relevant to the pathophysiology of ovarian dysfunction, as well as clinical intervention to treat infertility or to achieve contraception.

OVULATION AND MENSTRUATION

Menstruation is the periodic and cyclical discharge of blood, mucus and cellular debris from the uterine mucosa, which occurs due to progesterone withdrawal after ovulation in non-fertile cycles. It is initiated in response to changes in the hormonal production by the ovaries which themselves are controlled by the pituitary and hypothalamus. It takes place at approximately 28-day intervals between menarche (onset of menstruation) and menopause (cessation of menstruation).

Ovarian Cycle

The ovary has two functional roles. First gametogenesis and second hormonogenesis. During fetal life gonads contain 6-7 million oogonia at 16-20 weeks of gestation. Only 1-2 million survive to reach neonatal life. At puberty this number has depleted to only 300,000 to 500,000. Less than 500 of the original 6 million ovarian follicles will be selected to ovulate in the reproductive years. Two meiotic divisions are needed to produce haploid set of chromsones. The first meiotic divison begins at intrauterine life and the oogonia rest in diplotene stage. At the time of menarche recruited oocyte completes the first meiotic division at the time of ovulation. The completion of meiotic division 2 occurs at the time of fertilization releasing the second polar body.

The ovary contains thousands of primordial follicles. They are in a continuous state of development and atresia from birth through menopause. Ovarian follicles may be found in four basic conditions: At rest, growing, atretic or ready to ovulate as shown in Figure 3.1. In the process of oogenesis formation and maturation of the oocyte takes place. It is initiated with the growth of primordial follicle

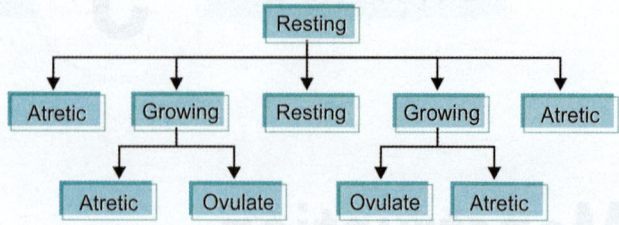

Fig. 3.1: Different types of follicles.

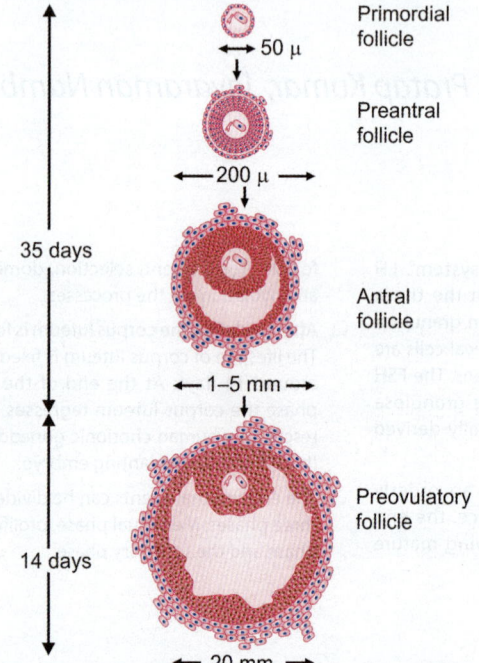

Fig. 3.2: Growth and different stages of follicle.

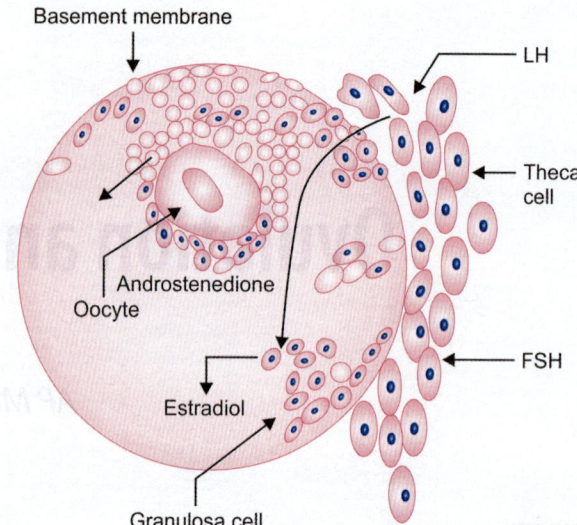

Fig. 3.3: FSH and granulosa cells; LH and theca cells—two cell, two gonadotropin system.

through the stages of prenatal, antral and preovulatory follicle (Fig. 3.2). Approximately 85 days are required for primordial follicle to grow and become a preantral stage. From preantral to preovulatory stage it takes 14 days, which occurs during follicular phase of ovarian cycle. The initial stage of follicular development is independent of hormonal stimulation. Development beyond preantral stage is stimulated by pituitary gonadotropins [(Follicular stimulating hormone FSH) and luteinizing hormone LH] which orchestrate the whole events of ovarian and menstrual cycle. In the absence of correct hormonal milieu, the follicles undergo atresia. Even though anatomically there are two ovaries, it functions as a single unit.

The hormonogenesis is functionally compartmentalized within the follicle as "two cell two gonadotropin system" as shown in Figure 3.3. In the preantral and antral follicles, LH receptors are present only on the theca cells and FSH receptors only on granulosa cells. In response to LH, the thecal cells are stimulated to produce androgens. The FSH induces aromatization in the granulosa cells, which converts the thecally-derived androgens into estrogen.

Androgen production within the follicle may also regulate the development of the preantral follicle. Low level of androgen enhances aromatization and increases estrogen production. In contrast high androgen production inhibits aromatization and produces follicular atresia. A delicate balance of FSH and LH is required for early follicular development. The ideal situation for the initial stage of follicular development is low LH level and high FSH level as seen in the early menstrual cycle.

The pelvic clock in the ovary, regulated by endocrine messages from hypothalamus-pituitary, is essential for successful reproduction and for generating a 28-day menstrual cycle. In a normal ovarian cycle typically only a single follicle containing a single oocyte usually reaches maturity. The hormonal milieu created and controlled by this follicle induce timed and specific changes within the cervix, fallopian tube, endometrium and hypothalamic-pituitary axis.

The ovarian cycle essentially consists of two phases: Follicular phase and luteal phase.

Follicular Phase

During the follicular phase, an orderly sequence of events takes place, the end results of which is one surviving mature follicle. The process occurs over a period of 10–14 days. The length of follicular phase may carry however.

The understanding of the endocrine dynamics of the folliculogenesis is essential for meaningful clinical intervention. The dynamics of this process have been characterized and divided into four phases (Figs. 3.4 and 3.5).

- Recruitment
- Selection
- Dominance
- Ovulation.

CHAPTER 3 Ovulation and Menstruation

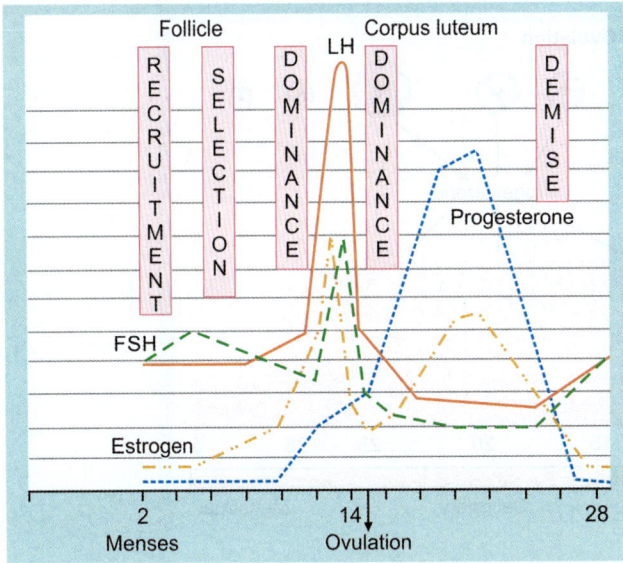

Fig. 3.4: LH, FSH, progesterone and estrogen levels in relation to growth of follicle.

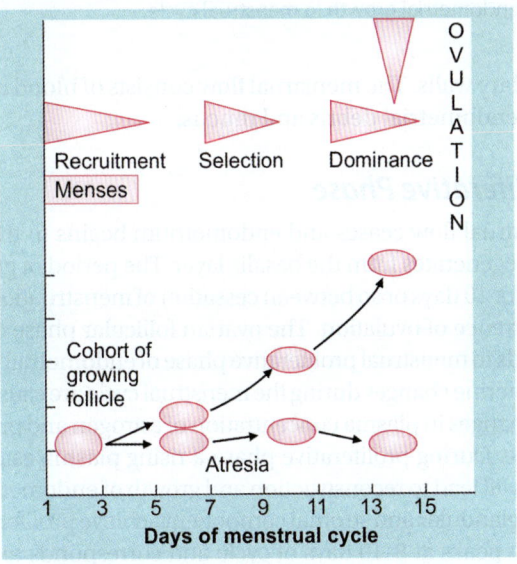

Fig. 3.5: The dynamics of folliculogenesis.

Recruitment
The process of recruitment begins at the end of the luteal phase of the previous cycle from the onset of menses to approximately day 5 to 7 of the current cycle. During recruitment multiple follicles are present that possess the ability to proceed to ovulation. But eventually only a single follicle will be able to utilize its hormonal milieu efficiently enough to sustain development until the interval of recruitment is completed. During recruitment, follicles in both ovaries actively grow and secrete estrogen.

Selection
Between day 5 and 7 of the current cycle, a single follicle becomes destined to ovulate. This is termed as selection of the dominant follicle. Selection of a dominant follicle creates an environment in which only it can adequately mature and reach ovulation.

Dominance
The interval of growth preceding ovulation but following selection is called dominance. The dominant follicle controls the endocrine milieu as it prepares itself, the reproductive tract, and hypothalamic-pituitary axis for ovulation.

Ovulation
One of the paramount events at the mid cycle is the LH surge which stimulates three major events.

1. Resumption of meiosis.
2. Luteinization of the granulosa and theca cells with increased production of progesterone.
3. Extrusion of the mature oocyte about 36 hours after the beginning of the LH surge.

Mechanism of ovulation
This involves proteolytic digestion of follicular wall (mediated by prostaglandins) leading to follicular rupture and extrusion of oocyte.

Unless fertilized the ovum survives only 12–24 hours and then disintegrates in the tube without leaving any trace.

Luteal Phase
After expulsion of oocyte, the granulosa and theca cells within the follicle convert from the production of estrogen and follicular peptides to the production of estrogen and progesterone. This process termed luteinization, actually begins prior to ovulation, but requires LH surge for completion.

The luteal function depends both qualitatively and quantitatively on normal development of the granulosa and theca cells during the preceding follicular phase. Inadequate proliferation of gonadal stromal cells during the follicular phase or incomplete luteinization during the early luteal phase results in decreased secretion of estrogen and progesterone. This in turn may cause altered function of the fallopian tube and endometrium, possibly resulting in abnormal gamete or embryo transport and decreased opportunities for implantation.

The lifespan of corpus luteum is fixed being around 14 days. At the end of the luteal phase the corpus luteum regresses unless rescued by human chorionic gonadotropin (hCG) from the implanting embryo. This is known as luteolysis.

Endometrial Cycle
The most obvious manifestation of a normal menstrual cycle is the presence of regular menstrual periods. Every month the uterus prepares for a pregnancy by generating a

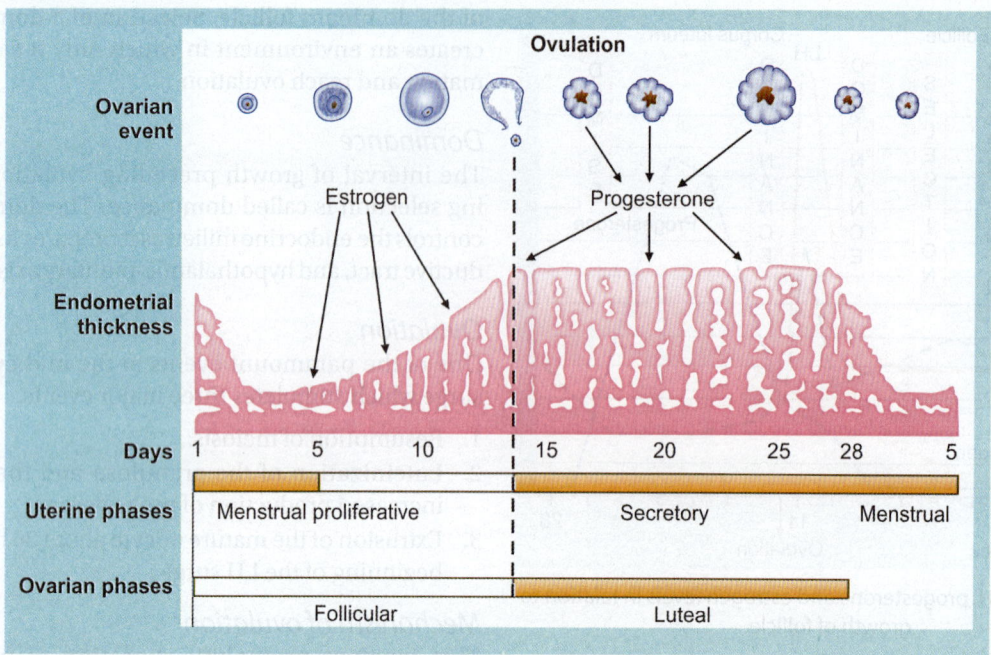

Fig. 3.6: Growth and atretion of follicle related to the endometrial growth in menstrual cycle.

thick bed of secretory endometrium for the implantation. Due to failure of fertilization of the oocyte or implantation, the menses starts. Hence, menstruation is described as "weeping of a disappointed uterus for a baby".

The endometrium is the superficial epithelium, which lines the uterine cavity. It has two principle components, the glandular epithelium and supporting stromal cells. During the menstrual cycle, the epithelium differentiates to form three functional zones. The basalis, spongiosum and stratum compactum.

The endometrial events can be divided into three phases (Fig. 3.6).
1. Menstrual phase.
2. Proliferative phase.
3. Secretory phase.

Menstrual Phase

The beginning of each endometrial cycle is characterized by complete shedding of the spongiosum and stratum compactum layers (day 1) during menstruation which lasts for 3 to 5 days. The fall in plasma progesterone and estrogen levels due to degeneration of corpus luteum leads to withdrawal of hormonal support of the endometrium, which causes menstruation. The first event is profound vasoconstriction of uterine blood vessels, which leads to decreased supply of oxygen and nutrients to endometrium. Disintegration starts in the entire lining except the basalis layer that will regenerate the endometrium in the next cycle. After the initial period of vasoconstriction, the endometrial arteriole dilates resulting in hemorrhage through vascular capillary walls. The menstrual flow consists of blood mixed with endometrial debris and mucus.

Proliferative Phase

Menstrual flow ceases and endometrium begins to thicken as it regenerates from the basalis layer. The period of growth lasts for 10 days or so between cessation of menstruation and occurrence of ovulation. The ovarian follicular phase corresponds to menstrual proliferative phase of endometrial cycle. The uterine changes during the menstrual cycle are caused by the changes in plasma concentration of estrogen and progesterone. During proliferative phase a rising plasma estrogen level will lead to reconstruction and growth of endometrium. Both glandular and stromal component achieve proliferation which peaks at 8–10 days of cycle and corresponds to peak estrogen level. During this phase, the endometrium grows from approximately 0.5 mm to 3–5 mm in height.

Secretory Phase

Soon after ovulation the endometrium begins to secrete various substances and the part of the menstrual cycle between ovulation and the onset of next menstruation is called secretory phase. The circulating progesterone which is secreted by the corpus luteum after ovulation acts upon the estrogen primed endometrium to convert it to actively secreting tissue. Its glands become coiled and filled with glycogen. The blood vessels become more numerous and densely coiled. Various enzymes are secreted in the glands and connective tissue. These changes are essential to make the endometrium a hospitable environment for an embryo.

FEEDBACK OSCILLATION OF THE HYPOTHALAMO-PITUITARY OVARIAN SYSTEM

The intermittent pulsatile secretion of gonadotropin releasing hormone (GnRH) produced by the hypothalamus is transported to the pituitary gland in the portal circulation. This pulsatile secretion of GnRH stimulates the pituitary gonadotropin (FSH and LH) secretion. These pituitary gonadotropins orchestrate the interplay of hormones from the pelvic clock.

The feedback oscillation that controls the rhythm of the menstrual cycle is better understood with the following sequence of three successive events (Fig. 3.4).

Follicular Growth Phase

Two to three days before menstruation the corpus luteum has regressed to almost total involution and the corpus luteum secretion of estrogen and progesterone decreases to the lowest level. This releases the hypothalamus and anterior pituitary from negative feedback effect of these hormones. Therefore, just before menstruation pituitary secretion of FSH begins to increase again and LH also increases slightly. These hormones recruit new ovarian follicles. There is progressive increase in secretion of estrogen from these follicles especially after the selection of the dominant follicle on day 5 to 7. During the first 11 to 12 days pituitary secretion of FSH and LH decreases slightly because of the negative feedback effect of the estrogen on anterior pituitary. Inhibin B secreted from granulosa cells also suppress FSH. This leads to withdrawal of FSH support from the other less developed follicle leading to atresia. The dominant follicle is capable of continued development in the face of falling FSH level. The increasing estrogen level is thought to trigger a marked increase in secretion of LH and to a lesser extent of FSH, which is followed by ovulation.

Preovulatory Surge of LH and FSH Causes Ovulation

At about 11 to 12 days after the onset of monthly cycle decline in the secretion of FSH and LH comes to an abrupt halt. High level of estrogen at this time (or beginning secretion of progesterone from follicle) causes peculiar positive feedback stimulatory effect on the anterior pituitary, which leads to terrific surge of secretion of LH and to a lesser extent of FSH surge. Sustained levels of Estrogen more than 200 pg/mL for more than 48 hours is needed for LH surge. High levels of LH leads to ovulation and subsequent development of corpus luteum. If no pregnancy occurs the corpus luteum degenerates and a new cycle begins. Estrogen, progesterone and inhibin A from corpus luteum suppresses pituitary hormones and a new cycle begins.

Postovulatory Secretions of Ovarian Hormones and Depression of Pituitary Gonadotropins

After ovulation corpus luteum secretes large quantities of both progesterone and estrogen. These hormones have a combined negative feedback effect on the anterior pituitary gland and hypothalamus to cause suppression of both FSH and LH secretion, decreasing them to the lowest level at about 3 to 4 days before menstruation.

The ovarian events, uterine events and the hormonal dynamics in normal menstruation is summarized in Table 3.1.

Table 3.1: Summary of ovarian events in menstrual cycle and its hormonal dynamics.

Days	Ovarian events	Endometrial events	Hormonal events
1–4	Recruitment: Cohort of follicles start growing	Endometrial lining sloughs	E and P are low Rise in FSH and LH
5–7	Selection: A single follicle is selected to ovulate	Endometrium proliferates	Rise in E because increase secretion from dominant follicle
8–12	Dominance: Atresia of all follicles except the dominant follicle. Dominant follicle thrives	Further stimulation of glands and stroma	Increased E and suppression of FSH (negative feedback)
13–15	Ovulation: Mediated by follicular enzymes and prostaglandins. Oocyte completes its first meiotic division	Changes to secretory endometrium	LH surge mediated by increased E (positive feedback)
15–25	Corpus luteum forms	Secretory endometrium	P and E are secreted which suppresses FSH and LH. No new follicle develops
25–28	Luteolysis: Corpus luteum degenerates. Recruitment of new follicles for next cycle	Endometrium begins to slough off due to withdrawal of estrogen and progesterone	Plasma E and P decreases which stimulates secretion of FSH and LH and a new cycle begins

(E: estrogen; P: progesterone)

PRACTICE POINTS

Clinical Features of Normal Menstruation

The physiologic spectrum of normal menses are as follows. The amount of flow is 30 mL. Duration of flow is 2 to 7 days. The cycle length can vary from 21 to 35 days. In healthy menstruation the blood which is discharged does not coagulate. Because normally the blood is coagulated as it is shed from the endometrium, but thereafter, it is liquefied by fibrinolytic activity (plasminogen activator). Hence, history of passing clots during menses indicates abnormally excessive bleeding (more than 80 mL). For all practical purposes, during reproductive age, regular menstruation means regular ovulation.

Clinical Correlation for Ovulation Induction

Ovulation induction with clomiphene citrate and injectable gonadotropins is used for management of infertility. Coordinating the onset and duration of these treatments with the status of developing cohort of follicles is necessary while managing patients with infertility.

Physiologic Basis for Use of Combined Oral Contraceptive Pills

The selection of the dominant follicle on day 5 is crucial time in the cycle. Exogenous estrogen administered even after the selection of the dominant follicle, disrupts the preovulatory development and induces atresia by decreasing the FSH level below the sustaining level. The combined oral contraceptive pills take the advantage of this physiologic mechanism for ovulation inhibition. Thus, the estrogen component suppresses FSH secretion and prevents the selection and emergence of a dominant follicle. The progestational component suppresses LH secretion thus preventing ovulation.

BIBLIOGRAPHY

1. Franscisco I, Gary DH. Mechanism of ovulation. Reproductive endocrinology: endocrinology and metabolism clinics of North America. 1992;21:19-38.
2. Fritz MA, Speroff. Clinical gynecologic endocrinology and infertility, 8th edition Lippincott Williams and Wilkins; 2011: 201-45.

CHAPTER 4

Gynecological History and Examination

Anna Gracia Perez-Bonfils, Edwin Chandraharan

Overview

- A detailed and thorough gynecological history and examination are essential to make the correct diagnosis.
- History taking should involve demographic details, history of presenting complaint, menstrual history, contraceptive history, gynecological history, past medical and surgical history, history of drug intake and allergies and social history.
- Examination should consist of a full general examination to exclude generalised disorders, systematic and abdominal examination, followed by a gynecological examination (i.e. a bimanual examination).
- In some cases (endometriosis or malignancy) a rectal and recotvaginal examinations may also be required prior to determining additional imaging and investigations.

INTRODUCTION

Solving the 'diagnostic puzzle' in clinical medicine involves taking a relevant history, carrying out a physical examination and requesting appropriate investigations to arrive at the correct gynecological diagnosis and to plan further investigations or treatment.

The traditional approach to gynecological examination has changed with the widespread use of the transvaginal ultrasound scan. A transvaginal probe is considered by some to be an extension of a gynecologist's fingers. One stop gynecology clinics are being created with facilities for transvaginal ultrasound scans with 'software packages' that make the process of diagnosis simpler. However, it is important to realize that there is no substitute for a good history and clinical examination.

Taking an elaborate history and examination of the patient is paramount. However, this process should be effective and should be done in the shortest possible time without losing its quality. Learning to ask direct questions after having listened to the patient, addressing patient's concerns and documenting all the relevant information, while awaiting her to get undressed for gynecological examination and performing an ultrasound examination as well as informing the findings and discussing the diagnosis with the patient might take time. With experience, a gynecologist should learn to achieve equilibrium between investing time to obtain a detailed and relevant history, performing medical examination and manage their time and resources appropriately. Moreover, with the widespread use of internet, the demand for information from patients has increased. In order to facilitate the art of history-taking and ensuring nothing important is overlooked; we have included a checklist at the end of the chapter.

Gynecological history and examination are important pillars of good clinical care.

A thorough and relevant history, coupled with a systematic examination would help in arriving at the correct diagnosis. It is the responsibility of the clinician to perfect the art of history-taking and to improve the skills and technique of clinical examination.

Taking a gynecological history requires additional skill, as one has to explore and inquire into personal and often intimate problems. Hence, developing a good rapport with the patient is of paramount importance. The onus is on the clinician to create a friendly and relaxed atmosphere, so as to enable the patient to build her trust and confidence and intimate questions should be avoided until the good rapport has been established. Patient's privacy and confidentiality should be respected always.

SECTION 1 General Gynecology

In order to facilitate gaining the patient's trust and confidence. It is strongly recommended that one should introduce him/herself and the members of the team by name and title before starting the consultation. One should not assume that the person who accompanies the patient has the right to have access to confidential information. Moreover, while asking questions it is desirable to make eye contact with the patient and to address questions directly to the patient whilst taking care to ensure cultural sensitivity.

There is no ideal model of history-taking. It is best to have an outline to ensure that relevant information is elicited in a systematic manner, so as to arrive at a set of differential diagnosis at the end of history-taking. A suggested outline is described below, but sometimes one has to be flexible, innovative and sensitive to the patient's feelings.

HISTORY-TAKING

Demographic Details

These include name, age and place of residence, which may help us to understand the patient's background and to identify some of the risk factors. It is mandatory to check that her details (name and date of birth) correspond to those in the medical record (paper or electronic patient information system).

Importance of age cannot be over-emphasized, as certain conditions are age-specific. Abnormal vaginal bleeding in a young woman is most likely to be dysfunctional uterine bleeding, pregnancy related causes or pelvic pathology such as fibroids or endometriosis. However, in a postmenopausal woman it is likely to be due to atrophic vaginitis or genital tract malignancies. Likewise parity may help us to understand the etiopathology for her symptoms as in genital prolapse or urinary incontinence.

Presenting Complaint

Patients should be encouraged to express in their own words the main purpose of their visit. Most of the times patients seek medical help with a specific symptom but sometimes the presenting symptoms may be vague, as in ovarian malignancy. Unfortunately, this often results in ovarian cancer being missed at an early stage. Moreover, it is vital to remember that patients do not always present with classical symptoms (i.e. 'textbook case') and that there may be multiple-pathology in the same patient. For example, 'perimenopausal symptoms' may be in fact be due to a combination of hyperthyroidism and estrogen deficiency. Diagnosing and treating the latter, while failing to appreciate the former may result in an unfavorable outcome.

If there are multiple symptoms, each of them should be further explored and is advisable to document them in order of severity.

History of Presenting Complaint

Elaborating the presenting complaint by considering the nature of the problem, onset, duration, possible etiological or predisposing factors, as well as complications, if any, is essential. A few examples relevant to gynecology are given below:

Abnormal Menstrual Bleeding

Any vaginal bleeding which a woman perceives as abnormal for her, should be considered significant. It is important to establish the nature of the patient's previous menstrual cycles. Quantification of the amount of blood loss by enquiring about the number of sanitary pads/tampons used, the passage of blood clots or flooding (staining the underwear) as well as symptoms of anemia, may help delineate the magnitude of the problem.

Hence, by enquiring about associated symptoms, it may be possible to arrive at a differential diagnosis (Box 4.1). It is important to determine the degree to which the problem affects the patient's quality of life, in terms of absence from work, social life and household duties. Symptoms of anemia such as breathlessness, tiredness, lethargy, headache or palpitations may suggest the severity of the menstrual disturbances.

Postmenopausal or intermenstrual bleeding would require a careful scrutiny to exclude genital tract malignancy.

Pelvic Pain

It is estimated that up to 20% of women may suffer from pelvic pain and this can significantly affect their quality of life. Details about the location and characteristics of pain (localized or diffuse), onset (acute or chronic), duration, progression (sudden or gradual), character (stabbing, colicky, dull-ache), radiation, aggravating and relieving factors as well as its relationship to the menstrual cycle, should be elicited (Box 4.2).

Abdominal Lump

This may arise from pelvi-abdominal lumps but also from the abdominal organs (e.g. bowel). It is important to enquire about when the lump was noticed (i.e. the duration), the rapidity of growth, presence of pressure symptoms and features of malignancy, which include cachexia and weight loss. Associated symptoms may give a clue to its origin

Box 4.1: Tips for differential diagnosis.

- Cyclical abnormal bleeding is likely to be related to the dysfunction of the menstrual cycle
- Intermenstrual or postcoital bleeding, especially, if they are associated with an abnormal discharge, may indicate a local pathology of the genital tract
- Associated symptoms like dysmenorrhea or dyspareunia may indicate an organic pelvic pathology such as pelvic inflammatory disease or endometriosis

CHAPTER 4 Gynecological History and Examination

Box 4.2: Common causes of pelvic pain.

- An acute pelvic pain associated with vaginal bleeding after a period of amenorrhea may indicate an ectopic pregnancy
  - Pain associated with menstruation (dysmenorrhea) may be suggestive of fibroids
  - Dysmenorrea associated with dyspareunia might be due to endometriosis or it may reflect an underlying chronic pelvic inflammatory disease (PID)
- Intermittent 'colicky' pain in between and during the period may be indicative of a submucous fibroid polyp, extruding through the cervix

Box 4.3: Differential diagnosis of abdomino-pelvic masses.

- Pelvic-fibroids, gravid uterus, ovarian cysts, tubo-ovarian masses, distended urinary bladder
- Extra-pelvic—vascular, gastrointestinal or urological

Box 4.4: Vulvovaginal masses.

- In a young woman: Bartholin's cyst/abscess/polyps
- Elderly woman: Cystocele/uterovaginal prolapse/rectocele/enterocele or carcinoma of the vulva

Box 4.5: Causes of abnormal vaginal discharge.

- Vulvovaginal candidiasis: Described as 'thick, curdy, white' and is often associated with itching and irritation
- Sexually transmitted infection: Abnormal vaginal discharge following a casual, unprotected intercourse
- Necrotic neoplastic lesion such as vulval cancer: A blood stained offensive discharge

(Box 4.3). For example, a bowel mass is likely to cause a disturbance in bowel function. Fibroids are likely to cause dysmenorrhea or menorrhagia.

Lump at the Vulva

Women often complain of 'something coming out down below' or sometimes a 'sense of pressure' inside the vagina which may be due to an uterovaginal prolapse. Predisposing factors like multiparity, chronic cough and chronic constipation may be present. It is vital to remember that many other disorders such as malignancy (e.g. carcinoma of the vulva in an elderly woman) and inflammation (Bartholin's cyst or abscess) may also present as 'lump at the vulva' (Box 4.4). Consideration of the age, predisposing factors and associated symptoms are paramount. It is not uncommon for patients to complain of disturbances in bowel or bladder function, as these organs are anatomically in close proximity to the genital tract. Sometimes, the presenting symptom may relate to the urinary tract (e.g. stress incontinence), while the underlying pathology may involve the genital tract (uterovaginal prolapse).

Abnormal Vaginal Discharge

It is important to appreciate that physiological vaginal discharge is normal. Increase in physiological discharge is likely during sexual excitation and during the 'mid-cycle' (i.e. periovulatory period). Pathological discharge may be secondary to an inflammatory, infectious or neoplastic process (Box 4.5). The amount of discharge, odor, color, itchiness and the presence of blood, etc. may help in understanding the underlying pathologic process during history-taking, so that appropriate examination and investigations may be carried out. In countries where routine cervical screening is not available, it is important to exclude a cervical malignancy.

Urinary Symptoms

Stress incontinence, urgency and urge incontinence, increased frequency of micturition and dysuria may be the presenting complaint, indicating the underlying pathology in the genitourinary tract. Rarely, patients may present with a 'true incontinence' (continuous dribbling or getting wet all the time due to a fistula), especially in advanced stages of cervical cancer.

Vague Symptoms

It is important to appreciate that all women may not present with 'classical' symptoms indicative of the underlying pathology. Women with ovarian cancer often present with 'vague' abdominal symptoms such as bloatedness, discomfort, 'acid-burn', lethargy and unfortunately, the diagnosis is often missed, leading to ovarian cancer presenting in late stages (hence, termed 'silent killer').

Climacteric Symptoms

These include hot-flushes, night sweats (vasomotor symptoms), depression, vaginal dryness and sexual dysfunction such as loss of libido. Although, they are most likely in the peri- or postmenopausal women, it is important to realize that they may indicate a non-genital tract pathology, such as thyroid dysfunction. Rarely, a woman with a premature ovarian failure may present with climacteric symptoms.

MENSTRUAL HISTORY

There is no substitute to eliciting a good menstrual history, as this may point to the underlying pathology. The age of menarche (age of commencement of periods), last menstrual period, regularity of the menstrual cycles, the duration and the amount of blood flow are important. Discomfort before, during and after periods, duration and interference with usual activities should be investigated.

A history of intermenstrual or postcoital bleeding should be elicited and enquiry regarding any post-menopausal bleeding or discharge is mandatory.

Box 4.6: Correlation between menstrual history and gynecological pathology.

- Early menarche and late menopause are associated with endometrial and breast cancer
- Infrequent periods (oligomenorrhea) and other symptoms like weight gain, excessive male-pattern of hair growth (hirsuitism) may indicate polycystic ovarian disease
- Recent changes in weight or personal circumstances (i.e. stress) may explain changes in menstrual cyclicity

Anovulatory cycles are often painless and irregular. In contrast, mid-cycle pain or spotting, primary dysmenorrhea and the presence of premenstrual symptoms may indicate 'ovulatory' menstrual cycles (Box 4.6).

CONTRACEPTIVE HISTORY

Contraceptive usage may be the cause of the presenting symptom. For example, a woman may present with irregular periods or amenorrhea, secondary to hormonal contraceptives. Conversely, a woman who has missed her pills and presents with a lump in the abdomen may in fact be pregnant. Previous history of tubal sterilization may arouse a suspicion of an ectopic pregnancy in a woman, who presents with pain and bleeding after a period of amenorrhea. Pelvic cramps may be associated with intrauterine contraceptive device (IUCD) and discontinuing the combined oral contraceptive pill may have resulted in heavy or prolonged periods.

PAST OBSTETRIC HISTORY

Previous obstetric history includes the details of previous pregnancies and their outcome, in a chronological order. Prolonged and/or instrumental delivery, multigravidity and short interpregnancy intervals predispose to uterovaginal prolapse or urinary incontinence. History of terminations of pregnancy or ectopic pregnancy may suggest a chronic pelvic inflammatory disease. Previous obstetric history may also influence future management: Conservative management may need to be instituted in a nulliparous woman with genital prolapse. Conversely, a radical management option like vaginal hysterectomy and repair could be offered to a woman who has completed her family.

PAST GYNECOLOGICAL HISTORY

Consideration should be given to past gynecological disorders or conditions as it may have predisposed to the current presenting complaint. Multiple fibroids may have necessitated a hysterectomy and subsequently the patient may complain of a lump at the vulva (i.e. vault prolapse).

When it comes to cervical screening the patient should be asked for the year of her last smear and if she has had any history of abnormal results in the past. Furthermore, considering her age and background the patient should be questioned about having received the vaccination for HPV and if indicated, information about it should be given.

PAST MEDICAL/SURGICAL HISTORY

Medical disorders may result in gynecological symptoms, such as disorders of the thyroid gland causing menstrual disturbances and diabetes mellitus causing vulvovaginal candidiasis. Taking a relevant medical history is also vital for planning future management, as a multidisciplinary input may be required. Patients with cardiovascular or respiratory disorders may require referral to an anesthetist prior to any surgical procedures.

When it comes to previous surgery as mentioned, a patient who presents with a lump in the vagina after an abdominal hysterectomy may have a vault prolapse. A patient complaining from amenorrhea following a vigorous curettage might be secondary to Ashermann's syndrome.

DRUG HISTORY/ALLERGIES

It is mandatory to ask for drug allergies and mark it very clear in the medical records. It is also important to record the dose and frequency of any drugs the patient is taking. If the woman is postmenopausal, inquiry about use of hormone replacement therapy (HRT) should be made.

Knowledge of drug usage may help the clinician understand the existence of underlying disorders, which may help avoid drug interactions (patients on antiepileptic drugs may have a higher failure rate with the combined oral contraceptive). There may be a cause-effect relationship as well (e.g. patients on anticoagulants presenting with menorrhagia).

Tamoxifen may cause postmenopausal bleeding due to endometrial hyperplasia.

SEXUAL HISTORY

Gynecological disorders may result in sexual problems or conversely, they may be a result of sexual activity. The onus is on the clinician to win the patient's trust and confidence, so as to elicit maximum information that may be helpful in the management. Age of first coitus, frequency of intercourse and presence of dyspareunia as well as information about sexual orientation and awareness of safe sex are important in further management.

Following menopause patients can experience dyspareunia and loss of libido secondary to estrogen deficiency and therefore it may be a frequent presenting complaint. Due to cultural factors, women with sexual disorders may present with pelvic or vaginal pain, hence, a sympathetic approach during history-taking, is essential.

SOCIAL HISTORY

Smoking habit and alcohol or illicit drugs consumption should be reflected in the history registering the amount and frequency of use.

Socioeconomic status, occupation, diet, access to transport and health care and the level of family support should be enquired.

Carcinoma of the cervix is typically associated with lower socioeconomic status, whereas, carcinoma of the endometrium may affect women of a higher socioeconomic class. One should remember that certain treatments might not be affordable or practical.

FAMILY HISTORY

Serious illnesses focusing in cancer should be noted with particular attention in first generation relatives (especially breast, ovarian and endometrium carcinoma). Also might be of interest is to ask about history of diabetes, venous thromboembolism, heart disease or hypertension.

SUMMARY

It is a good practice to summarize the relevant points at the end of taking a comprehensive history. This could be relayed back to the patient to confirm whether the information is accurate. Patient would then have an opportunity to correct any inaccuracies or to add any additional information.

GENERAL EXAMINATION

This is aimed at assessing the patient's general well-being and to detect any signs of systemic illness. Patient's mental status and disposition may give a clue to the underlying pathology, as stress, anxiety and body weight may have an effect on menstrual function. Body mass index (BMI) should be determined, if indicated. Apart from the standard 'PICKLE' (pallor, icterus, cyanosis, clubbing, lymphadenopathy and edema), thyroid gland and the breasts need to be examined. This should be followed by a systemic examination of the cardiovascular and respiratory systems, if clinically appropriate. Chronic respiratory disease may be the etiology of stress incontinence. A neurological examination is essential if a patient complains of incontinence or there is any evidence to suggest a neurological problem in the history. Referral to a neurologist may be appropriate in certain situations. Similarly, if a pituitary neoplasm is suspected to cause her menstrual irregularity, a visual field examination is mandatory.

ABDOMINAL EXAMINATION

Abdominal examination is an integral part of a gynecological examination. Pelvic organs enlarge cranially into the abdominal cavity and there may be abdominal signs secondary to a pelvic inflammatory process due to the anatomical continuity of peritoneum.

On inspection, any evidence of abdominal distension, paradoxical movement of the anterior abdominal wall with respiration, expansile cough impulse (suggestive of herniae) and the pattern of distribution of the pubic hair should be noted. Surgical scars, including laparoscopic scars should be noted and any evidence of incisional hernia should be elicited by asking the patient to cough. Rarely, endometriosis may affect the scar tissue (implantation endometriosis) or the umbilicus (weeping umbilicus). 'Sister Joseph's nodules' refer to metastatic deposits around the umbilicus, in advanced ovarian (or bowel) cancer.

Palpation should be performed in a systematic manner. Beginning by a superficial palpation and keeping constant eye contact to detect any areas of tenderness or pain, which should be palpated last.

If tenderness is present, then it is important to exclude the presence of guarding, rigidity and rebound tenderness, all of which are features of peritoneal irritation. These signs may be elicited in acute pelvic inflammatory disease, ectopic pregnancy or torsion, rupture or hemorrhage into an ovarian cyst.

Deep palpation is performed to confirm the findings of the superficial palpation and to obtain more details (Box 4.7). Any mass that is felt should be described in terms of its site, size, margins, shape, surface, consistency, tenderness and mobility. Generally, uterine masses have a horizontal mobility and limited vertical mobility, as the cervix is anchored by strong ligaments (cardinal and uterosacral) in the pelvis. A pedunculated, subserous

Box 4.7: Causes of tenderness on abdominal examination.

- Tenderness in both iliac fossae may indicate chronic pelvic inflammatory disease
- Unilateral tenderness may indicate ectopic pregnancy or ovarian cyst accidents, such as rupture, hemorrhage or torsion
- Pelvic inflammatory disease may cause tenderness in the right hypochondrial region due to perihepatic adhesions (Fitz-Hugh-Curtis syndrome)
- Usually, tenderness around the suprapubic region denotes a bladder or uterine pathology

fibroid may be an exception to this rule as it is free to move in all directions. Ovarian masses have free horizontal and vertical mobility. However, an adherent ovarian mass, as seen in endometriosis or advanced malignancy may have a restricted mobility. Abdominal palpation should also include palpation of the liver, spleen, para-aortic nodes and the kidneys.

Percussion is an important physical sign but nowadays with the widespread use of the ultrasonography, percussion might be losing the previously vital importance. It may help differentiate between a solid abdomino-pelvic mass (dull on percussion) from distended bowel (has a resonant note on percussion) and may help define the margins of an ill-defined mass. Percussion may help detect the presence of free fluid (hemoperitoneum in a ruptured ectopic pregnancy and ascitic fluid in ovarian neoplasms) inside the peritoneal cavity. Following clinical signs that are helpful in identifying the presence of minimal, mild, moderate and large amount of free fluid, respectively: The ('Puddle sign' <100 mL), 'shifting dullness' (<500 mL), 'horse-shoe dullness' (1L) and 'fluid thrill' (>2 L). However, in modern gynecological practice, these signs are increasingly becoming obsolete due to availability of ultrasound scan.

Auscultation is not an integral part of a routine gynecological examination, except to determine the presence of bowel sounds in an 'acute abdomen' (i.e. to exclude a bowel pathology or postoperatively, prior to commencing oral feeds).

GYNECOLOGICAL EXAMINATION

Aim of a gynecological or 'pelvic' examination is to examine the genital organs and to detect any abnormality. Patients often find this very embarrassing, stressful and overall an unpleasant experience. It is important to be sensitive and supportive and also respect a woman's right to dignity and privacy. An explanation for the reason for the examination and what it entails should be given (Fig. 4.1). Presence of a chaperone, quite relaxing environment as well as an empathetic clinician, may help allay anxiety and fear. It is likely that optimum information during a pelvic examination will be elicited when the patient is relaxed and comfortable. A tense, uncomfortable patient may contract her vaginal and abdominal muscles that may preclude further examination. Ideally, prior to start examination the patient should have emptied the bladder, except in cases of urinary incontinence.

POSITION

Patients are often examined in the dorsal position (i.e. they lie on their back with the legs flexed at the hip and knee joints). This position gives a good exposure of the perineum

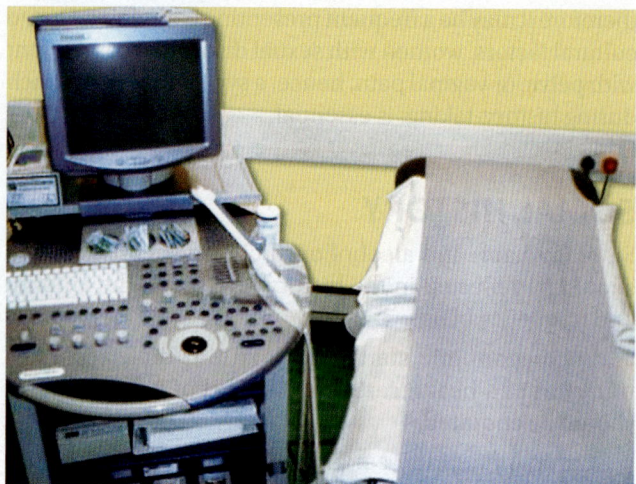

Fig. 4.1: Examination couch with facilities for immediate transvaginal scan in a 'Gynecology One Stop Clinic'.

and the introitus and facilitates use of Cusco's speculum. However, patients may feel too 'exposed' and hence, this may not be acceptable in some communities due to cultural reasons. An alternative is the lateral position with both knees flexed or its variant, the Sim's position (from the lateral position the inner—left—leg is kept extended whereas the outer—right—leg is flexed. Moreover, the left arm is flexed with the palms resting under the head and the patient's upper shoulder is rotated towards the couch). Both lateral and Sim position enables to study the vaginal walls and the Sim's speculum was initially used by Sim for the repair of vesicovaginal fistulae. It is also useful in the demonstration of enterocoele and uterovaginal prolapse (Fig. 4.1).

Lithotomy position with its various modifications is used especially when various procedures are carried out. This is a modified 'dorsal' position in which the feet are held in stirrups, with the thighs flexed and abducted to increase space and exposure.

TECHNIQUE OF BIMANUAL EXAMINATION

This is composed of three steps:

1. Inspection of the external genitalia
2. Visualization of the vagina and cervix using a speculum
3. Bimanual examination of the uterus and the adnexae.

Inspection of the External Genitalia

External genitalia should be inspected in a systematic manner. One useful suggestion is to start with labia majora and move inwards (i.e. describe the appearance of labia majora, minora, clitoris, urethral orifice, and the vestibule). The perineum, the perianal region and the anal verge should also be examined. This should be followed by opening the introitus with the thumb and the index finger of the left hand, placed at the junction of the upper two-thirds and lower third of the labia, to comment on the presence of any abnormal vaginal discharge or bleeding. Lower third of the vaginal walls could be examined and at this stage a rectocele or an urethrocele may be visible. This should be followed by asking the patient to cough and strain to demonstrate the presence of stress incontinence or uterovaginal prolapse, respectively.

Visualization of the Vagina and Cervix using a Speculum

Speculum examination should be carried out after choosing the appropriate type and size of speculum. Many specula have been designed to visualize the cervix and the upper vagina.

Cusco's bivalve speculum and Sim's speculum are the most commonly used. Modifications of Cusco's bivalve speculum have resulted in various sizes, including a virginial speculum and a 'self-retaining' mechanism. Nowadays disposable specula are broadly used, which need not be autoclaved or warmed and also have the advantage of being transparent which assist the inspection of the vagina's walls. Sim's speculum on the other hand is used in the Sim's position to visualize the anterior vaginal wall and in the repair of vesicovaginal fistulae. It is also used in the examination of the uterovaginal prolapse and in vaginal surgery, where more access and space is required.

Insertion of the Cusco's speculum is described below:

Speculum should be appropriately warmed if it is not disposable (Figs. 4.2A and B). A well-lubricated bivalve speculum is held in the right hand with the blades projecting between the index and middle fingers, while the main body of the speculum with the handle and the locking mechanism, rests on the palm. After parting the labia, it is helpful to ask the patient to strain, when inserting the speculum. This may aid the opening of the vaginal introitus as well as help to relax the patient by diverting her attention. It is important to keep both blades closed during insertion to avoid discomfort to the patient.

The handle was originally designed to face downwards as the speculum was designed to be used in the lithotomy position. However, if special gynecology 'detachable' examination beds are not available in the clinic setting, it is best to keep the handle superior, taking due care to keep the fingers and the lock mechanism away from the urethra or the clitoris. The angle of insertion should be along the axis of the vagina (45 degrees downwards) and the speculum should be advanced with gentle pressure on the posterior wall of the vagina, to open the vagina until it is not possible to advance it any further. The blades could then be opened to visualize the cervix.

Non-visualization of the cervix is often due to the mal positioning of the speculum and it may help to 'pull-back' a few centimeters prior to attempting to open it again. Cervix may be shifted anteriorly, against the symphysis pubis, if the uterus is acutely retroverted.

Care should be taken in postmenopausal women with genital tract atrophy as the cervix may be flushed with the vaginal wall which may have less rugosity.

Cervix is inspected for friability, lesions or discharge. Nulliparous patients generally have a conical, unscarred cervix with a small circular os, whereas multiparous patients' cervix is commonly bulbous, irregular and the os has a transverse configuration. It is important to describe the appearance of the cervix and if required, a cervical smear, high vaginal swabs (HVS) and endocervical swabs may be taken at this stage under direct vision (Figs. 4.3A and B). The Papanicolaou smear is designed to sample under direct vision desquamated cells from the transformation

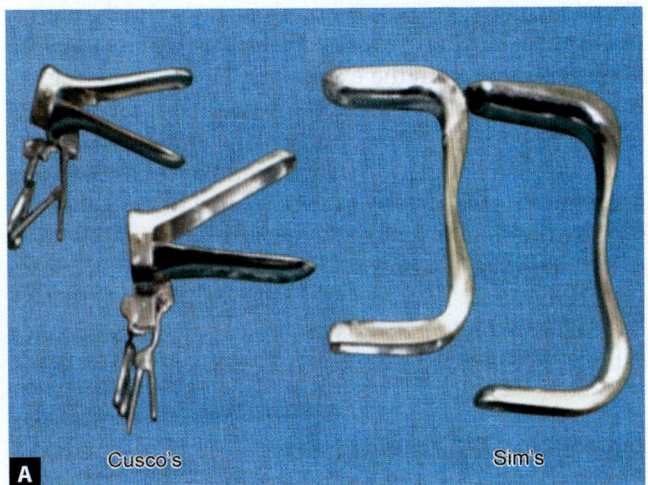
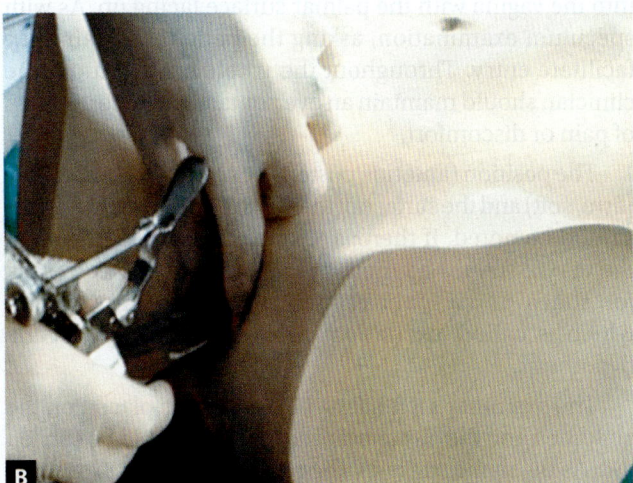

Figs. 4.2A and B: (A) Different types of specula and (B) insertion of Cusco's speculum.

SECTION 1 General Gynecology

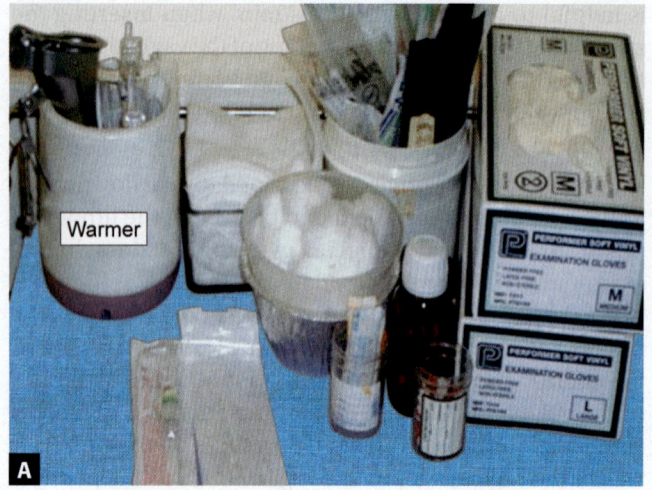
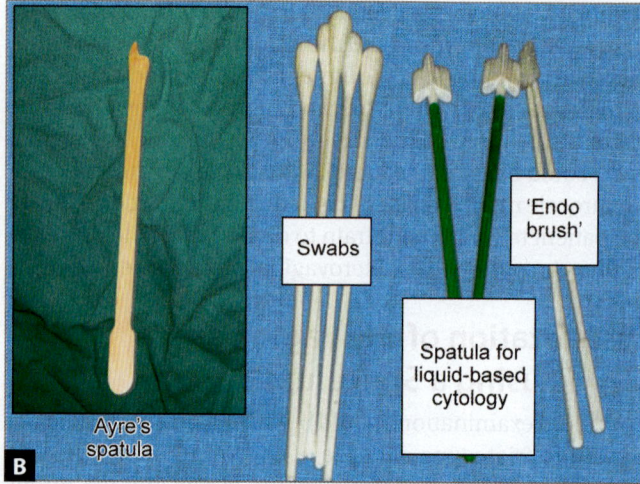

Figs. 4.3A and B: (A) Instruments needed for gynecological examination, including a warmer for Cusco's speculum and (B) spatulae for taking cervical smear.

zone of the cervix (the junction of the squamous cells lining in the vagina and the columnar cells lining in the endocervical canal).

During the removal of the speculum, it is important to observe the vaginal walls for any pathology as the speculum is withdrawn. If the blades are closed very early, they may cause entrapment of the cervix causing pain and discomfort. Hence, it should be removed gently under direct vision. The blades should be closed once the cervix disappears from the view and care should be taken to prevent the trapping of the vaginal wall between the blades.

BIMANUAL EXAMINATION OF THE UTERUS AND THE ADNEXAE

Bladder should be emptied prior to a bimanual examination. After separating the labia with the thumb and index finger of the left hand, two fingers of the right hand are introduced into the vagina with the palmar surface facing up. As with speculum examination, asking the patient to strain may facilitate entry. Throughout the whole examination, the clinician should maintain an eye contact to notice any sign of pain or discomfort.

The position (anterior, posterior or central), consistency (firm, soft) and the surface of the cervix (smooth or irregular) should be noted. If there is suspicion of pelvic infection, the cervix should be moved in lateral directions to seek for sharp pelvic pain related to cervical movement, which is called 'excitation pain' and will support the hypothesis.

The examiner's left hand should then be placed on the abdomen and the bimanual examination should be carried out. As the name suggests, the pelvic organs are examined between the abdominal hand and the fingers inside the vagina. The vaginal hand is often termed 'passive' and the abdominal hand 'active' because once the vaginal fingers are inserted, they are relatively kept stationary. The pelvic organs are 'pushed' with the vaginal hand towards the abdominal hand, which is moved towards the pelvis, so that they could be felt. Abdominal hand should be placed in the suprapubic region, while palpating the uterus. Once the size, direction (anteverted, retroverted, axial), mobility and tenderness of the uterus is determined, the vaginal fingers are moved to the right fornix of the vagina and the abdominal hand is moved to the right iliac fossa. Moving the adnexae towards the abdomen, from right iliac fossa, will enable the right adnexa to be felt between the abdominal hand and fingers positioned in the right fornix. The same procedure is repeated on the left side.

Uterine masses often move with the cervix and pushing the mass upwards would make the cervix move upwards from the vaginal fingers. A pedunculated subserous fibroid may be an exception to this rule as this may have a free mobility. Ovarian masses usually move separately in all directions as they are not anchored or attached to the uterus. In this case, moving the mass upwards would not displace the cervix away from the examining fingers in the vagina. However, adhesions between the ovarian mass and the uterus (e.g. endometrioma) may make it move en-masse. If the uterus is not felt, it may be retroverted. Therefore, it is important to perform the bimanual examination by placing the fingers in the posterior fornix of the vagina. Examination of the posterior fornix is also important in the detection of 'nodules' in the pouch of Douglas. This may indicate endometriosis or rarely ovarian malignancy (Bloomer's Shelf).

RECTAL EXAMINATION

This is occasionally appropriate if there is a suspicion of posterior wall prolapse as it allows discriminating between rectocele and enterocele and also it is a useful examination to assess the extent of malignant cervical disease. Gynecological disorders like endometriosis and malignancies of the ovary and the lower genital tract may involve the pouch of Douglas, rectal wall or mucosa. Examination of the tone of the anal sphincter is vital in patients with stress incontinence to exclude a neurological cause.

RECTOVAGINAL EXAMINATION

A rectovaginal examination may give additional information when pelvic organs are positioned in the posterior cul-de-sac or when examining for abnormalities in the rectovaginal septum and the parametrium, as these are often involved in pathological processes, such as, pelvic endometriosis or cervical cancer. As the name suggests, this is a 'combined' examination, in which the middle finger of the right hand is inserted into the rectum, whereas the index finger of the same hand is inserted into the vagina (Fig. 4.4). Normally, the rectal and vaginal fingers can be easily approximated without any difficulty. If the two fingers cannot be approximated together, it may indicate involvement of the parametrium in the disease process. If carcinoma of the cervix is suspected, this may indicate that the tumor may have spread to uterosacral and cardinal ligaments and hence, may help us in the clinical staging of the disease. If such a parametrial involvement extends up to the lateral pelvic wall, this may indicate Stage III B.

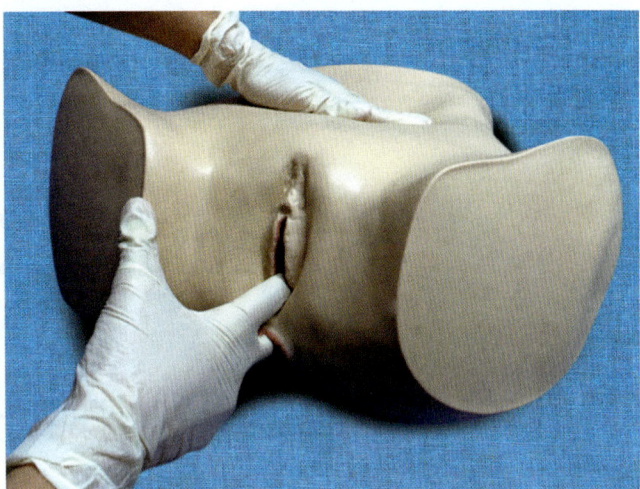

Fig. 4.4: Rectovaginal examination.

This implies that there is no 'tumor free space' between the cervix and the lateral pelvic wall and makes the patient unsuitable for surgery (radical hysterectomy). In ovarian malignancy, rectovaginal examination may give us a clue about the 'fixity' of the tumor and possible tumor deposits in the pouch of Douglas.

After having completed the history and proceeded with the examination, one might consider doing additional investigations such as a transvaginal ultrasound to gain further information to arrive at a diagnosis.

Checklist for Gynecological History and Examination
- Demographic details: Name, age, date of birth and occupation.
- Presenting complaint.
- History of presenting complaint: Onset, duration and progression with associated and aggravating factors.
- Menstrual history: Menarche, LMP, cycle duration and amount of flow. Abnormal genital tract bleeding (postmenopausal, intermenstrual or postcoital bleeding).
- Past obstetric history: Previous pregnancies and their outcomes.
- Past gynecological history: Fibroids, incontinence, prolapse. Last year of smear, was ever abnormal.
- Past medical/surgical history: Major illnesses and all surgeries. Any admission to hospital.
- Drug history/allergies: Dose and frequency of all drugs including history of allergy. Hormone replacement therapy
- Sex: Sexually active—superficial or deep dyspareunia.
- Contraceptive history: Hormonal or barrier methods.
- Social history: Smoking, alcohol, substance misuse.
- Family history: Inherited bleeding disorders, familial cancers.

Summarize History

Checklist of Gynecological Examination
- General examination: Blood pressure, pulse, PICKLE, thyroid, breast.
- Abdomen: Inspect, palpate, percuss and auscultate, if appropriate.
- Vaginal: Inspect vulva, visualization of the vaginal walls and cervix with a speculum.
- Bimanual examination, including cervical excitation.
- Perform an ultrasound scan (transvaginal scan is preferred).
- Arrive at a diagnosis or differential diagnosis based on history, clinical examination and results of investigations.
- Request additional investigations based on differential diagnosis.
- Summarize: Positive and important negative findings.
- Example: "68-year-old multiparous woman presented with a history of lump at the vulva. Pelvic examination confirmed a third degree uterovaginal prolapse with stress incontinence".

CHAPTER 5

Pediatric Gynecology

Pratap Kumar, Shyamala Guruvare, Arun Nagrath, Rupinder Kaur Ruprai

Overview

- Basic anatomy and gynecologic endocrinal milieu in pediatric group and at puberty.
- Disorders of sexual differentiation presenting at pediatric age requires multispecialty approach and careful assignment of sex after complete evaluation and considering the psychological and social impact.
- The development of progressive isosexual secondary sexual characteristics before the age of 8 years in girls and before the age of 9 years in boys is termed "precocious puberty". They can be Gn-dependent (central precocious puberty) or Gn-independent (peripheral precocious puberty).
- Ovarian cysts can occur in early childhood (3–8 years of age), but are more common in neonatal and adolescent periods.
- Labial adhesions result in partial to complete fusion of the labia minora.
- Vulvitis presents with vulvar discomfort or itching and urinary and/or anal signs.
- One should remember that it is important to gain the confidence of the child and make the process as pain-free as possible.
- Providing clear explanations of the problem assists in lowering the parents' anxiety and reassuring them that there are rarely any long-term consequences of these common problems.

INTRODUCTION

The gynecologic problems encountered in the pediatric population are unique to this age group and involve physician skills differing from those utilized with an adult population. It is important to understand the normal anatomy and physiology of the reproductive tract and genitalia in the prepubertal female in order to understand, evaluate, and manage the common problems seen in this age group.

NORMAL ANATOMY AND PHYSIOLOGY

At 5 to 6 weeks' gestation, the undifferentiated gonad is bipotential and is capable of differentiating into either a testis or an ovary.[1] Gonadal sex establishes under the influence of the chromosomal sex. The embryonic differentiation of the normal female genital tract begins in the presence of two normal X chromosomes and in the absence of the masculinizing Y chromosome. The Müllerian ducts fuse at the midline and subsequently migrate caudally to the urogenital sinus. In the female, the Wolffian duct system degenerates in the absence of testosterone. By 12 weeks' gestation the ovarian cortex begins to develop, with primordial follicles appearing at around 13½ weeks. At birth, the female infant has 1 to 2 million germ cells remaining.[2,3]

The fetal hypothalamic-pituitary-ovarian (HPO) axis is functioning at 12 weeks of age with unrestrained pulsatile release of embryonic hypothalamic gonadotropin-releasing hormone (GnRH). There is maturation of the HPO axis toward term with the development of a negative feedback to estradiol (E2).

Estrogen synthesis by the fetal ovary is low at term; however, the maternal estrogen, which readily crosses the placenta, estrogenises the neonate. From birth through the first 8 weeks of life, the female infant is under the influence of maternal estrogen. Placental separation at birth causes an elevation in follicle-stimulating hormone (FSH) and luteinizing hormone (LH) with a brief neonatal stimulation of the ovarian axis. Thus, the young female has two reasons for an estrogen effect on the genital mucosa:[3]

1. Effect of high maternal estrogen levels that crossed the placenta and
2. Stimulation of the child's ovaries by their own gonadotropins.

For the first one and a half years or so gonadotropins (Gn) continue to cause some ovarian stimulation and endogenous estrogen production.[4] Perinatal ovarian cysts have been described following delivery but resolve spontaneously as gonadotropin levels fall physiologically.[5] Beyond 18 months, until puberty, ovarian quiescence occurs due to the exquisite pituitary and hypothalamic sensitivity to even low levels of estrogen.[2]

Anatomical Findings in the Newborn

Until the first 8 weeks of life, the influence of maternal estrogen has a profound effect on the appearance of the female genitalia.

- Owing to the estrogenization, the labia minora are thick and sometimes longer than labia majora
- The mucosa is pink and covered with physiologic leukorrhea
- Clitoral hood is thick. The clitoris is often disproportionately enlarged
- Hymen is thick, pouting, and fimbriated, sometimes making the orifice and the urethral meatus difficult to visualize
- Vagina measures 4 cm in length. Vaginal mucosa is thick
- In the first 10 days of life, vaginal bleeding may be seen in the neonate.[3]

Maternal estrogen exposure may stimulate a mucoid discharge or a small amount of bloody vaginal discharge but these effects begin to recede in about 2 weeks. Higher estrogen levels promote the metabolism of glycogen in the cells, making the lower genital tract much more susceptible to monilial infections, but as estrogen levels fall the likelihood of monilial infections decreases. Discharge and vaginal bleeding persisting after 10 to 14 days is therefore not normal and should be investigated further.[6] Estrogen levels continue to fall until about 1½ to 2 years of age, although gonadotropins continue to cause some ovarian stimulation and endogenous production of estrogen during this time.

From the age of 3 until 8 or 9 years the estrogen levels are at their lowest and this influences the appearance of the female genitalia. With low levels of estrogen, the genital tissues become increasingly atrophic.

- The clitoral hood and the clitoris (the most prominent landmark in the prepubertal female's external genital area) age take on less prominence as the clitoris does not increase in size as do the other structures
- The urethral meatus is often quite small in the prepubertal child. Occasionally, the periurethral tissue becomes patulous and appears as an area of bright pink tissue.[3,4]
- The labia majora appear as normal skin circling around the more central genital structures. The labia minora are very thin, sometimes short, ridges of tissue that edge the vestibulum interiorly and course upward toward the midline, meeting just beneath the clitoris.[4] Below this, the urethra and vagina open. Unlike in the older female they do not provide coverage or protection for the vaginal opening
- Smegma—thick white substance noted in the anterior labia folds (should not be mistaken for leukorrhea).
- The vestibule, is the recessed mucosa that has as its landmarks the urethral meatus anteriorly and the vaginal orifice posteriorly. The vestibular sulcus is the base of the vaginal orifice and appears very erythematous due to the marked density of capillaries that surround this area and with minor trauma may lead to excessive bleeding[3,4]
- A normal clitoral glans in prepubertal child is 5 mm in length and 3 mm in transverse diameter on an average; it shows little variation after puberty[7,8]
- The hymen, which edges the vaginal orifice, varies in size and shape. The once thick, redundant hymen becomes thin and translucent with varying configurations. It may be:[2,9]
    - Annular (age 3—beginning of puberty)
    - Crescent-shaped (no hymenal suburethral tissue; age 3 to beginning of puberty)
    - Redundant (common in girls < 3 years) and irregular
    - Teardrop-shaped.

   The less common variations include:
    - Imperforate hymen
    - Microperforate
    - Septated hymen.

   Usually, correction of these variations is not necessary until the girl reaches puberty.[3]
- Until age 5, vaginal orifice measures 4–5 mm and from then until puberty, it measures 10 mm. It is important to note that the diameter of vagina can vary with the position of the child, degree of perineal relaxation, hymen shape and the level of estrogenization.[10,11]
- A child's vagina measure 5 cm in length.[8] Vaginal mucosa is red, thin (lack of estrogenization), and folded; it is quite sensitive to instrumentation (speculum/vaginoscope, etc).[8,12] The pH of the vagina is alkaline and consists primarily of columnar epithelium. Monilial infections, due to the low estrogen levels, vaginal discharge or bleeding is not a normal finding at this time
- The uterus grows progressively during fetal life. After birth, the uterine thickness and volume is relatively more than the prepubertal uterus, with endometrial and myometrial characteristics similar to that of adult uterus.[13] With withdrawal of maternal hormone, the size regresses and the size then remains constant until the age of 7 years.[14] From 7 years, there is a slow rate of increase in the uterine volume until appearance of

secondary sexual characteristics, after which there is a sharp acceleration during puberty.
- The cervix is small with a centered opening and is flushed with the vaginal vault (therefore, sometimes difficult to visualize). The prepubertal ratio of cervix to uterus is 2/3:1/3; alteration in this ratio generally presents as onset of precocious puberty.
- The ovaries are abdominal structures and gradual descent into the pelvis occurs with the onset of puberty.[2] The ovarian size increases throughout childhood in relation to the increase in size of antral follicles and stroma. Until the age of 6 years, these antral follicles measure <5 mm in size and in the early pubertal ovaries, these measure <9 mm (giving a PCOS like appearance). Any enlargement of the ovary can present as an abdominal mass with associated abdominal symptoms.

Examination of the Prepubertal and the Newborn

The Premenarchal Girls

Examination of the child: It begins with[15] plotting the height and weight on a growth chart, followed by checking the ears, neck, heart, and lungs. Sexual developmental stage of the breasts is noted. This is followed by abdominal and gynecological examination. Many of the problems encountered in the prepubertal patient are vulvar and lower vaginal in origin and not all will require visualization of the upper vagina and cervix.

Position and Technique(s)[15]

1. Supine with frog-legged position (supine, with legs flexed, knees apart and feet touching) or legs in stirrups.
2. Knee chest position can be used to try to visualize the upper vagina and cervix.

The external genitalia, hymen, and distal vagina can be visualized by the lateral spread technique where index fingers are placed on the posterior aspect of the labia and gentle downward-lateral traction is applied.

- Hymenal tags and periurethral grooves are normal findings
- Common lower tract abnormalities include: Hymenal and vaginal cysts, urethral prolapse, labial agglutination, vaginitis, foreign objects, imperforate hymen, and lichen sclerosis.[15]

Examination of the upper vagina and cervix is done for:
- Vaginal bleeding
- Persistent vaginal discharge
- Suspected foreign object
- Trauma
- Suspected vaginal tumor.

Bimanual examination is avoided as the estrogen status of the child in latency limits the examination. Insertion of the small finger for a rectal examination to evaluate the vagina and uterus is better tolerated.

Rectal examination is usually the last step, which helps in determining the existence and size of the cervix. It should measure about 5 mm in transverse diameter. Ovaries at this stage are too small to be felt. Any mass felt should be further investigated. Vagina can be palpated to look for foreign body or discharge.[8]

Examination under anesthesia and/or vaginoscopy may be required in only select cases such as tumor, foreign body and conditions where ultrasonography (USG) does not provide adequate information on source of vaginal bleeding/discharge.[12]

Collection of Specimens

Specimens (if necessary) should be obtained at the end of the examination. As the premenarchal vaginal mucosa is atrophic, obtaining specimens with dry cotton tip swabs can cause pain and bleeding. Therefore, swabs moistened with saline should be used. Specimens for cultures are indicated when there is:

- Vaginal discharge in absence of foreign body
- Suspicion of specific causes of vulvitis (infections by yeast, *Streptococcus*, etc.).

DISORDERS OF SEXUAL DIFFERENTIATION[16] AND SEXUAL AMBIGUITY[17]

Sex determination and sex differentiation are the two events that influence the phenotypic sex of an individual. It is the transcriptional regulators that determine the sex whereas the sex differentiation is dependent on hormones and their receptors. Disorders of sexual differentiation can be with or without ambiguous genitalia.

There are four major issues with intersexuality and the related disorders. They are: (1) etiological diagnosis, (2) assignment of gender, (3) indication for and timing of genital surgery, (4) the disclosure of medical information to the patient and his/her parents.[18]

Assignment of the gender of a newborn is an important responsibility of the obstetrician; wrong sex assigned at birth can have long-term psychosocial consequences. Until complete work-up is done and the etiology is found, sex assignment must not be made in cases with ambiguous genitalia; the parents need to be counseled effectively regarding the issue. The affected individual's desire, the feasibility of corrective surgeries and the net outcome related to sexual/fertility function also is taken into consideration while planning the management. The management would be at appropriate time and can be in terms of hormonal treatment and corrective surgeries. Hence, it is important that the treating team discusses these issues and plans with the parents.

- Examples of ambiguity:
  - Genital tubercle with development half way between that of penis and clitoris
  - Genital folds completely fused with bifid scrotum
  - Penis abnormally bent and buried inward
  - Posterior fusion of labia majora and single perineal orifice at the base of genital tubercle
  - True clitoral hypertrophy and oblong mass in the inguinal position with female phenotype.
- Objectives:
  - Thorough examination of general features and genitals
  - Investigations
  - Sex assignment-decision must only be made when sufficient information is available. This requires a multidisciplinary team of pediatric endocrinologists, obstetricians, radiologists, surgeons, geneticists, biologists, and pediatric psychiatrists.

Diagnosis

Step 1. Thorough physical examination, that begins by a methodical general inspection and careful genital inspection. Precise measurement of the penis is made; mean stretched penile length in the normal term newborn is 3.5 cm (± 0.5 cm).

Step 2. Note degree of ambiguity-define the extent of ambiguity by presence, number, size, symmetry and position of gonads if possible.

Step 3. Careful palpation to locate gonads below the genital folds/inguinal region:

- If gonads are absent: Female pseudohermaphroditism
- If gonad or gonads are palpable: Male pseudohermaphroditism
- In a masculinized female newborn, congenital adrenal hyperplasia (CAH) and undervirilized male newborn should be ruled out.

Step 4. Careful background history:

- Information on other siblings/family members with similar problem
- History of neonatal death
- Consanguinity
- Maternal ingestion of drugs/exposure to chemical environmental agents during pregnancy
- Questions about salt losing.

Step 5. Formulate a differential diagnosis[17] (Flowchart 5.11)

Step 6. Investigations:

- **Genetic:**
  - Buccal smears for Barr bodies (not reliable)
  - Karyotyping
  - Polymerase chain reaction (PCR) analysis of SRY gene on the Y chromosome (results available in one day).
- **Hormonal:**
  - Elevation of 17 hydroxyprogesterone (17 OHP) and plasma testosterone-CAH (due to 21 hydroxylase deficiency)
  - Basal plasma testosterone levels to evaluate Leydig's cell function
  - Testicular stimulation with hCG determines (1000 U/day of hCG for 3 days or 1500 U every 2 days for 2 weeks):
    - Functional value of testicular tissue (insufficient response of <3 ng/mL suggests gonadal dysgenesis)
    - Inborn error of testosterone biosynthesis by showing augmentation in precursors: 17 OHP, dehydroepiandrosterone (DHEA), androstenedione.
- **Peripheral androgen receptivity**—in all cases of under masculinized external genitalia associated with elevated testosterone secretion:
  - By clinical response of genital tubercle to exogenous testosterone (augmentation of <35 mm in phallic length in newborns with micropenis is insufficient); failure to respond → end-organ resistance to androgens).

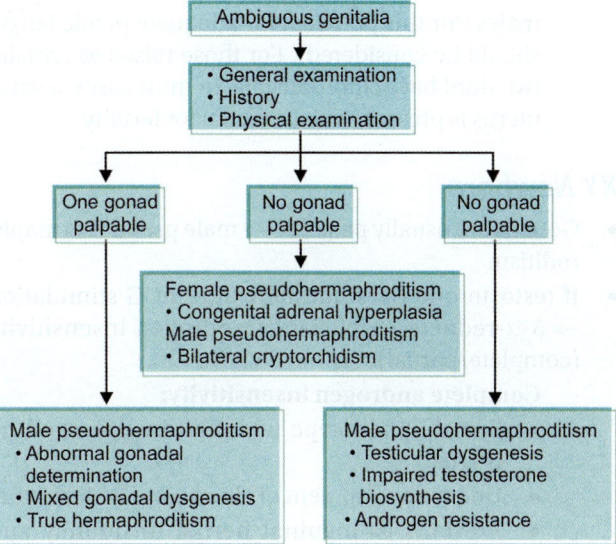

Flowchart 5.1: Differential diagnosis at completing of clinical examination.

- By measurement of concentration of receptor sites in external genitalia (concentration <300 fmol/mg of DNA → partial androgen insensitivity).
- Imaging:
  - Ultrasonography: Look for uterus and ovaries
  - Genitography: For level of implantation of vaginal cavity on the urethra.

Etiology of Ambiguous Genitalia

XX Newborn

Gonads are not palpable → female pseudohermaphroditism.

With SRY (–), causes of excessive androgen production include:

- Increased 17 OHP (fetal cause): CAH is the most frequent cause of androgen excess in female newborn.
- Normal 17 OHP: Excessive maternal production or exposure to androgen/progestins causes virilization of female fetus:
  - Exogenous steroids during pregnancy can cause posterior fusion of labia, clitoridal enlargement, and androgenization.
  - Danazol, because of its androgenic side effects.
  - Ovarian tumors—luteoma of pregnancy, arrhenoblastoma, hilar-cell tumor, ovarian stromal cell tumor, Krukenberg tumor.
  - Untreated maternal virilizing CAH.
- Placental aromatase deficiency: Placental aromatase protects the fetus from excess androgenization and a defect in the same leads to virilization in female offspring.

SRY +

- XX male
  - XX true hermaphrodite—has both testicular and ovarian tissue. Two-thirds of these are raised as males (for this potential for adequate penile length should be considered). For those raised as females two third have clitoromegaly. In most cases, a small uterus is present, with potential for fertility.

XY Newborn

- Gonads are usually palpable → male pseudohermaphroditism
- If testosterone rises normally after hCG stimulation → 5-α-reductase deficiency/androgen insensitivity (complete/partial).
  - **Complete androgen insensitivity:**
    - Female phenotype with blind vagina and no uterus
    - Under development of clitoris and labia minora
    - Presents as inguinal hernia in infancy and primary amenorrhea in puberty
    - Breast development is normal
    - Absent or scanty axillary and pubic hair
    - They develop female habitus.

    Treatment: Gonadectomy, ideally before puberty followed by estrogen therapy during puberty.
  - **Partial androgen insensitivity syndrome** has a spectrum of clinical phenotypes:
    - Wolffian duct that is developed to a variable extent
    - Simple hypospadiasis
    - Micropenis
    - Undervirilization and gynecomastia in adolescent boys.

    Management:
    - Individualized depending on degree of genital ambiguity, growth response of penis to testosterone and type of androgen receptor mutation
    - Female rearing is preferred as they are azoospermic and would otherwise require multiple reconstructive surgeries of external genitalia.
  - **5-α-reductase deficiency**
    - At birth—undervirilized phenotype with hypospadic phallus resembling clitoris, bifid scrotum that is labia like and urogenital sinus opening on the perineum. Testes can be either in the inguinal canal, labia majora, or scrotum. Wolffian duct is differentiated normally in vas deferens, epididymis, and seminal vesicles.
    - At puberty—virilization of external genitalia occurs along with acquisition of male genetic identity in these patients that are usually raised as females.

    Management: It depends on the phenotype findings and gender at time of diagnosis.
    - Gonadectomy should be performed early to prevent masculinization, along with vaginoplasty and clitoridal reduction
    - If diagnosed in puberty: One can consider raising child as male.

46 XY/XO Newborn

Diagnosis is mixed gonadal dysgenesis and characteristics include:

- A unilateral testis that is often intra-abdominal, a contralateral streak gonad, and persistent Müllerian structures. There are varying degrees of inadequate masculinization and such males are infertile. Affected patients are at risk of gonadal tumors, therefore, these should be removed, and patients should be reared as females.
- Distinction between mixed gonadal dysgenesis and Turner's syndrome with Y material is unclear.

Sex Assignment for Rearing

- The clinical examination provides an assessment of the degree of virilization and the presence of gonads.
- Biological assessments are mandatory for plasma 17 OHP and the SRY gene.
- Anatomic condition and functional abilities of genitalia; etiology of the genital malformation and family considerations should be kept in mind.

In cases of female pseudohermaphroditism, the newborn should always be declared to be of female sex. With normal ovaries and uterus, they are potentially capable of bearing children.

In cases of male pseudohermaphroditism, great care should be taken as major considerations are: Reconstructive surgery, probability of pubertal virilization, and response of external genitalia to exogenous and endogenous testosterone. The presence of testicular tissue is not an essential factor in this decision.

Disorders of sexual differentiation: summary of sex assignment and management plan

- Defect in 5 α reductase → male sex rearing because pubertal virilization will lead to penile development (although, it will be subnormal), normal pubic hair development, and the acquisition of male sexual identity
- Inborn errors of testosterone synthesis—when a vagina and uterus are present, female sex rearing is preferred since vaginoplasty can be done and especially if male reconstructive surgery appears highly unlikely
- Androgen resistance—female rearing
- True hermaphroditism—female sex assignment since ovarian function is preserved
- For male pseudohermaphroditism reared as girls—castration
- For male pseudohermaphroditism reared as boys—gonadal follow-up throughout life. Castration of XY intersex with testicular dysgenesis should be done, as there is a high chance of gonadal tumor.

VULVOVAGINAL DISORDERS

Labial Adhesions

Incidence: Labial adhesions occur in 1–38% of children aged from 13 months to 6 years.[19]

Labial adhesions result in partial to complete fusion of the labia minora.[20] The agglutination usually begins posteriorly and extends upward toward the clitoris, leaving a small opening anteriorly in most cases. The fused portion of the labia is usually identified by a thin line of demarcation or raphe.[21] Extreme cases of complete labial closure result in urinary retention, pruritus, and/or infection.

Etiology: It has been postulated that estrogen deficiency results in thinning of the superficial mucosal layers and any inflammation results in adhesions.

Treatment

- Spontaneous resolution can occur at puberty once estrogen is produced
- Application of estrogen cream to the fine thin raphe twice a day for 2 weeks followed by once daily application for 2 weeks. As estrogen cream can be systemically absorbed. Parents may notice transient breast development, and it is not advised to continue therapy for longer than 4 weeks
- For recurrence: A repeat course of treatment in 6 months to 1 year intervals is given
- Once separation of the labia has occurred, a thin coating of lubricant once daily is suggested to keep the area moist and prevent recurrence
- Surgical separation is done only if urinary problems result and estrogen therapy has failed
- Forceful manual separation is not advised as this causes pain and trauma to the child. In addition, recurrence is much more common.

Vulvitis

Vulvitis presents with vulvar discomfort or itching and urinary and/or anal signs. Symptoms can be persistent. Isolated erythematous areas can be seen. Lesions exclusively involve the vulva and there is no vaginal discharge, whereas, in vaginitis, there are both clinical vulvovaginal manifestations and a vaginal discharge due to an infection. Vulvitis is usually related to poor hygiene, irritants, and pinworms.

A careful history with regard to use of any possible irritant should be taken. Questions should be directed to the level of hygiene, urinary incontinence, frequency of diaper changes, and bathing habits.

Conditions that Cause Vulvitis

1. **Diaper dermatitis** is associated with exposure to urine and stool in infants but also in girls, who are developmentally delayed and wearing diapers. Based on localization of lesion and their shape, they are described as Y-diaper dermatitis, W-diaper dermatitis, mixed diaper dermatitis, Jacquet erosive diaper dermatitis and Lucky-Luke diaper dermatitis.
   Management:
   - Keep the area dry
   - Regular change of diapers
   - Application of petroleum based ointment that serves as a moisture barrier.
2. **Candidiasis:** It is rarely seen in the non-estrogenised prepubertal girl but is common in infants under the age of 2.[22] It presents as erythematous rash with raised, well-demarcated borders and satellite lesions.

Predisposing factors:
- It may follow a course of antibiotics in the infant
- Juvenile onset diabetes
- Immunosuppression.

Investigation: KOH preparation helps identify hyphae.

Treatment: Antifungal creams such as clotrimazole, miconazole or butaconazole applied twice a day to the affected area for 10–14 days or until rash is cleared.

3. **Group A β-hemolytic Streptococcus:** It is treated with an antibiotic therapy for 2 weeks and occasionally for longer periods of time (up to 4 weeks). Additional therapy consists of sitz baths with baking soda or colloidal oatmeal added one to two times daily. Soap should be avoided and the area can be dried thoroughly with a hair dryer on low heat or cool air. Hygiene must be emphasized along with thorough hand washing before and after using the toilet.

4. **Nocturnal pruritus:** Pinworms, or Enterobius vermicularis, are 1 cm long, thin white worms that can migrate from the anus to the vagina and cause severe nocturnal pruritus.

   Diagnosis: Inspection at night with a flashlight may show small thread like worms exiting the anus. Alternatively, a morning inspection with "Scotch tape" to the anal region can identify the eggs.[3]

   Treatment: Mebendazole 100 mg orally once and repeated in 1 week. It is advised to treat the entire family to prevent reinfection.

5. **Contact or allergic vulvitis:** This can lead to significant pruritis with scratching and excoriation.

   Offending agents: Poison ivy, topical creams, ointments and lotions, perfumed or colored toilet paper, bubble baths and soaps, adult or baby wipes, as well as laundry detergents, fabric softeners and dryer sheets, and bleach used to wash undergarments.

   Treatment:
   - Removal of the irritant
   - If itching is severe:
     - Oral hydroxyzine hydrochloride, 2 mg/kg/day divided into four doses
     - Application of topical hydrocortisone 2.5% twice a day for a week.

6. **Lichen sclerosus:** It presents as itching, irritation, soreness, bleeding, and dysuria.

   On examination: The vulva is characteristically white, atrophic, with parchment like skin and occasionally evidence of subepithelial hemorrhages, excoriations, fissures, and inflammation. It is usually symmetrically distributed (hourglass appearance) in the vulvar and perianal area.

   Diagnosis: In the prepubertal age group the diagnosis is made clinically.

   Treatment: Application of clobetasol cream 0.05% at nights to the affected area for 6 weeks. Follow-up should be scheduled at that time and if there is significant improvement, the dose is tapered progressively until it is being used only one time weekly at bedtime.[3]

7. **Nonspecific vulvovaginitis:** Vulvovaginal inflammation is the most common gynecological disorder of prepubertal girls and accounts for over 50% of visits to pediatric gynecological clinics.[23] Inflammation may involve the vulva, vagina, or both and can result from a variety of stimuli. Factors that contribute to nonspecific vulvovaginitis include:
   - Poor hygiene practices
   - Inadequate front-to-back wiping
   - Smaller labia minora, with a short anovaginal distance
   - Thinner vulvovaginal epithelium that is not well estrogenized and thus more prone to irritation
   - Foreign body such as toilet paper, small toys, or pieces of cloth, which may be inserted in the vagina by the child
   - Chemical irritants such as bubble baths, shampoos, or bath oils, and deodorant soaps
   - Dermatological conditions such as eczema and seborrhea
   - Chronic disease and altered immune status
   - Sexual abuse.

   Pathogenesis: It is not well-defined. It may be associated with an alteration of the vaginal flora with an overgrowth of fecal aerobes or an overabundance of anaerobes leading to symptoms of odor and discharge. *Escherichia coli* is often found on vaginal culture, suggesting poor hygiene; contamination with bowel flora may contribute to the problem.

   Symptoms of nonspecific vulvovaginitis include itching, dysuria, and discharge.

   Recommended vulvar hygiene measures include:
   - Use front-to-back wiping with warm water after a bowel movement
   - Avoid deodorant soaps, bubble baths, or lotions
   - Wear only white cotton underwear or if still in diapers, change soon after each urination or bowel movement
   - Use unscented toilet paper
   - Keep vulvar area clean and dry
   - Wash hands before and after use of toilet
   - Use mild bath soap
   - Remove wet bathing suits soon after exiting pool area.

   Occasionally, a child may be found to be in a "scratch and itch" cycle where the discharge and inflammation has led to pruritis and the subsequent scratching has led to bacterial infection.[3]

- Initially, sitz baths in lukewarm water with 2 tablespoons of baking soda, colloidal oatmeal, or Domeboro solution may soothe an acutely inflamed vulva
- Antibiotics are commonly used if secondary bacterial infection is suspected and include amoxicillin, amoxicillin/clavulinic acid, or cephalosporin for 7–10 days courses
- Topical estrogen cream once or twice a day for 7–14 days may promote healing if vulvovaginal denudation is suspected due to disturbed bacterial homeostasis
- Occasionally, a low-dose topical steroid (hydrocortisone 1% or 2.5%) will help relieve itching and inflammation.

8. **Infectious vulvovaginitis:** Specific vulvovaginal infections that occur in the prepubertal female are often from respiratory and enteric systems and, less frequently, sexually transmitted.
   Respiratory pathogens found in the vagina of young girls include:
   - *Hemophilus influenzae*
   - *Staphylococcus aureus*
   - Group A β-hemolytic streptococci
   - *Streptococcus pneumoniae* causing a yellowish to greenish purulent vaginal discharge
   - *Shigella flexneri*, an enteric pathogen, can cause a mucopurulent, sometimes bloody discharge following an episode of diarrhea in some young girls.

   Treatment: It is based on individual's microscopic report specific for the organism.

VAGINAL DISCHARGE

The newborn may experience some transient vaginal secretions resulting from maternal estrogen exposure in utero. This appears as clear mucous, whitish in color, or clear. On occasion, a bloody discharge is noted due to transient endometrial shedding. It often resolves within a few hours to days. Mucous secretions may appear again around the time of puberty as estrogen levels rise in the adolescent.

Premenarchal Vaginal Discharge

The hypoestrogenic hormonal milieu in a preadolescent child is a major factor contributing to the susceptibility of the vaginal mucosa to infection. The thin mucosa lacks cornification, has an alkaline pH, and is therefore more susceptible to invasion from pathogens. The premenarchal (with or without vulvovaginitis) vaginal flora contains both aerobic and anaerobic organisms.[24]

Vaginal discharge in children is a common gynecologic complaint and may be resistant to symptomatic and/or antibiotic treatment. Very copious discharge is a marker of unusual pathology.[25] In recurrent or unresponsive patients, an evaluation to rule out a foreign body is traditionally recommended.[26]

Common Sources for Vaginal Irritation or Discharge

- Fecal contamination from poor perineal hygiene
- Spread of respiratory bacteria from hand to perineal contact
- Local irritants such as bubble bath or nylon underwear.

Sexual Abuse as a Cause for Vaginal Discharge[3]

Evaluation is certainly warranted when organisms are found on cultures that are associated with sexual transmission.

- Genital infection with *Neisseria gonorrhoeae* is associated with a purulent thick yellow discharge along with vulvar erythema and edema
- *Chlamydia trachomatis* may present with vulvovaginitis, pruritis, and discharge. Infants born to mothers with chlamydia may carry the organism for up to 18 months[27]
- After 18 years, findings of chlamydia warrant a search for sexual abuse
- *Trichomonas* observed on saline wet mount is uncommon in an unestrogenized vagina and therefore, is rarely a cause of vaginitis in the prepubertal child.[23]

Other Causes of Vaginal Discharge

The child complaining of vaginal discharge may have some sand particles, pieces of toilet papers or other foreign bodies in vagina that might cause irritation and discharge.

Rarely, the discharge may be due to mucous polyps from cervix or even due to sarcoma botryoides; hence girls with persistent discharge may be subjected to examination under anesthesia to rule out these causes.

VIRAL INFECTIONS

- **Condyloma acuminata:** There anogenital warts are caused by the human papillomavirus (HPV).

  Presentation: Condyloma appears as white or fleshy, papilloma like tumors in the unestrogenized vulvar mucosa but have more verrucous characteristics of adult lesions on the perineum and perianal areas. As in the adult, certain subtypes of the HPV warts are potentially oncogenic.

Condyloma usually present as asymptomatic lesions and are noted by the parent or caregiver. Large lesions may present with a child complaining of pain on urination or defecation.

Mode of transmission:

- In children <2 years of age, mode of transmission generally, is vertical from mother to child during childbirth.
- After age 2, sexual abuse is a primary concern in children presenting with condylomatous lesions, as seen in one-third of cases. It is postulated that the incubation period may be markedly prolonged in cases where sexual abuse is not suspected or found.[28]

Treatment: Spontaneous resolution occurs often and so intervention is usually not required.[17] In the past, treatment was with trichloroacetic acid, podophyllin, cryotherapy or CO_2 laser vaporization therapy under anesthesia. However, more recently the imiquimod cream, an immune response modifier supplied in a cream base, has revolutionized therapy for external genital warts.[25] A thin layer of cream is applied to the wart(s) at bedtime and left on for 6 to 10 hours, after which it is washed off. Therapy is for 3 alternate days a week and continued until the warts are completely gone, or up to 16 weeks.

- **Molluscum contagiosum:** It is caused by pox virus localized in the genital area. Presents as 1 to 10 mm dome-shaped papule, flesh, or pearly colored with umbilicated center. It is a self-limiting disease. As treatment is often painful (curettage or cryotherapy), non-intervention is preferred.
- **Herpes and Zoster virus infection:** Genital herpes simplex virus (HSV) infections are rare in children.

URETHRAL PROLAPSE

Presentation: Urethral prolapse usually presents with unexplained bleeding, often thought to be vaginal. There is no recent history of vulvar trauma or pain.

On physical examination: Bright red, friable annular mass is seen just above the hymen surrounding the urethral opening.

Treatment: Estrogen cream to the area nightly for 1 to 2 weeks. If the prolapse does not resolve, a referral to an urologist is indicated.

FOREIGN BODIES

Incidence: It is 4–10% in the pediatric age group.[25]
Presentation: Unexplained bleeding, vaginal discharge, or genitourinary complaints may indicate the possibility of the presence of a foreign body. The vaginal discharge is often dark brownish in color and occurs daily, requiring the use of a panty liner by the child. The discharge is often malodorous.

Methods to rule out a foreign body

- Careful genital examination in the clinic
- Vaginal saline lavage
- Examination under anesthesia with vaginoscopy (also useful in identifying other etiologies of vaginal discharge and its ability to execute an extensive vaginal irrigation). Vaginoscopy in the operating room is the traditional method of assessment of foreign bodies in children unresponsive to improved perineal hygiene and medical therapy, such as antibiotics. The exam under anesthesia allows for a more thorough examination and for obtaining vaginal cultures and biopsies, if indicated.
- Pelvic ultrasound examination
- Plain abdominal X-ray
- Magnetic resonance imaging (MRI) in rare circumstances.

Treatment: Vaginal irrigation may wash out any loose pieces of toilet paper, but objects such as safety pins or parts of toys may require that the child be anesthetized to remove the foreign body. Following removal, sitz bath is recommended until the residual symptoms subside.

IMPERFORATE HYMEN

Issues related to imperforate hymen are discussed in Chapter 2 that deals with disorders of the development of the Müllerian system.

PRECOCIOUS PUBERTY[29]

The development of progressive isosexual secondary sexual characteristics before the age of 8 years in girls and before the age of 9 years in boys is termed "precocious puberty."[30] Increased growth is often the first change in precocious puberty. This is usually followed by breast development and growth of pubic hair. The rapid linear growth that characterizes precocious puberty is associated with premature and rapid skeletal maturation and fusion of the epiphyses. In many cases, this results in short adult stature compared with genetic height potential.

Precocity occurs in girls 5 times more frequently than boys and almost three quarters of precocity in girls is idiopathic.[31] Nevertheless, in the face of any precocious development, one should rule out a serious disease process in central or peripheral sites. The factors that regulate the hypothalamic-pituitary-ovarian (HPO) axis and modulate the timing of puberty remain elusive, but it is evident that some regulation is under genetic control. Identification of specific chromosomal abnormalities and gene mutations allows for diagnostic testing and enables the physician to offer accurate counseling of the recurrence risk for relatives.

Obesity at young ager is another risk factor found to be associated with precocious puberty. Higher body mass index (BMI) in girls as young as 36 months of age and higher rate of change of BMI between 36 months old and grade 1, a period well before the onset of puberty, are associated with earlier puberty.[32] Vice versa, researchers have also found that lower age at puberty is associated with obesity later in life.[33]

Classification[34,35]

There are two major classes of precocious puberty: Disorders that result from early reactivation of the HPO axis (referred to as Gn-dependent or central precocious puberty, CPP) and those that do not (referred to as Gn-independent precocious puberty). Most girls who present with precocious puberty have CPP, which results from the secretion of GnRH from the hypothalamus. Majority of girls have no discernible structural central nervous system (CNS) lesion and are thus said to have an "idiopathic" form of the disorder.

GnRH-dependent (True Precocity)

- Idiopathic   74%
- Central nervous system tumors   7%
  - Craniopharyngioma
  - Hypothalamic hamartoma
  - Optic glioma, astrocytoma, and others.
- Other CNS disorders
  - Static encephalopathy (secondary to infection, hypoxia, trauma, etc.)
  - Low-dose cranial radiation
  - Hydrocephalus
  - Arachnoid cyst
  - Septo-optic dysplasia.
- Secondary central precocious puberty (CPP)
  - After late treatment of congenital adrenal hyperplasia (CAH)
  - Hypothyroidism with elevated follicle stimulating hormone (FSH).

GnRH-independent (Precocious Pseudopuberty)

- Ovarian (cyst or tumor)   11%
  - Granulosa or theca-cell tumors
  - Simple follicular cyst
  - Estrogen-secreting tumors
- McCune-Albright syndrome   5%
- Adrenal feminizing   1%
- Adrenal masculinizing   1%
- Ectopic gonadotropin (Gn) production   0.5%

Other Disorders of Premature Sexual Maturation (Gn-independent)

- Premature thelarche
- Premature thelarche variant (slowly progressive precocious puberty/exaggerated thelarche)
- Isolated menarche

Particular attention should be given to the following possibilities:

- Drug ingestion
- Cerebral problems such as cranial trauma or encephalitis
- Retarded growth with symptoms of hypothyroidism
- Pelvic or abdominal mass.

GnRH-dependent Precocious Puberty

- There is a premature maturation of the HPO axis, resulting in production of Gn's and sex steroids. It runs in families and usually occurs very close to borderline age of 8 years. On the other hand, idiopathic precocious puberty does not run in families and occur much earlier in childhood. These diagnosis should be made only by exclusion and deserve long-term follow-up as cerebral abnormalities may not become apparent until adulthood.
- Clinical presentation of true precocity may not follow the usual progression of puberty. Adrenarche or menarche may be the first sign. There is normal reproductive life and it is not associated with premature menopause. Intellectual and psychosocial developments are also commensurate with chronological age rather than stage of puberty. The most serious effect is the resultant adult short stature.

GnRH-independent Precocious Puberty

GnRH-independent precocious puberty is characterized by increased production of gonadal steroids, causing the typical physical changes of puberty, in the absence of reactivation of the HPO axis.[29] This form includes conditions that mimic the effect of pituitary Gn on gonadal function, such as those in which there is secretion of Gn from nonpituitary sources:

- About 11% of girls with precocious puberty have an ovarian tumor. The tumor is usually an estrogen producing neoplasm or cyst. Bleeding is irregular and menorrhagic—clearly anovulatory. A pelvic mass is readily palpable in 80% of cases
- McCune-Albright syndrome (MAS) is characterized classically by the clinical triad of cutaneous hyperpigmentation (café-au-lait spots), polyostotic fibrous dysplasia, and isosexual precocious puberty.[36] In addition, this syndrome can be associated with ovarian cysts, growth hormone, and prolactin secreting

adenomas, hyperthyroidism, adrenal hypercortisolism, and osteomalacia. Premature menarche may be the first sign of the syndrome. However, these endocrine disturbances are not accompanied by increased plasma concentrations of the relevant trophic or stimulatory hormones. Thus, girls with precocious puberty caused by MAS have ovarian enlargement and follicular hyperplasia but have low serum levels of LH and FSH and a prepubertal response of LH to administration of GnRH.[37] Eventual fertility is unimpaired and adult height is usually normal.

- Autonomous benign ovarian follicular or luteal cysts. The cysts may enlarge, involute, and then recur so that signs of sexual precocity and vaginal bleeding remit and exacerbate.

Diagnosis of Precocious Puberty

Aims of Diagnosis
- Rule out life-threatening disease (includes neoplasms of the CNS, ovary, and adrenal)
- Define the progression of the process
- Rule out nonendocrine causes of vaginal bleeding (trauma, foreign body, vaginitis, genital neoplasm).

Differential Diagnostic Steps
Diagnostic confirmation is based on demonstration of pubertal levels of Gn and sex steroid secretion. Diagnosis of CPP is classically made when magnetic resonance imaging (MRI) is negative and a significant LH response occurs following GnRH stimulation that is 2 to 3 times higher than the prepubertal response.[38] Typically, stimulated LH levels rise to > 10 mIU/mL in CPP.[35] Physical examination should focus on determining whether the development reflects androgen action, estrogen action, or both.

Physical Diagnosis
- Record of growth, Tanner stages, height and weight percentiles
- External genitalia changes
- Abdominal, pelvic and neurological examination
- Signs of androgenization
- Special findings—McCune-Albright syndrome, hypothyroidism
- If the all signs of sexual precocity are present and basal or GnRH stimulated Gn's are in the pubertal range: Suspect a pituitary source of Gn
- When signs of sexual precocity are associated with accelerated growth and skeletal maturation in the absence of virilization: Suspect ovarian tumor or cysts
- If signs of sexual precocity are accompanied by virilization: Suspect an adrenal hyperplasia or a virilizing adrenal/ovarian tumor
- If breast and genital development, pubic hair growth, and vaginal bleeding are seen in a short child with a delayed bone age: Suspect primary hypothyroidism.

Laboratory Diagnosis
- Diagnostic evaluation should begin with an X-ray to assess bone age as a marker for sex steroid hormone action. When skeletal age is concordant with chronological age continued close observation could be done
- When secondary sexual characteristics are associated with an advanced bone age, measurements of: E2, DHEAS, testosterone, progesterone, 17-hydroxy progesterone, Gn's and thyroid hormones should be obtained, and a GnRH stimulation test is indicated to differentiate between CPP and peripheral precocious puberty
- In most cases, the diagnosis of GnRH-dependent precocious puberty warrants an USG of abdomen and pelvis and MRI or CT scan of the head.[39]

Treatment of Precocious Development

The objective of management and treatment of precocious puberty include:

- Diagnose and treat intracranial disease
- Arrest maturation until normal pubertal age
- Attenuate and diminish established precocious characteristics
- Maximize eventual adult height
- Avoidance of abuse, reduction of emotional problem. Contraception if necessary.

Long-term complications of true idiopathic precocious puberty include compromised adult height and psychosocial and behavioral issues. Adult height can be improved with treatment if treatment is instituted prior to epiphyseal closure.[40]

A number of therapies have been used to achieve these goals. These have included:

- Medroxyprogesterone and cyproterone acetate are not fully effective in inhibiting pubertal or skeletal maturation or improving adult height.
- Danazol
- GnRH agonists: Continuous, nonpulsatile presentation of GnRH to the pituitary Gn's induces a state of secondary hypogonadism.[41]

Treatment is maintained until the epiphyses are fused or until appropriate pubertal and chronological ages are matched:
  - Substantial regression of pubertal characteristic, amenorrhea, and reduction in growth velocity are

rapidly achieved and maintained within the 1st year of treatment
- The greatest improvement is obtained in children whose bone ages are relatively young at the onset of treatment. It does not substantially affect adult height in girls who enter puberty between 6 and 8.[42,43]
- Height outcome is not compromised in untreated slowly progressive variants of central precocious puberty. In rapidly progressing central precocious puberty in girls, GnRH agonists appear to increase final height by about 5 cm in girls treated before the age of 8, but there is no height benefit in those treated after 9 years.[44]
- Majority experience no increase in breast development, and a third show regression to an earlier Tanner stage. Some experience transient vaginal bleeding ~2-4 weeks after initiation of therapy due to estrogen withdrawal
- Growth can get suppressed to a subnormal velocity due to the decreased estrogen (suppressed by the analogue). Supplementation with mini-dose estrogen replacement is safe and effective (for at least 2 years) in maintaining normal prepubertal growth without acceleration of bone maturation or pubertal development.[45]
- GnRH agonist treatment is not effective for Gn-independent precocious puberty such as McCune-Albright syndrome, GnRH-independent sexual precocity or CAH. Treatment for MAS involves inhibiting the synthesis or action of sex steroids by inhibiting the synthesis of estrogen (aromatase inhibitors) and using a combination of drugs like cyproterone acetate, MPA, spironolactone, ketoconazole and testolactone
- Neurosurgical excision of hypothalamic, pituitary, cerebral or pineal tumors must be individualized in each patient
- For ovarian or adrenal tumor: Surgical excision is the treatment of choice
- For primary hypothyroidism: Give thyroid replacement
- For adrenal hyperplasia: Glucocorticoids (and mineralocorticoids if salt wasting is present) is the treatment of choice.

Forms of Precocious Puberty

- Precocious pubarche is most often a benign condition secondary to early adrenarche. In some patients, premature pubarche may predict the future development of chronic anovulation and androgen excess associated with polycystic ovarian syndrome.
- Premature thelarche usually occurs in the first 2 years of life (classical type), is self-limiting, and regresses before puberty. There is asymmetrical breast development with no other signs of sexual maturation; growth is normal. Approximately 10 to 15% of these girls develop CPP, but in the majority of patients, the breast bud is a transient event that warrants only close follow-up for the appearance of other pubertal signs.[46] It is typically associated with:
  - Some degree of FSH secretion
  - Antral follicular development
  - Ovarian function that is greater than normal.
- Thelarche variant represents a spectrum of conditions, which lie between premature thelarche and CPP. There is usually pubic hair development; growth prognosis is normal; and breast development arrests without advancing to full sexual maturation.
- Isolated menarche young girls have 6 weekly cyclical uterine bleeding without any other form of sexual maturation and have normal growth. Resolution can occur after 1 or 2 years.[34]

OVARIAN CYSTS

Ovarian cysts can occur in early childhood (3-8 years of age), but are more common in neonatal and adolescent periods. The incidence is <5% between birth and age 8. Small cysts are more frequent than large cysts.[47]

Types

- Functional cysts—due to ovarian gonadotropin stimulation and failure of follicular apoptosis
- Ovarian neoplasia
- Hormone secreting cysts can cause rapid pubertal development/precocious pseudopuberty (McCune-Albright syndrome)
- The onset of pubertal signs can be transient with breast development increasing during ovarian cyst formation and decreasing with spontaneous resolution
- Unilocular cysts <5 cm should be followed up conservatively with USG until they regress. Beyond 5 cm size, there is risk of torsion with rapid progression.

Clinical Presentation

- Asymptomatic cyst
- Painful abdominopelvic syndrome (acute/subacute): Associated with nonspecific signs (nausea, vomiting, urinary disorders)
- *Endocrine signs:* Marked by precocious development of sexual characteristics, associated with increased growth velocity and advanced bone maturation. Rapid breast development followed by metrorrhagia suggests pseudoprecocious puberty due to ovarian cysts. Café-au-lait spots and polyostotic dysplasia characterizes McCune-Albright syndrome.

Diagnosis

- *Pelvic ultrasonogram:* Note the size, shape and volume of cyst; thickness and regularity of wall; nature of cyst contents. Functional cysts are anechoic with thin, regular wall. Condition of contralateral ovary is also noted
- Color Doppler for vascularization of mass (e.g. hemorrhagic cyst can be echogenic but avascular)
- CT/MRI
- Hormonal E2, testosterone, and other androgens, LH and FSH. Hypersecretion of E2 with negligible LH and FSH that do not respond to stimulation with LHRH confirm autonomous independent Gn secretion and suggest secretory tumor
- Tumor markers a fetoprotein → embryonic carcinoma and immature teratoma.
- β hCG—choriocarcinoma and dysgerminoma
- Ca 125—can be high even in functional cysts.

Other Condition Associated with Cysts

- Acquired infantile hypothyroidism
- Adrenal disorder
- Benign teratoma
- Juvenile granulose cell tumors
- Sex cord—stromal and mixed germ cell tumors.

Management:

- Anechoic cyst: Monitor for 4 weeks to 6 months. An increase in size beyond this period or persistence warrants excision
- In cases of adnexal torsion or if the cyst is heterogeneous: Emergency surgery should be performed.
- Recurrence of secretory cyst is suggestive of McCune-Albright syndrome. Granulosa cell tumors are rare and associated with precocious pseudopuberty, therefore, these are treated surgically.

REFERENCES

1. Emans SJ, Grace E, Hoffer FA, Gundberg C, Ravnikar V, Woods ER. Estrogen deficiency in adolescents and young adults: impact on bone mineral content and effects of estrogen replacement therapy. Obstet Gynecol. 1990; 76:585-92.
2. Bradshaw K, George N, Moore A, Trump D. Mutations of the XLRS1 gene cause abnormalities of photoreceptor as well as inner retinal responses of the ERG. Doc Ophthalmol. 1999;98:153-73.
3. Kass-Wolff JH, Wilson EE. Pediatric gynecology: assessment strategies and common problems. Semin Reprod Med. 2003;21(4): 329-38.
4. Pokorny S. Pediatric and adolescent gynecology. Compr Ther. 1997;23:337-44.
5. Speroff L, Glass R, Kase N. Clinical gynecologic endocrinology and Infertility. 6th edition. Baltimore: Williams & Wilkins; 1999.
6. Baldwin DD, Landa HM. Common problems in pediatric gynecology. Urol Clin North Am. 1995;22:161-76.
7. Sane K, Pescovitz OH. The clitoral index: A determination of clitoral size in normal girls and in girls with abnormal sexual development. J Pediatr. 1992; 120:264-6.
8. Thibaud E. Gynecologic clinical examination of the child and adolescent. In: Sultan C (Ed) Pediatric and adolescent gynecology: evidence-based clinical practice. Endocr Dev Basel, Karger; 2004;7:1-8.
9. Pokorny SF, Kozinetz CA. Configuration and other anatomic details of the prepubertal hymen. Adolesc Pediatr Gynecol. 1998;1:97-103.
10. Gardner JJ. Descriptive study of genitalia variation in healthy, non-abused premenarchal girls. J Pediatr. 1992;120:251-7.
11. McCann J, Voris J, Simon M, Wells R. Comparison of genital examination techniques in prepubertal girls. Pediatrics. 1990;85:182-7.
12. Emans J. Office evaluation of the chilled and adolescent. In: Emans J, Laufer MM, Goldstein DF (Eds). Pediatric and adolescent gynecology. Philadelphia: Lippincott; 1998.
13. Porcu E. Imaging in pediatric and adolescent gynecology. In: Sultan C (Ed): Pediatric and Adolescent Gynecology. Evidence-based clinical practice. Endocr Dev. Baasel, Karger; 2004;7:9-22.
14. Orsini LR, Salardi S, Pilu G, Bovicelli L, Cacciari E. Pelvic organs in premenarchal girls: real time ultrasonography. Radiology. 1984;153:113.
15. Hewitt G. In-Training Section. Examining pediatric and adolescent gynecology patients. In: Strickland J (Ed). J Pediatr Adolesc Gynecol. 2003;16:257-8.
16. Lee PA, Houk CP, Ahmet F, Hughes IA, and in collaboration with participants in the international consensus conference on intersex organized by the Lawson Wilkinns Pediatric Endocrine Society and the European Society for Pediatric Endocrinology. Consensus statement on management of intersex disorders. Pediatrics. 2006;118:488-500.
17. Sultan C, Paris F, Jeandel C, Lumbroso S, Galifer RB, Picaud JC. Ambiguous genitalia in the newborn: diagnosis, etiology, and sex assignment. In: Sultan C (Ed). Pediatric and adolescent gynecology. Evidence-based Clinical Practice. Endocr Dev. Basel, Karger. 2004;7:23-38.
18. Ocal G. Current Concepts in Disorders of Sexual Development. J Clin Res Ped Endo. 2011;3(3):105-14.
19. Dominique Hamel-Teillac. Vulvovaginal disorders. In: Sultan C (Ed): Pediatric and adolescent gynecology. Evidence-based Clinical Practice. Endocr Dev Basel, Karger. 2004;7:39-56.
20. Christensen EH, Oster J. Adhesions of labia minora (synechia vulvae) in childhood: a review and report of fourteen cases. Acta Paediatr Scand. 1971;60:709-15.
21. Pokorny SF. Prepubertal vulvovaginopathies. Obstet Gynecol Clin North Am. 1992;19:39-58.

22. Sanfilippo JS, Muram D, Lee PA, Dewhurst J. Pediatric and Adolescent Gynecology. Philadelphia: WB Saunders; 1994.
23. Emans S, Laufer M, Goldstein D. Pediatric and Adolescent Gynecology. 4th edition. Philadelphia: Lippincott Williams & Wilkins; 1998.
24. Gerstner GJ, Grunberger W, Boschitsch E, Rotter M. Vaginal organisms in prepubertal children with and without vulvovaginitis. Arch Gynecol. 1982; 231:47.
25. Smith YR, Berman DR, Quint EH. Premenarchal vaginal discharge: findings of procedures to rule out foreign bodies. J Pediatr Adolesc Gynecol. 2002;13:227-30.
26. Widholm O. Genital bleeding during childhood. Pediatr Ann. 1981;1016.
27. Tyring S, Arany I, Stanley M, et al. A randomized, controlled, molecular study of condylomata acuminata clearance during treatment with imiquimod. J Infect Dis. 1998;178: 551-5.
28. McCune KK, Horbach N, Dattel BJ. Incidence and clinical correlates of human papillomavirus disease in a pediatric population referred for evaluation of sexual abuse. J Pediatr Adolesc Gynecol. 1993;6:20-4.
29. Carel J, Léger J. Precocious puberty. N Engl J Med. 2008; 358: 2366-77.
30. Plant TM. Puberty in primates. In: Knobil E, Neill JD (Eds). The physiology of reproduction. 2nd edition. New York: Raven Press; 1994:453-85.
31. Herman-Giddens ME, Slora EJ, Wasserman RC, et al. Secondary sexual characteristics in young girls seen in office practice: a study from the paediatric research in office settings network. Pediatrics. 1997; 99:505-12.
32. Lee JM, Appugliese D, Kaciroti N, et al. Weight status in young girls and the onset of puberty. Pediatrics. 2007;119(3): e624-30.
33. Currie C, Ahluwalia N, Godeau E, Nic Gabhainn S, Due P, Currie DB. Is obesity at individual and national level associated with lower age at menarche? Evidence From 34 Countries in the Health Behaviour in School-aged Children Study. J Adolesc Health. 2012;50(6):621-6.
34. Stanhope R, Traggiai C. Precocious puberty (Complete, Partial). In: Sultan C (Ed). Pediatric and adolescent gynecology. Evidence-Based Clinical Practice. Endocr Dev. Basel, Karger, 2004;7:57-65.
35. Kakarla N, Bradshaw KD. Disorders of pubertal development: precocious puberty. Semin Reprod Med. 2003;21(4):339-51.
36. De Sanctis C, Lala R, Matarazzo P, Balsamo A, Bergamaschi R, Cappa M. McCune-Albright syndrome: a longitudinal clinical study of 32 patients. J Pediatr Endocrinol Metab. 1999;12 (6): 817-26.
37. Holland FJ, Fishman L, Bailey JD, Fazekas AT. Ketoconazole in the management of precocious puberty not responsive to LHRH analogue therapy. N Engl J Med. 1985;312:1023-8.
38. Sathasivam A, Garibaldi L, Shapiro S, Godbold J, Rapaport R. Leuprolide stimulation testing for the evaluation of early female sexual maturation. Clin Endocrinol (Oxf). 2010;73(3):375-81.
39. Faizah MZ, Zuhanis AH, Rahmah R, Raja AA, Wu LL, Dayang AA, et al. Precocious puberty in children: a review of imaging findings. Biomed Imaging Interv J. 2012;8(1):e6.
40. Klein KO. Precocious puberty: Who has it? Who should be treated? J Clin Endocrinol Metab. 1999;84:411-4.
41. Fuld K, Chi C, Neely EK. A randomized trial of 1- and 3-month depot leuprolide doses in the treatment of central precocious puberty. J Pediatr. 2011;159(6):982-7.e1.
42. Hillard PJA. Menstruation in young girls: a clinical perspective. Obstet Gynecol. 2002;99:655-62.
43. Carel JC, Eugster EA, Rogol A, et al. Consensus statement on the use of gonadotropin-releasing hormone analogs in children. Pediatrics. 2009;123(4):e752-62.
44. Brown JJ, Warne GL. Growth in precocious puberty. Indian J Pediatr. 2006;73(1):81-8.
45. Lampit M, Golander A, Guttmann H, Hochberg Z. Estrogen mini-dose replacement during GnRH agonist therapy in central precocious puberty: a pilot study. J Clin Endocrinol Metab. 2002;87:687-90.
46. Bradshaw KD, Quigley CA. Disorders of pubertal development. In: Jameson JL (Ed). Principles of Molecular Medicine. Totowa, NJ: Humana Press;1998:569-80.
47. Millar DM, Blake JM, Stringer DA, Hara H, Babiak C. Prepubertal ovarian cyst formation: 5 years' experience. Obstet Gynecol. 1993;81:434-8.

CHAPTER 6

Adolescent Gynecology

Rupinder Kaur Ruprai

Overview
- Changes during normal puberty including clinical evaluaton of the adolescent girl are discussed.
- Condition affecting the pubertal delevelopment including precocious development and late development are discussed.
- Menstrual cycle and menstrual disorders are discussed ranging from amenorrhea to abnormal uterine bleeding with their management.
- Hyperandrogenism, its causes, evaluation and management are discussed.
- Various conditions such as premenstrual syndrome, abdomino-pelvic pain, endometriosis, ovarian enlargement causes, vulvovaginal complaints, cervical cytology, eating disorders, epilepsy, adolescent pregnancy, sexual abuse, atheletic adolescents, childhood cancer survivors and female cosmetic genital surgery is also briefly discussed.

INTRODUCTION

Adolescence, the transitional stage between childhood and adulthood (age 10-19 years) during which major physical and mental changes occur. It is usually defined by the rapid onset of biological and psychological growth and development. During transition through puberty, menstrual disorders become the most common complaint and mostly due to anovulation. Polycystic ovarian syndrome (PCOS) can develop in early puberty leading into adulthood with infertility, diabetes, and hirsutism requiring age-appropriate management. Recognition and prompt treatment in adolescents is key to prevent the future implications of consequences of endometriosis on future fertility.[1]

The initial visit to the gynecologist should occur between age 13-15 years.[2] Understanding the proper techniques for the initial examination is key to establishing a long-term relationship with this age group. During this visit, the practitioner's should make the patient as comfortable as possible providing education about sexuality, contraception immunizations, risk prevention, history of involuntary sexual experiences, eating disorders, screening for substance abuse and depression should be evaluated. Additionally, they should also take the opportunity to discuss the availability of the human papilloma virus (HPV) vaccine with adolescents.

After the initial gynecologic visit, which may or may not include a pelvic examination, annual/semiannual visits should be scheduled. A visit in each stage of adolescence may be advised in those that are not sexually active, i.e. early adolescence (13-15 years), middle adolescence (15-17 years), and late adolescence (17-19 years).

With adolescents, if possible, it is important to meet initially together with the teenager and her parents/guardian to explain the concept of confidentiality and privacy.

PUBERTY

Changes during Normal Puberty

Puberty is the slow transition from childhood to adult life characterized by growth acceleration and appearance of secondary sexual characteristics culminating in sexual maturity and attainment of reproductive capacity. In most, pubertal changes usually begin between age 8-13 years in girls,[3] influenced largely by genetic and environmental factors. Other influencing factors include geographic locations, leptin, nutrition, general health, and psychological factors.[4] For example, children closer to the equator, at lower altitudes, those in urban areas and mildly obese children start earlier than those in Northern latitudes, at higher elevations, in rural areas, and normal weight children, respectively. There is a good correlation between the time of menarche of mothers and daughters and between sisters.

The **endocrine changes** begin several years before physical changes manifest. The diurnal rhythms of serum luteinizing hormone (LH) and follicular stimulating hormone (FSH) already exist at 5–6 years of age, and serum levels increase before the onset of puberty suggesting that suggest that preparation for the onset of female puberty begins already in 5–6 year-old girls.[5] Initially, an increase in pulsatile secretion of LH (from pituitary gland) in response to an increase of pulsatile GnRH (from hypothalamus) at night occurs, and as puberty progresses, amplitude of nocturnal gonadatropin (Gn) pulse increases gradually changing to the adult pattern [maturation of the hypothalamic-pituitary-ovarian (HPO) axis]. These pulses then stimulate a rise in estradiol (E_2) levels. The cascade of events initiated by the release of pulsatile GnRH from prepubertal feedback and central negative inhibition results in increased levels of Gn's and steroids with appearance of secondary sexual characteristics and eventual adult function (menarche and later ovulation).

Inhibin Levels

- Inhibin A increases progressively from Tanner stage I into adulthood and is only detectable after menarche,[6] and is therefore a marker of ovulation.
- During menstrual cycle: Inhibin B levels are highest in early and late follicular phases, decrease in periovulatory phase, and are lower in mid- and end-luteal phases. Serum inhibin A levels are lowest in early follicular phase, increase significantly in late follicular phase with maximal levels in midluteal phase, with a subsequent decrease in end-luteal phase.[7]

Anti-Müllerian Hormone

- It is produced from gestational week 36 and onwards by granulosa cells of antral follicles. It reflects the follicle pool (ovarian aging) in adult women. Serum Anti-Müllerian Hormone (AMH) levels have relatively constant levels until age 35–40 years, followed by a decrease until menopause where it becomes undetectable. AMH shows only minor variation across the menstrual cycle.[8]
- The young ovary secretes higher mean AMH and inhibin B levels to the circulation. This is in contrast to the aging ovary which is characterized by low mean AMH and inhibin B levels, shorter menstrual cycle lengths, and minimal variation in AMH levels during the cycle, suggesting diminished ovarian reserve. Thus, AMH is considered a marker of ovarian reserve.[9]

Table 6.1: Tanner's Staging.

Stage	Breast development	Pubic hair
1.	Absence of breast bud	Nonsexual general body hair
2.	Presence of breast bud only	Long, coarse, pigmented hair, usually along labia majora
3.	Enlargement of entire breast mound	Greater concentration of coarse long hair extending to mons pubis
4.	Secondary areolar mound above primary mound	Abundance of coarse dark pubic hair on mons and labia
5.	Adult mature breast contour	Adult pattern and distribution of inverted triangle pattern extending to thighs

The progressive **physical changes** are described as 'Tanner' stages[10] as described in Table 6.1. The first noticeable change is the appearance of breast bud. Pubic hair begins about six months later. Secondary sexual characteristics appear in 95% of girls between age 8.5–13 years. Menstruation is a late feature where initial cycles are usually anovulatory and may be irregular. The average age for menarche is 12.8 years. Menstruation correlates with slowing down of the growth spurt.

Stages of Pubertal Development

On the average the pubertal sequence of accelerated growth and skeletal maturation, breast development, adrenarche and menarche requires a period of 4.5 years (range 1.5–6 years).[4] The first sign of puberty is an acceleration of growth followed by breast budding [*thelarche*, mean age 10.9 years). In a minority of cases, pubic hair growth (*pubarche*, mean ages 11.2 years)] is the initial event. Breast development follows a well-recognized sequence of events **Adrenarche** usually appears after the breast bud, with axillary hair growth 2 years later. **Menarche** is a late event (median 12.8 years), occurring after peak of growth has passed.[11] Menarche typically occurs within 2–3 years after thelarche (breast budding) at Tanner stage IV of breast development and is rare before stage III.

Vertical Growth

An adolescent girls growth spurt occurs 2 years earlier (at 11–12 years) than that of a boy, and reaches her growth peak about 2 years after breast budding and 1 year prior to menarche. Hormonal requirements for this increased growth velocity include growth hormone (GH) and gonadal estrogen. The pubertal growth spurt is associated with an increase in the circulating levels of GH and insulin like growth factor-I (IGF-I). Adrenal androgens are not involved.

Menarche occurs after the peak in growth velocity has passed. During the early pubertal period, maturation of the LHRH neurosecretory system causes an increase in mean FSH levels, followed by an increase in mean LH levels. The increase in Gn's stimulates ovarian estrogen secretion, which induces peripheral sexual changes and FSH suppression by a negative feedback. Periodic changes in increasing estrogen secretion leads to the first vaginal bleeding before any LH surge or ovulation occurs.[12] The menses following menarche are usually anovulatory, irregular and occasionally heavy. Anovulation lasts as long as 6–7 years after menarche.[13]

Summary of Pubertal Events

- FSH and then LH levels rise moderately before the age 10 and are followed by a rise in E_2. An increase in LH pulses is first seen only in sleep but gradually extends throughout the day.
- As gonadal estrogen increases (gonadarche), breast development, female fat distribution and vaginal and uterine growth occur. Skeletal growth rapidly increases as a result of initial gonadal secretion of low levels of estrogen, which increases the secretion of GH, which in turn stimulates the production of IGF-I.
- Adrenal androgen and to a lesser degree, gonadal androgen secretion cause pubic and axillary hair growth (adrenarche). Dehydroepiandrosterone sulfate (DHEAS) is the predominant marker of adrenarche in serum.
- At midpuberty, sufficient gonadal estrogen secretion proliferates the endometrium, and the first menses (menarche) occurs.
- Postmenarchal cycles are initially anovulatory. Sustained, predictable positive LH surge responses to E_2 are late pubertal events.

CLINICAL EVALUATION OF THE ADOLESCENT GIRL

Important Points in History Taking

Adolescents should be given an opportunity to speak privately with their physician without parental involvement. While parental involvement should be respected and encouraged, it must be balanced with the patient's right to privacy and confidentiality.

- Assumptions should not be made about sexual orientation or sexual experience. Questions must be asked in an open, non-judgmental way. History should include specific ages of adrenarche, thelarche, and menarche.
- The provider should be familiar with local regulations regarding a minor's rights to confidential care for contraception and sexually transmitted infections (STIs) and reporting requirements for suspected sexual abuse and suicide. The patient should be informed of these reporting requirements at the beginning of the interview.
- Each symptom should be questioned as to frequency, relationship to menstrual cycle, and ameliorating and provocative events.
- Menstrual history should detail amount, length, and frequency of flow. Questions more easily answered center on whether bleeding is so heavy that it cannot be contained in a pad or tampon, whether it requires both a pad and tampon, whether the patient must awaken at night to change or whether she soils her clothing.
- Explain the significance of symptoms such as molimina (e.g. mood swings, mastalgia, food cravings, headaches, fluid retention) and mild symptoms such as dysmenorrheal, which can reassure the patient that nothing is seriously wrong. Severe pain with menses, such as pain requiring absence from school, should be investigated.
- Frequent urinary tract infections/previous urologic surgery may be related to a gynecological problem.
- Enquire regarding vaccines, use of HPV vaccine, sexual activity, contraceptive use, smoking, alcohol, and drug use.

Gynecologic Clinical Examination

Objectives

- Clinical assessment
- Diagnosis and therapy
- Establishment of interpersonal relationship to support those especially with concerns of puberty, sexuality, and fertility.

Preparation for Examination

One must be familiar with the anatomy and physiology of genitalia before and during puberty. Prior to the gynecological examination, it is important to note and assure:

- A thorough explanation of the pelvic examination with the use of diagrams
- Must be preceded by a full medical assessment
- Conducted only after obtaining Consent
- Only the least invasive examination sufficient to assess the problem should be performed
- Examinations should not be omitted solely because of age of the patient
- Cultural issues should be respected.

It is important to inform her and her family of what will happen during the visit. Let the patient know whether a pelvic examination will not be needed at that visit. This will help to allay the patient's fears allowing for a more relaxed visit.

- Vital signs should be taken. Height, weight and age appropriate body mass index should be calculated
- Stature and posture should be noted
- Heart and lung examination should be performed
- Abdominal contour and scars will uncover previous surgery, hernias, and masses. Palpation of the liver, spleen, and kidneys; abdominal tenderness, rebound, or guarding should be noted.

Breast examination can elicit masses, cysts or nipple secretions. Tanner stage of breast development should be recorded.

- During the development phase, the breast is often firm upon palpation.
- The breast bud can be palpated before it actually appears. At this stage, examination can be tender. It appears as a small firm mound beneath an enlarged areola.
- Unequal breast size is a common finding in adolescents, reassure that this finding is normal. The onset of development between the two breasts can be unequal with a time lag of 3–12 month difference. With in 2–4 years form then, it reaches its fully developed size. During the developmental phase, the breast is firm but rarely sensitive.[14]
- Provide reassurance as common findings such as fibrocystic changes may be a source of worry for an adolescent. Unusual masses can be evaluated with an ultrasound. Mammogram is rarely indicated in an adolescent.

Pelvic examination is often not necessary at all (if without symptoms) or may be deferred to a subsequent visit. Table 6.2 lists indication for pelvic examination in adolescents. Asymptomatic patients who are not sexually active may delay their initial pelvic examination up to the age of 21. All adolescents should be reassured that the examination, although uncomfortable, is not painful and will not alter their anatomy/alter their "virginity." Examination of *external genitalia* may be all that is required, this should also be staged according to the Tanner classification.

- The *vulva* is estrogenized and there are physiologic secretions. The vulva axis has become horizontal. Vulva should be examined for lesions
- *Hymen* should be assessed for patency
- *Labia minora* have developed, become browner, and the *labia majora* usually cover the vulva
- *Vagina* measures on average 9.6 cm in length

- Single-digit bimanual examination or rectal examination can also be performed. Upon rectal examination the uterus is often laterally oriented to the left

Bimanual examination is indicated in adolescents with *gynecologic complaints* or *unexplained abdominal or pelvic pain*.

- For visual examination of vagina and cervix, provide an atraumatic examination. Use either Huffman adolescent speculum (for the not sexually active) that has 1.5-cm diameter and 11-cm length, or Pederson speculum (for the sexually active). In this age group, the genital tissues are estrogenized and vaginal introitus is more elastic which can allow speculum insertion.[15] The use of a finger applying pressure to the perineal area, away from the introitus, allows for lessening or diffusing of the sensation from the examination ("extinction of stimuli") and may be of benefit in those undergoing their first pelvic examination. Once a finger has been placed in this area, the insertion of a speculum may be easier. In nonactive adolescents, vaginoscopy must be limited to the identification of a tumor/foreign body if clinical examination and ultrasound were not able to provide the origin of a vaginal bleeding. This examination may need general anesthesia in some cases.[16]
- **For the sexually active adolescents:** Vaginal examination, speculum examination, PAP smear, and samples to look for genital infections should be done. After the initiation of intercourse, teenagers may choose to delay their cervical cytology screening up to 3 years. Annual Pap testing should be considered beginning with the initial visit in those with multiple partners/immunocompromised conditions and in whom follow-up is unlikely. Care should be taken to obtain sexually transmitted diseases (STD) screening with each new sexual partner.

Radiological tests may be performed when in suspicion of an abdominal mass, abdominal pain, or precocious

Table 6.2: Indications for pelvic examination in adolescents.

Common indications for pelvic examination	• Delayed puberty • Precocious puberty • Abnormal vaginal bleeding • Abdominal or pelvic pain • History of vaginal intercourse • Pathologic vaginal discharge • Suspicion of intra-abdominal pathology • Signs of virilization • Evaluation of abnormal genitalia • Sexual abuse
Indications for vaginal examination with the use of speculum	• Irregular bleeding • Menorrhagia • Vaginal discharge • Suspected sexually transmitted diseases (STD)

puberty. Pelvic ultrasonography (USG), computed tomography (CT), or a magnetic resonance imaging (MRI) scan can be scheduled if imaging is indicated.

CONDITIONS AFFECTING THE ADOLESCENT GIRL

Abnormal pubertal development includes a spectrum of disorders such as premature thelarche, premature adrenarche, precocious puberty (central and peripheral), adolescent polycystic ovarian syndrome (PCOS), functional ovarian hyperandrogenism, late-onset congenital adrenal hyperplasia (CAH), primary and secondary amenorrhea, and premature ovarian insufficiency.

Precocious Puberty

It is defined as the appearance of secondary sexual characteristics before age 8 years in girls and is divided into two broad categories, central and peripheral. Table 6.3 lists various clinical forms of precocious puberty.

1. **Central/Gonadotropin (Gn)-dependent puberty (CPP):** It caused by the activation of HPO axis. It is idiopathic (ICPP) in majority, and occasionally (10–20% cases),[17] it is secondary to organic causes (organic CPP) such as hamartomas, gliomas and hydrocephalus.
2. In 50–60% of the cases, only one secondary sex characteristic shows premature development and raises the diagnosis of premature thelarche, premature pubarche or isolated metrorrhagia.[17]
3. **Peripheral/Gonadotropin-independent puberty:** It is seen in 10%, is caused by abnormal steroid production in peripheral steroidogenic organs (adrenal/ovarian)

Table 6.3: Clinical forms of precocious puberty.

Central precocious puberty (CPP)	• Typical form • Extremely precocious puberty • Slowly progressing puberty • Spontaneously regressive puberty • CPP in adopted children • Familial CPP • CPP and genetic abnormality
Advanced puberty	• Simple advanced puberty • Advanced puberty and growth retardation • Advanced puberty after premature pubarche
Incomplete, partial or dissociated precocious puberty	• Premature thelarche • Premature pubarche • Isolated metrorrhagia

Peripheral precocious puberty: Precocious pseudopuberty	• Ovarian autonomy
	  – McCune-Albright syndrome, ovarian cyst
	  – Granulosa cell tumor
	• Adrenal tumor (feminizing)
	• Environmental pollution (pesticides)

which is not the result of sustained activation of the HPO-axis. Disorders of the ovarian/adrenals and secretion of sex steroids by tumors must be excluded. McCune-Albright syndrome causes precocious puberty in the presence of an isolated functional ovarian cyst. Ingestion of estrogens may also cause pubertal changes.

Isolated premature thelarche is benign, self-limiting, characterized by premature breast development, and no other clinical signs of sexual maturation. There are two types one type is, Classical, manifesting itself in the first year of life, following which it tends to resolve by 2 years of age and another type, that manifests itself after 2 years of age and tends to be more persistent. Breast development fluctuates over a period of time, it can disappear and reappear within months. Premature thelarche is characterized by overnight Gn secretion, but circulating E_2 levels are commonly undetectable by conventional immunoassays. A GnRH test demonstrates prepubertal LH rise, and a predominant FSH response. On ultrasound ovaries appear small but may contain large follicular cysts that vary in size in synchrony with the fluctuating breast development. No acceleration of linear growth is seen, and bone age is not advanced. However, this may progress into a true CPP in some cases. The distinction between CPP and premature thelarche may not be straightforward as intermediate slowly progressing forms (thelarche variant forms) exist. Flowchart 6.1 depicts the decision tree for adolescents with premature thelarche.

Isolated premature adrenarche is characterized by isolated pubic/axillary hair development before 8 years of age and may be associated with other cutaneous manifestations of androgen excess (microcomedonal acne, greasy hair and body odor). Behavioral changes are seen and bone age may be slightly advanced. Suspicion of adrenal pathology increases the more the bone age is advanced. Flowchart 6.2 depicts the decision tree for adolescents with premature pubarche.

Girls with precocious puberty should be investigated and treated by a pediatric endocrinologist. There is no role for the gynecologist in initial assessment, unless on rare occasions, examination under anesthesia is required by gynecologist to exclude local causes of vaginal bleeding.

DELAYED SEXUAL DEVELOPMENT

Absent puberty/primary amenorrhea may result from hypogonadotropic hypogonadism (HH) due to mutations in selected genes which account for only 20–30% of cases. Familial delayed puberty may be suspected based on family history once a 45,X karyotype, hyperprolactinemia or anorexia/ortorexia are excluded. Idiopathic HH results in low FSH and LH levels, and GnRH testing is of limited value.

It is usually associated with hypogonadism and patient may present as primary amenorrhea. Abnormal findings

Flowchart 6.1: Decision tree for premature thelarche.[17]

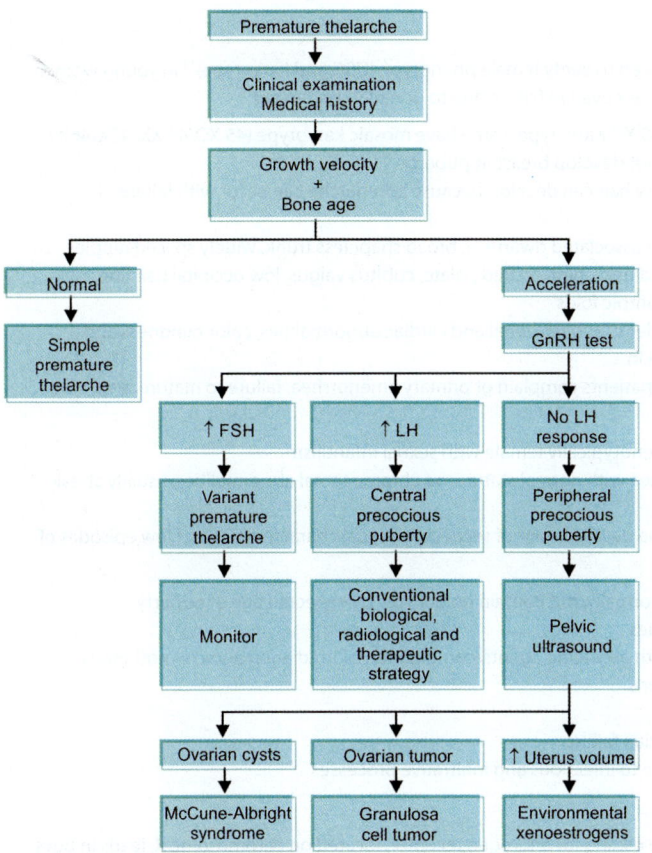

(FSH: follicle stimulating hormone; LH: luteinizing hormone; GnRH: gonadotropin releasing hormone)

Flowchart 6.2: Decision tree for premature pubarche.[17]

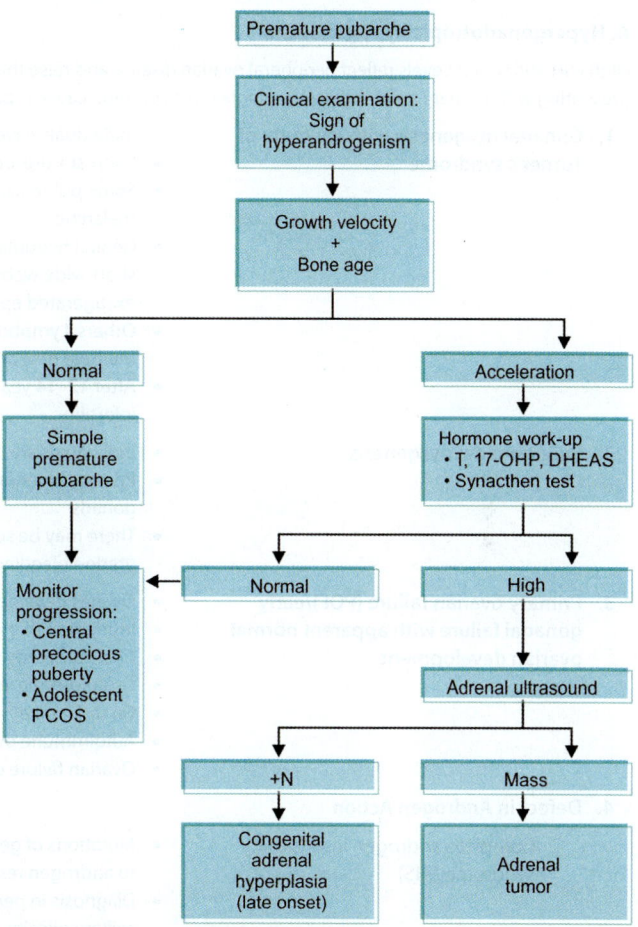

(PCOS: polycystic ovary syndrome)

on physical examination may suggest certain enzyme deficiencies but these conditions are very rare.

Delayed puberty constitutionally is characterized by positive family history, short stature, delayed secondary sexual characteristics and delayed epiphyseal maturation (on hand X-ray bone ageing). Other causes (Table 6.4) should be ruled out and puberty induced. Individuals with asynchronous development often present with failure to menstruate.

Delayed puberty includes absence of physical signs of puberty/failure to progress through puberty and is defined as:[18]

- Absence of thelarche by age 13
- Absence of menarche by age 16

An outline of evaluation of adolescents with delayed pubertal development is depicted in Flowchart 6.3.

TURNER'S SYNDROME

Turner's syndrome is the most common form of gonadal dysgenesis in females that leads to premature ovarian failure (POF). Incidence is 1 in 2,500 female live births. They also have an increased incidence of other associated anomalies and concerns with their cardiovascular systems.[21] Most patients are sterile with streak ovaries. However, 5–10% of Turner's mosaic patients undergo spontaneous pubertal development, and 2% of these are fertile.[22] Most patients require HRT to undergo pubertal development and protect their bones and heart. It is important to discuss contraception with spontaneously menstruating Turner's patients as their pregnancies are at risk for chromosomal problems and malformations.[23]

Adolescent girls may present with delayed menstruation with some pubertal development, an overview is given in Table 6.5.

CONGENITAL ADRENAL HYPERPLASIA

Majority (95%) childhood congenital adrenal hyperplasia (CAH) cases are of classic 21-hydroxylase deficiency (CYP21 mutation). Approximately 75% of these are salt wasters. Girls are usually virilized in utero and typically diagnosed in the neonatal period, due to clinical symptoms like failure to thrive, salt wasting (hyponatremic crisis) or

Table 6.4: Causes of delayed puberty/ Primary amenorrhea.

A. Hypergonadotropic hypogonadism		
High FSH and/ or LH Levels reflect peripheral ovarian disease and raise the need to verify female phenotype (USG and karyotype)[12] in young women presenting with primary amenorrhea, the single most common cause is primary ovarian failure due to gonadal dysgenesis[19]		
1. Gonadal dysgenesis with stigmata of Turner's syndrome		• Individuals have 45 XO Karyotype, some have mosaic karyotype (45 XO/46 XX, 45X/46XY) • Short stature, do not develop breast at puberty • Some pubic/axillary hair can develop because adrenarche can occur with failure of thelarche • Genital hypoplasia associated dwarfism, broad shapeless trunk, widely spaced nipples, short wide webbed neck, high arched palate, cubitus valgus, low occipital hair line, exaggerated epicanthic folds • Others: Lymphoedema at birth, renal and cardiac abnormalities, color blindness and multiple nevi on skin • After 12–14 years patients complain of primary amenorrhea, failure to mature, and infertility
2. Pure gonadal dysgenesis		• Individuals are phenotypically female with sexual infantilism • Primary amenorrhea with normal stature, no chromosomal abnormalities, usually streak gonads • There may be some development of secondary sexual characteristics and few episodes of uterine bleeding
3. Primary ovarian failure (POF)/early gonadal failure with apparent normal ovarian development		• Ovaries develop normally, but contain no oocytes by expected age of puberty • Irradiation of ovaries • Chemotherapy with alkylating agents/combination of irradiation and chemotherapy • Galactosemia in girls • Gn resistance • Autoimmune ovarian failure • Ovarian failure due to infectious and infiltrative processes
4. Defect in Androgen Action		
	i. Complete androgen insensitivity syndrome (AIS)	• Mutations of gene coding for androgen receptor, located on chromosome X, leads in boys to androgen resistance with resultant female external genitalia • Diagnosis in peripubertal period is suggested by primary amenorrhea with no pubian/axillary pilosity, normal breast development • LH is very high with adult male testosterone (T) level; FSH level is not elevated; E_2 is almost at a follicular phase level allowing breast development • Vaginal cavity is short and closed • USG: Absence of Müllerian and Wolffian structures and abdominal/inguinal testes that need to be removed • Estrogens complete feminization
	ii. 5α-reductase deficiency	• 5α-reductase converts dihydrotestosterone from T mutations cause 46, XY DSD with ambiguous external genitalia at birth—believed to be girls • Virilization occurs at puberty with a gender role change and without breast development • Ectopic testes are present as Wolffian-derivative organs • Plasma T is high normal with decreased DHT levels and high T/DHT ratio
5. Partial deletion of X chromosome		
	i. Deletion of part of **long arm of X** chromosome	Patients have sexual infantilism, normal stature, and no somatic abnormal and streak gonads
	ii. Deletion of **Short arm of X** chromosome	Similar to Turner's syndrome
B. Hypogonadotropic hypogonadism (Decreased FSH and LH levels, < 10 mIU/mL)		
1. **Constitutional delay**		Most common cause of delayed puberty. Low levels of LH and FSH normally present in the prepubertal years can be mistakenly presumed
2. **Isolated Gn deficiency**		Disorder of GnRH pulse generator rather than a failure of pituitary gland to produce Gn
	i. Kallmann syndrome	• Characterized by anosmia, hypogonadism, and color blindness • Gene defects lead to decreased GnRH neurons • Present with sexual infantilism, eunochoid habitus and primary amenorrhea

Contd...

Contd...

	ii. Prader-willi syndrome	Obesity, short stature, hypogonadism, small hands and feet, mental retardation and infantile hypotonia
	iii. Lawrence-Moon-Biedl syndrome	Post polydactyly, obesity, and hypogonadism
3.	Multiple pituitary hormone deficiency	• Usually hypothalamic in origin • If GH/ TSH concentrations are subnormal, growth in addition to pubertal development will be affected
4.	Tumors of hypothalamus and pituitary	• Craniopharyngioma, pituitary adenoma • Headache, visual disturbances, short stature, growth failure, delayed puberty, diabetes insipidus • Hyperprolactinemia
5.	Infiltrative processes (Langerhans cell type histiocytosis)	• Delayed puberty • Short stature • Diabetes insipidus
6.	Following CNS irradiation	• Partial/complete Gn deficiency
7.	Severe chronic illness	• Digestive disease, inflammatory bowel disease • Cystic fibrosis • Chronic renal disease • Major thalassemia • Sickle cell disease
8.	Anorexia nervosa	• Weight loss of <85% of ideal body weight results in hypothalamic GnRH deficiency • Significant weight loss and psychological dysfunction occurs simultaneously • If the disorder occurs in early in age, pubertal development may be delayed or interrupted
9.	Negative energy balance	• Undernutrition • Intensive exercise in young girls (athletes, ballet dancers, gymnasts)
10.	Following CNS irradiation	Partial/complete Gn deficiency
11.	Antidopaminergic and GnRH inhibiting drugs	Especially opiates
12.	Primary hypothyroidism	
13.	Cushing's syndrome	
14.	Severe hypothalamic amenorrhea	Rare
C. Primary Amenorrhea with Developed Secondary Sex Characteristics		
1.	Abnormalities of genitalia	
	i. Mullerian dysgenesis (Rokitansky-Kuster-Hauser syndrome)	• Characterized by agenesis of uterus and upper vagina with incidence of 1/4,500 females • Patient with normal growth, gonads and secondary sexual characteristics presents with primary amenorrhea • Associated renal anomalies in 30% and skeletal abnormality in 12–50%[20] • They have the potential to have their genetic children with use of a gestational surrogate
	ii. Imperforate hymen	• Patient may give history of vague abdominal pain with monthly exacerbations • Hydrocolpos/Hydrometrocolpos • Bulging hymen
	iii. Transverse vaginal septum	• Clinical features similar to those above; in some can be asymptomatic (depending upon level)
	iv. Distal obstruction	
2.	Hyperandrogenemia	
	• Mild adrenal hyperplasia with partial enzymatic blockage • PCOS with primary amenorrhea • Tumoral syndrome (ovarian/adrenal)	• Progressive hyperandrogenia/virilization (hirsutism, seborrhea, severe acne, alopecia and hyperclitoridism) • Measure androgens, LH and FSH, basal and ACTH-stimulated 17-OH-P • USG for ovarian evaluation

(LH: luteinizing hormone; USG: ultrasonography; FSH: follicle stimulating hormone; GH: growth hormone; TSH: thyroid stimulating hormone; Gn: gonadotropin; CNS: central nervous system; GnRH: gonadotropin releasing hormone; PCOS: polycystic ovary syndrome)

Flowchart 6.3: Evaluation of delayed/ interrupted pubertal development, including primary amenorrhea.

```
                        History and physical examination
                                      |
           ┌──────────────────────────┼──────────────────────────┐
           ▼                          ▼                          ▼
  Asynchronous development    Immature secondary sexual    Mature secondary sexual
  (breasts, pubic hair)            characteristics             characteristics
           |                          |                          |
           ▼                          ▼                          ▼
  Androgen in sensitivity          FSH, PRL            • Distal genital tract obstruction
           |                          |                 • Müllerian agenesis
           ▼                          ▼                          |
         ↑ FSH                   ↓ normal FSH                    ▼
           |                          |                        ↑ PRL
           ▼                          ▼                          |
       Karyotype          Pituitary function tests               ▼
           |                  Sellar X-ray/MRI              Check T₄, TSH
      ┌────┴────┐                  |                            |
      ▼         ▼              ┌───┴───┐                   ┌────┴────┐
   Normal    Abnormal       Normal   Abnormal          Normal TSH   ↑ TSH
      |         |              |        |                  |          |
      |         ▼              |        ▼                  |          ▼
      |  46X or 45XY           |    MRI/CT scan            |      Hypothyroidism
      |  Mosaic gonadal        |                           |
      |  dysgenesis            |                           |
      ▼                        ▼                           ▼
  46XX gonadal          • Constitutional delay       • Hypopituitarism
  dysgenesis            • Isolated Gn deficiency     • CNS tumor
  POF                   • Malnutrition
                        • Chronic illness
```

(FSH: follicle stimulating hormone; PRL: prolactin; MRI: magnetic resonance imaging; TSH: thyroid stimulating hormone; POF: premature ovarian failure, CNS: central nervous system)

Table 6.5: Delayed menarche with some pubertal development.

	Anatomic abnormalities	*Non-anatomic abnormalities*
Causes	1. **Mullerian anomalies** • Imperforate hymen • Transverse vaginal septum • Mayer-Rokitansky-Kuster-Hauser-syndrome	1. **Ovarian failure** • Genetic disorders • Autoimmune disorders • Galactosemia • Radiation and chemotherapy
	2. **Androgen insensitivity syndrome (AIS)** • Phenotypic females with complete congenital androgen insensitivity • Develop secondary sexual characteristics but do not have menses • Genotypically, are male XY but have a defect that prevents normal androgen receptor function	2. **Pituitary/Hypothalamic lesions** • Craniopharyngiomas • Germinomas • Tubercular/sarcoid granulomas • Dermoid cysts may prevent appropriate hormonal secretion • Pituitary gland may be destroyed by tumors (non-functioning/hormone secreting), infarction, and surgical/radiological ablations
	3. **Infections** • Tuberculosis • Schistosomiasis	3. **Altered hypothalamic GnRH secretion** • Chronic disease: Malnutrition, anorexia nervosa, exercise, stress, psychiatric disorders inhibit GnRH release thus altering menstrual cycle • Excess/insufficient hormones cause abnormal feedback and adversely affect GnRH secretion, e.g. hyperprolactinemia, Cushing disease, acromegaly
	4. **Absent endometrium** 5. **True hermaphrodites**	
Diagnosis	Most congenital abnormalities can be diagnosed by physical examination	Blood tests: • FSH • LH • TSH

Contd...

CHAPTER 6 Adolescent Gynecology

Contd...

	1. **Imperforate hymen:** Presence of a bulging membrane	
	2. **Mullerian anomaly:** USG or MRI	
	3. **Androgen insensitivity** • Pubic and axillary hair are absent • Karyotype	
	4. **Tuberculosis:** Endometrial cultures	
Treatment	1. **Imperforate hymen:** Make a cruciate incision to open vaginal orifice	Treat the underlying cause
	2. **Transverse septum:** Surgical removal is required	
	3. **Hypoplasia/Absent cervix:** Difficult to treat	
	4. **Absent/short vagina:** Progressive dilatations are usually successful in making it functional	
	5. **Complete AIS:** Testes should be removed after pubertal development to prevent malignant degeneration	

(GnRH: gonadotropin releasing hormone; USG: ultrasonography; MRI: magnetic resonance imaging; FSH: follicle stimulating hormone; LH: luteinizing hormone; TSH: thyroid stimulating hormone)

ambiguous genitalia. The internal genitalia are normal.[21] However, milder forms of CAH, **late-onset CAH,** present in childhood with varying degrees of virilization including pubic hair development. Late-onset CAH (CYP21 mutation) is diagnosed by an ACTH test during which 17-OH-P is significantly elevated. Thus, isolated premature adrenarche is an exclusion diagnosis that is relatively common, especially in overweight children and children born small for gestational age. Children born to mothers with PCOS may be at increased risk of premature adrenarche.

Puberty and Menstruation

- Pubertal development occurs normally if adequately treated from an early age. However, most CAH girls have delayed menarche.[24]
- If left untreated/under-treated with glucocorticoids, the child will enter puberty early with an advanced bone age. Likewise, if the disease is over-treated, puberty is often delayed and menarche can be absent.
- They have oligomenorrhea and anovulation, as LH surge is inhibited by steroid substrates. Some never ovulate normally, even on adequate replacement medication. Polycystic ovaries are also common, which produce more androgens and prevents ovulation.

Sexuality

They are more likely to have delayed heterosexual milestones as lesbians or to have bisexual imagery.[25] Negative body image, less sexual activity, and decreased sex drive[26] is seen due to high levels of progesterone in the follicular phase (acts like a biological minipill, preventing regular ovulation and decreasing libido).[27]

Table 6.6: Enzyme deficiency and abnormal physical examination.

17α hydroxylase deficiency, and hypokalemia	• Associated with either 46XX or 46XY • Uterus is present in individuals with 46XY (46XX) • Patients have primary amenorrhea, no secondary sexual characteristics, female phenotypes, hypertension
17-20 desmolase deficiency puberty	• Complete female phenotype in individuals with XY Karyotype • Uterus is present and sexual development does not occur at puberty
5α-reductase deficiency in XY individual	• Patient has amenorrhea and virilization at puberty • Has testes, no Müllerian structures

Other examples of enzyme deficiency and their characteristic features are listed in Table 6.6.

CYSTIC FIBROSIS

Cystic fibrosis (CF) is the most common serious autosomal recessive genetic disease with a mean age of survival of 28 years. These girls have normal secondary sexual development; however, puberty and menstruation may be delayed in severe disease. They have normal reproductive tracts with slightly decreased fertility[21] resulting from thick cervical mucus, poor nutritional status, severe respiratory disease, and increased incidence of anovulation. An increased incidence of stress incontinence (due to frequent coughing) is also seen.

- Combined oral contraceptive (COC) can exacerbate their respiratory tract, diabetes, malabsorption, and

Table 6.7: Treatment guidelines.

A. Hypergonadotropic hypogonadism		
1.	Turner's syndrome	• To increase final adult height—exogenous GH • For sexual maturation—low dose estrogen (0.3–0.625 mg) initiated at 12–13 years of age • To prevent endometrial hyperplasia—progestins (5–10 mg Medroxy progesterone acetate (MPA) for 12–14 days
2.	Pure gonadal dysgenesis	• Exogenous estrogens are beneficial for both 46XX and 46XY individuals • Surgical expiration in 46XY karyotype to prevent germ cell neoplasm
B. Hypogonadotropic hypogonadism		
1.	Constitutional delay	Exclude other causes
2.	Isolated Gn deficiency	• Pulsatile exogenous GnRH • For women not seeking pregnancy—replacement therapy with exogenous estrogen and progestin
3.	Multiple pituitary hormone deficiencies	Treatment accordingly
4.	Hypothalamus and pituitary tumors	• Surgical excision • Radiotherapy
5.	Chronic illness/ Malnutrition/ Anorexia	Adequate body weight and nutrition should be maintained
C. Eugonadism with anatomic abnormality of genital tract		
1.	Mayer-Rokitansky-Kuster-Hauser syndrome	Treatment is primarily by vaginoplasty **Frank technique/perineal dilation** • The only nonsurgical option, this technique is successful only in patients with a long rudimentary vagina. Patients apply progressive pressure to the perineum using a bicycle-seat stool to hold a dilator in place. Patient compliance is often poor due to discomfort **McIndoe's technique**[28] • The most common procedure used. The technique involves a split-thickness skin graft for vaginal replacement, a pocket created between the urethra and rectum, a cylindrical stent covered with the skin graft placed into the potential space and fixed by attaching cut edges of the skin incision to recreate the introitus. Stent is removed after 1 week and then reinserted by the patient every day and night for 3 months, followed by nightly insertion for 3 more months to prevent contraction • Disadvantages include scarring at the donor site, neovaginal stenosis, and the need for long-term dilation **William's vaginoplasty** • Uses a vulval flap to make a vaginal tube. This simple procedure does not damage the urethra or rectum • Disadvantages are dilation is needed for a lengthy period, and the neovagina has a physiologically abnormal angle **Rotational flap procedure** • These use the pudendal thigh, gracilis myocutaneous, labia minora, and other fasciocutaneous flaps. • Disadvantages include extensive skin scarring at the donor graft site and the need for patient diligence in post surgical dilation
2.	Distal obstruction—imperforate hymen	Simple excision or incision of membrane

(GH: Growth hormone)

hepatic dysfunction, if present, through the progestins, which increase the production and viscosity of respiratory tract mucus, impair glucose tolerance, and promote hyperplasia of goblet cells, causing increased intrahepatic cholestasis and cholelithiasis. Despite the concern with COC use, the overall experience has been favorable and without significant adverse events.

Table 6.7 lists the treatment guidelines for various causes of delayed puberty.

MENSTRUAL DISORDERS

Menstruation

In 98%, menstruation starts by age 15, with median age at 12.43 years. There is a correlation between body weight and age at menarche, with earlier menarche observed in obese girls. On the other hand, malnutrition, chronic disease, eating disorders and high levels of physical activity are associated with delayed initiation of menstrual periods.[29]

CHAPTER 6 Adolescent Gynecology

Early menarche is associated with early onset of ovulatory cycles and when it occurs before the age of 12, about 50% of cycles are ovulatory in the first year. In contrast, with late onset menarche it can take 8–12 years until cycles become fully ovulatory. In adolescents, mean duration of menses is 4.7 days, cycle is 21–40 days and average blood loss is 35 mL and a significant variability in postmenarchal menstrual cycles is common. In the 1st year following menarche, early menstrual cycles can range from 18–80 days, becoming frequent with variability from 20–40 days over the next 5 years.[30] During the first 2 postmenarchal years, most cycles are anovulatory. In majority (55–82%), it takes up to 24 months for onset of regular ovulatory cycles after menarche. After 24 months, 22% remain either anovulatory/oligoovulatory. The transition from anovulatory to ovulatory cycles results from "maturation of HPO axis" characterized by positive feed back mechanisms in which rising estrogen level triggers a surge of LH hormones and ovulation. In some, it may take up to 5 years to establish regular ovulatory cycles.[31]

Persistence of irregular menses after menarche may be indicative of PCOS. Heavy, prolonged and recurrent menstrual periods are not normal adolescent patterns of bleeding and may represent an underlying coagulation defect in about 20% of patients.[32] Heavy bleeding can also be due to acquired disorder of platelet dysfunction including immune thrombocytoplastic purpura (ITP), aplastic anemia, and leukemia. Thrombocytopenia is seen in 13% girls presenting with menorrhagia.[33] Table 6.8 lists the causes of abnormal vaginal bleeding.

Abnormal Uterine Bleeding

Abnormal uterine bleeding (AUB), especially the subtype dysfunctional uterine bleeding (DUB) is one of the most common problems, while dysmenorrhea is the most frequent one. Bleeding associated with organic causes such as pregnancy complications, clotting abnormalities, systemic diseases, reproductive tract's pathology, endocrine disorders and iatrogenic causes is defined as AUB.

Table 6.8: Causes of abnormal vaginal bleeding.

Vaginal or uterine abnormalities	
Endometriosis	
Hypothalamic disorders	
Dysfunctional uterine bleeding	
Trauma	• Coitus • Rape • Abuse
Foreign body	• Intrauterine device • Tampon, etc.
Infection	• Vaginitis (Trichomonas; gonorrhea) • Cervicitis (chlamydial infection results in postcoital bleeding) • Endometritis (tuberculosis) • Pelvic inflammatory disease • Sexually transmitted condylomata (human papillomavirus HPV of cervix/vagina)
Tumors	• Botryoid sarcoma • Polyps (uterine; cervical) • Ovarian cyst or tumor (mature teratoma; endometrioma) • Leiomyomatosis • Clear cell carcinoma of cervix/vagina (diethylstilbestrol) • Other ovarian malignancy and metastatic malignancy
Complications of pregnancy	• Threatened/spontaneous abortion • Ectopic pregnancy • Molar pregnancy • Self- or medically induced abortion
Coagulopathies	• Generalized coagulopathy • Thrombocytopenia (ITP, leukemia, lymphoma, aplastic anemia, hypersplenism) • Platelet dysfunction (von Willebrand's disease, Glanzmann's disease) • Clotting disorders (hemophilia; other coagulation factor deficiencies) • Uterine production of menstrual anticoagulants
Normal variation	• Midcycle ovulatory bleeding • Early postmenarcheal anovulation • Early postmenarcheal estrogen irregularities

Contd...

	Contd...	
Drugs	Exogenous steroids	
	Oral contraception	• Midcycle breakthrough bleeding • Relative luteal progesterone deficiency • Progestogens (oral agents, norplant, Depo-Provera) • Continuous estrogens
	Other drugs	• Danazol • Spironolactone • Anticoagulants • Platelet inhibitors • Chemotherapy drugs • Natural hormones from plant extracts (DHEA; dong quai; yam extract)
Systemic diseases		• Hyperthyroidism/hypothyroidism • Adrenal insufficiency • Cushing's syndrome • Diabetes mellitus • Chronic liver disease • Crohn's disease; ulcerative colitis • Chronic renal disease • Systemic lupus erythematosus • Ovarian failure • Hyperprolactinemia
Excess hormone	Androgen excess	• Exogenous androgens, PCOS • CAHs • Androgen-producing ovarian/ adrenal tumor
	Estrogen excess	• Granulosa-theca cell tumor of the ovary • Other tumors
Stress		• Emotional, chronic alcohol abuse • Physical stress, especially exercise, anorexia, bullemia
Ovulation disorders		• Short luteal phase • Prolonged luteal phase (Halban's disease) • Luteal progesterone insufficiency • Chronic anovulation

(DHEA: dehydroepiandrosterone; PCOS: polycystic ovarian syndrome; CAH: congenital adrenal hyperplasia)

Dysfunctional uterine bleeding (ovulatory or anovulatory) refers to endometrial bleeding that is prolonged, excessive, irregular and not attributable to any underlying structural or systemic disease.

Evaluation and Diagnosis

Firstly, exclude pregnancy-related hemorrhage. Bleeding disorders should be excluded, especially with AUB during first menstrual cycles. Almost 19% of adolescents with persistent menorrhagia requiring hospital admission have coagulation disorder, and more than 50% of these have thrombocytopenia, von Willebrand disease or leukemia.[34] von Willebrand factor's deficiency is a common hereditary bleeding disorder associated with AUB, with 65% reporting heavy bleeding at menarche.

Thorough history, physical examination and basic laboratory tests human chorionic gonadotropin (hCG), thyroid stimulating hormone (TSH), complete blood count, and coagulation studies guide in determining the cause. Other tests include culture for gonorrhea, chlamydial infection. USG for details of pelvic anatomy, ruling out pregnancy. MRI/CT can be used. Table 6.9 lists the outline of intial assessment.

Table 6.9: Laboratory assessment of the adolescent with dysfunctional uterine bleeding.[35]

Initial evaluation	• Complete blood count • Platelet count • Coagulation studies (including fibrinogen) • Hormonal assay: HCG, TSH, prolactin (PRL), FSH, LH, free T, and DHEAS
If bleeding is severe or prolonged or associated with menarche	• von Willebrand's factor antigen • Factor VIII activity • Factor XI antigen • Ristocetin C cofactor • Platelet aggregation studies
If the initial screen is abnormal then other tests should be performed	

(TSH: Thyroid stimulating hormone; hCG: human chorionic gonadotropin; PRL: prolactin; FSH: follicle-stimulating hormone; LH: luteinizing hormone; DHEAS: dehydroepiandrosterone)

Management

Management should be directed to treat the underlying condition and is based upon the degree of bleeding/anemia (Box 6.1). Primary target is to locate the source of bleeding and secondary to rule out all organic causes.

Treatment of patients with DUB should firstly focus to control bleeding and regulating menstruation. Anemia correction and iron stores replenishment is the second goal of the therapeutic strategy. In majority of cases, hormonal treatment is indicated.

- **Mild DUB**, menses are slightly prolonged or irregular, with hemoglobin >12 g/dL. Hormonal therapy is rarely indicated and patient reassurance and education about normal menstrual cycle are usually sufficient. Careful follow-up along with menstrual calendar.
- **Moderate DUB** is characterized by prolonged, profuse menses, impeding daily activities, or by a clearly shortened menses interval accompanied by mild anemia (hemoglobin >/= 10 g/dL). Treatment of choice includes the low-dose COC/cyclic progestogen for at least 3-6 months. Cyclic oral progestogen is administered for 10 days of every month inorder to stabilize the endometrium, preventing the action of unopposed estrogens. Iron deficiency anemia can be treated with supplemental oral iron therapy. NSAIDs reduce the flow by nearly 50%.
- **Severe DUB** with heavy bleeding and hemoglobin levels <10 g/dL usually require hospitalization. In hypovolemic patients, immediate resuscitation with intravenous fluids for volume expansion and possible transfusion are indicated. Exclude underlying bleeding disorders. Intramuscular MPA with COCs provide faster results in controlling heavy bleeding. Hemorrhage usually stops within 24 hours and continuation COCs alone is recommended. Dilation and curettage, is indicated in the rare cases where hormonal treatment is unsuccessful. A tablet of COCs containing high dose estrogen should be taken every 6 hours, along with an antiemetic for nausea. After a maximum of 8 doses during 48 hours, dose must be tapered over 3 days to one pill daily. Patient can begin new COCs pack with the same amount of estrogen for next 21 days taking one pill daily.

Tranexamic acid, antifibrinolytic, has no effect on blood coagulation parameters/dysmenorrhea. Dose of 1 g every 6 hours for first 4 days of cycle reduces menstrual blood by 40%. Other therapies (high progestogens orally/intramuscularly, GnRH agonists with add-back therapy and levonorgestrel IUDs) have little place in adolescent's DUB.[39] Summary of various treatment options is listed in Table 6.10.

Box 6.1: Management based upon the degree of bleeding/anemia.

Mild bleeding/anemia hematocrit (PCV) >33% or hemoglobin (Hb) >11 g/dL
- Treat with iron supplements and non-steroidal drugs at menses
- For contraception: Combined oral, transdermal, or intravaginal methods

Moderate bleeding (menses prolonged, heavy or interfering with daily activities, menses interval markedly shortened)/anemia
PCV: 27–33% or Hb: 9–11 g/dL
- Advise use of menstrual calendars
- Treat with antiprostaglandins
- COC should be used if the bleeding abnormality persists/if there are contraceptive concerns
- **Oral equine estrogen** 2.5 mg, for 21–25 days, followed by 10 mg of MPA, for last 7 days (This is started as the endometrium may be denuded and disordered)
- **Combination oral contraceptives (COC)** in accelerated dose, and later **for subsequent control** by **cyclical progesterone** (day 15–25, e.g. Medroxy progesterone acetate (MPA), norethindrone acetate) or **low dose COC** for 3–6 months. Cyclic oral progesterone is administered to check the unopposed estrogen and stabilize the endometrium.[36] Withdrawal of progesterone each month allows organized sloughing of the endometrium resulting in predictable menses during the perimenarchal anovulatory period. Pills may be given two times daily for one week, followed by 3 weeks of regular low dose.[37] Although, COC is prescribed to regulate the cycle, it may suppress the normal awakening of the HPO axis, which needs time to undergo the maturation process.

Severe bleeding anemia
PCV <27% or Hb <9 g/dL
The hemorrhage must be arrested and endometrium converted from proliferative to secretory phase using both estrogens and progestins
- **COC** once every 6 hours until bleeding decreases and then taper to complete a 21-day pill pack. This dosage of estrogen will require an antiemetic.[38] Later place on **COC** over the following 3 months
- **Intravenous conjugated estrogens (Premarin)** 25 mg every 4–6 hours until bleeding ceases (in most within 24 hours). Then taper to daily lower dose of COC without cycling until hemoglobin returns to normal. Later, give **COC** for 3–6 months before stopping.
- Alternatively, **oral equine estrogens**, 2.5 mg, can be continued for additional 20–25 days. **MPA** (10 mg) added for the last 7–10 days (allows for withdrawal menses after therapy after stabilizing the endometrium).

Young women with known bleeding disorders
Adjunctive therapy, in the form of **desmopressin acetate** or **antifibrinolytics** in addition to **hormonal therapy**[36]

Table 6.10: Summary of treatment options.

	Blood loss reduction	Pain relief	Cycle regulation	Contraceptive benefit
Tranexamic acid	50%	-	-	-
Mefenamic acid	20%	Anti-inflammatory, inhibits prostaglandin synthetase	-	-
Cyclical progestogen	80%	-	+	-
POP	-	-	-	+
COCP	>40%	50% reduction in menstrual cramping	+	+
Depo-Provera	70% amenorrhea by 12 months	+ secondary to amenorrhea	Yes, can cause amenorrhea, but 50% discontinuation due to irregular bleeding	+
Levonorgestrel IUS	65% amenorrhea/light bleeding by 12 months	+ effective treatment for dysmenorrhea and endometriosis	Yes, can cause irregular bleeding for first 3–6 months, then 65% amenorrhea/light bleeding	+

(POP: progestin only pill; COCP: combined oral contraceptive pill)

AMENORRHEA

Primary amenorrhea defined as absence of menstruation in 16 year old girls with developed secondary sexual characteristics, or in 14-year-old girls with no secondary sexual characteristics development. For girls with absent secondary sexual characteristics) the term 'delayed puberty' is more appropriate.[29] Due to a trend for earlier age at menarche, adolescent females with amenorrhea and normally developed secondary sexual characteristics should be evaluated by age 15. Evaluation is essential for adolescent girls presenting with amenorrhea within 5 years after thelarche (if thelarche occurs before age 10) and amenorrheic girls who are above the age 13 and have not yet developed secondary sexual characteristics.[40]

Secondary amenorrhea is defined as the cessation of menses once they have begun. It is the absence of menstruation for 6 months, for adolescents with previously irregular cycles or for those within first few years following menarche. For adolescents with formerly regular cycles of 21–45 days, it is the absence of 3/more subsequent menstrual periods.

Oligomenorrhea refers to menstrual cycles longer than 45 days. Most cases occur in the first decade after menarche mostly due to PCOS. It can present prior to secondary amenorrhea.

The causes of amenorrhea are classified as:[40]
1. Anatomic defects of the outflow tract
2. Primary hypogonadism
3. Hypothalamic causes
4. Pituitary causes
5. Endocrine gland disorders
6. Multifactorial causes

Causes

1. **Premature ovarian failure (POF):** It can occur in some genetic disorders, after radiation, chemotherapy, or surgical interference. It can also occur after infections, autoimmune disorders, galactosemia, cigarette smoking, etc.
2. **Pituitary/hypothalamic lesions:** Such as craniopharyngiomas, germinomas, etc. may prevent appropriate hormonal secretion. Hypopituitarism is with decreased secretion of ACTH and TSH as well as Gn's.
3. **Altered GnRH secretion:** It occurs in cases of chronic illness, starvation, psychological stress, drug abuse, and excessive exercise. Common disorders are Crohn's disease, malabsorption syndrome, cystic fibrosis, celiac disease, renal disease, and thalassemia.
   - In hyperprolactinemia, Cushing's disease and acromegaly, excess pituitary hormones are secreted that inhibit GnRH secretion.
   - In obesity, hyperandrogenism is seen.
4. **General disorders:** Asherman's syndrome can be caused by tuberculosis and schistosomiasis infections.

Evaluation and Diagnosis

A careful medical history should include information about any underlying systemic disease, family medical history and the age of menarche of the girl's mother. Presence of developed secondary sexual characteristics demonstrates that sexual steroids are produced and circulating. Particular attention should be paid to signs or symptoms of systemic diseases. Per rectum gynecological examination helps assess anatomy of internal genitalia, hematocolpos and/or hematometra.

CHAPTER 6 Adolescent Gynecology

In *primary amenorrhea with absent secondary sexual characteristics*, measure FSH and LH.
- Low/normal levels point to either constitutional delay of puberty, or hypothalamic/pituitary disorders.
- Elevated levels imply that the cause lies within the gonads. Further evaluation requires pelvic ultrasound for a clear view of anatomy of internal genitalia (especially presence or not of ovarian follicles). The next step is karyotype study which to rule out ovarian failure (ovarian insufficiency), gonadal dysgenesis, Turner syndrome and androgen insensitivity syndrome.

Progressively deteriorating cyclic abdominal pain with primary amenorrhea indicates genital tract obstruction. In *normal pubertal development and primary amenorrhea*, rectoabdominal gynecologic examination and pelvic ultrasound can reveal the existence of congenital anatomic defects of outflow tract.

Evaluation of *secondary amenorrhea* (Flowchart 6.4) should begin with pregnancy exclusion. Look for signs of hyperandrogenism, (acne, hirsutism, deepening of voice and clitoromegaly).
- If present, FSH, LH, T and DHEA-S must be measured. PCOS can be diagnosed with mild-moderate T elevation along with LH/FSH ratio above 2.
- If DHEA-S falls between 500–700 mg/dL, assess adrenal gland function with measurement of serum 17OH-P.
- DHEA-S >700 mg/dL suggest the cause of hyperandrogenism as late onset CAH.
- In *secondary amenorrhea with normal serum androgen levels*, despite the presence of clinical hyperandrogenism, progesterone challenge test should be performed to assess the levels of circulating estrogens and their effect on the endometrial function.

In *secondary amenorrhea with absence of clinical hyperandrogenism* measure FSH, LH, TSH and prolactin levels.

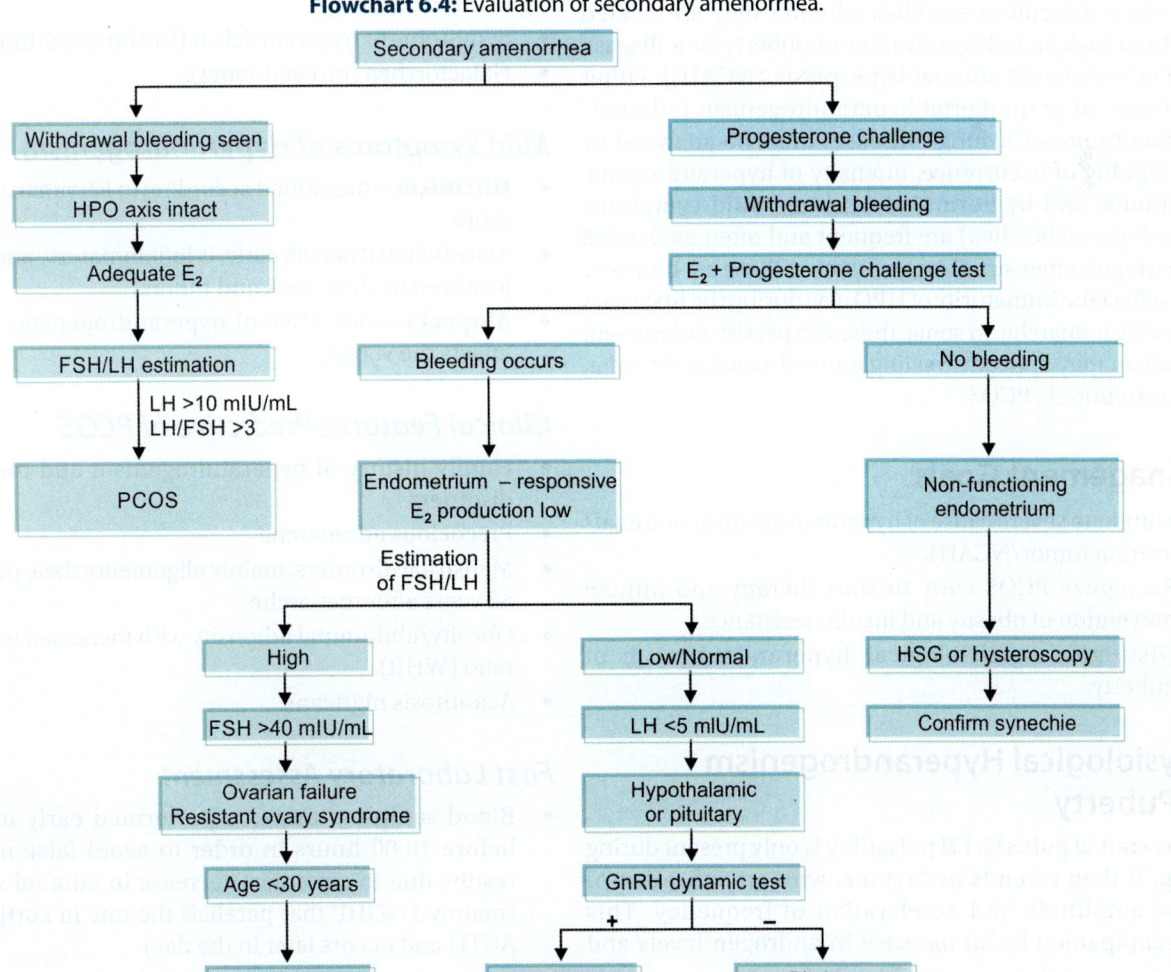

Flowchart 6.4: Evaluation of secondary amenorrhea.

- A significant elevation of PRL levels (>100 ng/mL) suggests pituitary adenoma, while mildly elevated PRL is usually the result of dysregulation in secretion inhibition mechanisms (antipsychotic drugs, hypothyroidism, pressure effect on the pituitary stalk). MRI of pituitary fossa should be performed in persistent, refractory, or excessive (>100 ng/mL) hyperprolactinemia to rule out lesions in the pituitary gland.
- If FSH and LH levels are persistently above normal range, with normal TSH and PRL levels, the most probable cause is ovarian failure.
- When FSH, LH, TSH and PRL are normal, progesterone challenge test must be performed. If there is no withdrawal bleeding, an estrogen-progesterone challenge test must be performed to ensure normal endometrial function.

HYPERANDROGENISM IN ADOLESCENT GIRLS

Symptoms of hyperandrogenism are mild in adolescents, it is often difficult to establish whether they are related to physiological androgenization of puberty or a disease [PCOS/nonclassic adrenal hyperplasia (NCAH)]. Other etiologies of peripubertal hyperandrogenism (adrenal/ovarian tumors/Cushing's disease) must be analyzed by the rapidity of occurrence, intensity of hyperandrogenic symptoms and by hormonal work-up. Mild symptoms (acne/hyperseborrhea) are frequent and often associated with irregular menstrual cycles. In most, these are transient and reflect the immaturity of HPO axis during the first years following menarche. In some, these can persist and worsen; hirsutism may appear revealing adrenal/ovarian disorder, most commonly PCOS.[41]

Management Goals

1. Eliminate severe cause of hyperandrogenism (adrenal/ovarian tumor/NCAH).
2. Recognize PCOS early to start therapy and initiate prevention of obesity and insulin resistance.
3. Distinguish physiological hyperandrogenism of puberty.

Physiological Hyperandrogenism of Puberty

At the start of puberty, LH pulsatility is only present during sleep. It then extends to daytime, with amplification of pulse amplitude and acceleration of frequency. This is accompanied by an increase in androgen levels and selective insulin resistance. This phenomenon results in a physiological hyperinsulinism.[42] The first menstrual cycles are frequently anovulatory characterized by higher serum levels of T, androstenedione (A) and LH, with mild hyperandrogenic symptoms. In most, these resolve within 1–2 years with regularization of menstrual cycles. In some they worsen with progressive constitution of PCOS (hirsutism, anovulation, increased plasma T, A and LH levels and ovarian enlargement). It is difficult to distinguish biologically and ultrasonically from those with 'physiological mini-PCOS' due to the normal maturational process of puberty. However, the association with oligomenorrhea should not be viewed as a normal feature of the first years following menarche.[43]

Diagnosis of Hyperandrogenism in Female Adolescents

Clinical Assessment

- Rapidly growing hirsutism, with signs of virilization (clitoromegaly, temporal balding, voice deepening, increasing muscle mass) are indicative of adrenal/ovarian tumor
- Symptoms of hypercorticism (Cushing syndrome)
- Galactorrhea (prolactinoma).

Mild Symptoms of Hyperandrogenism

- **Hirsutism**—quantified according to Ferriman-Gallwey score
- **Acne** (when it occurs early, is inflammatory, and mainly localized in chin, neck and thorax)
- **Alopecia**—indicative of hyperandrogenism when it affects the vertex.

Clinical Features Predictive of PCOS

- Family history of hyperandrogenism and menstrual disorders
- Precocious adrenarche
- Menstrual disorders, mainly oligomenorrhea, persisting >2 years after menarche
- Obesity/abdominal adiposity with increased waist/hip ratio (WHR)
- Acanthosis nigricans.

First Laboratory Assessment

- Blood sampling must be performed early morning before 10.00 hours in order to avoid false negative results due to circadian decrease in adrenal steroids (mainly 17-OHP that parallels the one in cortisol and ACTH and occurs later in the day)

- Investigate in early follicular phase to avoid false positive results due to steroid production from corpus luteum
- In amenorrheia/oligomenorrhea: Blood sampling should be performed after short sequence of progestin treatment
- Screening includes total T, DHEAS and 17-OHP.

Further Investigations

- **Adrenal/ovarian tumor**: Adrenal computed tomography (CT)/pelvic MRI
- **Nonclassical congenital adrenal hyperplasia (NCAH)** (basal 17-OHP >2 ng/mL): Perform ACTH test. This test is only useful when morning follicular unsuppressed 17-OHP level falls between 2–5 ng/mL (6–15 nmol/L)
- **Polycystic ovary syndrome (PCOS)**: Pelvic ultrasound and metabolic work-up are indicated.

Causes of Hyperandrogenism in Female Adolescents

Polycystic Ovary Syndrome

Intra-ovarian hyperandrogenism is the cardinal feature of PCOS. This disease stays quiescent until puberty because it hyperinsulinism needs pituitary LH to be expressed. However, LH does not have a central role in PCOS and elevated LH levels are not constant in patients with PCOS. A second event hyperinsulinism seems necessary. This metabolic defect is most likely genetic, it has a role in causing and/or propagating the disease. Hyperinsulinism may interfere early with pubertal maturation process at hypothalamic, pituitary, ovarian and adrenal levels, leading to a 'hyperpubertal state' and triggering a self-perpetuating process causing the outcome of puberty to be PCOS in genetically susceptible young women.

The clinical and biochemical features of PCOS can arise as a consequence of genetically determined hypersecretion of androgens by the ovary during in utero life.[44] The resulting hyperandrogenism results in 'programming' of the hypothalamic-pituitary unit to favor excess LH secretion during puberty and encourages preferential abdominal adiposity that predisposes to insulin resistance.

Clinical Aspects

Although very variable, phenotypic features of PCOS have three components, hyperandrogenic, anovulatory and dysmetabolic.

Hyperandrogenism

Consist of increased male-pattern hair growth, acne, seborrhea or alopecia, which reflect mild androgenic stimulation of the pilosebaceous unit. These symptoms frequently commence at the time of puberty, in some cases before puberty as 'precocious adrenarche' indicating early adrenal involvement.

Anovulation

Oligomenorrhea and secondary amenorrhea that often dates back to menarche. Primary amenorrhea is uncommon, (20%). These patients have no pubertal delay and are frequently overweight. The amenorrhea is reversible under short sequences of progestin treatment - 'normoestrogenic'/ 'type 2 anovulation'. Though 20% of patients with PCOS report normal menses, this does not mean that they ovulate each cycle.

Metabolic Syndrome

Obesity (BMI >25) is observed in 30–50%. Most become overweight just before/during puberty, a specific risk factor for subsequent development of PCOS. Obesity with fat distribution that favors the upper body (increased WHR), is associated with greater insulin resistance than if fat is in the lower body segment. Acanthosis nigricans (papular hypertrophic pigmented skin on nape of neck, axillae, chest and vulva), a non-specific marker of moderate to severe insulin resistance, is detected in 5–50%.

In order to prevent its long-term consequences, its best diagnosed early. Unfortunately, it is difficult to make the diagnosis in early puberty as most girls after menarche have anovulation, multiple small cysts in their ovaries, elevated LH and T levels, and decreased SHBG.[45]

The actual risk of an adolescent with a PCOS-like condition of developing adult PCOS is unknown.

- *In adolescents with anovulatory cycles and increased levels of T and A*, 70% get normal menstrual cycles after 5 years.[46] However, with very high levels of T and A as well as hirsuitism, the anovulatory cycles are likely to persist into adulthood.
- *In adolescents with anovulatory cycles and high LH levels 4 years after menarche*, 57% of patients continue to have anovulation and increased LH levels.[47]
- Adolescents who develop adult PCOS have irregular menstrual cycles and increased androgens and LH, but they rarely have increased insulin levels, unlike in adults, as girls in puberty have an increased sensitivity to insulin that later normalizes as they become adults.[48]

Menstruation

Many PCOS patients have irregular menstrual cycles or are amenorrheic. Physicians must ensure that these patients get menstrual cycles at least 4 times a year. If diet and exercise do not help regulate cycles, she must be given periodic progestins. Endometrial cancer can present in

PCOS patients in their 20s who have had years of unopposed endogenous estrogen. Alternatively, place them on the COC, but they must be warned that their irregular cycles will return when they discontinue the medication.[21]

Diagnosis
New Rotterdam definition,[49] at least two of the following three criteria are required:
- Oligo and/or anovulation (OA)
- Clinical and/or biochemical signs of hyperandrogenism (HA)
- Polycystic ovaries (PCO).

Hormonal Markers for PCOS
- Sensitivity and specificity of high LH in diagnosis of PCOS are low. It is not useful to look for elevated serum LH and/or exaggerated LH response to GnRH test and/or elevated LH/FSH ratio.
- In most cases, A and T levels are modestly and inconstantly elevated.

Ultrasound Definition of PCO and Anti-Müllerian Hormone
Rotterdam consensus:[49] It is 'either 12/> follicles measuring 2–9 mm in diameter in whole ovary and/or increased ovarian volume (>10 cm^3)'. In adolescent girls, follicle criterion is difficult, much less reliable by abdominal route, only the volume criterion should be used. Serum AMH can be used as surrogate to the follicle count.

Screening for Metabolic Syndrome
- **Clinical parameters:** Family history, body mass index, weight circumference, blood pressure, search for acanthosis nigricans
- **Biological parameters:** Glycemia, insulinemia, HDL-cholesterolemia, triglycerides
- Screen with oral glucose tolerance test (GTT)
- No tests for insulin resistance are necessary to make the diagnosis of PCOS nor are they needed to select treatments[49]
- **Increased WC and decreased HDL-C:** The most frequent metabolic abnormalities found in young PCOS[50]
- **Metabolic score ≥3** for diagnosis of metabolic syndrome does not seem appropriate for adolescents.[50]

The PCOS Phenotypes
The new definition of Rotterdam recognizes four phenotypes:
- HA+OA+PCO (full-blown syndrome)
- HA+OA
- HA+PCO (ovulatory PCOS)
- OA+PCO ('nonhyperandrogenic PCOS').

Nonclassic Adrenal Hyperplasia
The 21-OH-lase deficiency is responsible for oversecretion of 17-OHP. Gene mutations of cytochrome P450 C21, resulting in NCAH, reduce the activity of 21-OH-lase to 20–50%. This results in excessive accumulation of 21-OH precursors, mainly progesterone and 17-OHP, in the presence of normal stimulation by ACTH. This excess is partly converted to androgens, resulting in adrenal hyperandrogenism, without overt abnormality in the gluco- and mineralocorticosteroid pathways.

Clinical aspects
Before age 7–8 years, NCAH may mimic an idiopathic premature pubarche or a virilizing ovarian/adrenal tumor, especially when there are symptoms of precocious pseudopuberty, such as accelerated height velocity and clitoromegaly. No symptom of hyperandrogenism is specific for NCAH. Furthermore, NCAH may also be detected in individuals having mild symptoms such as acne. Therefore, the clinical presentation cannot be used for the diagnosis of NCAH. Clitoromegaly, male habitus and temporal baldness are infrequent findings, unless the patient suffers from undiagnosed simple virilizing CAH. NCAH is a progressive disorder since the prevalence of hirsutism increases with the patient's age.[51]

Diagnosis
Measure the morning 17-OHP level:
- Basal 17-OHP >2 ng/mL
- Poststimulation 17-OHP >12 ng/mL.

Other Causes
1. **Adrenal and ovarian tumors:** These causes are rare. Some extreme forms of PCOS, such as hyperthecosis, may also present with similar clinical and hormonal features.
2. **Cushing syndrome:** Some adrenal tumors may secrete high amounts of androgens and cortisol. It is wise to check 24-hour urinary free cortisol level, especially in obese patients with full-blown PCOS.
3. **Hyperprolactinemia:** PRL excess stimulates secretion of adrenal androgens, mainly DHEAS. Therefore, a mild hyperandrogenism frequently accompanies prolactinoma. Mild hyperprolactinemia frequently occurs in PCOS, but has no specific expression and often disappears spontaneously.
4. **Idiopathic hirsutism:** It is a diagnosis of exclusion. It is often observed Mediterranean/Hispanic ethnic background. It is thought to result from increased skin 5α-reductase activity.
5. **Drugs:** Anabolic steroids, nortestosterone-derived progestins, antiepileptic drugs, cortrosyn and metyrapone.

Treatment of Hyperandrogenism in Female Adolescents

Polycystic Ovary Syndrome

The treatment aims at interrupting androgen production and/or action.

- **Oral contraceptives** are the first line of therapy.
  - Arrest progression of hirsutism but does not lead to substantial improvement.
  - Lowers free T levels by reducing serum Gn levels, increasing SHBG levels, and modestly lowering DHEAS levels. COC with nonandrogenic progestin (desogestrel, gestodene, norgestimate, drospirenone or chlormadinone) is advisable.
- **Cyproterone acetate** is a potent progestin taken up by fat and released slowly. When given for 20 days every 4 weeks at 50-mg daily dose, it inhibits pituitary Gn secretion and acts as potent antiandrogen upon the pilosebaceous unit. An excellent response of hirsutism is seen in 90% of cases. It is administered with an estrogen to avoid irregular bleeding/amenorrhea due to endometrial atrophy. Natural E_2 (either percutaneously/orally, 2 mg/day for 1–20 days) is preferable to ethinyl E_2, which has more metabolic effects.
- **Spironolactone**, 50–100 mg bid, is effective. It is potentially teratogenic to fetal male genital development and may cause menstrual disturbance.
- In obese, **weight loss** is important.
- Insulin-sensitizing drugs in adolescence is an unsolved issue.

Nonclassical Adrenal Hyperplasia

- Long-term glucocorticoid therapy is controversial and is necessary only in adrenal hyperplasia on CT scan/pregnancy wish.
  - It aims to reduce adrenal hyperandrogenism. Very low doses of DXM are needed (0.25–0.5 mg at night).
  - Aim to normalize the morning 17-OHP plasma level.
  - The T or A plasma levels, rather than 17-OHP, should be monitored.
  - In case of pregnancy wish, progesterone serum level should be monitored during follicular phase inorder to avoid an anticervical mucus effect.
- **Cyproterone acetate** instead of DXM/ hydrocortisone is useful for hirsutism due to NCAH. It has a powerful antiandrogen effect on peripheral receptors that allows a more rapid and sustained improvement of hirsutism. Adverse effects with it are less than with glucocorticoids. The same applies to **spironolactone**.
- **Cosmetic treatments:** Should be encouraged.
  - Temporary methods: Bleaching, depilation, and epilation.
  - Permanent methods: Electrolysis or laser.

FUNCTIONAL OVARIAN HYPERANDROGENISM

Functional ovarian hyperandrogenism (FOH) is androgen excess in adolescent girls and is characterized by 17-OH-P hyper-responsiveness to GnRH stimulation/to hCG testing, and subnormal suppressibility of serum T by dexamethasone. FOH is often accompanied by functional adrenal hyper-responsiveness, which is characterized by 17-OH-P/DHEA hyper-responsiveness to ACTH.[6]

Evaluation of Basal Serum Hormone Levels (Table 6.11)

1. **FSH and LH** are glycoproteins of 20–30 different isoforms with varying biological activity. FSH, LH and hCG are composed of the α- and β-subunits of which the α-subunit is common, whereas β-subunits differ. In prepubertal girls, FSH levels are low, whereas LH levels are usually undetectable.[6] With the onset of puberty, Gn levels rise gradually in puberty until the adult cyclic pattern is obtained.
   - **FSH/LH ratio:** In prepubertal children, FSH levels are higher than those of LH (FSH/LH ratio >1), but half of healthy adolescent children have FSH/LH ratio <1. Thus, a random FSH/LH <1 in an adolescent girl is not pathological *per se*, whereas an increased follicular phase LH/FSH ratio is indicative of PCOS in cases of oligomenorrhea/hyperandrogenism. The LH/FSH ratio should not be used as part of the diagnostic criteria for PCOS.[49]

Table 6.11: Initial biochemical evaluation of hyperandrogenism.

Premature breast development	• Basal FSH, LH, E_2, SHBG, inhibin A and B • GnRH test (FSH, LH) • AMH (if granulosa cell tumor is suspected)	Urinary steroid profiling may additionally be useful in the above-mentioned conditions
Premature pubic hair	• Basal T, DHEAS, A, 17-OHP • ACTH test (cortisol, 17-OHP) • GnRH test (FSH, LH, 17-OHP)	
Hirsutism	• Basal T, DHEAS, Δ4-A, 17-OHP • ACTH test (cortisol, 17-OHP) • Fasting glucose, insulin, HbA1C (or preferably oral GTT)	
Primary amenorrhea/Premature ovarian failure	• Basal FSH, LH, E_2, SHBG, T, inhibin A, inhibin B, AMH, PRL • Karyotype	

(FSH: follicle stimulating hormone; LH: luteinizing hormone; E2: estradiol; SHBG: sex hormone binding globulin; GnRH: gonadotropin releasing hormones; AMH: anti-müllerian hormone; ACTH: adrenocorticotropic hormone; DHEAS: dehydroepiandrosterone; GTT: glucose tolerance test)

- **GnRH testing:** Basal LH and FSH is sufficient for some reproductive disorders, but a GnRH test is necessary for diagnosis of CPP. Luteinizing hormone-releasing hormone (LHRH; 100 μg) is injected intravenously, blood samples are drawn before and 30 minutes after the injection and analyzed for LH and FSH. The test is easy, can be performed in outpatient setting at any time during the day. The upper normal range of stimulated LH levels in prepubertal children may vary from 3.3 to 5–6 IU/L. Peak LH level >5 IU/L and/or stimulated LH/FSH ratio >0.66 IU/L are the cut off limits for a pubertal response during GnRH testing. Girls presenting with breast development and basal LH level above 0.3 IU/L are assumed to have CPP.[6, 52]

2. **Estrogens:** Primarily 17P-E2 and estrone, are produced in the ovarian granulosa cell following aromatization of their precursors A and T. Estrogen production is elevated during minipuberty and with the onset of puberty, whereas levels are typically below the detection limit in prepubertal children. In girls with premature thelarche, E_2 is usually below the detection limit, but clearly elevated compared to prepubertal children.[6]

3. **Sex hormone-binding globulin (SHBG):** E_2 is bound to SHBG, a minor part of circulating E_2 is in free biologically active form. SHBG is regulated by estrogens, androgens, thyroid hormones, insulin and liver function. It seems to reflect the degree of physiological insulin resistance seen in midpuberty.[53]

4. **Androgens:** DHEAS levels are low during childhood and start to increase before other hormonal changes of puberty take place (adrenarche). Levels are high in adrenal cortical tumors, whereas lesser elevations are seen in CAH, and moderate elevations are seen in precocious adrenarche.

5. **17-OH-Progesterone (17-OH-P):** It is produced by the adrenal and the ovary. In classical CAH (21-OH deficiency), 17-OH-P is elevated, whereas it is only marginally elevated in late-onset CAH.

6. **Urinary excretion of steroids:** Determination of steroid excretion rates in a 24-hour urine sample estimates the combined output of adrenal and gonadal steroid production. A 24-hour collection determines excretion rates (for diagnosis of Cushing/adrenal insufficiency), whereas spot urine diagnoses enzymatic defects in the steroidogenic pathway/tumors. Urinary steroid profiling is useful in a wide variety of clinical conditions:
   - *CAH due to 21-OH deficiency:* Elevated urinary levels of 17-hydroxypregnanolone, pregnanediol, and pregnanetriol
   - *CAH due to 11-OH deficiency:* Elevated urinary tetrahydro-11-deoxycortisol
   - *CAH due to 3β-HSD deficiency:* Increased urinary levels of DHEA, 16-OH-DHEA, pregnanetriol and 17-OH-pregnanetriol
   - *Children with adrenocortical tumors:* Markedly elevated urinary levels of DHEA
   - *Cushing's disease:* Urinary cortisol metabolites are increased
   - *Adrenal insufficiency:* Urinary cortisol metabolites are low/undetectable.

7. **Adrenocorticotropic hormone** (ACTH): It is elevated in adrenal insufficiency (or pituitary Cushing).
   - **ACTH testing:** A blood sample is drawn and 250 μg tetracosactrin IV bolus is injected. Blood samples are drawn 30 and 60 minutes later. The test is easy, can be performed at any time of the day, does not require fasting, and it can also be administered intramuscularly. Firstly, blood samples are used for cortisol measurements to rule out adrenal insufficiency. Secondly, steroidogenic metabolites (21-OHP, 11-OHP or DHEA) may be analyzed to evaluate possible CYP21, CYP11 or 3βHSD defects. A normal cortisol response during an ACTH test is a rise to >500 nmol/L (or rise of >250 nmol/L). Ongoing/ recent treatment with glucocorticoids interfere with cortisol measurements. Use of COC may result in high cortisol due to induction of corticosteroid binding globulin, and should be stopped for 4 weeks before ACTH testing.

PREMENSTRUAL SYNDROME

Premenstrual syndrome (PMS) is the cyclic appearance of one or more symptoms just prior to menses, to such a degree that lifestyle or work is affected followed by a period of time entirely free of symptoms. Approximately, 40% report significant problems related to their cycles and about 2–10% report a degree of impact on work or lifestyle. The most frequently encountered symptoms (usually in last 7–10 days of cycle) include:

- Abdominal bloating
- Anxiety
- Breast tenderness
- Crying spells
- Depression
- Fatigue
- Irritability
- Thirst and appetite changes
- Variable degrees of edema of the extremities

Diagnosis

Guidelines for diagnosis (American Psychiatric Association that called PMS as *luteal phase dysphoric disorder*) have the following criteria:

- **Symptoms** are temporally related to the menstrual cycle, beginning in the last week of luteal phase and remitting after onset of menses.

- **Diagnosis** requires at least five of the following and one of the symptoms must be either one of the first four:
  - Affective liability, e.g. sudden onset of being sad, tearful, irritable/angry
  - Persistent and marked anger/irritability
  - Marked anxiety/tension
  - Markedly depressed mood, feelings of hopelessness
  - Decreased interest in usual activities
  - Easy fatigability/marked lack of energy
  - Subjective sense of difficulty in concentration
  - Marked change in appetite, overeating or food craving
  - Hypersomnia/insomnia
  - Physical symptoms such as breast tenderness, headache, edema, joint/muscle pain, and weight gain.
- The symptoms interfere with work, usual activities, or relationships
- The symptoms are not an exacerbation of a psychiatric disorder.

Treatment

Before the diagnosis is established, women must log symptoms daily for at least two full cycles. At the same time patient must be screened for other psychiatric disorders. Women should be advised number of life style changes:

1. Elimination of caffeine from the diet
2. Smoking cessation
3. Regular exercise
4. Regular meals and a nutritious diet
5. Adequate sleep
6. Stress reduction by reducing responsibilities and by relaxation exercises like yoga.

Various Drugs Used in its Management

1. **Alprazolam:** 0.25 mg BD or TDS during the luteal phase is very effective. It has antidepressant, anxiolytic and smooth muscle relaxant properties.
2. **Fluoxetin:** 20–60 mg daily for 1–2 weeks preceding menstruation. It is a selective serotonin reuptake inhibitor.
3. **Evening primrose oil:** Provides linoleic and gamma linoleic acid (precursor PGE).
4. **Other drugs** include COC, Vitamin B_6, bromocriptine, monoamine oxidase inhibitors, synthetic progestational agents, spironolactone for bloating.
5. **GnRH agonist** treatment can produce hypogonadotropic hypoganadism, i.e. medical oophorectomy. Adding estrogen-progestin to avoid side effects of GnRH agonist diminishes the improvement in PMS symptoms.
6. **Medical and surgical oophorectomy:** A lasting response to surgical hysterectomy and oophorectomy in women unresponsive to medical therapy.

PELVIC PAIN AND RECURRENT ABDOMINAL PAIN

The pelvic pain can be:
- Acute
- Chronic
- Cyclic

In adolescents who present with chronic pelvic pain, the following systems should be considered with regard to the underlying cause of the problem:
- Gastrointestinal
- Genitourinary
- Musculoskeletal
- Gynecologic
- Psychological/psychiatric

Assessing the **character of pain** is very useful in analyzing the etiology (Table 6.12).

- Colic or severely cramping pain is commonly associated with contraction/obstruction of a hollow viscus such as an intestine/uterus
- Rapid onset of pain is more consistent with perforation of hollow viscus/ischemia
- Pain perceived over the entire abdomen suggests a generalized peritonitis.

DYSMENORRHEA

It is pain with menstruation usually cramping in nature and centered in the lower abdomen. It can be:

Primary: Menstrual pain without pelvic pathology.

Secondary: Painful menses associated with underlying pelvic pathology.

Primary Dysmenorrhea

Symptoms

It has a high prevalence in adolescence usually appears within 1–2 years of menarche, when ovulatory cycles are established and affects younger women, but may persist into 40s. Its severity is directly related to duration and amount of menstrual flow. The pain usually begins few hours before/just after the onset of menstrual period and may last up to 48–72 hours. It is similar to labor pain with suprapubic cramping, and may be accompanied by lumbosacral backache, pain radiating down the anterior thigh, nausea, vomiting, diarrhea, and rarely syncopal episodes. The pain is colicky in nature and is improved by

SECTION 1   General Gynecology

Table 6.12: Type and causes of abdominal pain in adolescents.

Type of pain	Causes	
Acute pain		

It is intense and characterized by sudden onset, sharp rise, and short course	• Gynecological disease/dysfunction	Acute infection:
		• Endometritis
		• Pelvic inflammatory disease (Acute salpingo-oophoritis)
		• Tubo-ovarian abscess:
		  – Rupture
		  – Torsion
		Adenexal disorders:
		• Hemorrhagic functional ovarian cysts
		• Torsion of adnexa
		• Twisted para ovarian cyst
		• Rupture of functional ovarian cyst/ovarian neoplasm

	• Gastrointestinal	• Gastroenteritis • Appendicitis • Bowel obstruction • Diverticulitis
	• Genitourinary	• Cystitis • Pyelonephritis
	• Musculoskeletal	Abdominal wall hematoma
	• Others	• Acute porphyria • Aneurysm
Chronic pain		

Defined as pain of >6 months duration	• Gynecological	• Endometriosis/adhesions
		• Salpingo-oopheritis:
		  – Subacute
		  – Chronic
		• Ovarian neoplasm's like teratomas

	• Gastrointestinal	• Recurrent appendiceal colic • Infectious diarrhea • Recurrent partial small bowel obstruction
	• Genitourinary	• Recurrent or relapsing cystouretheritis • Pelvic kidney
	• Musculoskeletal	
Cyclic pain		

Pain occurs at a definite time with a definite association to the menstrual cycle	Dysmenorrhea—most common cyclic pain	• Primary
		• Secondary:
		  – Imperforate hymen
		  – Transverse vaginal septum
		  – Cervical stenosis
		  – Uterine anomalies (bicornuate uterus, blind uterine horn)

	Mittelschmerz syndrome	

abdominal massage, counter pressure, movement of body, by COC use and previous vaginal deliveries.

Signs
The suprapubic region may be tender. Bowel sounds are normal and there is no upper abdominal tenderness or rebound tenderness. *On bimanual examination,* there is uterine tenderness, however pain with movement of cervix, or palpation of adenexal structures is absent. The pelvic organs are normal in primary dysmenorhea.

Pathology
It is due to myometrial contractions induced by high concentration of prostaglandin, originating in secretory endometrium. There is higher uterine tone with high amplitude contractions resulting in decreased uterine blood flow and high vasopressin concentrations.

Diagnosis
Confirm the cyclic nature of pain and rule out underlying pelvic pathology. During the pelvic examination:

- Size, shape, mobility of uterus
- Size and tenderness of adnexal structures
- Nodularity/fibrosis of uterosacral ligaments and rectovaginal septum should be assessed
- Cervical studies for gonorrhea and chlamydia
- Complete blood count with erythrocyte sedimentation rate (ESR) to rule out subacute salphingo-oophoritis.

Management
- **Prostaglandin synthase inhibitors**: Should be taken just before/at onset of pain every 6-8 hours, for first few days of menstrual flow. The fenamates (mefenamic acid) and propionic acid derivatives (ibuprofen, naproxen, ketoprofen) are very effective in treatment of dysmenorrhea.
- **Combined oral contraceptives** are a good choice for combining contraception with beneficial effect on dysmenorrhea, menstrual flow, and menstrual irregularity.
- It inhibits ovulation, leading to suppression of endometrial tissue growth and, secondary, to reduction of menstrual flow below normal levels.
- It leads to concomitant drop of menstrual prostaglandins' levels, therefore, lessening menstrual flow along with decrease of prostaglandins that reduces uterine motility and ischemia and thus uterine cramping pain.
- If dysmenorrhea is not relieved by NSAIDs/COC, **laparoscopy** should be considered to rule out endometriosis, Pelvic inflammatory disease (PID), Müllerian duct anomalies.

Secondary Dysmenorrhea

It is defined as pain during menstruation associated with underlying pathology. Any menstrual pain arising >3 years after menarche is considered pathologic. Chronic pelvic/low abdominal pain, beginning one/two days prior menses, irregular/heavy menstrual patterns, dyspareunia and bowel symptoms are signs usually associated with an underlying organic pathology. If often begins 1-2 weeks before menstrual flow and persists until few days after cessation of bleeding. In adolescents it can be because of:

- Endometriosis
- Pelvic inflammatory disease
- Imperforate hymen
- Transverse vaginal septum
- Cervical stenosis
- Uterine anomalies (Bicornuate uterus, blind uterine horn)

Other infrequent causes during adolescence:
- Uterine retroversion in fixed position
- Stenosis of cervical channel
- Intrauterine devices without progestin-containing system
- Uterine fibroids
- Endometrial or endocervical polyps
- Adenomyosis
- Pelvic venous congestion.

Management

Treatment of underlying cause is the mainstay of management. These patients do not much benefit by NSAIDs and COCs. Laparoscopy is the single most useful diagnostic procedure because most adolescents have minimal or mild stages of endometriosis. Cervical and vaginal cultures, pelvic ultrasonography, MRI, hysterosalpingography and hysteroscopy can be helpful in the evaluation.

ENDOMETRIOSIS

Endometriosis should be suspected in adolescents aged younger than 18 years with recurrent dysmenorrhea refractory to NSAIDs and COCs (incidence as high as 70%).[54] Patients typically present with pelvic pain and worsening symptoms at a time close to their menses. The use of a pain diary is helpful to document the patient's symptomatology. Most have normal findings on examination, some may exhibit tenderness with out evidence of any mass/nodularity. Diagnostic laparoscopy can confirm the diagnosis. Early diagnosis and treatment is crucial to prevent progression of symptom relief.

Treatment is usually conservative, with a combination if medical (NSAIDs, continuous COCs, progestins, danazol and GnRH analogs) and surgical intervention (laser ablation and adhesiolysis). The best mode of treatment remains a topic of debate.

- When comparing continuous with cyclic oral contraceptive therapy, a 2-year prospective study noted continuous to be more efficacious.[55] Symptomatic improvement was noted with use of 20–30 micrograms of ethinyl E_2 over a 6–9 month period in 75–100% of patients, and it is felt to be the best initial therapy for endometriosis after laparoscopic diagnosis and management.[56]
- Danazol is androgen derived and minimal data supports its efficacy in adolescents.
- Progestin-only protocols are still an option and include oral as well as depot preparations. Long-term use of depomedroxyprogesterone acetate leads to bone demineralization, which seems to recover after discontinuation.
- It is acceptable in patients aged 18 years or older to be offered an empiric course of GnRH agonist.[57] With long-

term use (>6 months), there is an associated bone loss and therefore add-back therapy (progestin) should be given to minimize this effect.
- If there is persistence of symptoms, operative laparoscopy is appropriate. The goal of surgical treatment is to remove visible areas of endometriosis and restore normal anatomy by lysis of adhesions if present.

Chronic Pelvic Pain in the Adolescent

Chronic pelvic pain is defined as lower abdominal pain lasting 3–6 months or longer.[58] It occurs commonly in the adolescent and can be a diagnostic and therapeutic challenge.

Role of Laparoscopy

The early use of diagnostic laparoscopy in refractory cases of chronic pelvic pain can lead to a more precise diagnosis when less invasive methods fail. It helps diagnose endometriosis or other specific pelvic pathology. Negative findings provide reassurance that pelvic structures are normal.

Causes of Chronic Pelvic Pain in the Adolescent

Classically, the causes of pelvic pain are divided into:
- Acute versus chronic
- Gynecologic versus nongynecologic

Acute pelvic pain starts over a short time (few minutes - days), whereas CPP is defined as cyclic/acyclic pelvic pain that persists for at least 3–6 months, requires medical/surgical evaluation and intervention, and can cause functional disability.[59] Common causes include PID, undertreated dysmenorrhea, hemorrhaghic corpus luteum cysts, endometriosis and pelvic adhesions.

Specific Etiologies, Diagnosis and Treatment

Acute pelvic pain
1. **Ectopic pregnancy**: A high index of suspicion for pregnancy in the adolescent remains warranted when she presents with acute/chronic pelvic pain. In a normal intrauterine pregnancy, she may experience pain due to round ligament strain, 'morning sickness' with the associated nausea and abdominal pain, or as a result of a urinary tract infection. More serious causes include threatened/incomplete miscarriage, rupture of corpus luteum cyst, ectopic pregnancy, septic miscarriage with peritonitis and acute urinary retention due to a retroverted gravid uterus or an impacted ovarian cyst in the pelvis.

2. **Ovarian torsion—a surgical emergency:** Torsion in adolescents more often occurs in absence of an associated adnexal mass and is due to increased mobility of the vascular pedicle. The pain occurs suddenly, commonly on the right side, acute enough to wake them from sleep/keep them from falling asleep. Occasionally, ovary may intermittently twist, resulting in intense pain that resolves completely between episodes; this may occur during sexual intercourse, with change of position/movement. It can be difficult to diagnose clinically because of nonspecific symptoms (pain, nausea, vomiting) and delay in treatment can lead to ovarian necrosis. If suspected, Doppler imaging should be done. A more conservative approach after detorsion of ovaries remains preferable to surgical removal, unless ovary is clearly necrosed and not viable. When size of the abdominopelvic mass is <75 mm, laparoscopy and detorsion, aspiration of a benign-appearing cyst, and upholding of ovary in the abdominal cavity, is safe and effective in children and adolescents.[58]

3. **Appendicitis** is the most common cause of nongynecologic acute pelvic pain. Patients typically present with fever, leukocytosis, nausea, vomiting, and periumbilical pain, which gradually moves to the right lower quadrant. The presentation may result in delay in diagnosis due to overlap of other similar gynecological condition symptoms (23.6–26.6%).[58] USG with graded compression is useful for diagnosing appendicitis, and the lack of ionizing radiation and a high positive predictive value (95%) make it the recommended first-line investigation in adolescents. The treatment is appendectomy with adjunctive antibiotics perioperatively.

Causes of Acute and Chronic Pelvic Pain

Nonemergent gynecologic causes
1. **Sexually transmitted infections (STIs) and vulvovaginitis** is fairly common among adolescents, and are often associated with pelvic pain. Between ages of 14–19, STDs occur more frequently in girls than boys by a ratio of 2:1 (due to deficiency in progesterone, as a result of, HPO instability, which results in increased vulnerability of female genital tract to infection). These diseases are caused by bacterial, viral, fungal or protozoal infection. Besides HIV and hepatitis B, most common infections include Chlamydia, *N Gonorrhoeae,* HPV, herpes simplex virus (HSV), and syphilis. Prolonged infection with *N. gonorrhoeae* or *C. trachomatis* may lead to chronic pelvic pain, tubal scarring, and infertility (5 fold higher),[60] even without the classic signs of PID. It is critical that sexually active teenagers presenting with pelvic pain be evaluated for STI and treated empirically.

2. ***Pelvic inflammatory disease:*** This is presents in girls that are sexually active. It is a polymicrobial disease, which can involve combination of endometritis, parametritis, oophoritis, and tubo-ovarian abscess, with adhesions potentially connecting to bowel. Subacute PID is relatively common, and refers to undiagnosed 'silent' state of chronic inflammation that goes unreported and/or undetected. It can be just as damaging to the tubes as acute form. PID is highly correlated with sexual activity at younger age, several sexual partners, non-use of barrier contraception, and infection with *C. trachomatis* and *N. gonorrhoeae*. The incidence is inversely proportional to age, with highest rates in 15–19-year-olds. High levels of estrogen exposure in early-middle adolescence leads to cervical ectopy with relatively large transformation zone of exposed columnar epithelium that may facilitate the attachment of *C. trachomatis* and *N. gonorrhoeae*. It should be suspected in all presenting with pelvic pain/cervical motion tenderness. However, many do not demonstrate classic symptoms. Laparoscopic evaluation is the gold standard for diagnosis. Add transvaginal scan in cases where a tubo-ovarian abscess is suspected/the examination is unclear. Treatment includes broad-spectrum antibiotics. Empiric treatment should be started immediately in women at risk if they are experiencing pelvic/lower abdominal pain, no other cause for the illness other than PID can be identified, and if cervical motion tenderness, uterine tenderness, or adnexal tenderness is present. If treatment is delayed, infection can result in pyosalpinx and/or tubo-ovarian abscess necessitating radiologic/surgical drainage.
3. ***Dysmenorrhea*** is defined as mild-to-severe cramping pain in the lower abdomen that occurs during and/or prior to menses. It is the most common gynecologic complaint among adolescent and young adult females with a reported prevalence from 40–90%.[61,62] The majority is primary (or functional), associated with a normal ovulatory cycle. The rate of dysmenorrhea increases age and is attributable to establishment of ovulatory cycles. Primary dysmenorrhea usually presents with symptoms 6–12 months following menarche, when ovulatory cycles begin. Lower abdominal cramping is the most common symptom, many suffer from other prostacyclin-mediated symptoms such as nausea, headache, vomiting, diarrhea, and fatigue. Symptoms typically accompany the start of menstrual flow/occur within few hours before/after onset, and last for first 24–48 hours. Girls with severe dysmenorrhea have cramps that begin before the onset of menses and persist for up to 7 days; this subset should be evaluated for endometriosis. In secondary dysmenorrhea common causes include endometriosis, Müllerian anomalies and congenital malformations (e.g. imperforate hymen), cervical stenosis, and pelvic infections. This is seen in 10% and is more likely associated with chronic pelvic pain, midcycle pain, dyspareunia, and metrorrhagia.
   - Nonsteroidal anti-inflammatory drugs (NSAIDs)—the most common pharmacologic treatment - inhibit cyclo-oxygenase. The resulting lower level of prostaglandin leads to less vigorous contractions of uterus, and less discomfort. NSAIDs should be avoided in perioperative patients, those with gastrointestinal bleeding/ulcers, renal disease, clotting disorders, and allergies to NSAIDs. In the nonsexually active adolescent, therapy is mentioned in Table 6.13.
   - For the sexually active adolescent, COC remain the first-line therapy and third-line therapy for nonsexually active teens not responding to NSAIDs.
   - If symptoms do not improve with 3 months of NSAIDs plus COC, consider continuous hormone therapy. Those with persistent pain despite continuous hormone therapy for 3 months should be evaluated by laparoscopy to identify underlying organic causes such as endometriosis, adhesions, or an obstructive pelvic anomaly.
   - In moderate-to-severe pain for whom NSAIDs and COC are contraindicated: Tramadol hydrochloride tablets—centrally acting analgesic that binds to μ-opioid receptors and inhibits reuptake of norepinephrine and serotonin. Prescribed as 50-mg pills, 1–2 tablets every 6 hours, not to exceed 8 tablets in 24-hour period.
4. ***Endometriosis:*** The true incidence among adolescents remains unknown, but identified in >50% of teenagers with chronic pelvic pain and dyspareunia[63,64] and in 70% with pelvic pain not responding to NSAIDs and COC.[65] Adolescents can present with either acyclic or cyclic pelvic pain, and are unlikely to present with classic triad of dysmenorrhea, dyspareunia, and infertility. Have a high index of suspicion in adolescents with cyclical pain, especially if it radiates to back/lower extremities/is accompanied by gastrointestinal symptoms such as abdominal pain, nausea, diarrhea, and constipation. Findings can range from normal to generalized pelvic tenderness, some tenderness in uterosacral ligaments, nodularity, or palpable masses (though endometriomas are uncommon in <20 years of age). Rectovaginal examination may reveal focal

Table 6.13: NSAIDs for treatment of dysmenorrhea.

Ibuprofen	400 mg	Every 6 hours
Naproxen sodium	550 mg	Every 12 hours
Mefanimic acid	500 mg	Loading dose
	Then 250 mg	Every 6 hours

tenderness in the posterior cul-de-sac/nodularity of uterosacral ligaments. Laparoscopy is the gold standard for diagnosis and staging of endometriosis. Larger implants can be identified with radiologic imaging. Initial medical treatment for endometriosis consists of low-dose, monophasic COC continuously. The goal is to avoid endometrial proliferation and to prevent endometrial implants from bleeding. Other therapies include medroxyprogesterone acetate (MPA) and GnRH-agonists (nafarelin/leuprolide). Aromatase inhibitors (target ovarian and extraovarian sources of estrogen production), and selective progesterone receptor modulators, may also be useful.[66–68]

5. ***Ovarian cysts:*** Functional (follicular and corpus luteal) ovarian cysts are a common cause of acute pelvic pain when associated with acute intracystic hemorrhage/rupture. The abrupt onset of pain can be severe and localized, or more diffuse and non-specific. Majority (even large ones) do not cause pelvic pain. Secondary dysmenorrhea caused by simple ovarian cysts usually resolves spontaneously after two/three menstrual cycles, and therefore should be managed conservatively. Although COC are commonly prescribed to these patients, hormonal therapy does not improve the regression rates of ovarian cysts.[69] For a cystic mass of 7 cm/less, observation for 6-weeks followed by re-examination will confirm resolution of most cystic masses.[71] Cysts that are large, persist over several cycles, or contain solid components require surgical excision.

6. ***Pelvic adhesions:*** The role of pelvic adhesions in pelvic pain is controversial.[70,71] It appears that some adhesions are associated with pain and some are not.[72] Adhesions may be more likely to play a role when they limit mobility of intraperitoneal organs. Majority of pelvic adhesions in adolescents are secondary to PID/appendicitis. Pelvic adhesions are found in only 12.8% of adolescent patients with pelvic pain.[63,73] There is currently lack of consistent support that adhesiolysis is useful.[74,75] Laparotomy should be avoided because adhesions formation can take place more commonly than after laparoscopy.

7. ***Interstitial cystitis:*** Incidence of 39% among adolescent females with pelvic pain, dysmenorrhea, dyspareunia, and urinary symptoms is seen.[76] Bladder syndrome is characterized by pelvic pain and chronic irritative voiding symptoms which may be aggravate prior to/during menses (urinary frequency and urgency, nocturia, suprapubic pain, bladder pain often relieved by voiding, and pelvic/abdominal pain). Diagnosis requires:[77]
    – Pain and chronic irritative voiding symptoms
    – Characteristic findings on cystoscopy [low bladder capacity on hydrodistension, postdistension capillary hemorrhages (glomerulations), terminal hematuria, or ulcerations of bladder mucosa (Hunner's ulcers)]
    – Absence of other urinary pathology/disease processes.

Young women presenting with chronic pelvic pain, urinary symptoms and dyspareunia, should be considered for bladder cystoscopy and hydrodistension along with diagnostic laparoscopy.

Nongynecologic Causes of Chronic Pelvic Pain

1. **Irritable bowel syndrome (IBS):** The most common cause of nongynecologic chronic pelvic pain among adolescents (15–20%).[78] It is defined as chronic abdominal pain (usually in lower segment) associated with a change in consistency/frequency of stools, relieved by defecation. They may also complain of passage of mucus/abdominal bloating. These symptoms should be present for at least 12 weeks and not necessarily consecutively for past 12 months.[79] It is a diagnosis of exclusion. Medical management (directed at alleviating the symptoms) includes antispasmodics, fiber bulking agents, antidiarrheals, psychological, and behavioral interventions (cognitive-behavioral therapy, psychotherapy, hypnosis, relaxation training, and family or group therapy).

2. **Psychosocial causes** accounts for some cases of CPP in the adolescent. Parental stress/recent divorce, sexual abuse can result in somatic symptoms including headaches and abdominal and/or pelvic pain can be manifested in a teenager as chronic pelvic pain. There is an association between negative emotions (anxiety and depression) and pelvic pain. Techniques including biofeedback, relaxation training, or ongoing counseling may be useful to ameliorate/control pain completely, using mind over body. Some may improve with adjunctive psychological therapy/with intensive pain programs.

OVARIAN ENLARGEMENTS IN ADOLESCENT GIRL

Ovarian masses, cystic and solid, may occur at any age. They can be non-neoplastic or neoplastic.

Non-Neoplastic Enlargement of the Ovary

Follicular cyst: This is the most frequent type. It arises from the ovarian follicles through the process of atresia folliculi with death of the ovum. They appear as tiny, often microscopic cysts lined by one or more layers of granulosa cells and are found in considerable numbers even in normal ovaries. They may attain the size of 8–10 cm and can then become of clinical importance producing discomfort in the pelvis.

Nevertheless these can spontaneously regress in most instances, are transient and thus self-limiting. When symptoms like amenorrhea are prolonged, administering oral MPA 10 mg three times a day over 5–7 days generally induces menstruation.

Neoplastic Enlargement of Ovary

An ovarian tumor in adolescents is more often malignant than benign. Most of germ cell tumors (60%) occur in young girls. A list of various tumor markers elevated in various conditions is listed in Table 6.14.

1. **Dysgerminoma:** In adolescents its occurrence is 40–45%. It presents with abdominal pain. In 90%, menstrual history is normal. In younger age group, its recurrence is most likely.
2. **Endodermal sinus (Yolk sac) tumor:** It is rare and thought to originate from multipotential embryonal tissue as a result of selective differentiation of yolk sac structures. It characteristically presents with papillary projections composed of a central core of blood vessels enveloped by immature epithelium. Most present with abdominal pain and pelvic mass. It responds to chemotherapy with good survival rate.
3. **Choriocarcinoma:** Rarely seen in a pure form. It is generally a part of a mixed germ cell tumor. It secretes large quantities of hCG hormone, which forms an ideal tumor marker in the diagnosis and management. The tumor is highly malignant and metastasizes by bloodstream to the lungs, brain, bones, and other body viscera.
4. **Embryonal cell carcinoma:** It is a rare, highly malignant tumor accounting for 5% of all germ cell tumors that occurs in prepubertal girls. It secretes both a fetoproteins and hCG. It is associated with symptoms of precocious puberty and menstrual irregularities.
5. **Granulosa cell tumor:** It is a sex cord stromal tumor with feminizing functioning mesenchymoma. These tumors are composed of cells closely resembling the granulosa cells of the Graffian follicles. The clinical features depend on the estrogenic activity of the tumor with only larger ones causing pain and abdominal swelling. It can result in precocious puberty with development of secondary sexual characteristics, hypertrophy of the breast and external genetalia, pubic hair and myohyperplasia of the uterus. The endometrium shows an estrogenic anovulatory pattern. Removal of the tumor causes regression of all these manifestations.

Androgen-producing adrenal tumors are characterized by rapidly progressing puberty, and high serum T levels (>5–6 nmol/L). Adrenal tumors are extremely rare in children, and may be combined with symptoms of Cushing.

Concern with use of COC in adolescents with ovarian tumor: In adolescents with malignancy, the added risk for venous thromboembolism (VTE) in the presence of prothrombotic states (e.g. COC) is unknown, but may be increased.[80,81]

1. Female adolescents with malignancy often are treated with COC. An association between hormonal therapy and VTE is well-established. Presence of a central venous line is also a major risk factor for development of VTE.[82,83]
2. The mature hemostatic system may be the cause of adolescents having an increased incidence of VTE compared to other younger children.[84]

The mechanism of COC-associated VTE is not known but is probably due to its estrogen component. However, recent studies have found that the progestin component also has an effect on VTE risk as third-generation COC confer a two- to three-fold greater risk of VTE than second generation COC, which contain a different progestin component.[85]

Table 6.14: Serum tumor markers.

Marker	Associated tumor
CA 125 CA 19.9	Epithelial tumors (especially serous) Immature teratoma (rare)
A-fetoprotein (AFP)	• Endodermal sinus tumors • Embryonal carcinomas • Mixed germ cell tumors • Immature teratoma, • Polyembryoma (rare)
Human chorionic gonadotropin (hCG)	Choriocarcinoma Embryonal carcinomas Mixed germ cell tumors Polyembryoma Dysgerminoma (rare)
Carcinoembryonic antigen (CEA)	Serous tumors, Mucinous tumors
Lactate dehydrogenase (LDH)	Dysgerminoma, Mixed germ cell tumors
Estradiol (E_2)	Thecomas Adult granulosa cell tumors
Testosterone (T)	Sertoli cell tumors Leydig (hilus) cell tumors
F9 embryoglycan	Embryonal carcinoma, yolk sac tumor Choriocarcinoma Immature teratoma
Inhibin	Granulosa-theca cell tumor
Müllerian inhibiting substance (MIS)	Granulosa-theca cell tumor

VULVOVAGINAL COMPLAINTS

Pruritis vulvae: It is an itching sensation with a desire to scratch vulva. This may (Table 6.16) or may not (Table 6.15) be associated with vaginal discharge.

The various **causes associated with vaginal discharge** are:
- *Candida albicans:* Accounts for 80% of cases of pruritis vulva
- *Trichomonas vaginalis*

Vaginal discharge: May be physiological or pathological (Table 6.16).

CERVICAL CYTOLOGY, HISTOLOGY, AND HUMAN PAPILLOMAVIRUS

Those involved with the care of teenagers should be well-versed on the new recommendations for cervical and histologic management of cervical disease as well as the indications, risks, and benefits of the HPV vaccine.

Table 6.15: Causes not associated with vaginal discharge.

General disease	Diabetes, jaundice, uremia, cirrhosis, hemochromatosis
Nutritional	Iron deficiency anemia, Vitamin A and B_{12} deficiency, achlorhydria
Allergy	Drugs, soap, detergents, antiseptics, deodorants, dusting powder, wearing tight synthetic undergarments, condoms, spermicidal agents
Parasitic infections	Pediculosis, scabies
Vulval diseases	Condyloma acuminate, granulomas Behcet's syndrome, Paget's disease, vulvar cancer
Cervical causes	Cervicitis, erosion causing excessive mucoid discharge
Anal disease	Thread worm infestation
Urinary diseases	Bacilluria, acidic urine, incontinence, glycosuria
Psychological	Psychoneurosis due to stress
Generalized/localized	Dermatitis, psoriasis, eczema

Table 6.16: Causes of vaginal discharge.

Physiological discharge	Normal increased amount vaginal discharge as seen at time of ovulation (ovulation cascade from cervix)	• Premenstrual phase • Pregnancy • Sexual excitement (outpouring of Bartholin's secretions)

	Leukorrhea: Increased amount of normal vaginal discharge	• At birth, due to stimulation of uterus and vagina by placental estrogens
		• At puberty
		• Increase in glandular elements in the cervix as in case of cervical erosion/ectopy
		• Vaginal adenosis
		• Estrogen-Progesterone COC use
		• Regular douching of vagina (washes away natural secretions and protective lactobacilli)
		• Active or passive congestion of pelvic organs especially cervix as seen in:
		  – Prolonged ill health
		  – Anxiety states and neurosis
		  – Sedentary occupation
		  – Standing for long periods in hot atmosphere

Pathological discharge	Inflammatory discharge	Vulvovaginitis: • *Gonococcus* • *Trichomonas vaginalis* • *Candida albicans* • Bacterial vaginosis • Nonspecific organisms in childhood and old age
		Cervicitis: • *Gonorrhea* • Chlamydia • Anerobic organisms • Puerperal infection
		Endometritis: • Puerperal • Senile
		Secondary infection of wounds
		Abrasions
		Burns
		Chemical injuries
	Neoplasms	Urinary and feculent discharge due to presence of fistula
	Rarely, intermittent emptying of hydrosalpinx, discharge of ascitic fluid through fallopian tubes and uterus	

CHAPTER 6 Adolescent Gynecology

Table 6.17: Recommendations for Adolescents' Cervical Cytology and Histology Management by American Society for Colposcopy and Cervical Pathology (ASCCP).

Diagnosis		Recommendation
Atypical squamous cells of undetermined significance (ASCOS) (no HPV testing)		Repeat cytology in 12 months
Atypical squamous cells cannot exclude high grade (ASC-H)		Colposcopy
Low-grade squamous intraepithelial lesion (LSIL) (no HPV testing)		Repeat cytology in 12 months
High-grade squamous intraepithelial lesion (HSIL)		Colposcopy
Atypical glandular cells (AGC)		Colposcopy (may need to refer to a specialist)
Cancer		Refer to specialist
Dysplasia	Mild dysplasia	Repeat cytology in 1 year
	Moderate dysplasia	Repeat colposcopy and cytology in 4–6 months
	Severe dysplasia or carcinoma in-situ (CIS)	Treat per guidelines

Adolescents are a special population with significant differences in their management of abnormal cytology and histology (Table 6.17). New guidelines have determined that, given the high prevalence of HPV as well as the high rate of spontaneous resolution in these patients, it is recommended that this population not have an HPV test in the presence of low-grade squamous intraepithelial lesion (LSIL)/ atypical squamous cells of undetermined significance (ASC-US). If the human papillomavirus (HPV) test is performed, then the result should not be used for deciding upon colposcopy, and patients should be observed with annual cytology for up to a period of 2 years. These guidelines hold true as long as the results are not consistent with a high-grade squamous intraepithelial lesion (HSIL), in which case a colposcopy is recommended. In those with HSIL, the management does not change.[86-88]

- *For mild and moderate dysplasia*: Observe and repeat test as the first line of management, rather than using ablative/excisional procedures.
- *Severe dysplasia*: Requires treatment.

The availability of the HPV vaccine provides prevention rate of more than 90% with HPV types 6, 11, 16, and 18 (quadrivalent) and 16 and 18 (bivalent) in patients not previously exposed to HPV.[89,90]

The duration of protection seems to be longer than 4 years, but the exact duration of protection is still not known. Details on ideal age of initial dosing, use in boys, and boosters, are still not clear.

MÜLLERIAN ABNORMALITIES

These present as cyclic abdominal pain, dyspareunia, amenorrhea, pelvic mass, infertility, endometriosis, dysmenorrhea, menometrorrhagia, pelvic pain, and urinary tract anomalies.

- *Imperforate hymen*: Primary amenorrhea, cyclic abdominal pain and bulging hymenal tissue; no uterine malformations. Treatment is removal of hymenal tissue and attaching vaginal mucosa to hymenal ring.
- *Transverse vaginal septum*: Presentation is similar to imperforate hymen but may also be associated with uterine malformations. Treatment is resection of the septum and reanastomosis of upper and lower segments of vaginal mucosa.
- *Vaginal atresia*: Treatment is by creating a neovagina using vaginal dilators or split skin rafts as described above.

Obstructive abnormalities are more likely to be associated with pelvic pain and endometriosis, and there may be associated hematosalpinx, hematometra, or hematocolpos. Uterine abnormalities associated with outflow tract obstruction causing pain include:

- *Bicornuate uterus with noncommunicating rudimentary horn*: Treated with laparoscopic resection of noncommunicating horn
- *Uterine didelphys with obstructed Heim vagina and ipsilateral renal agenesis*: Treated with resection of wall of obstructed vagina.

Diagnosis

- History and examination
- USG or MRI
- Laparoscopy
- Hysteroscopy.

EATING DISORDERS

The incidence peaks in the 13–18 year age group. These patients present with amenorrhea, oligomenorrhea, or infertility. Oligomenorrhea may be caused by overeating. Eating disorders can also exacerbate an underlying menstrual problem as seen in PCOS.

- *Prognosis*—follows the rule of thirds: 1/3 recover completely, 1/3 have persistent lifelong concerns about their weight, and 1/3 have a chronic relapsing illness where death occurs in 2–5%.[91]

- **Menstruation**: Oligomenorrhea and amenorrhea can result due to weight gain or loss, caloric restriction, excessive exercise, or psychogenic stress. A weight 10% below the normal for the patient's height can delay menarche from the expected time by causing hypothalamic dysfunction. Likewise, gain or drop in weight from the baseline can cause menstrual changes that are usually anovulatory.
- **Sexuality**: COC do not work well in this population, as their induced vomiting does not allow consistent hormonal levels to prevent ovulation. Thus, we see a high rate of therapeutic abortions in the bulimics.

ATHLETIC ADOLESCENTS

The female athlete triad consists of amenorrhea, an eating disorder, and osteopenia. A caloric deficit leads to a disruption in the pulsatile release of GnRH, resulting in low levels of Gn's and secondarily reduced levels of estrogen and progesterone, leading to amenorrhea and osteopenia.[91]

- There is a higher incidence of delayed menarche and menstrual dysfunction in girls who start intensive athletic training and dieting before menarche/early postmenarchal period.[92] Amenorrhea varies from 6–43% depending on the intensity of the exercise (intensity is a more important factor than total time). A shortening of cycle length is frequently observed in exercising females.[93]
- **Osteopenia**: The vast majority of bone mass is acquired by the end of the 2nd decade of life. Adolescent athletes who are amenorrheic are osteopenic in their early adult years.[94] Bone mineral density (BMD) should be measured after 6 months of amenorrhea and if osteopenia is found, hormonal treatment should be started, such as COC with calcium supplementation (current recommendation for adolescents is 1,500 mg/day).

EPILEPSY

Epilepsy is the most common neurological disorder seen in reproductive years with a prevalence of 1%. Seizure disorders that continue into adolescence often remain into adulthood.[21]

- **Menstruation**: Seizure disorder may be exacerbated with menarche in 37% of patients. Up to 50% of epileptic women, have seizures that occur at predictable times in the menstrual cycle, with 70% in the premenstrual time when estrogen and progesterone are high.[95]

- **Combined oral contraceptives**: These are often used in epileptics to regulate menstrual cycle, but seizure medications decrease the effectiveness of low-dose COC.

CHILDHOOD CANCER SURVIVORS

Cytotoxic cell damage is progressive and irreversible in the ovary, where the number of germ cells is fixed and cannot be regenerated. Gonadal function is more likely to be preserved if treatment occurs prepubertal. Strategies to decrease ovarian damage from cancer treatments include substitution of alkylating agents, cyclical rather than continuous regimens, surgically tacking the ovaries out of radiation field, ovarian suppression during treatment (with COC, GnRH agonists, GnRH antagonists), and cryopreservation of ovarian tissue before treatment.

- **Radiation**: Prepubertal abdominal or pelvic radiation exposure can cause delayed menarche. Permanent ovarian failure occurs if the ovary receives >1,000 rads of radiation.[96] Premature menopause is more common if the teenager received radiation therapy in addition to chemotherapy.[97] Ovary decreases in size with loss of follicles, and FSH levels are found in the menopausal range.
- **Chemotherapy**: Chemotoxic agents act on primordial follicles by inducing apoptotic changes in the pregranulosa cells and causing follicle loss. The alkylating agents (cyclophosphamide, melphalan, and chorambucil) are the most harmful to undeveloped oocytes (4.5 fold risk), whereas antimetabolites and plant alkaloids are safer for the ovary.[98]

ADOLESCENT PREGNANCY

Other than abortion as an outcome of this, other problems of concern include aggression during course of pregnancy, addictive behavior, and congenital malformations. Teenagers that are pregnant consistently have less prenatal care, they are more likely to smoke, and they deliver infants with lower birth weights. Besides the numerous pregnancy related complications, early parenthood tends to curtail opportunities for education and employment, hampering social and cultural development.

TERMINATION OF PREGNANCY

Termination of pregnancy in an adolescent girl is a serious problem from medical, legal, and social angles. If a girl below 18 years becomes pregnant, she cannot give a valid consent of MTP under MTP out and consent of parent/legal guardian is required for MTP on a girl <18 years of age. Any abortion that is not performed in accordance of MTP Act amounts to illegal abortions.

88. Wright TC Jr, Massad LS, Dunton CJ, Spitzer M, Wilkinson EJ, Solomon D, et al. 2006 consensus guidelines for the management of women with abnormal cervical cancer screening tests. Am J Obstet Gynecol. 2007;197:346-55.
89. Harper DM, Franco EL, Wheeler C, Ferris DG, Jenkins D, Schuind A, et al. Efficacy of a bivalent L1 virus-like particle vaccine in prevention of infection with human papillomavirus types 16 and 18 in young women: a randomised controlled trial. Lancet. 2004;364:1757-65.
90. VillaLL, CostaRL, PettaCA, AndradeRP, AultKA, Giuliano AR, et al. Prophylactic quadrivalent human papillomavirus (types 6, 11, 16, and 18) L1 virus-like particle vaccine in young women: a randomised double-blind placebo-controlled multi-centre phase II efficacy trial. Lancet Oncol. 2005;6:271-8.
91. Gidwani G, Rome E. Eating disorders. Clin Obstet Gynecol. 1997; 40(3):601.
92. Hergenroeder A. Bone mineralization, hypothalamic amenorrhea, and sex steroid therapy in female adolescents and young adults. J Pediatr. 1995; 126(5):683.
93. Allen D. Effects of fitness training on endocrine systems in children and adolescents. In: Advances in Pediatrics. New York, Mosby Inc., 1999, p. 41-66.
94. Warren M, Steihl A. Exercise and female adolescents: effects on the reproductive and skeletal systems. JAMWA. 1999; 54(3):115.
95. Penovich P. The effects of epilepsy and its treatment on sexual and reproductive function. Epilepsia. 2000; 41(2):553.
96. Schover L. Psychosocial aspects of infertility and decisions about reproduction in young cancer survivors: a review. Med Pediatr Oncol. 1999; 33:53.
97. Chatterjee R, Goldstone A. Gonadal damage and effects on fertility in adult patients with haematological malignancy undergoing stem cell transplantation. Bone Marrow Transplant. 1996; 17:5.
98. Blumenfeld Z, Avivi I, et al. Preservation of fertility and ovarian function and minimizing chemotherapy induced gonadotoxicity in young women. J Soc Gynecol Invest. 1999; 6(5): 229.

52. Carel JC, Eugster EA, Rogol A, et al. Consensus statement on the use of gonadotropin-releasing hormone analogs in children. Pediatrics. 2009;123: e752-62.
53. Sørensen K, Aachmann-Andersen NJ, Petersen JH, Hilsted L, Helge JW, Juul A. Sex hormone-binding globulin levels predict insulin sensitivity, disposition index and cardiovascular risk during puberty. Diabetes Care. 2009;32:909-14.
54. Gidwani G. Endometriosis is more common than you think. Contemp Ob/Gyn. 1989; 33:75.
55. Vercellini P, De Georgio O, Aimi G, Panazza S, Uglietti A, Crosignani PG. Menstrual characteristics in women with and without endometriosis. Obstet Gynecol. 1997;90:264-8.
56. Moghissi K. Medical treatment of endometriosis. Clin Obstet Gynecol. 1999;42:620-32.
57. Endometriosis in adolescents. ACOG Committee Opinion No. 310. American College of Obstetricians and Gynecologists. Obstet Gynecol. 2005;105:921-7.
58. Hicks CW, Rome ES. In: Sultan C (Ed). Pediatric and adolescent gynecology. Evidence-Based Clinical Practice. 2nd, revised and extended edition. Endocr Dev. Basel: Karger; 2012; 22: 230-50.
59. ACOG Committee on Practice Bulletins – Gynecology. ACOG practice bulletin No 51: chronic pelvic pain. Obstet Gynecol. 2004;103:589-605.
60. Westrom L, Mardh P, et al. Acute pelvic inflammatory disease. In: Sexually Transmitted Diseases. 2nd edition. New York: McGraw-Hill Co; 1987.
61. Andersch B, Milsom I. An epidemiologic study of young women with dysmenorrhea. Am J Obstet Gynecol. 1982;144:655-60.
62. Klein JR, Litt IF. Epidemiology of adolescent dysmenorrhea. Pediatrics. 1981;68:661-4.
63. Goldstein DP, deCholnoky C, Emans SJ, et al. Laparoscopy in the diagnosis and management of pelvic pain in adolescents. J Reprod Med. 1980;24:251-6.
64. Reese KA, Reddy S, Rock JA. Endometriosis in an adolescent population: the Emory experience. J Pediatr Adolesc Gynecol. 1996;9:125-8.
65. Laufer MR, Goitein L, Bush M, et al. Prevalence of endometriosis in adolescent girls with chronic pelvic pain not responding to conventional therapy. J Pediatr Adolesc Gynecol. 1997;10:199-202.
66. Ailawadi RK, Jobanputra S, Kataria M, et al. Treatment of endometriosis and chronic pelvic pain with letrozole and norethindrone acetate: a pilot study. Fertil Steril. 2004;81:290-6.
67. Amsterdam LL, Gentry W, Jobanputra S, et al. Anastrazole and oral contraceptives: a novel treatment for endometriosis. Fertil Steril. 2005;84:300-4.
68. Chwalisz K, Perez MC, Demanno D, et al. Selective progesterone receptor modulator development and use in the treatment of leiomyomata and endometriosis. Endocr Rev. 2005;26:423-38.
69. Steinkampf MP, Hammond KR, Blackwell RE. Hormonal treatment of functional ovarian cysts: a randomized, prospective study. Fertil Steril. 1990;54:775-7.
70. Alexander-Williams J. Do adhesions cause pain? Br Med J (Clin Res Ed). 1987;294:659-60.
71. Duffy DM, diZerega GS. Adhesion controversies: pelvic pain as a cause of adhesions, crystalloids in preventing them. J Reprod Med. 1996;41:19-26.
72. Cheong Y, William Stones R. Chronic pelvic pain: aetiology and therapy. Best Pract Res Clin Obstet Gynaecol. 2006;20:695-711.
73. Goldstein DP, deCholnoky C, Leventhal JM, et al. New insights into the old problem of chronic pelvic pain. J Pediatr Surg. 1979;14:675-80.
74. Peters AA, van Dorst E, Jellis B, et al. A randomized clinical trial to compare two different approaches in women with chronic pelvic pain. Obstet Gynecol. 1991;77:740-4.
75. Swank DJ, Swank-Bordewijk SC, Hop WC, et al. Laparoscopic adhesiolysis in patients with chronic abdominal pain: a blinded randomised controlled multi-centre trial. Lancet. 2003;361:1247-51.
76. Rackow BW, Novi JM, Arya LA, et al. Interstitial cystitis is an etiology of chronic pelvic pain in young women. J Pediatr Adolesc Gynecol. 2009;22:181-5.
77. Hanno PM, Landis JR, Matthews-Cook Y, et al. The diagnosis of interstitial cystitis revisited: lessons learned from the national institutes of health interstitial cystitis database study. J Urol. 1999;161:553-7.
78. Hyams JS, Burke G, Davis PM, et al. Abdominal pain and irritable bowel syndrome in adolescents: a community-based study. J Pediatr. 1996;129:220-6.
79. Rasquin-Weber A, Hyman PE, Cucchiara S, et al. Childhood functional gastrointestinal disorders. Gut. 1999;45(suppl 2):II60-8.
80. Revel-Vilk S, Chan AK, Bauman M, et al. Prothrombotic conditions in an unselected cohort of children with venous thromboembolic events. J Thromb Haemostas. 2003;1:915.
81. Nowak-Gottl U, Junker R, Kreuz W, et al. Risk of recurrent venous thrombosis in children with combined prothrombotic risk factors. Blood. 2001; 97:858.
82. Massicotte MP, Dix D, Monagle P, et al. Central venous catheter related thrombosis in children: analysis of the Canadian Registry of Venous Thromboembolic Complications. J Pediatr. 1998; 133:770.
83. Monreal M, Alastrue A, Rull M, et al. Upper extremity deep venous thrombosis in cancer patients with venous access devices–prophylaxis with a low molecular weight heparin (Fragmin). Thromb Haemost.1996; 75:251.
84. Andrew M, Vegh P, Johnston M, et al. Maturation of the hemostatic system during childhood. Blood. 1992; 80:1998.
85. Vandenbroucke JP, Rosing J, Bloemenkamp KW, et al. Oral contraceptives and the risk of venous thrombosis. N Engl J Med. 2001; 344:1527.
86. Evaluation and management of abnormal cervical cytology and histology in the adolescent. ACOG Committee Opinion No. 330. American College of Obstetricians and Gynecologists. Obstet Gynecol. 2006;107:963-8.
87. Wright TC Jr, Massad LS, Dunton CJ, Spitzer M, Wilkinson EJ, Solomon D, et al. 2006 consensus guidelines for the management of women with cervical intraepithelial neoplasia or adenocarcinoma in situ. Am J Obstet Gynecol. 2007;197: 340-55.

18. Gracia CR, Driscoll DA. Molecular basis of pubertal abnormalities. Obstet Gynecol clin N Am. 2003;30:261-77.
19. Reindollar RH, Byrd JR, McDonough PG. Delayed puberty: an update study of 326 patients. Transactions of the American Gynecological and Obstetrical Society. 1989; 8:146-62.
20. Griffin JE, et al. Congenital absence of the vagina: the Mayer-Rokitansky-Kustner-Hauser Sydrome. Ann Int Med. 1976; 85:224.
21. Elford KJ, Spence JEH. Mini-Review-the forgotten female: pediatric and adolescent gynecological concerns and their reproductive consequences. J Pediatr Adolesc Gynecol. 2002; 15:65-77.
22. Hovatta O. Pregnancies in women with Turner's syndrome. Ann Med. 1999; 31:106.
23. Tarani L, Lamperiello S, et al. Pregnancy in patients with Turner's syndrome: six new cases and review of literature. Gynecol Endocrinol. 1998;12:83.
24. Brook CG. The management of classical congenital adrenal hyperplasia due to 21-hydroxylase deficiency. Clin Endocrinol. 1999; 33:559.
25. Money J, Schwartz M. Dating, romantic and nonromantic friendships and sexuality in 17 early treated adrenogenital females aged 16–25. In: PA Lee, LP Plotnick, AA Kowarski (Eds). Congenital Adrenal hyperplasia. Baltimore:University Park Press, pp. 419-31.
26. Kuhnle U, Bollinger M, et al. Partnership and sexuality in adult female patients with congenital adrenal hyperplasia. J Steroid Biochem Mol Biol. 1993; 45:123.
27. Helleday J, Siwers B, Ritzen E, et al. Subnormal androgens and elevated progesterone levels in women treated for congenital virilizing 21-hydroxylase deficiency. J Clin Endocrinol Metab. 1993;76:933.
28. Edmonds DK. Congenital malformations of the genital tract and their management. Best Pract Res Clin Obstet Gynaecol. 2003; 17(1):19-40.
29. Deligeoroglou E, Creatsas G. In: Sultan C (Ed). Pediatric and adolescent gynecology. Evidence-based Clinical Practice. 2nd, revised and extended edition. Endocr Dev. Basel:Karger, 2012; 22:pp 160-70.
30. Treloar A, Boynton R, Behn B, et al. Variation of the human menstrual cycle through reproductive life. Int J Fertil. 1967; 12(1):77.
31. Rimsza M. Dysfunctional uterine bleeding. Pediatr Rev. 2002; 23:227-33.
32. Claessens EA, Cowell CA. Acute adolescent Menorrhagia. Am J Obstet Gynecol. 1981;139(3):277-80.
33. Beven JA, Maloney KW, Hillery CA, et al. Bleeding disorders: a common cause of menorrhagia in adolescents. J Pediatr. 2001;138(6): 856-61.
34. Claessens EA, Cowell CA. Dysfunctional uterine bleeding in the adolescent. Pediatr Clin North Am. 1981;28:369-78.
35. Strickland JL, Wall JW. Abnormal uterine bleeding in adolescents. Obstet Gynecol Clin North Am. 2003;30:321-35.
36. Chuong CJ, Brenner PF. Management of abnormal uterine bleeding. Am J Obstet Gynecol. 1996; 175(3):787-92.
37. Speroff L, Glass RH, Kase NG. Dysfunctional uterine bleeding. In: clinical gynecologic endocrinology and infertility. 6th edition. Baltimore: Lippincott, Williams and Wilkins; 1999. p.575-93.
38. Matytsina LA, Zoloto EV, Sinenko LV, Greydanus D. Dysfunctional uterine bleeding in adolescents: concepts of pathophysiology and management. Prim Care. 2006;33:503-15.
39. Kriplani A, Kulshrestha V, Agarwal N, Diwakar S. Role of tranexamic acid in management of dysfunctional uterine bleeding in comparison with medroxyprogesterone acetate. J Obstet Gynaecol. 2006;26:673-8.
40. The Practice Committee of the American Society for Reproductive Medicine: Current evaluation of amenorrhea. Fertil Steril. 2008;90 (suppl 3): S219-25.
41. Sophie Catteau-Jonard, Christine Cortet-Rudelli, Chloé Richard-Proust, Didier Dewailly. In: Sultan C (Ed) Pediatric and Adolescent Gynecology. Evidence-Based Clinical Practice. 2nd, revised and extended edition. Endocr Dev. Basel: Karger, 2012; 22: 181-93.
42. Ibanez L, Potau N, Carrascosa A. Insulin resistance, premature adrenarche, and a risk of the polycystic ovary syndrome (PCOS). Trends Endocrinol Metab. 1998;9:72-7.
43. van Hooff MH, Voorhorst FJ, Kaptein MB, Hirasing RA, Koppenaal C, Schoemaker J: Endocrine features of polycystic ovary syndrome in a random 14 population sample of 14–16 year old adolescents. Hum Reprod. 1999;14:2223-9.
44. Abbott DH, Dumesic DA, Franks S. Developmental origin of polycystic ovary syndrome – a hypothesis. J Endocrinol. 2002;174:1-5.
45. Rosenfield RL, Ghai K, Ehrmann DA, et al. Diagnosis of polycystic ovary syndrome in adolescence: comparison of 76 Elford and Spence: the forgotten female adolescent and adult hyperandrogenism. J Pediatr Endocrinol Metab. 2000; 13(5):1285.
46. Apter D, Vihko R. Endocrine determinants of fertility: serum androgen concentrations during follow-up of adolescents in the third decade of life. J Clin Endocrinol Metab. 1990; 71:970.
47. Venturoli S, Porcu E, Flamigni C. Polycystic ovary syndrome. Curr Opin Pediatr. 1994; 6:388.
48. Van Hoof M, Voorhorst F, et al. Polycystic ovaries in adolescents and the relationship with menstrual cycle patterns, luteinizing hormone, androgens, and insulin. Fertil Steril. 2000; 74(1):49.
49. Revised 2003 consensus on diagnostic criteria and long-term health risks related to polycystic ovary syndrome (PCOS). Hum Reprod .2004;19:41-7.
50. Dewailly D, Contestin M, Gallo C, Catteau-Jonard S. Metabolic syndrome in young women with the polycystic ovary syndrome: revisiting the threshold for an abnormally decreased high-density lipoprotein cholesterol serum level. BJOG. 2009;117:175-80.
51. Moran C, Azziz R, Carmina E, Dewailly D, Fruzzetti F, Ibanez L, et al. 21-Hydroxylase-deficient nonclassic adrenal hyperplasia is a progressive disorder: a multicenter study. Am J Obstet Gynecol. 2000;183:1468-74.

SEXUAL ABUSE

Clinicians should be familiar with the locally mandated reporting laws while examining a sexually abused child/adolescent. Young children do not always present with physical signs of injury as the abuse may have occurred some time ago, or there may not have been actual attempt to penetrate the vagina. Behavioral symptoms vary for each individual. Sleep disturbances with nightmares may be seen. Also, children who perform sexual acts on others are often found to have a history of abuse. Physical symptoms may include enuresis, encopresis, dysuria, vaginal bleeding, and pelvic/abdominal pain. Collection of forensic evidence should be handled by an experienced practitioner with recognition of the emotional needs of the child as well as the legal requirements.

FEMALE COSMETIC GENITAL SURGERY

Female cosmetic genital surgery (FCGS) is not unusual for adolescent girls to have concerns over the appearance of the genital area and request "corrective" surgery. There has been an increasing trend towards FCGS over the last decade. This often consists of reducing or removing the labia minora (labial reduction surgery, labioplasty), but may include surgery to the clitoris or clitoral hood. Careful discussion establishing reasons for concern, and background knowledge of normal female anatomy are important. An examination of the labia will offer reassurance that everything is normal. Labia minora may appear more prominent due to lack of labia majora fat pads, which develop later. If pubic hair has been removed this may also make the labia more apparent. Surgery on normal labia is not indicated for the alleviation of anxiety. Its good practice to counsel the adolescent in person and defer any corrective surgery till after the age of 18 years.

SUMMARY

Failure to address both the physical concerns and their reproductive implications can have profound lifelong consequences, especially if the reproductive desires cannot be fulfilled. Not every condition encountered can be rectified, but with sensitive physiological management, appropriate treatment, and the use of new reproductive technologies, most of these patients with early gynecological concerns can live normal sexual and reproductive lives.

REFERENCES

1. Sanfilippo J, Lara-Torre E. Obstet Gynecol. 2009; 113:93-47.
2. American College of Obstetricians and Gynecologists. A guideline for women's health care, 2nd edition. Washington, DC: ACOG; 2002.
3. Plant TM. Puberty in primates. In: Knobil E, Neill JD (Eds). The physiology of reproduction, 2nd edition. New York: Raven Press; 1994;453-85.
4. Lalwani S, Reindollar RH, Davis AJ. Normal onset of puberty, Have the definitions of onset changed? Obstet Gynecol Clin N Am. 2003;30: 279-86.
5. Juul A, et al. In: Sultan C (Ed). Pediatric and adolescent gynecology. Evidence-based clinical practice. 2nd edition, revised and extended edition. Endocr Dev. Basel: Karger, 2012;22:24-39.
6. Juul A, Scheike T, Pedersen AT, Main K, Pedersen LM, Skakkebæk NE. The impact of endogenous sex steroids on serum growth hormone, insulin-like growth factor (IGF)-I, IGF binding proteins (IGFBP-1 and -3) levels and urinary GH excretion during menstrual cycle in normal women. Human Reprod. 1997;12:101-6.
7. Sehested A, Juul A, Andersson AM, Petersen JH, Müller J, Skakkebæk NE. Serum inhibin A and inhibin B in healthy prepubertal, pubertal and adolescent girls and adults women: relation to age, stage of puberty, menstrual cycle, FSH, LH and estradiol levels. J Clin Endocrinol Metab. 2000;85:1634-40.
8. Sowers M, McConnell D, Gast K, Zheng H, Nan B, McCarthy JD, etal. Anti-Müllerian hormone and inhibin B variability during normal menstrual cycles. Fertil Steril. 2010;94:1482-6.
9. Hagen CP, Aksglaede L, Sørensen K, Main KM, Boas M, Cleemann L, etal. Serum levels of anti-Müllerian hormone as a marker of ovarian function in 926 healthy females from birth to adult- hood and in 172 Turner syndrome patients. J Clin Endocrinol Metab. 2010;95:5003-10.
10. Marshall WA, Tanner JM. Variations in patterns of pubertal changes in girls. Arch Dis Child. 1969;44:291-303.
11. Kakarla N, Bradshaw KD. Disorders of pubertal development: precocious puberty. Semin Reprod Med. 2003;21(4): 339-51.
12. Fenichel P. Delayed puberty. In: Sultan C (Ed). Pediatric and adolescent gynecology. Evidence-based clinical practice. Endocr Dev. Basel:Karger, 2004;7: 106-28.
13. Gan SM, Bailey SM. Genetic and maturational process. In: Falkner F, Tanner JM (Ed). Human growth1: principles and prenatal growth. New York: Plenum; 1978;pp.307-30.
14. Thibaud E. Gynecologic clinical examination of the child and adolescent. In: Sultan C (Ed). Pediatric and adolescent gynecology. Evidence-Based clinical Practice. Endocr Dev Basel: Karger, 2004; 7: pp 1-8.
15. Hewitt G. In: Strickland JJ(ed). Training Section. Examining pediatric and adolescent gynecology patients. Pediatr Adolesc Gynecol. 2003;16:257-8.
16. Sultan C (Ed). Pediatric and adolescent gynecology. Evidence-based clinical practice. 2nd, revised and extended edition. Endocr Dev. Basel:Karger, 2012; 22: pp 1-10.
17. Sultan C (Ed). Pediatric and adolescent gynecology. Evidence-based clinical practice. 2nd, revised and extended edition. Endocr Dev. Basel: Karger, 2012; 22: pp 84-100.

CHAPTER 7

Dysmenorrhea

PK Shah, Keshav Pai

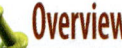 **Overview**

- Mainly primary dysmenorrhea (without cause) and secondary type of dysmenorrhea (with causes) are seen.
- Nonsteroidal anti-inflammatory drugs or prostaglandin synthetase inhibitors (PSIs) form the mainstay of treatment of primary dysmenorrhea.
- Oral contraceptive pills of the combined variety are the best agents in order to convert ovulatory cycles into anovulatory ones.
- If there are conditions causing secondary dysmenorrhea, it has to be tackled according to the condition.

INTRODUCTION

This Chapter deals with dysmenorrhea which is one of the commonest gynecological disorders affecting women in the reproductive age group. Dysmenorrhea is defined as pain associated with menstruation.

It describes various types of dysmenorrhea with their risk factors and etiology. The management protocol has been schematically represented using flow charts, describing various medical and surgical methods. Dysmenorrhea is preventable to some extent and the preventive measures have also been listed. A brief mention has been made of the recent advances made in the management of this disorder and various differential diagnosis of this condition. The aim of this Chapter is to enable the student to have a concise and complete overview of this menstrual disorder.

The term dysmenorrhea is derived from a Greek word: *Dys*—difficulty, *Menorrhea*—monthly flow.

Thus, meaning difficulty in monthly flow and practically implying difficult or painful menstruation.

DEFINITION

It is defined as pain associated with menstruation.

It is a major cause of absenteeism from work amongst women thus decreasing efficiency and quality of life among affected women.[1] International Classification of Diseases (ICD) uses 2014-ICD-10-CM Diagnosis Code N94.6 to specify the diagnosis.

INCIDENCE

Dysmenorrhea is one of the commonest gynecological complaints among women, but the exact incidence is difficult to estimate. Pain is a subjective symptom and cannot be accurately estimated by an outside observer, since different women may perceive pain with different severity and tolerance. It is now estimated that almost 50% of all women experience some degree of dysmenorrhea while 10% are incapacitated by it.

RISK FACTORS FOR DYSMENORRHEA

The following are some of the proposed risk factors for dysmenorrhea:

Menstrual Factors[2]

1. *Early menarche*: A study conducted on adolescent girls revealed that early age of menarche was associated with a higher incidence of dysmenorrhea.
2. *Long and heavy menstrual flow*: It was also seen that women with long and heavy cycles had more severe dysmenorrhea.

Parity
The incidence of dysmenorrhea is lower in multiparous women. It was seen that the incidence of primary dysmenorrhea decreased after the first delivery. It was also found to be decreased in terms of severity.

Diet
Lower consumption of fish, eggs and fruits are believed to increase the incidence of dysmenorrhea but the association is not clearly established.[3]

Exercise
Various types of exercises were advocated to reduce dysmenorrhea. It was also seen that among athletes the incidence of dysmenorrhea was lower, probably due to anovulatory cycles. But good evidence for that explanation is lacking.[4]

Cigarette Smoking
Heavy smoking was found to be associated with decreased duration of bleeding but increased duration of dysmenorrhea. Thus, duration of dysmenorrhea was increased in heavy smokers with no effect on cycle length.[5]

Psychological
Emotionally dependent and overprotected girls are more likely to develop dysmenorrhea. It is also more commonly seen in girls whose mothers suffered from dysmenorrhea, since the mother becomes overzealous and apprehensive around the time of menarche of her daughter which thereby makes the young girl more conscious, aware and paranoid of her forthcoming menses. Rather than being the cause of the pain, it is more likely that the psychological factors modify the pain causing depression and anxiety.[6]

CLASSIFICATION OR TYPES
A. **Primary or spasmodic dysmenorrhea:** Synonyms—essential/intrinsic/functional. It is defined as painful menstruation in the absence of pelvic pathology.
B. **Membranous dysmenorrhea:** It is actually a type of spasmodic dysmenorrhea characterized by the passage of an endometrial or decidual cast.
C. **Secondary dysmenorrhea:** Painful menses secondary to underlying organic disease of the pelvic organs.

Primary Dysmenorrhea
Etiology
There are various theories for the etiology of primary dysmenorrhea and are as follows:[1,7,8]

The Prostaglandin Theory
This is the most widely accepted theory suggested by Pickles as early as the 1960s. He extracted the smooth muscle stimulant from menstrual fluid which was identified as a mixture of prostaglandins.

Prostaglandins are derived from arachidonic acid. The three main prostaglandins concerned with menstruation are:
- $PGF_{2\alpha}$
- PGE_2
- PGI_2

The main effects of the prostaglandins on dysmenorrhea are as follows:
- $PGF_{2\alpha}$ is a potent vasoconstrictor and causes increased myometrial contractility.
- PGE_2 increases the sensitivity of the nerve endings.
- PGI_2 causes vasodilatation, decreases prior to menstruation leading to ischemia.

Thus, there is enough evidence to suggest that prostaglandins play an important role in the etiology of dysmenorrhea:
- Both PGE_2 and $PGF_{2\alpha}$ are present in high quantities in menstrual fluid
- The established actions of both PGE_2 and $PGF_{2\alpha}$ have been mentioned earlier
- Prostaglandin synthetase inhibitors are found to relieve dysmenorrhea, decrease menstrual fluid prostaglandin concentration and decrease uterine contractility.

Hormonal or Endocrine Theory
Dysmenorrhea is characteristically seen in ovulatory cycles where progesterone plays a key role.

The evidence to support this theory is seen in the following facts:
- Anovulatory cycles are usually painless and that is why primary dysmenorrhea starts 1 to 2 years after menarche
- Oral contraceptive pills which abolish ovulation improve dysmenorrhea dramatically
- Prostaglandin concentrations are higher in the secretory phase.

Progesterone plays an important role. It is believed that prostaglandin synthesis by the endometrium requires priming by progesterone but the mechanism is not clear.

It is also seen that high doses of estrogen relieve dysmenorrhea and decrease uterine contractility. Thus, it is established that steroid hormones play a role in causing dysmenorrhea but the exact mechanism is not clearly understood.

Vasopressin, which is found in menstrual fluid, is also a potent vasoconstrictor.

Recent evidence suggests vitamin D deficiency could have a role in primary dysmenorrhea.[9]

Myometrial Contractility

It is well-known that the myometrium contracts in order to shed the endometrial lining during menstruation. MRI findings revealed marked changes during cycle days 1–3. Thickness of inner low signal intensity myometrial layer and endometrial distortion were significantly associated with pain degree.[10] The myometrial contraction thus puts a stretch on the uterine nerve fibers thus causing pain.

Myometrial Ischemia

In a normal menstrual cycle there is vasodilatation during the secretory phase which increases the tortuosity of the spiral artery. The spiral arteries are the main sources of blood supply to the endometrium.

Just prior to the menses the spiral arteries undergo vasoconstriction. The decrease in uterine blood flow causes ischemia. Ischemia is a known cause of pain and thus this theory compares dysmenorrhea to the pain of angina.

Cervical Obstruction

In the earlier years cervical stenosis was believed to be the single most important cause of dysmenorrhea.

Abnormal uteri like septate or bicornuate may be associated with narrow cervices but normal uteri in patients with dysmenorrhea revealed no hysterosalpingographic evidence of cervical narrowing. Thus, this theory is less likely to be the cause of dysmenorrhea in anatomically normal uteri.

Psychological

Psychological cause for dysmenorrhea was earlier believed to be the single etiological factor for dysmenorrhea. Later psychological and physiological dysmenorrhea were believed to be mutually exclusive causes. In modern day practice, we understand that though dysmenorrhea is proven to be a physiological disorder, psychological factor do play an important role. It is now believed that psychological factors modify pain or its intensity rather than causing it. Thus, a severe recurring pain can easily cause depression in any woman especially when it alters efficiency.

Thus, girls with lower threshold for pain can be completely incapacitated in comparison to women with a higher threshold for pain.

A Combination of the Above

This is the actual theory of dysmenorrhea wherein pain is a result of the concerted occurrence of two or more factors for, e.g. hormones are precursors of prostaglandins which alter myometrial contractility and thus pain is caused. The psychological factors may play a part in all of the above.

Pathogenesis

The pain pathway for dysmenorrhea is as follows:

Sympathetic fibers pass from the uterus through the posterior roots of T10, T11, T12 and L1 and from the cervix through S2, S3 and S4.[8]

Thus, uterine pain is referred to the cutaneous distribution of lower abdominal wall in front, groins, upper and medial aspects of the thighs nearly to the knees and posteriorly to the sacral area and buttocks while that from the cervix to the lower sacral area and buttocks.

Clinical Features[11]

History

Age: Usually seen among younger women up to 25–30 years.

Time of onset: 2 to 3 years after menarche thus corresponding to the beginning of ovulation.

Duration of pain: It starts just prior to the menses lasting for 2 days.

Type of pain: Cramping pain in the above described areas.

Examination

General and abdominal examination: Usually normal.

Local examination: Essentially normal pelvic organs.

Management of Dysmenorrhea[1]

It can broadly be classified as general and specific measures and is given in Flowchart 7.1. The management options can be selected based on the severity of dysmenorrhea and is given in Table 7.1.

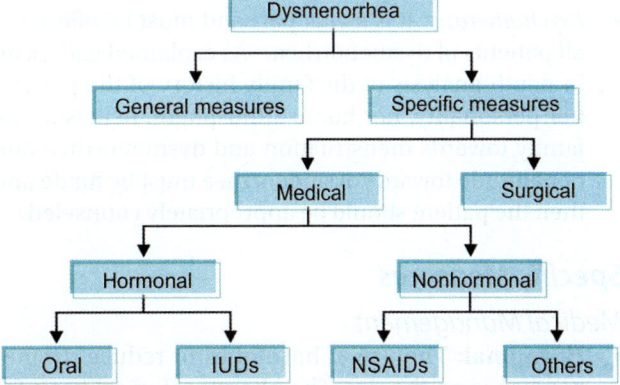

Flowchart 7.1: Management of dysmenorrhea.

(IUD: intrauterine device; NSAIDs: nonsteroidal anti-inflammatory drugs)

Table 7.1: Severity of dysmenorrhea.

Mild	Moderate	Severe or incapacitating
• Psychotherapy	• NSAIDs	• OC pills
• Counseling to allay anxiety	• OC pills	• Conjugated estrogens
• Occasionally NSAIDs		• Surgery
• Laxatives		

(OC: oral contraceptives; NSAIDs: nonsteroidal anti-inflammatory drugs)

General Measures

These include:

- *Improvement in nutritional state and dietary changes*: A healthy and nutritious diet is a prime factor in the betterment of general health. Thus the inclusion of fruits, eggs and fish in the diet of the patient may help to alleviate the pain of dysmenorrhea to some extent. Recent literature advocates the use of phytoestrogens, i.e. estrogens derived from plant and vegetable sources like soyabeans, chick peas, etc. to reduce dysmenorrhea.
- *Regular exercise*: Various remedial exercises were advocated for dysmenorrhea like floor polishing movements, bending, twisting, swaying and rowing movements and other similar routines. These must be done for at least 15 minutes daily between and during the periods. These can be done in addition to or instead of various games.
- *Explanation regarding the condition and reassurance*: This plays an extremely important role in the management of dysmenorrhea and should be included as an essential component in the treatment plan. The patient must be reassured that dysmenorrhea is not a sign of abnormal reproductive organs or future infertility. One should explain the normal menstrual cycle, its physiology and the cause of dysmenorrhea. She must be told that it is a physiological symptom (except in cases of secondary dysmenorrhea) that could be relieved.
- *Palliative measures like laxatives and hot baths*: These are believed to cause pain relief by increasing the blood supply and thus taking away the ischemic element as the cause of dysmenorrhea.
- *Psychotherapy*: It is a vital part and must be offered to all patients of dysmenorrhea—As explained earlier, an in depth analysis of the family history of the patient, her personality, her home atmosphere, beliefs in the family towards menstruation and dysmenorrhea and her attitude towards dysmenorrhea must be made and then the patient should be appropriately counseled.

Specific Measures

Medical Management

- **Hormonal:** The use of hormones to reduce dysmenorrhea is on the rise. The pharmacological basis for the use of hormones is simply that anovulatory cycles are not associated with dysmenorrhea. Thus, conversion of an ovulatory cycle into an anovulatory one is the principle of treatment using hormones.
    - *Oral hormonal therapy*: Oral contraceptive pills of the combined variety are the best agents in order to convert ovulatory cycles into anovulatory ones. It serves a dual purpose for women with dysmenorrhea and also requiring contraception. They are usually started on the 3rd day of the cycle and continued for 21 days. Recently conjugated estrogens are also being promoted, especially in women suffering from progestogenic side effects like acne, bloating, etc. with the combined pill. Low dose oral contraceptive pills could be used as a single agent or in combination with analgesics for treatment of primary dysmenorrhea.[12]
    - *Intrauterine device (IUD)*: Progestasert, which is a progesterone containing IUD, was being advocated for the treatment of dysmenorrhea but it was discontinued since it was accompanied with increased incidence of ectopic pregnancy. The principle of action of this IUD is that the progesterone is maintained in low concentrations and the prostaglandin concentration will be reduced. It may cause anovulation. Levonorgestrel intrauterine system (LNG-IUS) has also been cited as useful in reducing symptoms of dysmenorrhea.[13]
- **Nonhormonal:**
    - *NSAIDs*:[14] Nonsteroidal anti-inflammatory drugs or prostaglandin synthetase inhibitors (PSIs) form the mainstay of treatment of primary dysmenorrhea. Amongst the NSAIDs the following are important:
        - Fenamates:
            - Tablet mefenamic acid 250–500 mg 3 to 4 times a day
            - Tablet flufenamic acid 100–200 mg 3 times a day
            - Tablet tolfenamic acid 133 mg 3 times a day
        - Tablet indomethacin 25 mg 3–6 times a day
        - Tablet ibuprofen 200–400 mg 4 times a day
        - Tablet naproxen sodium 275 mg 4 times a day

        NSAIDs can be started just prior to menses and continued for 5 days.

        The doses are as mentioned above but may be altered as required.
    - Others:
        - *Calcium antagonists:*[15] Calcium antagonists—relax the uterine muscle and reduce pain but they cause bradycardia and hypotension. The common ones used are nifedipine, verapamil and diltiazem.
        - *Beta adrenergics:*[15] These increase the endometrial flow and thus decrease ischemic pain. Among them, only terbutaline has been found to be more effective than placebo. The high incidence of side effects confirmed that this is not a practical approach.

Surgical Management

The surgical management could be conservative or radical, but are not commonly advocated except in severe cases.

Conservative Surgeries[8]
1. Dilatation of the cervix is especially helpful in cases of cervical stenosis.
2. Injection of alcohol into the pelvic plexus is rarely practiced.

Radical Surgeries
Cotte's operation or presacral sympathectomy

Resection of the hypogastric nerve where it lies in front of the fourth and fifth lumbar vertebrae. The management depends on the severity of dysmenorrhea.

There are various alternative modalities which are currently available:
- *Heat fomentation*: Application of heat over the painful areas especially the back, lower abdomen and thighs often produces relief
- *Microwave diathermy*:[16] It has been tried in women suffering from severe dysmenorrhea not responding to other medical line of management and has proved to be successful in relieving the same
- *Acupuncture and acupressure*: They often prove to be helpful especially in women who have a strong psychological factor and those who have a strong faith in alternative remedies
- *Yoga*: This provides some form of exercise and at the same time allays anxiety by relaxation thus helping to relieve dysmenorrhea
- *Ayurveda and homeopathy*: This century is seeing a lot of alternative types of medicines in practice on the rise. Thus, these two major sciences have also proved successful in treating dysmenorrhea.

Membranous Dysmenorrhea
It is a type of spasmodic dysmenorrhea with passage of endometrial cast.

Etiology
Unknown, but is proposed to be due to a hypersecretory endometrium thus leading to thick endometrium which is eventually shed as large fragments or casts.

Histologically, the cast is decidua with blood clot.
- *Patient profile*: Usually, a young patient and the periods are heavy associated with colicky pain
- *Treatment*: It is the same as that for primary dysmenorrhea.

Secondary Dysmenorrhea
Synonyms—extrinsic, congestive or organic dysmenorrhea.

Etiology
Painful menses secondary to the following underlying organic diseases of the genital tract.

1. Uterine abnormalities

   Congenital:
   - Redundant uterine horn
   - Imperforate hymen
   - Cryptomenorrhea.

   Accessory and cavitated uterine masses (ACUM) with functional endometrium, an under-diagnosed entity being more frequent than previously thought is a significant cause of severe dysmenorrhea and recurrent pelvic pain in young women.[17]

   Acquired:
   - Uterine fibroids
   - Endometrial polyps
   - Adenomyosis.

2. Infections: Pelvic inflammatory disease of any etiology.
3. Endometriosis: It is one of the commonest causes of secondary dysmenorrhea.
4. Foreign bodies: Intrauterine device.
5. Iatrogenic: Cervical stenosis following surgery like cone biopsy.

Clinical Features
Age: Usually seen among older women in the 3rd to 4th decade.

Time of onset: Usually follows initial years of normal painless cycles.

Duration of pain: Onset few days prior to menses and continues throughout the cycle and even after cessation of menses.

Type of pain: Continuous dull aching or dragging type of pain.

On Examination
General: Look for anemia.

Abdomen: Presence of a mass or doughy abdomen in cases of tuberculosis.

Per vaginum: Enlarged uterus or uterine mass altered mobility of the uterus, forniceal tenderness due to adhesions or forniceal mass, e.g. chocolate cysts.

Management
Investigations
Routine investigations like complete blood count to look for anemia or any evidence of infection seen as leukocytosis or raised erythrocyte sedimentation rate.

Urine microscopy to rule out any urinary tract infection.

Flowchart 7.2: Summary of management of dysmenorrhea.

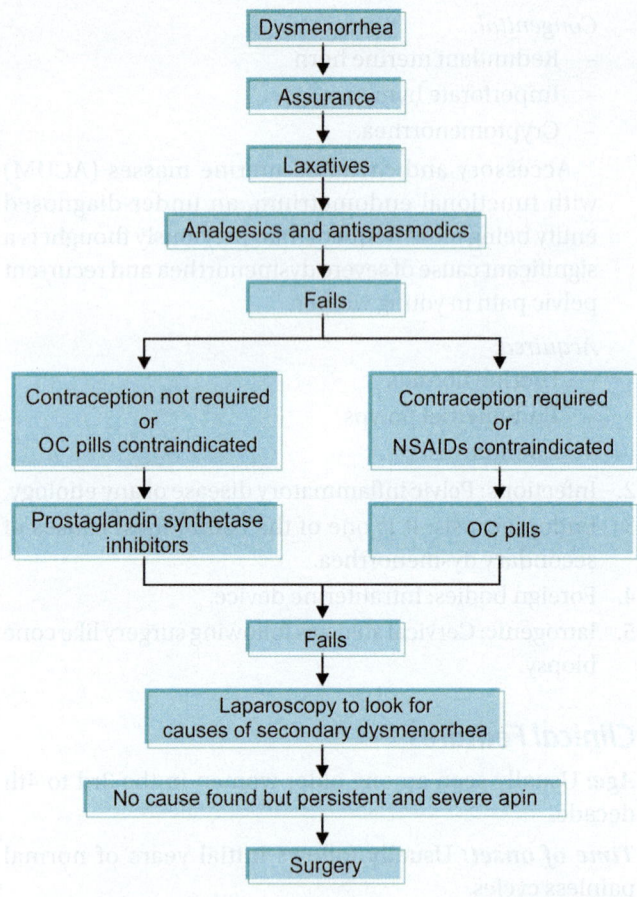

Stool examination for worm infestation or amoebiasis causing colitis.

Specific Investigations
- Ultrasonography to look for any pelvic mass, ectopic pregnancy (positive urine pregnancy test), uterine anomaly or chocolate cysts.
- Hysteroscopy for small polyps which maybe missed on routine pelvic examination
- Dilatation and curettage for endometrial pathology like carcinoma endometrium, tuberculosis of the endometrium, cervical stenosis or uterine polyp
- Laparoscopy for pelvic adhesions, uterine anomalies, infections or ovarian mass.

Treatment
Treatment of the cause and symptoms (Flowchart 7.2):
1. Medical—NSAIDs and OC pills.
2. Surgical
   - Laparoscopic adhesiolysis for pelvic adhesions
   - Cystectomy in cases of ovarian cysts including chocolate cysts
   - Hysteroscopic septum resection in case of septate uterus
   - Myomectomy for fibroids
   - Hysteroscopic polypectomy in case of uterine polyps.

Differential Diagnosis
- Chronic pelvic pain due to gastrointestinal tract disease
- Ectopic pregnancy
- Premenstrual tension
- Mittelschmerz pain or ovulation dysmenorrhea
- Arthritic pain.

RECENT ADVANCES
- Laser or laparoscopic presacral neurectomy
- Mirena
- Vitamin D deficiency could have a role in primary dysmenorrhea.
- Accessory and cavitated uterine masses (ACUM) is a significant cause of severe dysmenorrhea in young women

CONCLUSION
Thus, the management of dysmenorrhea starts from the correct diagnosis of the condition, differentiation between primary and secondary dysmenorrhea and whether there is need for contraception. Once the correct diagnosis has been made the patient must be reassured and appropriate therapy started. Laparoscopy should be advocated in patients not responding to medical treatment for more than six months to one year. Thus, dysmenorrhea is no longer believed to be a psychological problem but often physiological and at times due to pathology which deserves treatment due to its ability to alter efficiency and quality of life for a woman.

REFERENCES
1. Parsons. Primary dysmenorrhea. Textbook of Gynecology, 2nd edition, Saunders (WB). 1978;325-29.
2. Lumsden MA. Dysmenorrhea. Progress in obstetrics and gynecology, Elsevier Health Sciences. 1994,5:276-89.
3. Browne M. Dysmenorrhea. Postgraduate obstetrics and gynecology, 3rd edition, London; Butterworth.1974, 89-99.
4. Shahr-jerdy S, Hosseini RS. Effects of stretching exercises on primary dysmenorrhea in adolescent girls. Biomedical Human Kinetics. 2012;(4):127-32.

5. Hornsby PP, Wilcox AJ, Weinberg CR. Cigarette smoking and disturbance of menstrual function. Epidemiology. 1998;9(2): 193-96.
6. Lawlor CL, Davis AM. Primary dysmenorrhea. Relationship to personality and attitudes in adolescent females. J Adolesc Health Care. 1981;1(3):208-12.
7. Shaw R. Disorders of Menstruation. Shaw's textbook of Gynecology, 12th edition, New Delhi; Churchill Livingstone, 1999; 227-9.
8. Dawood YM. Dysmenorrhea. Clinical Obstet and Gynecol. 1983;26(3):719-27.
9. Lasco A, Catalano A, Benvenga S. Improvement of primary dysmenorrhea caused by a single oral dose of vitamin D: results of a randomized, double-blind, placebo-controlled study. Archives of Internal Medicine. 2012;172(4):366-7.
10. Kataoka M, Togashi K, Kido A. Dysmenorrhea: Evaluation with Cine-Mode-Display MR Imaging—Initial Experience; Radiology. 2005;235(1):124-31.
11. Kistner. The menstrual cycle. Kistner's Gynecology, 6th edition, USA; Harcourt Brace and Co., 1995;44-6.
12. Harada T, Momoeda M, Terakawa N. Evaluation of a low-dose oral contraceptive pill for primary dysmenorrhea: a placebo-controlled, double-blind, randomized trial. Fertility and Sterility. 2011; 95(6):1928-31.
13. Gupta HP, Singh U, Sinha S. Levonorgestrel intrauterine system: a revolutionary intrauterine device. J Indian Med Assoc. 2007;105(7):380, 382-5.
14. Novak. Pelvic pain and dysmenorrhea. In: Berek J (Eds). General Gynecology, 6th edition, Williams and Wilkins. 1996;408-14.
15. Dutta. Dysmenorrhea and other disorders of menstrual cycle. Textbook of Gynecology, 4th edition, Kolkata; Central Books 1997; 168-71.
16. Vance AR, Hayes SH, Spielholz NI. Microwave diathermy treatment for primary dysmenorrhea; PhysTher. 1996;76(9): 1003-08.
17. Acién P, Bataller A, Fernández F. New cases of accessory and cavitated uterine masses (ACUM): a significant cause of severe dysmenorrhea and recurrent pelvic pain in young women; Hum Reprod. 2012;27(3):683-94.

CHAPTER 8

Abnormal Uterine Bleeding

PK Sekharan

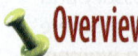

Overview

- Abnormal uterine bleeding (AUB), especially heavy menstrual bleeding (HMB) is a major health concern for women of reproductive age, affecting her physical, social, emotional and economic quality of life. Work up for diagnosis for AUB should exclude pregnancy states and malignancy. With proper evaluation, majority of these patients can be managed by medical treatment and can avoid major surgical intervention like hysterectomy. The new classification system introduced by FIGO-the PALM-COIN system, will help to standardize the outcome of management of AUB.

INTRODUCTION

Abnormal uterine bleeding (AUB) is a deviation from normal menstrual parameters, deviation in frequency, regularity, duration and volume. AUB is the new internationally agreed terminology for abnormal menstrual pattern. Nearly one-third of the gynecology outpatient visits of women of reproductive age will be for seeking medical advice for abnormal uterine bleeding.[1] Abnormal uterine bleeding can result from a wide variety of systemic and local causes or may be due to medications. The common etiologies in nonpregnant women are structural uterine pathology (e.g. fibroids, endometrial polyps, and adenomyosis), anovulation, disorders of hemostasis, or neoplasia. The importance of AUB relates to its major impact on women's quality of life, productivity, and utilization of healthcare services. Till recently many women had undergone hysterectomy for AUB without any organic pathology and by proper evaluation many such cases could be treated by medical management.

NORMAL MENSTRUAL BLEEDING

Menstruation should be described in terms of frequency, regularity, duration and amount of flow. The frequency of menstruation is measured by the number of days from the first day of one menstrual period to the first day of the next, and the normal range is 24–38 days and >38 days is considered as infrequent. The regularity of menses quantifies the cycle to cycle variation in frequency over a 12-month time frame. Duration of menstrual flow is 4–8 days and more than 8 days is considered as prolonged periods. Normal menstrual loss is based on the Scandinavian study,[2] a population-based study wherein the menstrual, blood loss was objectively measured using the alkaline-hematin technique. Average blood loss is 40 mL, with 90% of women having a blood loss less than 80 mL. Therefore, heavy menstrual bleeding is objectively defined as a loss of more than 80 mL per cycle. In the clinical setting, where a woman's perception of heaviness and its impact on her social, physical, and economic quality of life are of much greater importance, and is important in defining the amount of menstrual bleeding. The term menorrhagia to denote excess menstrual blood loss is replaced by heavy menstrual bleeding (HMB).

THE NEW CLASSIFICATION OF AUB

A woman of reproductive age presenting with abnormal uterine bleeding may be having many disorders or pathologic entities, as structural anomalies, ovulatory disorders, coagulopathies and even malignancy. In order to have uniformity in diagnosis and management of abnormal uterine bleeding in non-pregnant women of reproductive age, the International Federation of Gynecology and Obstetrics (FIGO) Menstrual Disorder Group introduced the PALM-COEIN system of classification.[3-7]

FIGO Classification of AUB

The FIGO classification system is divided into nine categories, denoted by the easy to remember acronym PALM-COEIN. The PALM component represents structural entities that can be visualized by ultrasound, hysteroscopy, or histology, and includes **P**olyps, **A**denomyosis, **L**eiomyomas (fibroids) and **M**alignancy and pre-malignant conditions. COEIN represents non-structural abnormalities, comprising **C**oagulopathies, **O**vulatory disorders, **E**ndometrial causes, **I**atrogenic causes and those that are **N**ot-otherwise classified.

PALM-COEIN CLASSIFICATION-FIGO

POLYP	**C**OAGULOPATHY
ADENOMYOSIS	**O**VULATORY DYSFUNCTION
LEIOMYOMA	**E**NDOMETRIAL
MALIGNANCY & HYPERPLASIA	**I**ATROGENIC
	NOT YET CLASSIFIED

PALM—Structural

1. Polyps (AUB-P): An abnormal protrusion of the endometrium, polyps may be endometrial or cervical. Polyps may be diagnosed using ultrasound saline sonohysterography and/or hysteroscopy but may require histological assessment to confirm they are benign.
2. Adenomyosis (AUB-A): Adenomyosis is the presence of endometrial tissue within the myometrium and traditionally necessitates a histological diagnosis from hysterectomy specimens. Ultrasonography/MRI may be used for diagnosis.
3. Leiomyoma (AUB-L): By ultrasound, leiomyoma are grouped according to whether they are submucus, intramural or subserus.
4. Malignancy and pre-malignant conditions (AUB-M): Consequences of a diagnosis of malignancy or atypical hyperplasia necessitate their consideration in each patient, particularly if there are predisposing risk factors such as obesity or chronic anovulation (e.g. polycystic ovarian syndrome).

COEIN—Non-Structural

1. Coagulopathies (AUB-C): Disorders that interfere with coagulation will lead to AUB in about 10% of patients with heavy menstrual bleeding and may due to Von Willebrand disease. History of heavy menstrual bleeding since menarche, easy bruising, excess bleeding during dental extraction and history of post-partum hemorrhage are suggestive of coagulation disorders.
2. Ovulatory dysfunction (AUB-O): More common at extremes of reproductive age. Higher incidence in obese women and patients with hypothyroidism and polycystic ovarian syndrome.
3. Endometrial causes (AUB-E): Women with regular cycles having heavy menstrual bleeding without any structural abnormality and coagulation disorders are likely to be having local endometrial factors leading to defective hemostasis, delayed endometrial repair or impaired local vasoconstriction. There is no definitive diagnostic testing for AUB-E, but one by exclusion.
4. Iatrogenic causes (AUB-I): When AUB develops during the use of Intrauterine Systems, contraceptive pills, injections, implants, gonadotropin-releasing hormone therapy, aromatase inhibitors, selective estrogen receptor modulators, or progesterone receptor modulators, the woman is categorized as having AUB-I. By convention, when HMB occurs after the use of anticoagulants (e.g. warfarin, heparin), the woman is categorized as having AUB-C.
5. Not-otherwise classified (AUB-N): To allow for undiscovered, poorly defined, inadequately researched and/or extremely rare causes of AUB, the FIGO classification system includes a 'not-otherwise classified' category.

Classification of Leiomyoma (Fig. 8.1)

- Those that are intracavity with no myometrial involvement and attached to the endometrium by a narrow stalk are designated as type 0.
- If the tumor is within the endometrial cavity, with less than half of the largest diameter within the myometrium, it is categorized as type 1.
- If the tumor is visible in the endometrial cavity but half or greater of the largest diameter is in the myometrium, it is called type 2.
- Fibroids that abut the endometrium but do not distort the cavity are categorized as type 3.
- Those that are completely within the myometrium—meaning that there is myometrium interposed between both the serosa and the endometrium—are categorized as type 4 (or intramural).
- Types 5–7 are categorized by their relationship with the uterine serosa with type 5 lesions distorting the serosa but with half or more than of their largest diameter being within the myometrium, while type 6 lesions have less than half of the diameter within the myometrium.
- Type 7 lesions are attached to the uterus by a stalk.
- Type 8 includes 'others' such as cervical and parasitic leiomyomas.

SM—Submucosal	0	Pedunculated intracavitary
	1	<50% intramural
	2	>50% intramural
O—Other	3	Contacts endometrium; 100% intramural
	4	Intramural
	5	Subserosal ≥ 50% intramural
	6	Subserosal <50% intramural
	7	Subserosal pedunculated
	8	Other (specify, e.g. cervical, parasitic)
Hybrid leiomyomas (Impact both endometrium and serosa)		Two numbers are listed separated by a hyphen. By convention, the first refers to the relationship with the endometrium while the second refers to the relationship to the serosa. One example is below
	2–5	Submucosal and subserosal, each with less than half the diameter in the endometrial and peritoneal cavities, respectively.

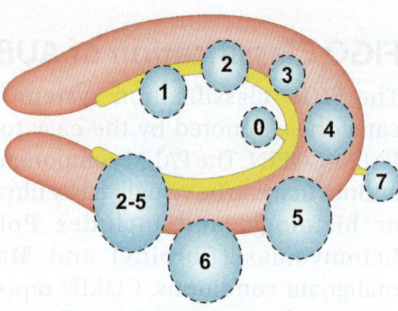

Fig. 8.1: Classification of leiomyoma.

Source: Malcolm GM, Critchleyc HOD, Michael, Fraser IS. FIGO classification system (PALM-COEIN) for causes of abnormal uterine bleeding in non-gravid women of reproductive age. Int J Gynaecol Obstet. 2011;113:3–13.
Submucus: (0) Pedunculated intracavitary, (1) ≤ Submucus, (2) ≥ 50% Intramural.
Other: (3) Intramural but contacts endometrium, (4) Intramural, (5) Subserous ≥ 50% intramural (6) Subserous <50% intramural, (7) Subserous pedunculated, (8) Other (e.g. cervical).

SALIENT FEATURES OF PALM-COEIN CLASSIFICATION

- The PALM-COEIN classification for AUB does not include abnormal bleeding related to pathologic conditions of the lower genital tract
- The term dysfunctional uterine Bleeding used as diagnosis when there was no systemic or locally discernible structural cause is abandoned. Such patients generally will have one or a combination of coagulopathy, disorder of ovulation, or primary endometrial disorder, may be a primary or secondary disturbance in local endometrial hemostasis
- The term menorrhagia used in excess menstrual bleeding is replaced by heavy menstrual bleeding (HMB)
- As per NICE guidelines[8] - "Heavy menstrual bleeding (HMB) is defined as excessive menstrual blood loss which interferes with a woman's physical, social, emotional and/or economic quality of life. It can occur alone or in combination with other symptoms". This definition is accepted as it is not easy to measure the actual menstrual blood loss. It is the woman's perception that what she considers as heavy bleeding.
- Metrorrhagia uterine bleeding at irregular intervals, particularly between the expected menstrual periods is replaced by intermenstrual bleeding.
- Chronic AUB is defined as bleeding from the uterine corpus that is abnormal in volume, regularity, or timing; is present for most of the prior 6 months; and may not require immediate intervention.
- Acute AUB is defined as an episode of heavy bleeding requiring immediate intervention
- Not yet classified causes include rare or ill-defined conditions: chronic endometritis, arteriovenous malformations, and myometrial hypertrophy.
- The full notation of classification would include the entire acronym AUB PALM-COEIN with the abnormalities noted, whereas the abbreviated notation would include only the abnormalities. As an example, if the patient on investigation found to have a submucus fibroid as a cause for abnormal bleeding—classification will be AUB—$P_0A_0L_1smM_0$–$C_0O_0E_0I_0N_0$. An abbreviation is also accepted like—AUB-L_{1SM}.

Acute AUB is an episode of bleeding in a woman of reproductive age, who is not pregnant, that is of sufficient quantity to require immediate intervention to prevent further blood loss. By comparison, chronic AUB is defined as bleeding from the uterus that is abnormal in frequency, duration and/or volume and has been present for the majority of the previous 6 months. Intermenstrual bleeding is defined as bleeding between clearly defined cyclic and predictable menses, and includes random episodes as well as predictable episodes occurring at the same time each month.

EVALUATION OF ABNORMAL UTERINE BLEEDING

Although, the patient's perception of the bleeding is not quantifiable, it is important for the management of the problem. Ultimately, the woman's experience and the impact on her quality of life determine the intervention which may be required. Heavy menstrual bleeding is the most common complaint of AUB. It has been defined as "excessive menstrual blood loss which interferes with the woman's physical, social, emotional, and/or economical quality of life. It can occur alone or in combination with other symptoms."[8]

History and Physical Examination

A detailed history and physical examination will help to establish the cause of the abnormal bleeding, to direct further investigations and to decide on the management. Menstrual history as regards to regularity, amount, duration of flow, intermenstrual bleeding, postcoital bleeding, and premenstrual symptoms and pain may give the clue regarding anovulatory bleeding or ovulatory bleeding, cervical lesions and polyps. Regular heavy menstrual bleeding with pelvic pain can be due to adenomyosis or submucus fibroids. Anovulatory bleeding is characterized by heavy bleeding following a short period of amenorrhea and is seen among patients at adolescent age or at perimenopausal age or in patients with PCOS. There is risk of endometrial hyperplasia and endometrial cancer.

Further details regarding sexual life, contraception, use of intrauterine devices, chance of being pregnant, symptoms suggestive of thyroid disorders and hyperprolactinemia, history of other drug intake, use anticoagulants, and history of systemic diseases and its treatment should also be elicited. History of heavy menstrual bleeding with menarche and personal or family history of abnormal bleeding indicates testing for coagulation disorders.

Physical Examination

A thorough physical examination including the general examination, examination of the abdomen with bimanual pelvic examination should be carried out. Per vaginal examination may be avoided in unmarried girls instead a per rectal examination may help to find out any organic condition.

Investigations

- Complete blood count.
- Pregnancy should be excluded in suspected cases by urine pregnancy test/serum βhCG.
- TSH, T3, and T4 with suspicion of thyroid dysfunction.
- Testing for coagulation disorders is done in women with human menopausal gonadotropin (HMG) since menarche and history of excess bleeding with minor surgical procedures.

Imaging Studies

Ultrasound scanning is indicated when there is suspicion of structural abnormalities, failure of conservative management, suspicion of malignancy and in patients older than 45 years.

Transvaginal Sonography

After a transabdominal survey scan, all patients with AUB should have a detailed Transvaginal sonography. It allows detailed assessment of anatomical abnormalities of the uterus and endometrium.[9] In addition, pathologies of the myometrium, cervix, tubes, and ovaries may be assessed. This investigative modality may assist in the diagnosis of endometrial polyps, adenomyosis, leiomyoma, uterine anomalies, and generalized endometrial thickening associated with hyperplasia and malignancy.

Saline Infusion Sonohysterography

In saline infusion sonohysterography (SIS) 5 to 15 mL of saline is instilled into the uterine cavity during transvaginal sonography which improves the diagnosis of intrauterine pathology. In cases of uterine polyps and fibroids, SIS allows for greater discrimination of location and relationship to the uterine cavity.[10-12] As a result, SIS can also obviate the need for MRI in the diagnosis and management of uterine anomalies.[13]

Hysteroscopy

Hysteroscopy done in cases of abnormal uterine bleeding will help to visualize the cavity pathology like endometrial thickening or polyps, submucus fibroids, müllerian anomalies like septate and bicornuate uterus, retained intrauterine devices and retained products of conception. It can be used simultaneously for directed biopsy of abnormal looking endometrium and removal of polyps.

MRI

MRI can assess the myometrial pathology better than ultrasonography and help to map the site of fibroids before planning myomectomy and embolization. Adenomyosis will be better evaluated by MRI than by ultrasonography. As per the NICE guidelines MRI should not be used as the first line diagnostic tool in abnormal uterine bleeding.[9]

Endometrial Sampling

Endometrial sampling is indicated in:
- Women over 40 years, who fail to respond to medical treatment
- Women with significant intermenstrual bleeding

- Suspicious of cavity pathology on imaging
- In patients with risk factors for endometrial cancer
- Endometrial study is also indicated in women with AUB with infrequent cycles with heavy bleeding as in anovulatory cycles and in obese patients with PCOS
- All women age 45 years or older with abnormal uterine bleeding to rule out endometrial cancer or a premalignant lesion.

Dilatation and curettage (DC) is still being used as a method of endometrial sampling though office procedures are available. Patients with prolonged bleeding can have temporary relief after dilatation and curettage. An endocervical sample may be taken before dilatation. The sample is blind and therefore will miss a focal lesion. Hysteroscopic directed sampling is recommended in the situation of a focal lesion found on ultrasound.[14]

The development of equipment for office-based endometrial sampling has mostly replaced the dilatation and curettage. Pipelle endometrial suction curette and Vabra aspirator can get adequate endometrial samples for evaluation. Continuation of bleeding with a normal report on such sample would necessitate the hysteroscopy directed biopsy.

MANAGEMENT

If history, examination and investigation suggest no evidence of any structural abnormality, pharmaceutical therapy using hormonal or nonhormonal agents could be started after discussing with the patient. Patients with acute HMB require agents that will control bleeding quickly. Although most women with acute AUB can be managed on an outpatient bases, acute bleeding occasionally will be severe enough to require hospitalization and emergency treatment. Some patients will require stabilization with IV fluids and blood transfusion. Acute anovulatory bleeding can be treated with estrogen, estrogen-progestin or progestin alone.

High Dose Progestin Therapy for Acute AUB

Acute severe anovulatory bleeding can be effectively treated with high dose progestin alone using medroxyprogesterone acetate 10–20 mg twice daily, megesterol acetate 20–40 mg twice daily, norethindrone 5 mg twice daily. Treatment should be continued for one with the high dose followed by one daily dose for three weeks. High dose progestin treatment induces stabilizing predecidual changes in a thickened, vascular and fragile endometrium. Progestin withdrawal will result in the so-called "medical curettage". Thereafter cyclic progesterone treatment or an estrogen-progesterone COC pill can be given for long-term management.

Munro et al. (2006)[15] reported the result of a randomized controlled trial with oral medroxyprogesterone acetate and combination of oral contraceptives for acute uterine bleeding. Medroxyprogesterone acetate was given in a dose of 20 mg three times a day for one week and then 20 mg daily for three weeks. OC containing 1 mg norethindrone and 35 µg ethinyl estradiol three times a day for week followed by 1 daily for three weeks was given to the control group. Cessation of bleeding had occurred in 88% of the OC group and 76% of those receiving medroxyprogesterone acetate, with a median time to bleeding cessation of 3 days for both groups.

Though depot-medroxyprogesterone acetate is less effective for management of acute bleeding, Ammerman et al. (2013)[16] in a pilot study has shown that depot-medroxyprogesterone acetate 150 mg IM combined with 3 days of oral medroxyprogesterone acetate 20 mg every 8 hours for 9 doses is an effective outpatient therapy for acute abnormal uterine bleeding.

Estrogen Therapy for Acute Heavy Bleeding

When acute heavy bleeding result in a thin denuded endometrium, high dose estrogen therapy is the initial treatment. Estrogen stimulates endometrial re-epithelialization and proliferation. There is only one randomized study by DeVore GR et al. (1982)[17] who reported the effectiveness of high dose estrogen for control of acute heavy bleeding. Bleeding stopped in 72% of patients who received intravenous Premarin and in 38% who received placebo. 25 mg conjugated equine estrogen (Premarin) is given intravenously every 4 hours up to 24 hours and bleeding will be controlled within 8 hours. Then oral premarin 2.5 mg is given 6th hourly and tapering to once daily for one week. Medroxyprogesterone acetate is added for two weeks to stabilize estrogen stimulated endometrial growth.

Other Treatments for Heavy Menstrual Bleeding

Pharmaceutical treatment should be considered where no structural or histological abnormality is present, or for fibroids less than 3 cm in diameter which are causing no distortion of the uterine cavity.

Nonsteroidal Anti-inflammatory Drugs (NSAIDs)

Elevated levels of prostaglandin E2 and prostaglandin F2-α have been demonstrated within the uterine tissues of women with heavy menstrual bleeding.[18] There is further evidence of deranged hemostasis (abnormal clotting) as the ratio of prostaglandin E2 to F2 and the ratio of prostacyclin to thromboxane A2 are elevated. NSAID reduce prostaglandin levels by inhibiting the enzyme cyclo-oxygenase and reduces blood loss by 20–40% and to a greater extent in those with excessive bleeding. In a Cochrane review including 17 randomized trials, NSAIDs reduced menstrual blood loss by 33–55% when compared with placebo, without a significant difference in adverse effects.[19] Mefamamic acid was most commonly studied and the usual dosage was 500 mg three times a day from onset of menses for four or five days or until menstruation ceased. Naproxen was given 500 mg twice a day for three to five days to get the therapeutic effect while Ibuprufen was effective in controlling the bleeding at a dose of 200–400 mg three times a day. NSAIDs have the added advantage of giving relief from dysmenorrhea. Significant differences in efficacy between different NSAIDs have not been demonstrated but the risk of gastrointestinal side effects was significantly less in the mefanamic acid group when compared with the naproxen group. Treatment with NSAIDs may be considered as the first line treatment for ovulatory bleeding with heavy menstrual bleeding and no demonstrable pathology. Clinical trials comparing NSAIDs to other medical agents have found them to be less effective in objectively reducing menstrual blood loss than tranexamic acid, the combined oral contraceptive pill, danazol, or the LNG-IUS.[20,21]

Antifibrinolytic Agents

An increase in the levels of plasminogen activators has been found in the endometrium of women with heavy menstrual bleeding compared to those with normal menstrual loss.[22] Plasminogen activators are a group of enzymes that cause fibrinolysis. Plasminogen activator inhibitors have, therefore, been promoted as a treatment for heavy menstrual bleeding. Tranexamic acid is an antifibrinolytic agent (or plasminogen activator inhibitor) that reversibly binds to plasminogen to reduce local fibrin degradation without changing blood coagulation parameters.

Tranexamic acid was approved by FDA in 2009 for the treatment of HMB. The dose is 1–1.5 g 3–4 times daily during periods. In placebo-controlled trials, Tranexamic acid has been shown to be effective in AUB with an overall reduction in menstrual blood loss between 40% and 59%.[23]

Cochrane review has shown that antifibrinolytics are more effective than NSAIDs, oral luteal phase progestogens and ethamsylate in reducing heavy menstrual bleeding. There is a 25–50% reduction from baseline in menstrual blood loss for participants treated with tranexamic acid when compared to these medical therapies.[23]

Ethamsylate

This is hemostatic agent act by increasing the platelet adhesiveness and aggregation. Use of ethamsylate shows varying effect and may achieve up to 20% reduction in bleeding. Ethamsylate is less effective in controlling HMB and NICE guideline does not recommend its use in HMB.[8]

Combined Oral Contraceptive Pills

Combined oral contraceptive pill (OCP) is effective in controlling heavy menstrual bleeding in unexplained menorrhagia and in patients with adenomyosis and fibroid to a lesser extent. Long-term use can reduce the blood loss to 40–70%. Combined OCPs have the additional benefit of reducing dysmenorrhea and providing contraception. Combined OCPs can also be used in control of acute heavy bleeding as mentioned earlier (Munro 2006). NICE guideline 44(2007) states that it is appropriate to use combined OCPs for control of HMB if pharmacological therapy is appropriate. Cochrane review suggests that there is no difference in effectiveness between combined OCPs and NSAIDs.[24]

Oral Progestins

In patients with HMB due to anovulatory cycles with unopposed estrogen stimulation of endometrium, progestins, norethindrone 5 mg three times a day or medroxyprogesterone 10 mg daily for 10 days will result in controlled withdrawal bleeding. Ovulatory menorrhagia will not respond to luteal phase progesterone. They may respond to continued use of progestins from day 5 to 26, but with more side effects. NICE do not recommend luteal phase progestins for control of HMB.

Cochrane database review 2008 states that progestogens administered from day 15 or 19 to day 26 of the cycle offer no advantage over other medical therapies such as danazol, tranexamic acid, NSAIDs and the progesterone-releasing intrauterine system in the treatment of menorrhagia in women with ovulatory cycles. Progestogen therapy for 21 days of the cycle results in a significant reduction in menstrual blood loss, although women find the treatment less acceptable than using intrauterine levonorgestrel. This regimen of progestogen may have a role in the short-term treatment of menorrhagia.[25]

Gonadotropin-releasing Hormone Agonists (GnRHa)

Treatment with long-acting GnRHa can achieve short-term relief from HMB and can be used effectively as a preoperative adjunct in women waiting for myomectomy, endometrial ablation or hysterectomy. Due to the estrogen deficiency symptoms it can produce, the treatment is limited to 6 months. In severe anemia, GnRHa can be given for 6 months at 3.75 mg dose monthly or 11.25 mg every three months. Due to the cost factor and the side effects, it is not recommended for long-term use.

Levonorgestrel-releasing Intrauterine System (LNG-IUS)

LNG-IUS (Mirena) has a reservoir with 52 mg levonorgestrel mixed with polydimethylsiloxane which control the rate of hormone release 20 μg per day. Menstrual blood loss in women with heavy menstrual bleeding can be reduced by 75 to 95% due to progesterone induced decidualization of the endometrium.

Cochrane Database of Systematic Reviews 2005[26] summarizes that the levonorgestrel-releasing intrauterine device (LNG-IUS) is more effective than cyclical norethisterone (for 21 days) as a treatment for heavy menstrual bleeding. Women with an LNG-IUS are more satisfied and willing to continue with treatment but experience more side effects, such as intermenstrual bleeding and breast tenderness. The LNG-IUS results in a smaller mean reduction in menstrual blood loss than endometrial ablation but there is no evidence of a difference in the rate of satisfaction with treatment. Women with an LNG-IUS experience more progestogenic side effects compared to women having TCRE for treatment of their heavy menstrual bleeding but there is no evidence of a difference in their perceived quality of life. The LNG-IUS treatment costs less than hysterectomy but there is no evidence of a difference in quality of life measures between these groups.

DANAZOL AND GESTRINONE

Use of danazol and gestrinone in control of HMB is limited because of its androgenic side effects.

Iron Therapy

Anemia due to HMB should be treated with oral iron therapy which will improve the sense of well-being.

Surgical Management of Heavy Menstrual Bleeding

Most women with heavy menstrual bleeding will have control of HMB with medical management. However, nearly 50% of women with HMB would have had hysterectomy within 5 years of their referral to a gynecologist, and at least 30% of the uterus removed will be anatomically normal.[27] Though hysterectomy ensures 100% effective treatment of HMB, it is a major operation with significant morbidity. As an alternative to hysterectomy, various endometrial ablative procedures were developed which gives satisfactory improvement, but later on many of them will require hysterectomy for a cure.

Endometrial Ablation/Resection

Endometrial ablation is used to control heavy menstrual bleeding when

- Bleeding has not responded to other treatments.
- Patient not desirous of further childbearing.
- Patient prefer not to have a hysterectomy to control bleeding.
- Other medical problems prevent a hysterectomy.

Endometrial destruction or ablation involves the removal of endometrial tissue. The endometrium has great powers of regeneration and to suppress menstruation successfully it is essential to remove the full thickness of this lining together with the superficial myometrium, including the deep basal glands. The deep basal glands are believed to be the primary foci for endometrial regrowth. This tissue may be removed under direct hysteroscopic view either by excision with an electrosurgical loop or by ablating the endometrium with some form of thermal energy of sufficient power to produce necrosis of the full thickness of the endometrium when applied to its surface.

The first generation endometrial ablation techniques require advanced hysteroscopic skills and longer operating times. These first generation techniques include Nd-YAG laser, Rollerball ablation and transcervical resection of the endometrium (TCRE). They all require direct hysteroscopic visualization. The expectation was that these first-generation ablation methods would become an alternative to hysterectomy but, analyses of recent hospital statistics in the UK suggest that first generation endometrial ablation has failed to have an impact on hysterectomy numbers.[28] The first generation ablation techniques require expertise and were associated with more complications.

Subsequently, second-generation non-hysteroscopic techniques have been developed, which are considered easier to perform, equally effective and safe. They can potentially be used in outpatient settings. The techniques use thermal energy, cryosurgery, electrosurgery and microwave energy.

Thermal Balloon Ablation

Several thermal balloon ablation systems are currently used worldwide. These are Cavaterm plus system, Thermablate Endometrial Ablation System and Thermachoice III Uterine Balloon Therapy System.

Thermachoice III Uterine Balloon System is a software-controlled devise to ablate endometrial tissue using thermal energy. After cervical dilatation of 5.5 mm, the Thermachoice device is introduced into the uterine cavity and 5% dextrose water is instilled into the silicon bag at the tip. The fluid is heated to 87°C and circulated for 8 minutes.

All hot liquid balloon devices do not require hysteroscopy and complication rates are low. Thinning of the endometrium by pharmacological agents or dilatation and curettage prior to the procedure improves the success rate.

After resection or ablation 70–80% of women experience significantly decreased flow, and 15–35% of them will experience amenorrhea. As time passes on more and more failures occur due to regeneration of the endometrium. After 5 years, up to 15% may require hysterectomy for a cure.

Authors of Cochrane database of systematic reviews (2013)[29] on endometrial resection and ablation techniques for heavy menstrual bleeding concluded that:

- Endometrial destruction by first or second-generation techniques should be considered for all women with normal uteri who wish to reduce their heavy menstrual bleeding and wish to retain their uterus.
- The potential for second-generation methods to be performed under local anesthesia is a considerable advantage and should be considered in cases where general anesthetic may be having more risk.
- There is sufficient evidence to confirm that, on average, second generation techniques are technically more simple and quicker to perform than first-generation techniques, while satisfaction rates and reduction in heavy menstrual bleeding are similar. However, technical difficulties have not yet been completely resolved.

Hysterectomy

Hysterectomy gives 100% cure of abnormal uterine bleeding. Hysterectomy is not the first line management of HMB and is considered only when:

- Other treatment options have failed, are contraindicated or are declined by the woman
- The woman no longer wishes to retain her uterus and fertility
- The patient accepts amenorrhea and who has been fully informed requests for it
- The route of hysterectomy preferably be vaginal if possible or else laparoscopic or abdominal
- Healthy ovaries should not be removed at the time of hysterectomy especially in women under the age of 45 years
- Ovaries should only be removed only with the informed consent of the women having understood its impact on her future health including the need for hormone replacement therapy.

REFERENCES

1. Spencer CP, Whitehead MI. Endometrial assessment re-visited. Br J Obstet Gynaecol. 1999;106:623.
2. Hallberg L, Hogdahl AM, Nilson L, Rybo G. Menstrual blood loss: a population study. Acta Obstet Gynecol Scand. 1966;45:320-51.
3. Munro MG, Critchley HO, Fraser IS. FIGO menstrual Disorders Working Group. The FIGO classification of causes of abnormal uterine bleeding in the reproductive years. Fertil Steril. 2011;95:2204-8.
4. Fraser IS, Critchley HO, Broder M, Munro MG. The FIGO recommendations on terminologies and definitions for normal and abnormal uterine bleeding. Semin Reprod Med. 2011; 29:383-90.
5. Munro MG, Critchley HO, Fraser IS. The flexible. FIGO classification concept for underlying causes of abnormal uterine bleeding. Semin Reprod Med. 2011;29:391-9.
6. Munro MG, Critchley HO, Broder MS, Fraser IS; FIGO Working Group on Menstrual Disorders. FIGO classification system (PALM-COEIN) for causes of abnormal uterine bleeding in nongravid women of reproductive age. Int J Gynaecol Obstet. 2011;113:3-13.
7. Munro MG, Critchley HO, Broder MS, Fraser IS. FIGO classification system (PALM-COEIN) for causes of abnormal uterine bleeding in nongravid women of reproductive age. Int J Gynaecol Obstet. 2011;113:3.
8. National Collaborating Centre for Women's and Children's Health; National Institute for Health and Care Excellence. NICE guideline CG44: heavy menstrual bleeding. London: Royal College of Obstetricians and Gynaecologists, 2007. Available at: http://www.nice.org.uk/CG44.
9. Vercellini P, Cortesi I, Oldandi S, Moschetta M, DeGiorgi O, Crosignani PG. The role of transvaginal ultrasonography and outpatient diagnostic hysteroscopy in the evaluation of patients with menorrhagia. Hum Reprod. 1997;12:1768-71.
10. Wolman I, Jaffa A, Hartoov J, Bar-Am A, David M. Sensitivity and specificity of sonohysterography for the evaluation of the uterine cavity in perimenopausal patients. J Ultrasound Med. 1996;15:285-8.
11. Widrich T, Bradley LD, Mitchenson AR, Collins RI. Comparison of saline infusion sonography with office hysteroscopy for the evaluation of the endometrium. Am J Obstet Gynecol. 1996;174:1327-34.
12. Farquhar C, Ekeroma A, Furness S, Arroll B. A systematic review of transvaginal ultrasonography, sonohysterography and hysteroscopy for the investigation of abnormal uterine bleeding in premenopausal women. Acta Obstet Gynecol Scand. 2003;82:493-504.
13. Abnormal Uterine Bleeding in Pre-Menopausal Women, SOGC CLINICAL PRACTICE GUIDELINE No. 292, May 2013, JOGC. 2013,35:5.

14. Huang GS, Gebb JS, Einstein MH, Shahabi S, Novetsky AP, Goldberg GL. Accuracy of preoperative endometrial sampling for the detection of high-grade endometrial tumors. Am J Obstet Gynecol. 2007;196:243.e1-e5.
15. Munro MG, Mainor N, Basu R, Brisinger M, Barreda L. Oral medroxyprogesterone acetate and combination oral contraceptives for acute uterine bleeding: a randomized controlled trial. Obstet Gynecol. 2006;108:924-9.
16. Ammerman SR, Nelson AL. A new progestogen-only medical therapy for outpatient management of acute, abnormal uterine bleeding: a pilot study. Am J Obstet Gynecol. 2013;208: 499.e1-5.
17. DeVore GR, Owens O, Kase N. Use of intravenous Premarin in the treatment of dysfunctional uterine bleeding—a double-blind randomized control study. Obstet Gynecol. 1982;59:285-91.
18. Willman EA, Collind WD, Clayton SC. Studies on the involvement of prostaglandins in uterine symptomatology and pathology. BJOG. 1976;83:337-41.
19. Lethaby A, Augwood C, Duckitt K, Farquhar C. Nonsteroidal anti-inflammatory drugs for heavy menstrual bleeding. Cochrane Database Syst Rev. 2007;4:CD000400.
20. Fraser IS, McCarron G. Randomized trial of 2 hormonal and 2 prostaglandin-inhibiting agents in women with a complaint of menorrhagia. Aust N Z J Obstet Gynaecol. 1991;31:66-70.
21. Reid PC, Virtanen-Kari S. Randomised comparative trial of the levonorgestrel intrauterine system and mefenamic acid for the treatment of idiopathic menorrhagia: a multiple analysis using total menstrual fluid loss, menstrual blood loss and pictoral blood loss assessment charts. BJOG. 2005;112:1121-5.
22. Gleeson NC. Cyclic changes in endometrial tissue plasminogen activator and plasminogen activator inhibitor type 1 in women with normal menstruation and essential menorrhagia. American Journal of Obstetrics & Gynecology. 1994;171(1):178-83.
23. Lethaby A, Farquhar C, Cooke I. Antifibrinolytics for heavy menstrual bleeding. Cochrane Database of Systematic Reviews 2000, Issue 4. Art. No.: CD000249. DOI: 10.1002/14651858.CD000249.
24. Farquhar C, Brown J. Oral contraceptive pill for heavy menstrual bleeding. Cochrane Database of Systematic Reviews 2009, Issue 4. Art. No.: CD000154. DOI: 10.1002/14651858. CD000154.
25. Lethaby A, Irvine GA, Cameron IT. Cyclical progestogens for heavy menstrual bleeding. Cochrane Database of Systematic Reviews 2008, Issue 1. Art. No.: CD001016. DOI: 10.1002/14651858.CD001016.
26. Lethaby A, Cooke I, Rees MC. Progesterone or progestogen-releasing intrauterine systems for heavy menstrual bleeding. Cochrane Database of Systematic Reviews 2005, Issue 4. Art. No.: CD002126. DOI: 10.1002/14651858.CD002126.
27. Roy SN, Bhattacharya S. Benefits and risks of pharmacological agents used for the treatment of menorrhagia. Drugs Saf. 2004; 27:75-90.
28. Reid PC. Endometrial ablation in England - coming of age? An examination of hospital episode statistics 1989/1990 to 2004/2005. European Journal of Obstetrics, Gynecology, and Reproductive Biology. 2007;135:191-4.
29. Lethaby A, Penninx J, HickeyM, Garry R ,Marjoribanks J. Endometrial resection and ablation techniques for heavy menstrual bleeding. Cochrane Database of Systematic Reviews 2013, Issue 8. Art. No.: CD001501. DOI: 10.1002/14651858. CD001501.

CHAPTER 9

Amenorrhea and Oligomenorrhea

B Kanchana Devi, N Pandiyan

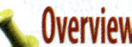
Overview

- Menstrual abnormalities may occur because of endocrine disorders of ovulation, endometrial pathologies or due to systemic conditions.
- In primary amenorrhea, evaluation of secondary sexual characteristics is done to estimate the degree of pubertal development. Normal secondary sexual development appropriate for age may indicate normal ovarian function and the cause for amenorrhea could be 'delayed menarche' or uterine pathology. Imperforate hymen should also be considered.
- Poor or absent secondary sexual development with normal genitalia by clinical examination and ultrasonography may indicate 'delayed puberty' or hypogonadism. Serum FSH estimation would help in diagnosing and differentiating hypogonadotropic from hypergonadotropic hypogonadism.
- The commonest cause of secondary amenorrhea is pregnancy. The other common cause is polycystic ovarian disease—though, it often produces oligomenorrhea. Hyperprolactinemia and tuberculosis of the genital tract are also to be considered.

INTRODUCTION

Amenorrhea and oligomenorrhea are common gynecological problems. Thirty percent of women attending the gynecology outpatient department at a large teaching hospital had these menstrual disturbances. Amenorrhea and oligomenorrhea, though not disabling conditions, can be disturbing to the woman who is used to having regular menstrual cyclicity. They may also be indicators of other sinister disabling conditions. Proper evaluation of the cause of amenorrhea is essential for its rational management. We will now briefly outline the physiology of menstruation. A clear understanding of the physiology is essential for the proper planning and treatment of amenorrhea and oligomenorrhea.

PHYSIOLOGY OF MENSTRUATION

Menstruation is the periodic physiological shedding of the endometrium. During the follicular phase of the ovulatory cycle, the growing follicle secretes estrogens, which acts on the endometrium inducing proliferative changes. With ovulation, the follicle is transformed into a corpus luteum and the progesterone from the corpus luteum induces secretory changes in the endometrium in preparation for nidation. When pregnancy fails to take place the endometrial lining is shed and is recognized as menstruation. Normal menstruation has a cyclicity of 28 days +/- 4 days. The blood loss is about 80 mL and mild crampy pains accompany the blood flow.

Menstrual abnormalities can occur because of endocrine disorders of ovulation, endometrial pathologies or due to systemic conditions.

The commonly encountered menstrual abnormalities are:
- Amenorrhea—absence of menstruation
- Oligomenorrhea—infrequent menstruation
- Hypomenorrhea—scanty menstruation
- Polymenorrhea—frequent menstruation
- Menorrhagia—excessive menstruation
- Dymenorrhea—painful menstruation
- Metrorrhagia—midcycle bleeding.

Endocrine Causes of Menstrual Abnormalities

The cyclical release of a fertilizable oocyte is the main function of the female reproductive system. This requires synchronized action of the higher cortical centers, hypothalamus, pituitary, ovary and endometrium. Asynchrony of this axis may lead to menstrual abnormalities and amenorrhea.

Endometrial Pathology Causing Menstrual Abnormalities

Infections of the endometrium—particularly endometrial tuberculosis, may cause menstrual abnormalities and amenorrhea.[1,2] Endometrial tuberculosis may cause menometrorrhagia in early stages and amenorrhea in advanced stages.

Systemic Diseases

Severe systemic illnesses by causing generalized ill health and severe weight loss may lead to menstrual abnormalities and particularly amenorrhea. A critical body mass is essential for normal hypothalamo-pituitary ovarian and menstrual function. Coagulation disorders and hematological disorders may cause menorrhagia.

Amenorrhea

Definition: Absence of menstruation for 6 months or longer in woman with regular cycles or for a period of 3 cycle lengths or longer in woman with irregular cycles is called as amenorrhea.

Amenorrhea is physiological under the following conditions:

1. Prepubertal/Premenarcheal
2. Pregnancy
3. Lactation
4. Postmenopausal.

Physiology of Menarche

The age of onset of menarche has steadily declined over the last century and has now stabilized. Onset of menarche is related to critical body fat of 30%. The current trend of early onset of menarche is attributed to improved nutrition and better living standards.

The higher cortical centers exhibit constant inhibitory control over the hypothalamo-pituitary-ovarian axis. When a critical body mass is reached, the inhibitory control is lost and this permits the generation of GnRH pulse from the pulse generator in the hypothalamus. The release of GnRH leads to release of FSH/LH from the pituitary and further development of the ovarian and endometrial axis. In the early post-menarcheal years this circuit is not mature and may lead to anovulatory cycles. There is enough data to indicate that endogenous opioid have a crucial inhibitory role in the control of gonadotropin secretion.[3]

Primary Amenorrhea

When a girl has not attained menarche by the age of 18 years she is said to have primary amenorrhea.

Commonly primary amenorrhea is idiopathic.

Other Causes

Primary amenorrhea can be caused by:

1. Endocrine causes.
2. Endometrial causes.
3. Systemic causes.

Endocrine causes: Lesions of the higher centers and those involving the hypothalamus may lead to defects in GnRH pulse generation, causing disruption in the hypothalamo-hypophyseal axis. This would lead to failure of gonadotropin production and hence, cause secondary ovarian failure leading to amenorrhea. The classic example of this condition is Kallmann's syndrome. Patients with Kallmann's syndrome, besides amenorrhea also have defects in their olfactory neurons, and hence have anosmia/hyposmia. Defects in the olfactory sulci in the brain have been demonstrated at MRI.[4] Hypothalamic dysfunction may also be a post-encephalitic sequel.

- Pituitary lesions particularly those involving the non-gonadotroph cells may lead to pressure effect on the gonadotroph leading to decreased gonadotropin production. Prolactinomas causing hyperprolactinemia may impair pituitary function both by pressure effect and by interfering with the GnRH pulse generation. Pituitary destruction as occurs with Sheehan's syndrome may lead to pituitary failure, non-production of gonadotropins and hence, amenorrhea.

  Conditions like primary hemochromatosis, Wilson's disease, thalassemia major may affect pituitary gonadotrophs leading to hypogonadism and amenorrhea.

- Primary ovarian failure either due to chromosomal disorders like Turner's syndrome or due to premature ovarian failure may lead to non-production of gonadal steroids and consequently amenorrhea.[5]

Endometrial pathologies: Endometrial pathology usually causes secondary amenorrhea. Very rarely this could contribute to primary amenorrhea. Vigorous curettage of the uterine cavity may lead to adhesions between the uterine wall (synechiae) leading to amenorrhea.[6]

Genital tract tuberculosis, though primarily tubal, often extends to the endometrium, causing menorrhagia in early days and amenorrhea in the advanced stages due to destruction of the endometrium and sub-endometrial layers.

Endometrial receptor defects may lead to inadequate proliferation of the endometrium and poor or inadequate secretory changes causing menstrual abnormalities, oligomenorrhea and amenorrhea.

In Müllerian agenesis, the uterus and upper vagina are absent and hence, the girls present with primary amenorrhea. Due to normally functioning ovaries, normal secondary sexual characters are found.

Transverse septum of the vagina and imperforate hymen should also be considered. Though they present with primary amenorrhea, they actually have cryptomenorrhea.

Systemic diseases: Many chronic illnesses like chronic liver failure and chronic renal failure lead to significant ill health, weight loss and to amenorrhea. Chronic renal failure also leads to elevation of prolactin levels and this may cause amenorrhea. Significant weight loss of any etiology, including eating disorders like anorexia nervosa may lead to amenorrhea.[7]

Clinical Approach to Primary Amenorrhea (Flowchart 9.1)

In a girl presenting with primary amenorrhea, a detailed personal history, sibling history, family history, clinical examination and a few relevant investigations will help in establishing a proper diagnosis and aid in appropriate management.

History of developmental delay in milestones may point to lesions in the higher centers. Consanguineous marriage among parents may suggest inherited disorders causing primary amenorrhea.

History of mother or sisters attaining menarche late may point to constitutional, familial 'delayed menarche'.

Past history of trauma to the head or encephalitis may suggest a post-traumatic, post-encephalitic sequel.

History of pulmonary tuberculosis may indicate genital tract tuberculosis as the cause of the amenorrhea.

History of cyclical abdominal pain, urinary retention may point towards outlet obstruction.

Clinical examination is done to evaluate the state of nourishment, height and weight of the child and for evidence of other systemic diseases. Malnourished children have a greater risk of primary amenorrhea and delayed puberty. Evaluation of secondary sexual characteristics is done to estimate the degree of pubertal development. Normal secondary sexual development appropriate for age may indicate normal ovarian function and the cause for amenorrhea could be 'delayed menarche' or uterine pathology. The clinical presentation and management has been discussed in the earlier chapter.

Estimates of serum, FSH, LH, prolactin and estradiol will help in identifying the site of lesion and in planning future management. All the hormone investigation may not be essential for all the patients.

Peripheral blood karyotyping may help in identifying Turner's syndrome, Turner mosaic and testicular feminization syndrome.

Galactosemia may be a rare cause of primary amenorrhea due to ovarian dysfunction.[8]

Clinical Features of Some Common Conditions Associated with Primary Amenorrhea

Turner's syndrome is the most common cause of primary ovarian failure and primary amenorrhea. In the classical condition the ovaries are dysgenetic and present as streak gonads. The gonadotropin levels are markedly raised.[9]

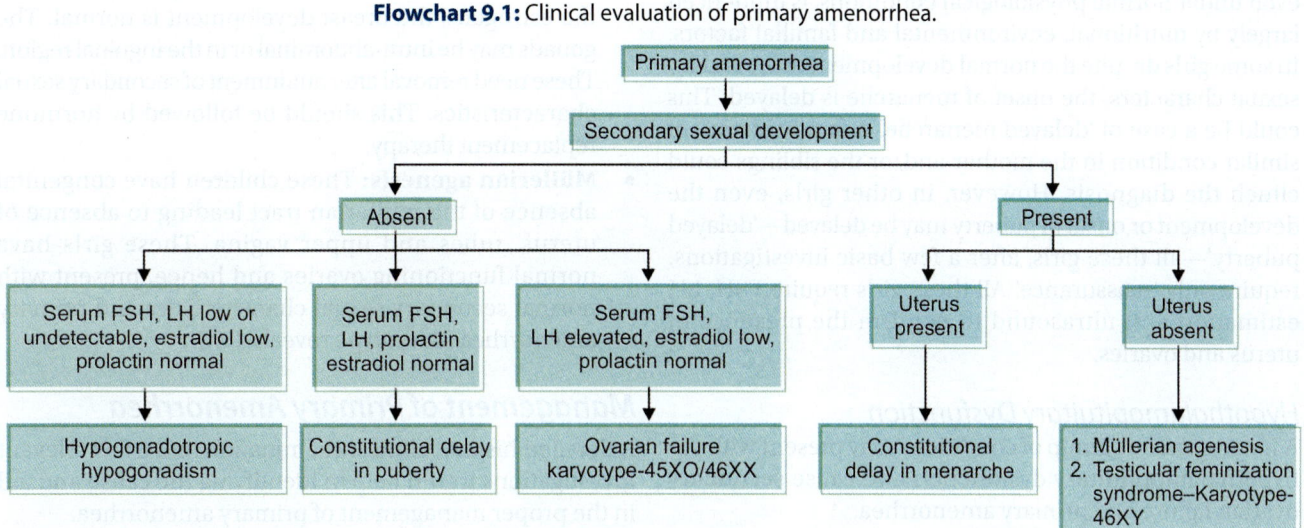

Flowchart 9.1: Clinical evaluation of primary amenorrhea.

Turner's syndrome occurs in around 1 in 2500 births and the usual karyotype picture is 45X. Mosaic forms are also common with karyotype picture presenting 45X/46XX, 45X/46XY, or with partial deletion of one arm of the X chromosome.

The presence of Y chromosome may be dangerous as they may have testes and these children may require gonadectomy to prevent the risk of gonadoblastoma or dysgerminoma.

The classical features of Turner's syndrome include:

1. Short stature
2. Web neck
3. Lymphoedema
4. Shield chest with widely spaced nipples
5. Scoliosis
6. Wide carrying angle
7. Short metacarpals
8. Soft, curling nails
9. Low set ears, low hairline, micrognathia and high arched palate.
10. Coarctation of the ankle
11. Horseshoe kidney
12. Strabismus
13. Ptosis
14. Multiple naevi.

All the features may not be present in all the patients. However, most patients present with varying combinations of these elemental features.

A high index of suspicion is essential for prepubertal diagnosis of the condition and proper management of these children.

Constitutional Delay

The onset of puberty and the occurrence of menarche, even under normal physiological conditions, is influenced largely by nutritional, environmental and familial factors. In some girls despite the normal development of secondary sexual characters, the onset of menarche is delayed. This could be a case of 'delayed menarche'. A family history of similar condition in the mother and/or the siblings could clinch the diagnosis. However, in other girls, even the development or onset of puberty may be delayed—'delayed puberty'—all these girls, after a few basic investigations, require only 'reassurance'. All these girls require FSH, LH estimation and ultrasound to confirm the presence of uterus and ovaries.

Hypothalamopituitary Dysfunction

A heterogeneous group of conditions may present with the hypothalamopituitary dysfunction and cause secondary ovarian failure and primary amenorrhea.

Inflammatory lesions or tumors of the hypothalamus-pituitary region may lead to decreased secretions of FSH and LH and to ovarian failure. Lesions of the pituitary, like craniopharyngioma and hydrocephalus, may cause such a condition.

The syndromes associated with hypogonadotropic hypogonadism are:

- **Laurence-Moon-Biedl syndrome:** This is an autosomal recessive disorder characterized by obesity, retinitis pigmentosa, mental retardation, polydactyly and hypogonadism.
- **Prader-Willi syndrome:** It presents with hypotonia, mental retardation, characteristic facies, obesity and hypogonadism.
- **Kallmann's syndrome or olfactory genital dysplasia:** Patients present with primary amenorrhea due to defect in the hypothalamic pulse generator and consequently hypopituitarism and hypogonadism. Incomplete/complete agenesis of the olfactory bulbs may lead to anosmia/hyposmia. It is inherited as an autosomal dominant trait.
- **Androgen insensitivity syndrome:** Children with this condition though genetically male with a karyotype of 46XY, are almost always raised as girls in view of the female phenotype. Often the girls present in their late teens with good secondary sexual development and primary amenorrhea. The condition is an X-linked recessive disorder where the primary defect is the 'insensitivity of the androgen receptor'. The gonads are testes, which are functional and produce normal amounts of testosterone and müllerian inhibiting substance. Therefore, these girls do not have uterus, tubes and upper vagina. Due to androgen insensitivity, secondary sexual characteristics and the external genitalia have a female configuration. As there is adequate conversion of testosterone to estrogens and due to exposure to unopposed action of the estrogens, the breast development is normal. The gonads may be intra-abdominal or in the inguinal region. These need removal after attainment of secondary sexual characteristics. This should be followed by hormone replacement therapy.
- **Müllerian agenesis:** These children have congenital absence of the müllerian tract leading to absence of uterus, tubes and upper vagina. These girls have normal functioning ovaries and hence, present with normal secondary sexual characteristics and primary amenorrhea. Karyotype reveals 46XX.

Management of Primary Amenorrhea

A detailed history, clinical examination and a few relevant investigations would help in identifying the cause and aid in the proper management of primary amenorrhea.

CHAPTER 9 Amenorrhea and Oligomenorrhea

Table 9.1: Management of primary amenorrhea.

Condition	Clinical features	Investigations	Management
Delayed puberty/menarche	Poor or absent or normal secondary sexual development	Normal serum FSH, LH and prolactin	Reassurance
Turner's syndrome	Poor or absent secondary sexual development. Uterus and tubes present, streak gonads	Elevated serum FSH, LH and normal prolactin. Karyotype-45XO or Mosaic-46XX/45XO	• Estrogen and progesterone for normal secondary sexual development and oocyte or embryo donation for conception • Rarely, normal sexual development, menstruation and conception have been reported
Müllerian agenesis	Normal secondary sexual development. Poorly developed or absent tubes, uterus and upper vagina. Ovaries normal	• Normal serum FSH, LH and prolactin • Karyotype-46XX	• If fertility is desired, surrogacy would be the choice • In some women with rudimentary Müllerian structures uterine reconstruction has been done and pregnancies have been reported
Testicular feminization syndrome	Normal secondary sexual development. Absent uterus, tubes and upper vagina. Absent axillary and pubic hair. Inguinal swellings (hernia) may be present which may contain the testes	• Normal serum FSH, LH and prolactin • Karyotype-46XY	• Gonadectomy after normal pubertal development • Fertility cannot be restored • May function as women with normal sexual function. Some women may require vaginoplasty
Genital tuberculosis	If postpubertal—normal secondary sexual characters. If prepubertal—before the development of secondary sexual characters and if ovaries are involved—poor or absent secondary sexual development	• Normal FSH, LH, prolactin. Karyotype-46XX • Endometrium—tuberculosis • Laparoscopy—tuberculosis	• Antituberculosis treatment may re-establish the cycle in many women • Pregnancies by IVF have been reported in cases where the tubes were damaged
Hypothalamic amenorrhea as in Kallmann's syndrome or other hypothalamic lesions	Poor or absent secondary sexual characters	• Low or undetectable serum FSH, LH • Normal prolactin. Karyotype-46XX	• Estrogen/progestogen for restoration of secondary sexual characters • GnRH pulsatile infusion for induction of ovulation and restoration of fertility. Gonadotropins can also be used for induction of ovulation

History of consanguinity amongst parents and/or history of similar problems among siblings may all point to a genetic origin. History of delayed milestones, past history of head trauma or encephalitis may suggest a central cause for the 'primary amenorrhea'.

Short stature, web neck and increased carrying angle with cardiac defects with no secondary sexual development may point to Turner's syndrome. Normal secondary sexual characteristics with a blind vagina may indicate 'Testicular Feminization Syndrome' or 'Müllerian agenesis'. Patients with testicular feminization syndrome also present with absent axillary and pubic hair.

Normal secondary sexual characteristics with normal internal and external genitalia may indicate 'delayed menarche'.

Poor or absent secondary sexual development with normal genitalia by clinical and ultrasonography may indicate 'delayed puberty' or hypogonadism. Serum FSH estimation would help in diagnosing and differentiating hypogonadotropic from hypergonadotropic hypogonadism.

The treatment of primary amenorrhea depends upon the cause, what is desired at that point in time and what is possible under prevailing conditions (Table 9.1).

Secondary Amenorrhea

If a woman who has previously menstruated spontaneously, does not menstruate for 6 months or longer or for 3 cycle lengths or longer, she is considered to have 'secondary amenorrhea' (Table 9.2). In practice many patients with

Table 9.2: Management of secondary amenorrhea.

Condition	Clinical features	Investigations	Management
Polycystic ovarian disease	Anovulation, amenorrhea, oligomenorrhea, +/– hirsutism, +/– obesity	USG—bilateral enlarged ovaries; volume >10 cc, follicles > 12 of < 9 mm, clinical/biochemical hyper-androgenism[10]	Life-style modification, induction, of ovulation or combined oral contraceptive pill
Hyperprolactinemia	Luteal phase defects, galactorrhea, amenorrhea and hypogonadism	• Serum prolactin is elevated • Serum TSH elevated when hyperprolactinemia is due to hypothyroidism • CT scan/MRI for evidence of prolactinoma	• Thyroxine if the hyperprolactinemia is due to hypothyroidism • Bromoergocryptine in patients with hyperprolactinemia • Transsphenoidal microsurgery in selected cases
Sheehan's syndrome or postpartum pituitary necrosis	Failure of lactation. Other features of hypopituitarism	• Low serum FSH, LH, prolactin, progesterone • May also have low TSH, ACTH	• Estrogen/progesterone therapy for restoration of menses • Gonadotropins for induction of ovulation

primary amenorrhea are given inappropriate hormonal treatment and made to menstruate and are subsequently wrongly diagnosed as 'secondary amenorrhea'.

Causes

The most common cause of secondary amenorrhea is pregnancy. The other causes are:

1. Polycystic ovarian disease—though it often produces oligomenorrhea.
2. Hyperprolactinemia.
3. Tuberculosis of the genital tract.
4. Postpartum hemorrhage, postpartum collapse, pituitary necrosis and Sheehan's syndrome.
5. Post-pill amenorrhea.
6. Asherman's syndrome: Vigorous curettage of the endometrium leads to uterine adhesions and fibrosis.

The clinical evaluation of secondary amenorrhea is given in Flowchart 9.2.

Polycystic Ovarian Disease

Most patients with polycystic ovarian disease present with varying periods of amenorrhea/oligomenorrhea followed by menorrhagia. However, some patients may have only anovulation with no irregularity in menstrual pattern.

The diagnosis is based on clinical findings, biochemical features and ultrasonographic findings. The management is dependent on patient's presenting feature—infertility or irregular cycle.

Hyperprolactinemia

Hyperprolactinemia may lead to anovulation and amenorrhea.

Milder forms of hyperprolactinemia are often due to hypothyroidism.[11] Moderate elevation can be due to 'hyperplasia or neoplasia'.

Hyperprolactinemia regardless of its etiology may produce varying degrees of ovulatory disturbances and amenorrhea.

Mild elevation may produce 'luteal phase defects' and moderate elevation may cause anovulation and amenorrhea.

Prolactinomas are almost always benign. They present clinically with galactorrhea, amenorrhea and if large with pressure symptoms. The diagnosis is based on history, clinical findings, laboratory findings and CT/MRI parameters. The management depends on the cause of hyperprolactinemia and the desire for childbearing.

When hypothyroidism is the cause of hyper-prolactinemia correction of hypothyroidism leads to correction of hyperprolactinemia.

In moderate and severe hyperprolactinemia, medical management is the first-line of management. Bromoergocryptine is the drug of choice. In patients intolerant to bromoergocryptine or not responding to bromoergocryptine, Cabergoline can be used.

In some patients, particularly those with macro adenoma and pressure symptoms, trans-sphenoidal microsurgery may have to be undertaken. Patients with hyperprolactinemia on medical management may have to take it for a long time, sometimes for several years.

Tuberculosis of the Genital Tract

Tuberculosis is a major killer disease in many developing countries including India. Genital tuberculosis is not uncommon. Tuberculosis of the genital tract primarily involves the tubes, but subsequently spreads to the endometrium. Women with genital tuberculosis develop tubal damage and block, which is usually not amenable to surgery. Destruction of the endometrium by tuberculosis leads to amenorrhea. Effective treatment of tuberculosis may help in regeneration of the endometrium in some

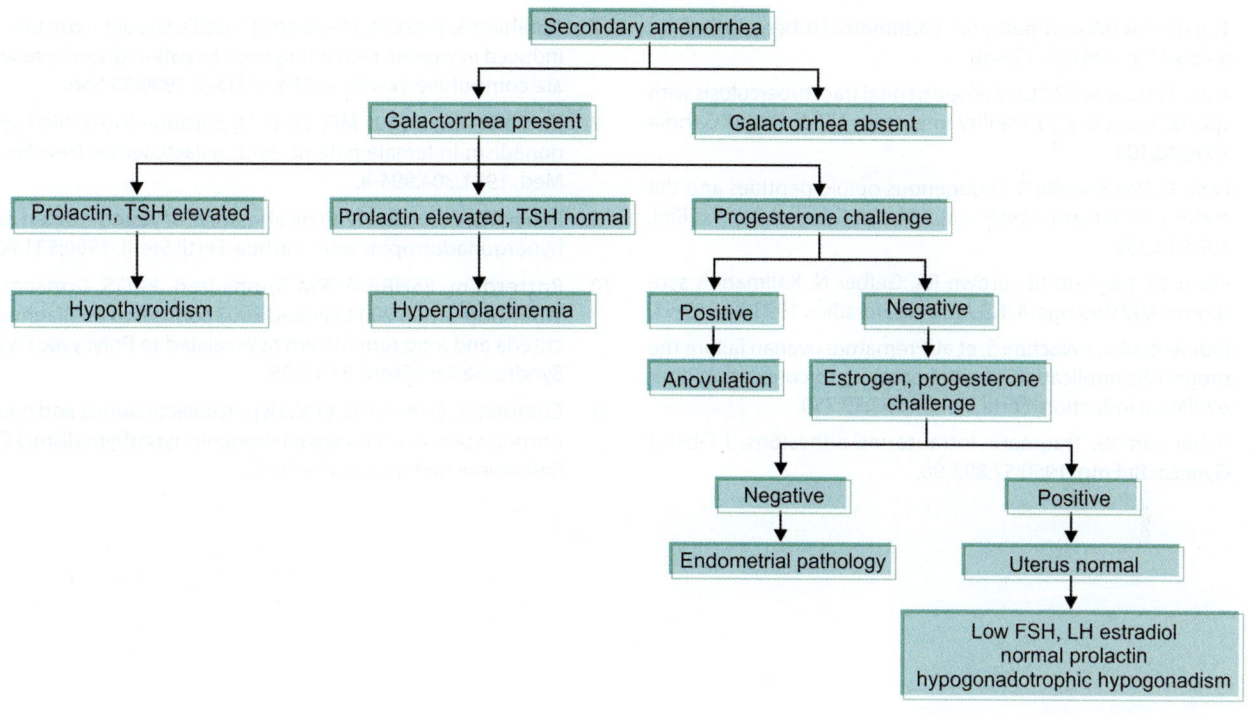

Flowchart 9.2: Clinical evaluation of secondary amenorrhea.

women, but others may continue to be amenorrheic with poor prognosis for menstrual function and fertility.

Tubal tuberculosis often leads to irreparable tubal damage and even in women in whom menstrual function has been restored, IVF may be the only option left for restoration of fertility.

Postpartum Pituitary Necrosis—Sheehan's Syndrome

In some women who suffer from postpartum hemorrhage and collapse, the pituitary may undergo necrosis leading to hypopituitarism. This often involves all the trophic hormones from the anterior pituitary, but it could also be gonadotropin specific. This could lead to hypogonadotropic hypogonadism and amenorrhea. These patients respond well to gonadotropin therapy. Menstrual function can be restored by estrogen/progestogen therapy.

Oligomenorrhea is mostly due to anovulation. Spells of oligomenorrhea may precede amenorrhea. These patients require evaluation for hypothalamopituitary dysfunction.

Asherman's Syndrome

Endometrial damage caused by the procedures like repeated and vigorous curettage leads to fibrosis and adhesions damaging the functional layer of endometrium leading to amenorrhea.

These women do not respond to progesterone treatment and do not resume menstruation on combined hormonal replacement also.

Doing a *Hysterosalpingography or Hysteroscopy* can clinch the diagnosis. Adhesiolysis by hysteroscopy may help in re-establishing the cycles.

The treatment of amenorrhea depends upon the cause and whether the patient requires re-establishing menstrual cyclicity or desires fertility.

Combined oral contraceptives pill given cyclically would re-establish menstrual cyclicity.

Induction of ovulation with clomiphene, cyclofenil, tamoxifen, or gonadotropin would help in restoring fertility in many of these women.

In some women, during the spells of amenorrhea there may be a build-up of endometrium leading to menorrhagia subsequently. This is called as 'oligomenorrhagia'.

Prognosis

Amenorrhea and oligomenorrhea can be effectively treated in most women with these menstrual disorders. However, it is important to understand the basic pathophysiology of the condition and treat appropriately. The treatment depends also on the patients presenting complaint and her desire for childbearing.

REFERENCES

1. Tripathy SN (Mrs), Tripathy SN. Endometrial tuberculosis. J Ind Med Assoc. 1987;85:136-40.
2. Misra R, Sharma SP, et al. Female genital tract tuberculosis with special reference to sterility in eastern UP. Jr O and G India 1996;46:104.
3. Ferin M, VandeWeile R. Endogenous opioid peptides and the control of menstrual cycle. Eur J Obstet Gynecol Reprod Biol. 1984;18:365.
4. Knorr JR, Ragland RL, Brown RS, Gelber N. Kallmann's syndrome: MRI findings. AJNR Am J Neuroradiol. 1993;14:845-51.
5. Blumenfeld Z, Halachmi S, et al. Premature ovarian failure the prognostic application of autoimmunity to conception after ovulation induction. Fertil Steril. 1993;59:750.
6. Asherman JG. Traumatic intrauterine adhesions. J Obstet Gynecol Br Emp. 1950;57:892-96.
7. Abraham S, Mitra M, Llewellyn-Jones D. Should ovulation be induced in women recovering from an eating disorder or who are compulsive exercisers? Fertil Steril. 1990;53:566.
8. Kaufman FR, Kogut MD, et al. Hypergonadotrophic hypogonadism in female patients with galactosemia. New Engl J Med. 1981;304:994-8.
9. Rebar RW, Connolly HV. Clinical features of young women with hypergonadotrophic amenorrhea. Fertil Steril. 1990;531:804.
10. Rotterdam ESHRE/ASRM-Sponsored PCOS Consensus Workshop Group 2004.Revised 2003 consensus on diagnostic criteria and long term health risks related to Polycystic Ovary Syndrome Fert-Steril. 81:14-25.
11. Contreras P, Generini G, et al. Hyperprolactinaemia and galactorrhea; spontaneous versus iatrogenic hypothyroidism. J Clin Endocrinol metab. 1981;53:1036.

CHAPTER 10

Reproductive Health

WC Maina, Sambit Mukhopadhyay

Overview

- Reproductive health is an issue of global importance and an integral part of United Nations millennium development goals.
- Global efforts aimed at improving reproductive health include, but are not limited to, promoting gender equality, empowering women, reducing maternal mortality rate, improving access to contraceptive services, tackling the obesity epidemic, reducing the impact of infections, provision of safe abortion and discouraging female genital mutilation.
- Globally maternal mortality rate has declined by 47% over the last 2 decades.[1]
- Worldwide, the number of people newly infected with HIV continues to fall, dropping 33% from 2001 to 2011 and malaria deaths fell by an estimated 26% from 2000 to 2010.[2]
- Gender equality and empowering of women is being promoted globally through access to education, jobs and representation of women in parliament.
- Developing countries continue to experience significant challenges in provision of reproductive health due to economic, social and political factors.

INTRODUCTION

Reproductive health is recognized as an important global issue in the millennium development goals. Significant progress has been achieved since 2000 but further improvements are needed beyond 2015, especially in developing countries. Improving access to education, promoting gender equality, empowering women and, provision of accessible and affordable services is central to promoting reproductive health. This Chapter discusses the main factors that influence reproductive health.

ADOLESCENT HEALTH

The WHO defines adolescent as a person between 10 and 19 years of age. In 2005, there were 1.21 billion adolescents in the world. Population in this age group is estimated to continue to increase until the year 2040, to finally reach 1.23 billion.[3] India has the largest proportion of adolescents in the world. The 2011 census of India revealed that adolescents constitute 20.9% of the total female population.[4]

Adolescence is the period of transition from childhood to adulthood. During these years, following puberty, young people gradually mature to become adults, but do not generally assume the privileges, roles and responsibilities commonly associated with adulthood. Nonetheless, this is the age when most people begin to explore their sexuality and have sexual relationships. Endocrine changes also trigger emotional and psychological development. A sense of identity develops and this is influenced to some extent by peer groups and family background.

There are more than 500 million adolescent girls currently living in developing countries.[5] Each year an estimated 16 million women 15–19 years old give birth.[6]

Sexual activity during adolescence increases the risk of sexual and reproductive health problems. These include unsafe abortion, sexually transmitted infections including HIV and, sexual coercion and violence. A meta-analysis and review of pregnancy complications in developing countries revealed that teenagers were at increased risk of maternal anemia, preterm birth and cesarean delivery.[7] Up to 65% of women with obstetric fistula develop this as adolescents. Reassuringly, rates of adolescent pregnancy have fallen considerably in most countries in the past two to three decades. In India, the adolescent fertility rate (births per 1000 women ages 15–19) has fallen steadily from a high of 116.10 in 1997 to 77.00 in 2011.[8]

A multitude of factors contribute to the sexual and reproductive health problems of adolescents. These include lack of knowledge about safe sexual practice, poor access to reproductive health services and inability to negotiate safe sex with the male partner. Sexual violence against girls remains a common problem. Early childbearing results in lost educational and career opportunities. Fear prevailing among policy makers or public leaders that sexual education will encourage sexual activity and the resulting lack of educational measures prevent adolescents from making informed choices regarding their reproductive health.

Globally, according to United Nations Population Fund (UNFPA), comprehensive and correct knowledge about HIV among young men and young women has increased slightly since 2003- but at only 34%, the number of young people with this comprehensive knowledge is only slightly greater than one third of UN General Assembly Special Sessions target of 95%.[5]

The global sex survey conducted in 2004 highlighted the state of adolescent health in Europe.[9] There is a trend towards declining age at sexual debut (Table 10.1). The age when respondents first received sex education varied from 11.3 years to 15.4 years.

Addressing the sexual and reproductive health needs and problems of adolescents is a crucial element of the World Health Organization (WHO) Global Reproductive Health Strategy (RHS).[10] Governments throughout Europe are planning and adopting RH strategies with emphasis on and inclusion of adolescents. HIV/AIDS and sexuality education is being implemented in countries where previously absent. In most developing countries, the sexual and reproductive health needs of adolescents are either poorly understood or not fully appreciated.

Table 10.1: Average age at first intercourse in 16–20 years olds in Europe.[9]

Country	Age at first intercourse
Iceland	15.7
Germany	16.2
Austria	16.3
Netherlands	16.4
Sweden	16.4
Denmark	16.5
Finland	16.5
Norway	16.5
United Kingdom	16.7
Bulgaria	17.1
France	17.1
Israel	17.1
Belgium	17.2
Macedonia	17.2
Slovenia	17.2
Hungary	17.3
Switzerland	17.3
Czech Republic	17.5
Ireland	17.5
Croatia	17.6
Italy	17.6
Serbia and Montenegro	17.6
Spain	17.7
Greece	17.8
Poland	17.9
Slovakia	18

FEMALE GENITAL MUTILATION

Female genital mutilation (FGM) is defined as the partial or total removal of the female external genitalia for non-medical reasons. According to recent UNICEF data, more than 125 million girls and women have experienced some form of FGM in the 29 countries in Africa and the Middle East where the harmful practice is common. FGM is mostly carried out on young girls sometime between infancy and age 15. Because of migration and the movement of refugees, the issue of female genital mutilation is now a global concern. The practice is increasingly seen in European countries; Canada, Australia and the USA. The WHO has outlawed it on the grounds that it is a violation of human rights.[11] The practice has been banned in many parts of the world but not eradicated.

FGM has no health benefits. It involves removing and inflicting damage to healthy and normal female genital tissue, and consequently interferes with important female functions. The WHO classifies female genital mutilation into four distinct types (Box 10.1).[12] The most common type of female genital mutilation is excision of the clitoris and labia minora, accounting for up to 80% of all cases; the most extreme form is infibulations, which constitutes about 15% of all procedures. It is rare for women to survive the mutilation procedure without complications and it leaves permanent physical and psychological scars. Types III and IV FGM are the most likely to cause major complications. Acute complications include hemorrhage, shock and death; infection, such as tetanus and septicemia; retention of urine from pain and direct mechanical obstruction; injury to the urethra, vagina, perineum or rectum; and urinary and fecal incontinence. Long-term complications are shown in Box 10.2.[13]

Approximately, one woman dies of genital mutilation-related complications every ten minutes. This is almost half

Box 10.1: WHO classification of female genital mutilation.[12]

- Clitorodectomy: Partial or total removal of the clitoris and, in very rare cases, only the prepuce
- Excision: Partial or total removal of the clitoris and the labia minora with or without excision of the labia majora
- Infibulation: Narrowing of the vaginal opening through the creation of a covering seal. The seal is formed by cutting and repositioning the inner, or outer, labia, with or without removal of the clitoris.
- Other: All other harmful procedures to the female genitalia for non-medical purposes, e.g. pricking, piercing, incising, scraping and cauterizing the genital area.

Source: Reproduced with permission from WHO

Box 10.2: Long-term complications from female genital mutilation.[13]

- Keloid formation from slow, incomplete wound healing leading to deposition of excess connective tissue and vulval granulation
- Para-clitoral cysts
- Sexual dysfunction and marital disharmony resulting from painful intercourse
- Anorgasmia from repeated difficulty in penetration and absence of the clitoris
- Recurrent urinary tract infection (from the collection and stagnation of urine in the vagina allowing bacteria to enter the urethra)
- Renal failure
- Hematocolpos from retention of menstrual flow
- Incontinence resulting from a damaged urethra
- Pelvic inflammatory disease and infertility as a result of chronic infections
- Vesicovaginal or rectovaginal fistula (after prolonged labor and delivery)
- Transmission of HIV and hepatitis from the use of non-sterile instruments
- Psychological disorders

Source: Reproduced with permission from Rashid M, et al. The Royal College of Obstetricians and Gynaecologists. 2007.

that from malaria, which causes some 1 million fatalities per year, yet it is not even a recognized medical condition. The most important step in educating health practitioners is to include this in the international classification of diseases. The World Health Organization has initiated strategies aimed at eliminating the practice.[12] An example is education of health workers in countries where the practice is common and promoting their active involvement as advocates against FGM. The review by Rashid et al.[13] is an important step in educating practitioners involved in the care of pregnant women in the developed world. This review has highlighted substandard care in obstetric management of these women in the developed world. Medical and nursing staff are unfamiliar with the procedure, as well as the culture and the traditions of the immigrant communities. It is recommended that management includes psychological support, antenatal assessment of the external genitalia, advice on the importance of good nutrition, monitoring for urinary tract infections and antenatal defibulation.

There are many strategies that have been adopted internationally to eliminate FGM. In December 2012, the UN General Assembly adopted a resolution to eliminate the practice. WHO, in 2010, published a global strategy to stop health care providers from performing FGM. It is a serious criminal offence in the UK with a maximum penalty of 14 years in prison for anyone found guilty of the offence. The decrease in the prevalence of FGM in most countries suggests that interventions have had a positive impact.

OVERWEIGHT AND OBESITY

Overweight and obesity are defined as abnormal or excessive fat accumulation that may impair health. The prevalence of overweight and obesity is commonly assessed by using body mass index (BMI), defined as the weight in kilograms divided by the square of the height in meters (kg/m^2). A BMI over 25 kg/m^2 is defined as overweight and a BMI over 30 kg/m^2 as obese. The BMI is shifting upwards in many populations. Adult prevalence rates of obesity vary considerably by country from 1.1% to 74.0% with 28 countries having rates above 30%.[14]

Obesity has reached epidemic proportions globally, with the number of overweight and obese people rising from 857 million in 1980 to 2.1 billion in 2013.[15] In developing countries, women have higher rates of obesity than men, while the opposite is true in developed countries. Obesity affects all age groups including children, adolescents and adults. More than 40 million children under the age of 5 were overweight or obese in 2012.[16] The key causes are genetics, epigenetics and consumption of energy-dense foods high in saturated fats and sugars, and reduced physical activity.

Obesity has a great number of negative health, social and economic consequences. Mortality and morbidity rates are higher among overweight and obese individuals than lean people. Recent studies have shown that people who were undernourished in early life and then become obese in adulthood, tend to develop conditions such as high blood pressure, heart disease and diabetes at an earlier age and more severe form than those who were never undernourished.[17-21] Obesity and overweight pose a major risk for chronic diseases, including type 2 diabetes, cardiovascular disease, hypertension and stroke, and certain forms of cancer. A more important aspect of obesity is the regional distribution of excess body fat. Mortality and morbidity vary with the distribution of body fat, with the highest risk linked to excessive abdominal fat (central obesity). Central obesity is related to a number of diseases, including cardiovascular disease, and non-insulin dependent diabetes mellitus (NIDDM). The importance of central obesity is clear in

SECTION 1 General Gynecology

populations such as Asian who tend to have relatively low BMIs but high levels of abdominal fat, and are particularly prone to NIDDM, hypertension and coronary heart disease.

In the UK, obesity in women of childbearing age is rising. Data from health survey for England (2004)[22] revealed that 12.1% of women aged 16–24, 16.9% of women aged 25–34 and 24% of women aged 35–44 had BMI greater than 30 kg/m². This has important implications for the reproductive health of women. There is an increased risk of menstrual disorders in women who are obese such as oligomenorrhea, amenorrhea and irregular menstrual cycles. Endometrial hyperplasia is more common, both pre- and postmenopausally, in women who are obese as androgens produced by the adrenal glands are converted into estrogens (estrone) in adipose tissue by aromatase. The risk of breast and endometrial cancer is increased. The relationship between obesity and endometrial cancer has been known for many years. Increased risk of endometrial cancer is noted in diabetes, polycystic ovary syndrome and hypertension, all of which have relationship to increased BMI. Endometrioid carcinomas which constitute around 80% of endometrial cancers are considered to be more estrogen-dependent and, associated with hyperlipidemia and obesity. Maternal obesity is associated with many risks to the pregnancy, with increased risk of miscarriage, gestational diabetes, pre-eclampsia, thromboembolism, operative delivery, perinatal mortality and macrosomia.[7] Obese women are more likely to experience subfertility. Figure 10.1 illustrates the medical complications of obesity.

The International Obesity Task Force (IOTF) was established in 1996 to tackle the global epidemic of obesity.[23] The IOTF aims to achieve action on the prevention and management of overweight and obesity and endeavors to create an environment that encourages and supports the development of appropriate public health policies and programs for prevention and management of obesity.

Fertility Control

In the past 50 years, the world has experienced an unprecedented increase in population growth (Fig. 10.2). Low-income countries still have the world's highest birth rates.

In low-income countries more than a third of the population is under age 15 compared with less than a fifth in high-income countries. Between 1980 and 2030, the population of low- and middle-income countries will more than double, to 7 billion, compared with 1 billion for high income countries. Rapid population growth rates can make it difficult for countries to raise standards of living and protect the environment because the more people there

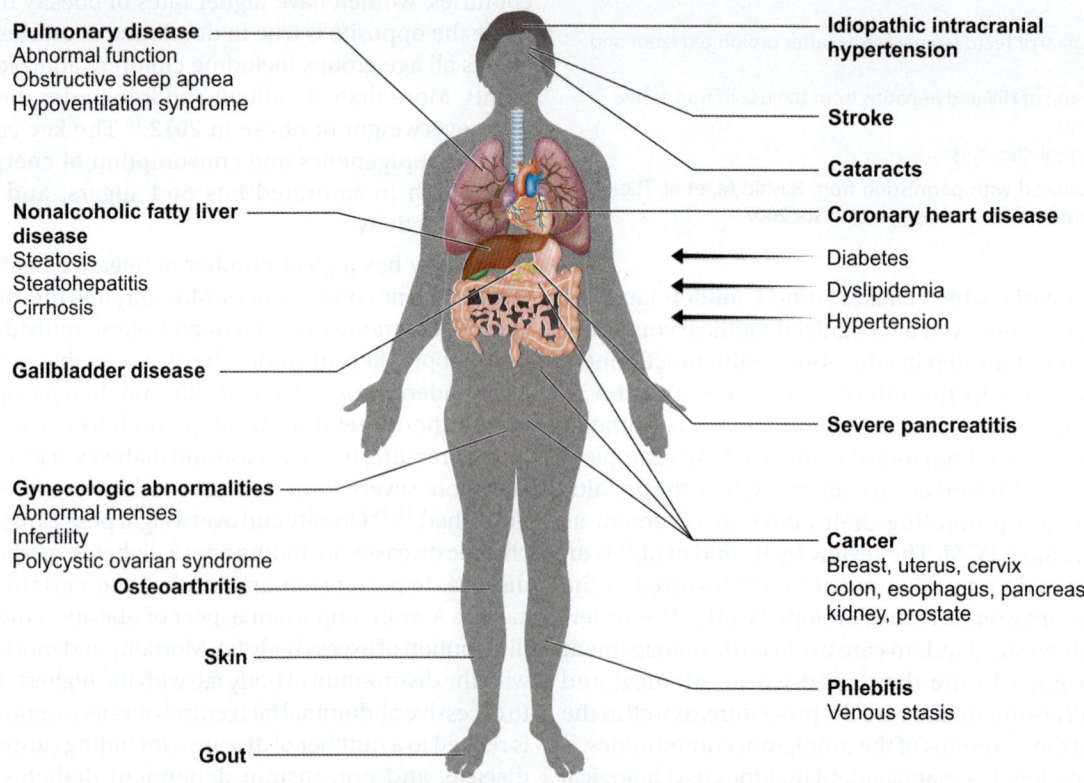

Fig. 10.1: Medical complications of obesity.

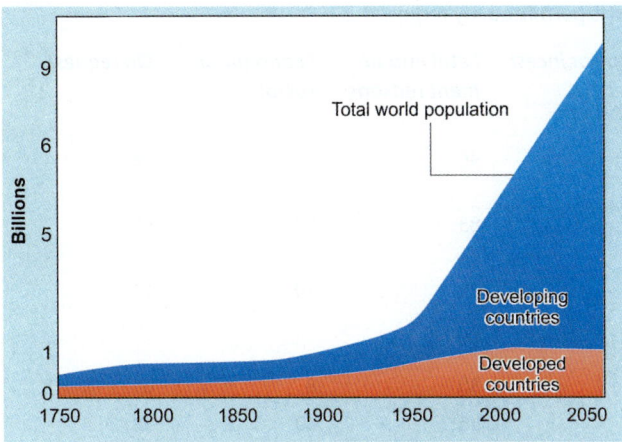

Fig. 10.2: World population 1750–2050.[24]

are, the greater the need for food, health care, education, houses, land, jobs, and energy. This will impact negatively on the reproductive health of women. Increased access to immunization and disease eradication programs has seen population growth rate in low- and middle-income countries decrease.

Experience shows that there are three successful strategies to reduce fertility rates. People should have greater access to primary health care and family planning services. Secondly, they should receive a basic education, especially girls and women. Finally, they should have access to government services that help protect them when they are sick, old or unemployed.

In recent decades, there have been tremendous advances in the development of safer and more effective contraceptives, and in the provision of affordable and accessible family planning services. Yet millions of individuals and couples around the world are unable to plan their families as they wish. It is estimated that over 120 million couples do not use contraceptives, despite wanting to space or limit their childbearing. In addition, many women who use contraceptives nevertheless become pregnant. This may be due to lack of services or barriers to their access. Services may be of poor quality and choice of methods may be limited or inappropriate. There may be broader social issues such as individual's lack of knowledge, power imbalance within couples, and sociocultural, religious and gender barriers.

In seeking to ensure that the maximum numbers of people are able to access the services they need, the department of reproductive health[15] focuses on four objectives. Firstly, it aims to increase the availability of high quality services. Secondly, it aims to broaden the range of safe, effective, acceptable and affordable family planning and infertility technologies and interventions that is available to all women and men. Thirdly, it aims to strengthen the capacity of national health systems to ensure the availability of high-quality and sustainable family planning programs and services in resource poor settings. Finally, it aims to promote an environment at international level that is supportive of family planning.

UNSAFE ABORTION

Unsafe abortion is a persistent, preventable pandemic. According to WHO, an estimated 22 million unsafe abortions took place worldwide in 2008, almost all in developing countries where abortion is highly restricted by law or if legally permitted, safe abortion is not easily accessible. Abortion rates are over 30 per 1000 in Eastern Africa, Middle Africa and South America.[25]

Deaths due to unsafe abortion remain close to 13% of all maternal deaths but account for a higher proportion of maternal deaths in Latin America (17%) and Southeast Asia (19%). About half of all deaths from unsafe abortion are in Asia, with most of the remainder in Africa. Unsafe abortion-related deaths have, however, reduced to 47000 in 2008 from 56000 in 2003.[25] Millions of women are estimated to suffer major abortion-related morbidities.[26] Of these, more than 3 million suffer from the effects of reproductive tract infection and nearly 1.7 million will develop secondary infertility. In developing countries the risk of death is estimated at 1 in 270 unsafe procedures. Despite its significance, it remains one of the most neglected global public health problem.

Leading causes of death are hemorrhage, infection, and poisoning from substances used to induce abortion. Unsafe abortion can result in complications such as sepsis, anemia from hemorrhage, cervical tear, pelvic abscess, uterine perforation with peritonitis, injury to gut, chemical vaginitis, vaginal laceration and vesicovaginal fistula. Chronic complications can include chronic pelvic pain, pelvic inflammatory disease and infertility. Legalization of abortion at request is a necessary step towards reducing the burden of unsafe abortion. When abortion is made legal, safe, and easily accessible, women's illness related to complications of abortion are dramatically reduced.

In developed countries where abortion is legal, it has become one of the safest procedures with minimum morbidity and a negligible risk of death. However, in some countries such as India, where abortion has been legal for decades, access to competent care remains restricted because of other barriers. Abortion is a crime in many countries. Examples include Chile, Honduras, El Salvado, Nicaragua and the Vatican. Portugal voted to legalize abortion up to 10 weeks of gestation in February 2007. In Kenya, abortion is legal only to save the mother's life but there are 300,000 unsafe abortions per year accounting for 50% of the countries maternal mortality.[27] Table 10.2 outlines the conditions under which abortion is legally permitted in various countries.[18]

Table 10.2: Percentage of countries by legal grounds on which abortion is permitted, by region.[25]

Country or region	To save the woman's life	To preserve physical health	To preserve maternal health	Rape or incest	Fetal impairment reasons	Economic or social	On request
All countries (n = 193)	98	67	65	49	46	34	28
Developed regions (n = 48)	98	90	88	85	85	79	69
Developing regions (n = 145)	97	60	57	37	32	19	15
Africa (n = 53)	100	58	55	30	30	8	6
Asia[1] (n = 45)	100	67	62	49	56	40	38
Europe (n = 43)	98	88	85	84	86	79	70
Other developed countries[2] (n = 5)	100	100	80	100	80	80	60

[1] Japan, Australia and New Zealand have been excluded [2]
Source: Reproduced with permission from WHO

The availability of modern contraception can reduce but never eliminate the need for abortion. In several countries of Central and Eastern Europe, abortion rates declined rapidly with the establishment of family planning services and increase in the availability of contraception. All patients seeking abortion or treatment of a complication should be offered contraceptive counseling and a choice of appropriate methods. Results of many studies in Latin America and Africa have shown that after having an abortion, patients will accept contraception at high rates. Where contraception is inaccessible or of poor quality, many women will seek to terminate unintended pregnancies, despite restrictive laws and lack of adequate abortion services. Prevention of unplanned pregnancies by improving access to quality family planning services must therefore be the highest priority, followed by improving the quality of abortion services, where legal, and of post-abortion care.

The advent of the vacuum aspiration in the 1960s revolutionized the primary prevention of complications in developing countries. Vacuum aspiration is safer than sharp curettage, and the WHO recommends vacuum aspiration as the preferred method for uterine evacuation before 12 weeks of pregnancy. The combined use of mifepristone and misoprostol has become the standard WHO recommended medical regimen for early medication abortion, and is better than either drug alone. However, mifepristone can be expensive and is not available in much of the world, whereas misoprostol is cheap and widely available. Regimens with misoprostol alone as an abortifacient have varied widely, with reported success rates ranging between 87 and 97%. Improved access to misoprostol has been associated with improved women's health in developing countries.

Treating the complications of unsafe abortion overwhelms impoverished health care services and diverts limited resources from other critical health care programs. The burden of abortion to society due to restrictive laws in many countries and inadequate services is likely to persist for many decades.

PELVIC INFLAMMATORY DISEASE AND SEXUALLY TRANSMITTED INFECTIONS

According to WHO, more than 1 million people acquire an sexually transmitted infection (STI) each day and an estimated 500 million people become ill with one of 4 STIs: chlamydia, gonorrhea, syphilis and trichomoniasis. More than 530 million people become ill with the virus that causes genital herpes (HSV2). More than 290 million women have the human papilloma virus (HPV) infection.[28] STIs can have serious consequences such as mother-to-child transmission of infections and chronic diseases such as pelvic inflammatory disease (PID). The exact incidence of PID is unknown because the disease cannot be diagnosed reliably from the clinical signs and symptoms alone. PID and STIs are responsible for considerable morbidity worldwide, both directly and by increasing the risk of transmission of human immunodeficiency virus (HIV).

PID accounts for one of the main causes of acute gynecological admission. Factors associated with PID include young age, low socioeconomic class and lower educational attainment.

Pelvic inflammatory disease carries a high morbidity: About 20% of infected women become infertile, 20% develop chronic pelvic pain, and 10% of those who conceive develop ectopic pregnancy. Therefore, education and promoting safe sexual health, especially for the younger age group is of paramount importance. Early diagnosis and prompt treatment with antibiotics can prevent sequelae of PID. Drug resistance, especially for gonorrhea, is a major threat to reducing the impact of STIs internationally. The detailed treatment of PID and STIs is discussed elsewhere in this book.

CHILDBIRTH AND MATERNAL MORTALITY

Millennium development goal number 5 is aimed at improving maternal health by reducing maternal mortality ratio by three quarters (between 1990 and 2015) and achieve (by 2015) universal access to reproductive health. The maternal mortality ratio dropped by 45% between 1990 and 2013, from 380 to 210 deaths per 100,000 live births.[1] All regions have made progress in this respect. In Eastern Asia, Northern Africa and Southern Asia, maternal mortality has declined by about two-thirds. The proportion of deliveries in developing regions attended by skilled health personnel rose from 56 in 1990 to 68% in 2012. The maternal mortality ratio in developing regions is still 14 times higher than in developed regions. The rural-urban gap in skilled care has narrowed. More women are receiving antenatal care. In developing regions, antenatal care increased from 65% in 1990 to 83% in 2012. Only half of women in developing regions receive the recommended amount of health care they need. Fewer teens are having children in most developing regions. The largest increase in contraceptive use in the 1990s was not matched in the 2000s. The need for family planning is slowly being met for more women, but demand is increasing at rapid pace. Official development assistance for reproductive health care and family remains low. WHO global reproductive health strategy (2004) is aimed at accelerating progress towards attainment of these international development goals and targets.[10]

Reproductive health conditions, including HIV/AIDS, are the leading cause of death and illness in women of reproductive age (15–44 years of age) worldwide. Worldwide an estimated 250 million years of reproductive life are lost every year as a result of reproductive health problems. The poor disproportionately bear the consequences of poor reproductive health, especially impoverished women and young people. There are glaring disparities in access to reproductive health care between rich and poor, within and among countries.

Complications during pregnancy and childbirth are a leading cause of death and disability among women of reproductive age in developing countries. An estimated 529,000 women died from complications of pregnancy and childbirth in 2000. An estimated 8 to 20 million suffer serious morbidity each year. A mother's death has devastating consequences to the children left behind. Virtually all maternal deaths (99%) occur in developing countries. Ninety-five percent of all maternal deaths occur in Asia and Africa. Less than 1% occurs in the developed world due to availability of life saving care.[20]

Hemorrhage and hypertensive disorders are major contributors to maternal deaths in developing countries. Hemorrhage is the leading cause of maternal mortality in Africa, accounting for 34% of maternal deaths, and also in Asia, where it accounts for 31% of maternal deaths.[29] Over 80% of maternal deaths are due to direct causes and the rest are due to indirect causes such as anemia and malaria.

Neonatal death rates closely follow the figures for maternal mortality. Over 50% of infant deaths occur during the neonatal period, nearly two-thirds of which occur during the first week of birth. These are mostly due to perinatal causes.

CONCLUSION

Reproductive health of women should be a national priority for each country. There is a wide disparity in maternal health indices between developing and developed countries. Interventions should start in the adolescent period. With increasing literacy, better earnings and empowerment, women will be in a better position to make appropriate reproductive choices. Access to quality health service for all pregnant women and infants should be made available. Reduction in maternal and perinatal mortality should be the topmost priority for any national health strategy. Collaboration between government and non-governmental organizations (NGOs), and health professionals is needed to achieve the unmet need of many women and their babies.

Most maternal deaths in developing countries are preventable through adequate nutrition, appropriate health care, including access to family planning, the presence of a skilled birth attendant during delivery and emergency obstetric care.

REFERENCES

1. Goal 5. Improve maternal health. United Nations millennium development goals. (http://www.un.org/millenniumgoals/pdf/Goal 5_fs.pdf -accessed July 2014).
2. Goal 6. Combat HIV/AIDS, malaria and other diseases. United Nations millennium development goals. (http://www.un.org/millenniumgoals/pdf/Goal_6_fs.pdf- accessed July 2014).
3. World population prospects: The 2004 revision. New York, United Nations, 2005.
4. Census of India. (http://censusindia.gov.in/- accessed July 2014).
5. United Nations Population Fund. Adolescents and youth. (http://unfpa.org/public/home/adolescents/pid/6485- accessed July 2014).
6. Adolescent health. World Health Organization. (www.who.int/entity/maternal_child_adolescent/topics/maternal/adolescent_pregnancy/en/- accessed July 2014).
7. School TO, Hediger ML, Belsky DH. Prenatal care and maternal health during adolescent pregnancy: A review and meta-analysis. Adolesc Health. 1994;15(6):444-56.
8. India-adolescent fertility rate. (http://www.indexmundi.com/facts/india/adolescent-fertility-rate- accessed July 2014).
9. Global sex survey 2004. (http://www.durex.com-accessed November 2007).
10. Reproductive health strategy to accelerate progress towards the attainment of international development goals and targets. Geneva, World Health Organization, 2004 (Document NO. WHO/RHR/04.S).
11. World Health Organization. Female genital mutilation- a joint WHO/UNICEF/UNFPA statement. WHO, Geneva, 1997.
12. Female genital mutilation. World Health Organization. Fact sheet No 241. (http://www.who.int/mediacentre/factsheets/fs241/en/-accessed July 2014).
13. Rashid M, Rashid MH. Obstetric management of women with female genital mutilation. The Obstetrician and Gynaecologist. 2007;9:95-101.
14. Central Intelligence Agency. The world fact book. Adult prevalence of obesity. (https://www.cia.gov/library/publications/the-world-factbook/rankorder/2228rank.html-accessed July 2014).
15. Marie NG, Emmanuela Gakidou, et al. Global, regional, and national prevalence of overweight and obesity in children and adults during 1980–2013: a systematic analysis for the Global Burden of Disease Study 2013. The Lancet. 2014; DOI: 10.1016/S0140-6736(14)60460-8.
16. Overweight and obese. World Health Organization. Fact sheet No. 311. (http://www.who.int/mediacentre/factsheets/fs311/en/- accessed September 2014).
17. Sawaya AL, Martins P, Hoffman D, Roberts SB. The link between childhood undernutrition and chronic diseases in adulthood: a case study of Brazil. Nutr Rev. 2003;61(5 Pt 1):168-75.
18. Victoria CG, Adair L, Fall C, et al. Maternal and child undernutrition study group. Maternal and child undernutrition: consequences for adult health and human capital. Lancet. 2008:371;340-57.
19. Sawaya AL, Martins PA, Grillo LP, et al. Long-term effects of early malnutrition on body weight regulation. Nutr Rev. 2004:62; 127-33.
20. Sawaya AL, Sesso R, Florencio TM, et al. Association between chronic undernutrition and hypertension. Matern Child Nutr. 2005:1;155-63.
21. Sawaya AL, Martins PA, Baccin Martins VI, et al. Malnutrition, long-term health and the effect of nutritional recovery. Nestle Nutr Workshop Ser Pediatr Program. 2009:63;95-105.
22. Health survey for England 2004. London: Department of Health; 2006.
23. The global challenge of obesity and the International Obesity Task Force. (http://www.iuns.org/affiliated_bodies/international-obesity-task-force-iotf-accessed September 2014).
24. World population growth. World Bank. (http://www.worldbank.org/depweb/beyond/beyondco/beg_03.pdf-accessed-September 2014).
25. Unsafe abortion. Global and regional estimates of the incidence of unsafe abortion and associated mortality in 2008. Sixth edition. World Health Organization. (http://whqlibdoc.who.int/publications/2011/9789241501118_eng.pdf?ua=1-accessed-August 2014).
26. Grimes DA, Benson J, Sigh S, et al. Unsafe abortion: the preventable pandemic. The Lancet. Sexual and reproductive health series, October, 2006.
27. Kent A. Snippets: What's new in other journals? BJOG. 2007; 114:1451-2.
28. Sexually transmitted infections. Fact sheet No. 110. World Health Organization. (http://www.who.int/mediacentre/factsheets/fs110/en/-accessed September 2014).
29. Khan KS, Wojdyla D, Say L, et al. WHO analysis of causes of maternal death: A systematic review. Lancet. 2006;367: 1066-74.

CHAPTER 11

Endometriosis and Adenomyosis

Siti Zawiah Omar

Overview

- Endometriosis is a "Disease of Enigma", remaining a challenging condition for clinicians, patients and researches.
- Its clinical presentation is variable; the most reliable diagnostic test is laparoscopy.
- The etiology, pathophysiology and progression is still poorly understood.
- Problems still exist in determining who and when to treat and for how long following the diagnosis.
- Adenomyosis, although considered a variant of endometriosis, is different because of its behavior. It causes excessive per vaginal bleeding, and is unresponsive to hormonal therapy or endometrial curettage.

INTRODUCTION

Endometriosis is a relatively common and potentially debilitating condition affecting women of reproductive age. It is defined as the presence of endometrial-like tissue outside the uterus, which induces a chronic, inflammatory reaction.[1]

Endometriosis can be asymptomatic, but those with symptoms generally present early in reproductive life and improve after menopause. Symptomatic endometriosis can result in long-term adverse effects on personal relationships, quality of life, and work productivity.

OCCURRENCE

The prevalence of endometriosis in the general population is not known, but it is estimated that 2–10% of women in the reproductive age group have endometriosis. Interestingly, endometriosis is noted in 5–15% of women undergoing gynecologic laparotomies.[2]

ETIOLOGY

The etiology of endometriosis is unknown, although there have been many theories[3,4] to explain the various manifestations of endometriosis and the different locations where the endometriotic implants can be found.

Sampson's Retrograde Menstruation

This retrograde menstruation theory proposes that endometrial fragments transported through the fallopian tubes at the time of menstruation and subsequently implant on the pelvic peritoneum and the organs surrounding it. Endometriosis is also found in women with genital tract anomalies where there is obstruction to the menstrual flow.

Meyer's Coelomic Epithelium (Müllerian) Transformation

The Müllerian metaplasia theory proposes that endometriosis results from the metaplastic transformation of peritoneal mesothelium into endometrium and may be due to hormonal stimuli or inflammatory irritation.

Genetic and Immunological Factors

There appears to be an increased incidence in first-degree relatives of patients with endometriosis and a higher prevalence among oriental women and a low prevalence in women of Afro-Caribbean origin. It is suggested that genetic and immunological factors may alter the susceptibility of a woman to develop endometriosis.

Vascular and Lymphatic Spread

Embolization via vascular and lymphatic channels has been demonstrated and explains the finding of endometriosis in distant sites such as the lung and the pleural cavity.

CLINICAL MANIFESTATIONS

Symptoms (Table 11.1)

The severity of the patient's symptoms does not necessarily correlate with the extent of the disease. Thus, a patient may have minimal disease with severe dysmenorrhea or no symptoms but still have severe endometriosis.

Dysmenorrhea and *pelvic pain* are the most common symptoms.

Typically, the pain begins prior to the onset of the menses, increases in intensity during the flow and gradually improves with the cessation of menses.

The pelvic pain of endometriosis can be acute or chronic. Pain can be felt either in the lower abdomen, the lower back or the perineum.

Tenesmus may be a feature if the disease involves the rectovaginal septum.

Dyspareunia of endometriosis is felt deep within the vagina and is a common symptom but is usually not volunteered by the patient unless specifically enquired by the clinician.

Abnormal per vaginal bleeding may occur with endometriosis. Menses may be irregular, heavy or inter menstrual bleeding may occur.

Table 11.1: Symptoms of endometriosis in relation to sites of involvement.

Site	Symptoms
Female reproductive system	• Dysmenorrhea • Pelvic pain • Lower abdominal pain/discomfort • Dyspareunia • Abnormal per vaginal bleeding • Infertility
Urinary system	Cyclical hematuria
Gastrointestinal system	• Tenesmus (pain on defecation) • Cyclical rectal bleeding
Umbilicus	Cyclical pain and/or bleeding
Respiratory system/thorax	• Recurrent pneumothorax/hemothorax • Cyclical hemoptysis

Endometriosis is associated with *subfertility* and up to 50% of women with endometriosis have difficulty conceiving.

Endometriosis occurring outside the pelvic cavity is rare.

Physical Examination

Endometriosis may present with minimal signs or acutely as in the case of a ruptured endometrioma. Abdominal examination may identify areas of tenderness or a palpable abdominal mass (endometrioma or chocolate cyst) arising from the pelvis.

Vaginal examination may reveal a globular enlarged uterus or a fixed retroverted uterus. Presence of tender nodular indurations along the uterosacral ligaments is pathognomonic/characteristic of endometriosis.

Rarely, endometriotic spots may be seen in the vagina or on the cervix.

A rectovaginal examination may identify a mass or nodule in the rectovaginal septum.

INVESTIGATIONS

Transvaginal ultrasound may detect endometriomas and the typical finding described as "kissing ovaries" with echogenic material within situated behind the body of uterus. Ultrasound is of limited value for detection of small endometriotic deposits.

Other imaging modalities are of limited value except for magnetic resonance imaging (MRI) which may help in presurgical planning of resection of the rectovaginal septum nodule.

To date no individual serum marker has been found to specifically correlate with symptoms of endometriosis.

Measurement of Serum CA-125

Women with endometriosis often have a high (>35 U/mL) level of serum CA-125. It is nonspecific as a diagnostic tool but is sometimes useful in monitoring the response of disease with treatment and subsequent follow-up.

Laparoscopy

Laparoscopy remains the main confirmatory diagnostic tool; besides it has the therapeutic advantage of carrying out concurrent surgical diathermy and/or surgical excision of endometriotic lesions. Endometriotic lesions at laparoscopy are typically described as "powder burn"; these are small brown/black puckered lesions (Fig. 11.1). Other features that can be seen are white fibrous lesions or a chocolate cyst (endometrioma) (Fig. 11.2).

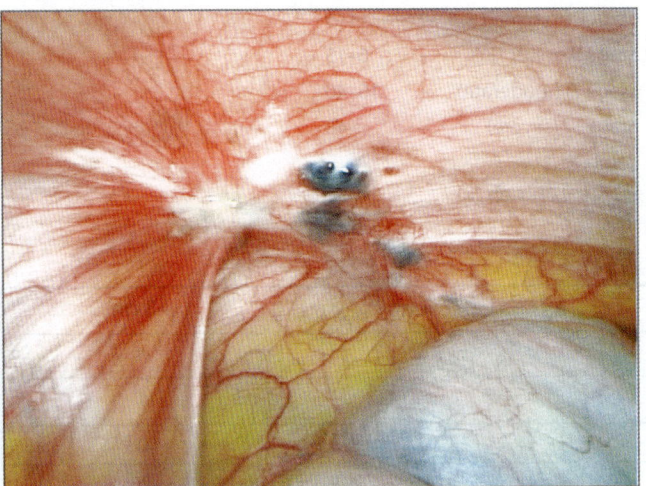

Fig. 11.1: Laparoscopy view of pigmented and non-pigmented endometriotic lesion (powder burn—brown or black lesion).

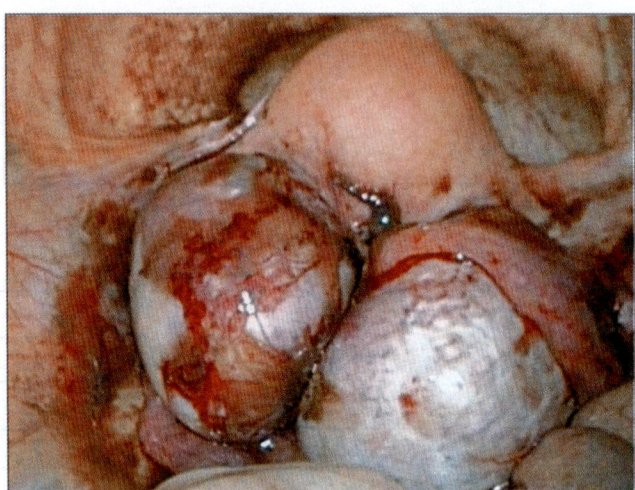

Fig. 11.2: Endometrioma or chocolate cysts.

STAGING

Staging the disorder helps physicians formulate a treatment plan and evaluate response to therapy. According to the American Society for Reproductive Medicine, endometriosis may be classified as stage I (minimal), II (mild), III (moderate), or IV (severe), based on number, location, and depth of implants, and presence of endometriomas and filmy or dense adhesions (Table 11.2).

Documentation of laparoscopic and or laparotomy findings (Fig. 11.3) can also help in management of cases currently and incase of recurrence of disease in the future.

MANAGEMENT[5,6]

Patients with endometriosis present a challenge to physicians not only from the diagnostic but also treatment point of view. It is difficult to achieve a complete cure; it has a tendency to recur. Often coexistent diseases, such as irritable bowel/constipation, may be present and these may affect the quality of life.

Table 11.2: Staging of endometriosis.

Stage	Classification	Description
I	Minimal	A few superficial implants
II	Mild	More and slightly deeper implants
III	Moderate	Many deep implants, small endometriomas on one or both ovaries, and some filmy adhesions
IV	Severe	Many deep implants, large endometriomas on one or both ovaries, and many dense adhesions, sometimes with the rectum adhering to the back of the uterus

Box 11.1: Treatment strategies for endometriosis.

- Pelvic pain
- Infertility
- Pelvic masses/endometriomas

Box 11.2: Factors to consider when individualizing therapy for endometriosis.

- Severity of symptoms
- Extent of disease and location
- Desire for fertility
- Age
- Medication side effects
- Surgical complications
- Cost

Treatment should, therefore, be individualized. This should be tailored taking into account her age, severity of symptoms, extent of disease and the desire for future childbearing (Boxes 11.1 and 11.2).

Medical Therapy

Analgesics

Nonsteroidal anti-inflammatory drugs (NSAIDs) are potent analgesics helpful in reducing severity of dysmenorrhea and pelvic pain. Its use is for symptom control only and has no effect on curing the disease.

Combined Oral Contraceptive Agents

Combined oral contraceptive (COC) is a good choice for women with minimal or mild pain who also want to prevent pregnancy. This works primarily by inhibiting ovulation. Clinicians can consider prescribing a combined hormonal contraceptive, as it reduces endometriosis-associated

SECTION 1 General Gynecology

Patient's Sticker		Stage I (minimal)	–	1–5
		Stage II (mild)	–	6–15
		Stage III (moderate)	–	16–40
		Stage IV (severe)	–	>40
		Total		

Laparoscopy/Laparotomy

Date performed: _____

	Endometriosis	< 1 cm	1-3 cm	>3 cm
Peritoneum	Superficial	1	2	4
	Deep	2	4	6
Ovary	R Superficial	1	2	4
	Deep	4	16	20
	L Superficial	1	2	4
	Deep	4	16	20
	Posterior cul-de-sac obliteration	Partial		Complete
		4		40
	Adhesions	<1/3 enclosure	1/3–2/3 enclosure	>2/3 enclosure
Ovary	R Filmy	1	2	4
	Dense	4	8	16
	L Filmy	1	2	4
	Dense	4	8	16
Tube	R Filmy	1	2	4
	Dense	4*	8*	16
	L Filmy	1	2	4
	Dense	4*	8*	16

*If the fimbriated of the fallopian tube is completed enclosed, change the point assignment to 16.

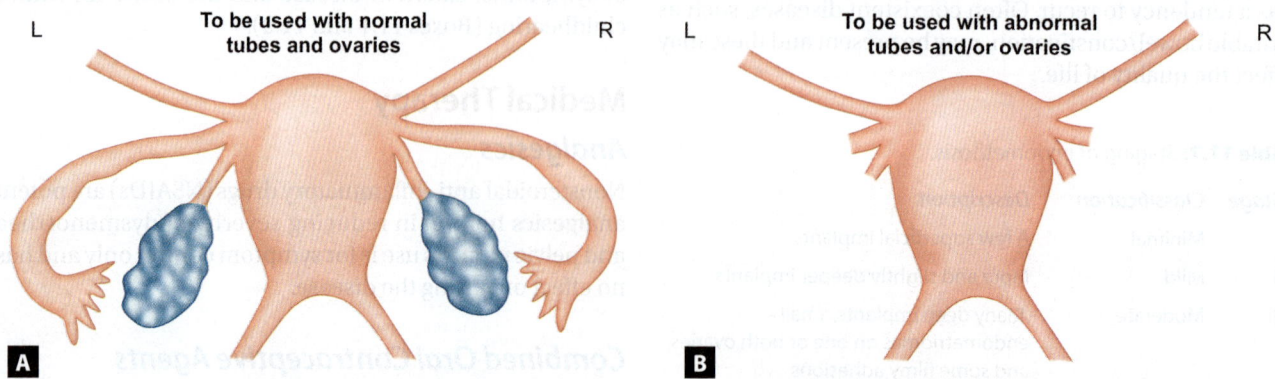

Figs. 11.3A and B: Modified American Fertility Society classification of endometriosis.

dyspareunia, dysmenorrhea and non-menstrual pain.[7] oral contraceptives (OCs) may retard the progression of disease but evidence is conflicting. If pain does not respond well to cyclic therapy, switching to continuous OC administration may be effective.

Non-oral estrogen-progestin contraceptives such as the ring or patch may also be effective but have not been studied extensively.

Dienogest

Dienogest is a progestin with several beneficial properties that enable it to be a treatment targeted for endometriosis. It has a high specificity for progesterone receptors and demonstrates anti-androgenic properties. At an oral dose of 2 mg/day, dienogest completely inhibits ovulation, but estradiol levels remain within the suggested 'therapeutic window' for endometriosis treatment.

In a dedicated clinical study program in over 600 women with endometriosis,[8] dienogest has been shown to be well-tolerated, and to provide highly effective pain relief with significant lesion reduction. Hypoestrogenic effects such as hot flushes, reduced bone mineral density, dryness of vagina, and reduced libido were not observed in this study. There was no associated interference of lipid metabolism.

Gonadotropin Releasing Hormone Agonist

Gonadotropin releasing hormone agonist (GnRH) agonist may be considered for treatment of moderate to severe pain, associated with endometriosis. Randomized trials[9] have shown that GnRH agonist is more effective than placebo and is as effective as other medical therapy for relieving pain and reducing the size of endometriotic implants. With add-back therapy, side-effects are better tolerated than those with progesterone or danazol.

GnRh agonist is administered either by daily nasal spray or intramuscular injection every month or every three months (depending on the preparation). Treatment is continued for approximately 6 to 9 months. The *disadvantages* include cost, loss of bone mineral density and intolerable hypoestrogenic side effects.

OTHER OPTIONS

Another option that's available is **Danazol**; this is a synthetic 17 alpha ethinyltestosterone derivative. It is used to suppress symptoms of endometriosis if fertility is not a present concern.

It's been specifically approved for the treatment of endometriosis and it works by creating a hyperandrogenic and hypoestrogenic state, which then creates a hostile environment for the growth of endometriotic lesions.

However, it can cause significant side effects that may result in patients not tolerating the medication very well; these include weight gain, muscle cramps, acne, seborrhea, decreased breast size, hirsutism, clitoral hypertrophy and hoarseness of the voice. In view of these side effects, it is only prescribed for 6–9 months.

Aromatase inhibitors, such as *letrozole* and *anastrozole*, have been used to treat deep seated endometriosis in combination with OCPs, progestogens or GnRH analogues. They appear to work by regulating the estrogen formation locally in the endometriotic lesions, as well as in the ovary and the brain. Side effects such as headache, stiffness or joint pain, nausea, diarrhea and flushing limits their use.

Gestrinone, an anti-progestogen, is now not commonly used due to its androgenic side effects.

SURGICAL TREATMENT

Indications for Surgical Intervention

The indications include the diagnosis of unresolved pelvic pain, symptoms that are severe and refractory to medical treatment, an advanced or in an anatomic position that is causing problems to other organs such as bowel, bladder or kidneys and in emergencies such as rupture of an endometrioma, bowel obstruction, etc.

Approaches to Surgical Treatment

1. Conservative surgery refers to excision or ablation of lesions at the time of laparoscopy or laparotomy.
2. Definitive refers to hysterectomy with or without bilateral salpingo-oophorectomy.

When performing surgery for ovarian endometrioma, surgeons should perform cystectomy instead of drainage and coagulation, as cystectomy reduces endometriosis-associated pain.

Hysterectomy should only be performed in patients who have persistent, refractory symptoms of endometriosis, those who are not interested in future childbearing and have had previously failed medical therapy and have had at least one conservative treatment procedure. The performance of bilateral salpingo-oophorectomy at the same time is only indicated if reducing the risk of reoperation down the line due to recurrence of endometriosis symptoms outweigh the risks of premature menopause.

This procedure may not completely exclude the possibility of symptom recurrence down the line.

Laparoscopy

Laparoscopy remains a safe and well-tolerated procedure in the hands of an experienced surgeon. As long as the best practice techniques are followed closely, there is a very good success rate. However, incomplete treatment can happen if disease is not recognized at the time of surgery because of non-visibility or technicality resulting in persistent symptoms and recurrent disease.

Hysterectomy Bilateral Salpingo-oophorectomy

When considering hysterectomy and bilateral salpingo-oophorectomy, the surgical approaches can be laparotomy, laparoscopy or a vaginal approach. This depends on the extent of the disease and the presence or absence of adhesions or involvement of adjacent organs. The procedure does not 100% guarantee relief of symptoms, but the chance is very high as endometriosis is said to be hormonally dependant. The probability of pain after hysterectomy is 15% and the risk of pain worsening is 3–5%. Bilateral salpingo-oophorectomy is very rarely considered for patients younger than 40 years of age because of the associated risk of early menopause.

Surgery for deep endometriosis is possible and effective, but is associated with significant complication rates, particularly when bowel surgery is required.[5]

The reported total intraoperative complication rate is 2.1% and total postoperative complication rate is 13.9%. Patients would be better referred and managed in a tertiary referral center with experienced gynecologists and multidisciplinary backup of colorectal surgeon and urologist whenever the need arises.

Various anti-adhesion agents have been used and proven effective for adhesion prevention.[5] Surgeons should not perform laparoscopic uterosacral nerve ablation (LUNA) as an additional procedure to conservative surgery to reduce endometriosis-associated pain.[10] Although, presacral neurectomy (PSN) is effective to reduce endometriosis-associated midline pain, it requires a high degree of skill and is a potentially hazardous procedure.

ENDOMETRIOSIS AND INFERTILITY

Endometriosis is associated with subfertility and up to 50% of women with endometriosis have difficulty conceiving naturally. The cause and effect of endometriosis on subfertility remains controversial. Although, it is known that without intervention, women with more severe disease are less likely to conceive. There are conflicting results regarding the reproductive outcomes associated with subfertile women with varying severity of endometriosis undergoing assisted reproductive technology (ART).

A systematic review and meta-analysis[11] shows that women with endometriosis undertaking ART have a similar live birth rate, a lower clinical pregnancy rate, and lower mean number of oocytes retrieved per cycle when compared with those without endometriosis. Although, women with less severe disease (American Society of Reproductive Medicine I–II) have a similar reproductive outcomes compared with those with no endometriosis, women with more severe disease (American Society of Reproductive Medicine III–IV) had a 30% lower live birth rate, 40% lower clinical pregnancy rate, and lower mean number of oocytes retrieved when compared with women with no endometriosis.

With regard to the effect of surgery, one study showed some evidence of benefit for treating less severe endometriosis before ART (American Society of Reproductive Medicine I–II). Given that this is the only available study comparing groups of women who had surgical treatment with those who had no treatment, this result needs to be interpreted with caution. The nature of the study does not allow a high level of recommendation and does not imply laparoscopy should be performed in all asymptomatic patients before ART only to diagnose and treat less severe endometriosis to improve the result of the ART treatment. Our subgroup analysis,[11] however, suggests that surgical treatment before ART in women with more severe endometriosis (American Society of Reproductive Medicine III–IV) is associated with a lower live birth rate, clinical pregnancy rate, and mean number of oocytes retrieved. Hence, there is insufficient evidence to recommend surgery routinely before ART.

The mechanisms accounting for a poorer reproductive outcome in women with endometriosis are largely unknown. The disease process, with a largely inflammatory component, can directly affect the oocyte quality, quantity, and the endometrial receptivity. Surgical removal of the disease just before ART, although beneficial for the reduction of symptoms and the reduction of the bulk of endometriotic disease, can damage ovarian tissue, diminish ovarian reserve, and induce adhesion formation and reformation.

ADENOMYOSIS

Introduction

Adenomyosis, although considered a variant of endometriosis, is different because of its behavior. Adenomyosis was first described by Rokitansky in 1860 and then clearly defined by von Recklinghausen in 1896. It causes chronic bleeding which is unresponsive to hormonal therapy or endometrial curettage.

It is a condition characterized by the benign invasion of endometrial glands and stroma into the myometrium of the uterus. Often this is an incidental finding on pathologic examination of hysterectomy specimens. It tends to occur in older multiparous women. About 15% of patients with adenomyosis have associated pelvic endometriosis.

Symptoms

Most women are asymptomatic; those who suffer from this condition complain of dysmenorrhea and menorrhagia. Pain is said to be due to prostaglandin release and local inflammatory changes that may disrupt the vasoconstriction of the arterial arcade supplying the endometrium. Deep thrust premenstrual dyspareunia can also be a symptom.

Signs

The uterus is generally felt globularly enlarged or bulky uterus on pelvic examination. Occasionally, if significantly enlarged, it can also be felt on abdominal palpation. Premenstrual tenderness on palpation may be present.

Investigation

The gross features of adenomyosis on *ultrasound* examination include irregular myometrial cystic spaces predominantly involving the posterior uterine wall; an enlarged uterus with a widened posterior wall; an eccentric endometrial cavity; and decreased uterine echogenicity without lobulations, contour abnormality, or mass effects (which is more commonly seen with leiomyomas) (Fig. 11.4).

Sometimes, there is loss of the junctional zone on ultrasound images, which is a subtle sign. A focal region of adenomyosis, an adenomyoma, can sometimes be seen. These lesions are more subtle than leiomyomas.

Sonograms may also show an ill-defined margin between the normal myometrium and the abnormal myometrium, as well as an elliptically shaped myometrial abnormality. However, the occurrence of adenomyosis cannot be consistently differentiated from the presence of leiomyomas by using transabdominal ultrasonography (TAUS).

Magnetic resonance imaging (MRI) is the more definitive investigation of choice as it provides excellent images of the myometrium, endometrium and adenomyosis. Although, it is more expensive than ultrasonography, MRI can be employed in cases with indeterminate sonographic results for adenomyosis or in patients who are undergoing uterine-sparing surgery for leiomyomas.

Thin-section, high-resolution MRI scans obtained with a pelvic multicoil array are optimal for diagnosing adenomyosis. The uterine zonal anatomy is best seen on T2-weighted images.

Variations in the normal thickness of the inner myometrium, or junctional zone, have been reported, with a mean thickness of 2–8 mm. Widening of this junctional zone has been associated with adenomyosis (Fig. 11.5). Furthermore, the thickness of a normal junctional zone changes with the menstrual cycle, while the thickness of diffuse adenomyosis does not.

The MRI appearance of adenomyosis can, however, change in response to hormonal stimulation and treatment. Findings from an MRI study suggested that the altered junctional zone should be at least 12 mm to avoid a high false-positive rate in the diagnosis of adenomyosis. These authors noted that myometrial contractions can appear as adenomyosis.[12]

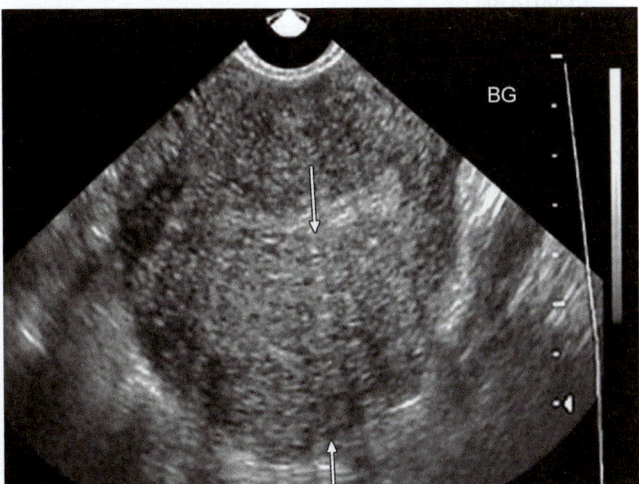

Fig. 11.4: Transvaginal sonogram of an enlarged uterus with a thickened posterior myometrium (arrows).

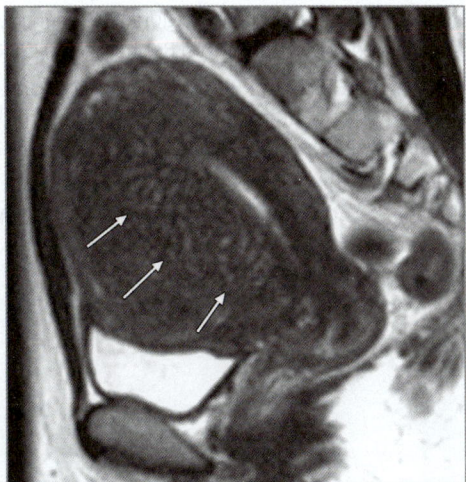

Fig. 11.5: Sagittal magnetic resonance image of an enlarged uterus with a thickened anterior myometrium. T2-weighted image without gadolinium enhancement shows a widened junctional zone of 23 mm (arrows) and focal high signal intensity (arrowheads).

The reported accuracy of MRI for diagnosing adenomyosis is high. Its sensitivity and specificity are 80–100%, with an overall accuracy of 85–90.5%.

Treatment

The treatment of adenomyosis depends on the symptoms. Any history of abnormal per vaginal or heavy bleeding in women above 35 years of age should be investigated by endometrial biopsy or cervical dilatation and endometrial curettage with or without hysteroscopy (depending on availability) to rule out malignancy.

Conservative management with NSAIDs and hormonal control of the endometrium are mainstays of therapy. COCs, dianogest, vaginal ring and levonorgestrel IUD can be used to reduce cyclic blood loss and dysmenorrhea.

Hysterectomy may be indicated for failure of medical therapy and in symptomatic women who have completed family.

CONCLUSION

- Endometriosis should be considered in the differential diagnosis of any reproductive age women presenting with abdominopelvic pain, adnexal masses or infertility.
- Accurate diagnosis and management:
  - Requires careful consideration of the patient's history and physical examination.
  - Should not be solely based on imaging or initial response to empiric therapy.
  - Other pelvic organ or tissues involvement and related symptoms will need appropriate attention.

REFERENCES

1. Kennedy S, Bergqvist A, Chapron C, D'Hooghe T, Dunselman G, Greb R, et al. ESHRE Special Interest Group for Endometriosis and Endometrium Guideline Development. ESHRE guideline for the diagnosis and treatment of endometriosis. Hum Reprod. 2005;20:2698-704.
2. Eskenazi B, Warner ML. Epidemiology of endometriosis. Obstet Gynecol Clin North Am. 1997;24:235-58.
3. Burney RO, Giudice LC. Pathogenesis and pathophysiology of endometriosis. Fertil Steril. 2012;98(3):5119.
4. Jump up^ van der Linden PJ. Theories on the pathogenesis of endometriosis. Human Reproduction (Oxford, England). 1996;11 (Suppl 3): 53-65. doi:10.1093/humrep/11.suppl_3.53. PMID 9147102.
5. Dunselman GA, Vermeulen N, Becker C, Calhaz-Jorge C, D'Hooghe T, De Bie B, et al. ESHRE guideline: management of women with endometriosis. Hum Reprod. 2014;29:400-12.
6. D' Hooghe TM, Hill JA, In: Berek JS (Ed). Berek and Novak's Gynaecology, 14th edition. Philadelphia: Lippincot Williams and Wilkins. 2007, pp 1137-84.
7. Vercellini P, Frontino G, De Giorgi O, Pietropaolo G, Pasin R, Crosignani PG. Continuous use of an oral contraceptive for endometriosis-associated recurrent dysmenorrhea that does not respond to a cyclic pill regimen. Fertil Steril. 2003;80: 560-3.
8. Strowitzki T, Marr J, Gerlinger C, Faustmann T, Seitz C. Dienogest is as effective as leuprolide acetate in treating the painful symptoms of endometriosis: a 24-week, randomized, multicentre, open-label trial. Human Reproduction. 2010;25(3): 633-41.
9. Brown J, Pan A, Hart RJ. Gonadotrophin-releasing hormone analogues for pain associated with endometriosis. Cochrane Database Syst Rev. 2010:CD008475.
10. Proctor M, Latthe P, Farquhar C, Khan K, Johnson N. Surgical interruption of pelvic nerve pathways for primary and secondary dysmenorrhoea. Cochrane Database Syst Rev. 2005: CD001896.
11. Hamdan M, Omar SZ, Dunselman G, Cheong Y. Influence of endometriosis on assisted reproductive technology outcomes: a systematic review and meta-analysis. Obstet Gynecol. 2015;125:79-88.
12. Novellas S, Chassang M, Delotte J, et al. MRI characteristics of the uterine junctional zone: from normal to the diagnosis of adenomyosis. AJR. 2011;196:1206-13.

CHAPTER 12

Pelvic Inflammatory Disease

Siya Sharan Sharma, Sucheta Jindal

Overview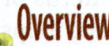

- When natural barriers to PID is absent there is increased incidence of PID.
- Endosalpingitis and exosalpingitis causes different pathology.
- PID can present as acute and chronic.
- However, the correct treatment will resolve a good number of problems.
- Sequelae of PID can have long-term effects on fertility and chronic abdominal pain.

INTRODUCTION

Pelvic inflammatory disease (PID) implies inflammation of the upper genital tract involving the uterine cavity, fallopian tubes, and the ovaries resulting in endometritis, salpingitis, oophoritis, tubo-ovarian abscess (mass) parametritis and pelvic peritonitis.

The PID lesions are usually bilateral since infection is ascending or blood born, though at times it may be unilateral. PID is caused by the microorganisms either colonizing in the endocervix or enter into the cervix from exterior via vagina and later ascending to the endometrium and fallopian tube.

NATURAL BARRIERS TO PID

Before describing the etiological factors the normal protective mechanism of female genital tract should be understood. Natural barriers to the ascent of pathogenic organisms from the vagina to the fallopian tube include (Box 12.1):

Box 12.1: Natural barriers to PID.

- Intact hymen
- Acidity of vaginal secretions inhibits the growth of bacteria
- Narrow cervical canal with alkaline mucus plug
- Downward ciliary movements of endometrial and cervical lining discouraging the ascent of non-motile organisms

VULNERABILITY TO PID

These natural protective mechanisms are impaired and render the genital tract more vulnerable to infection (Box 12.2).

ETIOLOGICAL FACTORS OF PID (TABLE 12.1)

1. **Sexually transmitted diseases (STDs) organisms:** The most common (60–75%) cause of PID is sexually transmitted diseases. Commonly PID is caused by *Neisseria gonorrhoeae* in 30% of these, and *Chlamydia trachomatis*.[1] These pathogens ascend along with mucosa and may be with sperm, to the pelvis to

Box 12.2: Vulnerability to PID.

- During menstruation
- Pregnancy: After miscarriage and termination of pregnancy (alternatively termed as abortion), delivery, and manual removal of placenta due to:
  – Widening of cervical canal and opening of internal os
  – Shedding of the protective epithelium of endometrium and cervical canal
  – Raw surface present in the uterine cavity and cervical canal
  – Vaginal pH is increased and become alkaline
- Intrauterine manipulations like dilatation and curettage
- Intrauterine contraceptive devices (IUCD) application without strict asepsis

SECTION 1 General Gynecology

Table 12.1: Organisms responsible for PID.

Common	• Neisseria gonorrhoeae • Chlamydia trachomatis
Occasional	• Gardnerella vaginalis • Mycoplasma hominis or genitalium • Tubercular bacillus • Escherichia coli
Rare	• Haemophilus influenzae • Group A Streptococci • Pneumococci

cause salpingo-oophoritis. Endogenous vaginal microorganisms as *Gardnerella vaginalis* is often cause PID.[2] The infection by anaerobic organisms is greatly favored by blood loss, anemia, and tissue damage as seen in septic hemorrhage.

2. **Postabortal and post-delivery (Puerperal) sepsis**: This is the second most common cause of the PID. The incidence of PID in about one third of the all patients is due to this factor. An illegal and septic abortion by untrained persons is the common factor. After delivery in some cases manual removal of placenta may induce ascending infections.
3. **Operative procedures**: Minor surgical procedures such as dilatation and curettage, hysterosalpingography, and sonosalpingography, may cause acquired ascending infection resulting in PID.
4. **Intrauterine contraceptive devices (IUCD)**: IUCD users are in no way having higher incidence of PID. If the asepsis is maintained during IUCD insertion and the IUCD users maintain hygiene, the incidence of PID is not more.

Pathology of Acute PID

Exterior of the Fallopian Tube (Exosalpingitis)

The fallopian tube is swollen, edematous, and congested or hyperemic with dilated vessels on the serosal surface. Serous exudation is usually seen around the tube. From the fimbrial end, seropurulent discharge is the strongest feature in favor of salpingitis. Peritoneal surface may be congested in the pelvis.

Interior of the Fallopian Tube (Endosalpingitis)

In ascending infection, the mucosa is the first one to be affected. The mucous membrane inflammation with edema, redness and deciliation is the initial stage of salpingitis. Submucosa is infiltrated with leukocytes and plasma cells. The inflammatory exudate is discharged into the lumen. The inflammatory response leads to breach of mucosal surface and adhesions are formed between mucosal folds of the tube. This leads to narrowing and finally blockage of the tube resulting into the infertility. The inflammation extends to the serosal surface in later stage.

In early part of this inflammatory process fimbrial end remains open, and allows the seropurulent secretions to be discharged into the peritoneal cavity. The collection of this pus may lead to **pelvic abscess**. In later part of the disease, fimbria get adherent to each other by fibrinous adhesions and fimbriae are drawn into the tube leading to closure of fimbrial opening. With continuous secretion of such exudates the ampullary portion of the tube is distended. The formation of retort shape **pyosalpinx** follows. Once ovaries are involved with tube a **tubo-ovarian mass** is formed where both tube and ovary are entangled in adhesions. The pyosalpinx or TO mass becomes adherent to posterior surface of the uterus or broad ligament involving ovaries, sigmoid colon, and loops of small intestine. Tubal wall appears thickened and tense. In advanced stages and untreated cases of PID, pelvic and general peritonitis may occur associated with paralytic ileus and rarely sub-diaphragmatic, perinephric abscess, and even septicemia.

Usually, infection through cervix and endometrium causes endosalpingitis affecting inner lumen of tube and fimbriae, leading to pyosalpinx or hydrosalpinx. While it is interesting to note that in some patients, specially after abortion or vaginal delivery, infection through cervix spreads via lymphatics to parametrium and broad ligament causing parametritis. Finally this reaches to outer aspect of tube causing exosalpingitis.

Pathology of Chronic PID (Tubo-ovarian Mass)

This form of disease is the continuation of the acute form if the infection fails to resolve completely due to inadequate antibiotic treatment or reinfection. This may result in tubo-ovarian mass formation, which may present as (Flowchart 12.1):

1. Hydrosalpinx
2. Chronic pyosalpinx
3. Tubo-ovarian cyst
4. Chronic interstitial salpingitis.

Hydrosalpinx

In PID hydrosalpinx, which is bilateral, is the end result of previous acute salpingitis. Fimbrial end is closed and fimbriae are drawn into the tube. It is retort shape clear fluid collection in the ampullary part of the tube. Outer surface appears smooth; wall is thin and translucent. Commonly, it is adherent to surrounding structures but occasionally if it is mobile it may undergo torsion causing acute pain abdomen.

CHAPTER 12 Pelvic Inflammatory Disease

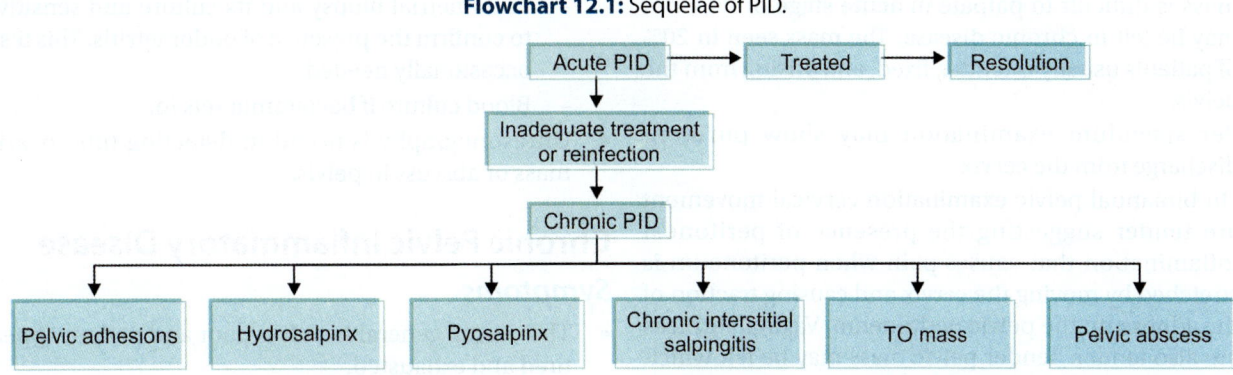

Flowchart 12.1: Sequelae of PID.

Chronic Pyosalpinx

Pyosalpinx is thick walled and surrounded by dense adhesions. The granulation tissue replaces the inner wall. Usually, it obliterates pouch of Douglas (POD) where it is densely adherent.

Tubo-ovarian Cyst

In this condition, a hydrosalpinx or pyosalpinx communicates with the ovarian cyst such as follicular cyst or ovarian abscess.

Chronic Interstitial Salpingitis

The wall of fallopian tube is thickened and fibrotic but there is no dilatation of tube due to pus or fluid. Usually adhesions are present in pelvis.

CLINICAL FEATURES OF PID

The pelvic inflammatory disease is common in young sexually active women population. Chlamydial infection remains asymptomatic or produces minimal symptoms, and therefore, the infection goes unnoticed and untreated, but the damage it causes to the tube is extensive leading to adhesions, fibrosis and tubal blockage (Box 12.3).

One previous episode of PID predisposes the woman to the another episode of PID in 12%, two episodes of PID increase the risk to 35% and three episodes to as much as 75%.[3]

Acute Pelvic Inflammatory Disease

Symptoms
- The commonest symptom is acute abdominal pain. The pain is in lower abdomen and difficult to pinpoint. Pain may be felt in upper part of abdomen if peritonitis is present.

Box 12.3: Summary of clinical criteria for the diagnosis of PID.

- Symptoms
  - Not necessary for diagnosis
- Signs
  - Uterine, cervical or adnexal tenderness
  - Leukorrhea and/or mucopurulent endocervicitis
- Additional/laboratory investigations
  - Endometrial biopsy and culture and sensitivity showing evidence of endometritis.
  - Elevated C reactive protein or ESR
  - Temperature higher than 38 °C
  - Leukocytosis
  - Positive test for gonorrhea or chlamydia
- Specific tests
  - Sonography of pelvic organs to search for TO mass or adnexal mass.

- It is accompanied by high temperature and vomiting may occasionally be present.
- There may be history of deep dyspareunia and vaginal or cervical discharge specially in associated STDs.
- Menstrual problems include intermenstrual, post- coital bleeding or menorrhagia, which is due to endometritis and congestion of the pelvis.
- In cases of pelvic abscess diarrhea may develop with passage of small loose stools due to rectal irritation.
- In some women associated urinary tract infection is present giving rise to increased frequency of micturition and dysuria.

Signs
- She may appear ill with high temperature ranging 103–104°C.
- Tachycardia and tachypnea are associated findings.
- Dehydration is present and tongue is dry and coated.
- Abdominal examination reveals distention, tenderness, and rigidity specially in lower abdomen. Direct or rebound abdominal tenderness may be present. TO

mass is difficult to palpate in acute stage of PID, but may be felt in chronic disease. The mass seen in 20% of patients usually is tender, fixed, and arising from the pelvis.
- Per speculum examination may show purulent discharge from the cervix.
- On bimanual pelvic examination cervical movement are tender suggesting the presence of peritoneal inflammation that causes pain when peritoneum is stretched by moving the cervix and causing traction of the adnexa on the pelvic peritoneum. Vaginal fornices are also tender. Tender pelvic mass may be felt which has restricted mobility. This mass usually is posterior and close to uterus. If pelvic abscess is present there will be fluctuating tender swelling in the pouch of Douglas, bulging in posterior fornix.

It is invariably found that there are wide variations in many symptoms and signs among these patients, and this is the reason for the difficult diagnosis of acute PID. Many women with PID exhibit subtle or mild symptoms that are not readily recognized as PID. Consequently, delay in diagnosis and therapy probably contributes to the inflammatory sequelae in upper genital tract.[4]

Laboratory Investigations

- Blood:
  - Hemoglobin and PCV—usually within in normal parameters.
  - Total and differential leukocyte counts—TLC is increased and neutrophils are more in acute phase of infection while lymphocytes are increased in chronic infections.
  - Erythrocyte sedimentation rate (ESR) is raised.
  - C-reactive protein levels are elevated characteristically to 20–30 mg/dL or more.
  - Blood urea and electrolytes.
  - Test for gonorrhea and chlamydia should also be performed.
- Wet smear microscopy: Evaluation of high vaginal and endocervical secretions is important in reaching to the correct diagnosis of PID. In women with PID, an increased number of polymorphonuclear leukocytes may be detected in a wet mount of the vaginal secretions or in the mucopurulent discharge.[5]
- Culture and sensitivity:
  - Endocervical and high vaginal swabs are taken and cultured for both aerobic and anaerobic organisms.
  - Urethral swab culture is also done if gonorrhea is suspected.
  - For chlamydial infection endocervical swab is taken, this is inoculated on relevant culture.
  - Endometrial biopsy and its culture and sensitivity to confirm the presence of endometritis. This test is occasionally needed.
  - Blood culture if bacteremia sets in.
- Ultrasonography is useful in detecting tubo-ovarian mass or abscess in pelvis.

Chronic Pelvic Inflammatory Disease

Symptoms

- The overall general health is poor and patient appears tired and exhausted.
- History of the previous pelvic infections is the clinching feature in the diagnosis.
- Constant lower abdominal pain is the main complaint. This pain is worsened prior to and during menstruation.
- Low backache and dyspareunia are accompanying features due to pelvic mass in POD.
- Occasionally vaginal discharge may be present usually due to cervicitis.
- Menstrual problems including menorrhagia, polymenorrhagia, and congestive dysmenorrhea are present due to pelvic congestion.
- Infertility may be a complaint if tubes are blocked.
- Rectal irritation and accompanying diarrhea is also seen in few patients due to pelvic abscess.

Signs

- Vaginal discharge is seen coming through the external os. Cervical movement is tender.
- Adnexal and forneceal tenderness and thickening are also present.
- Uterus generally is retroverted with limited mobility. Some times it is difficult to define the uterus separately from adnexa or pelvic mass due to dense pelvic adhesions and fixity of the pelvic organs. This condition is known as "Frozen Pelvis".
- The Fitz-Hugh-Curtis syndrome comprises right upper quadrant pain associated with perihepatitis and adhesions, which occur in some women with PID.

Differential Diagnosis

- **Acute appendicitis**: Pain is central around the umbilicus and later radiates to right iliac fossa. Nausea and vomiting is severe and present in most women with appendicitis while in 50% of those with PID. Cervical movement pain will occur in about 25% of women with appendicitis.[6] Temperature is not too high.
- **Ectopic pregnancy**: Pain abdomen may be more on one side and irregular uterine bleeding with or without amenorrhea are characteristic. Painful

cervical movement is also present. Temperature is not high. Signs of internal hemorrhage may be present. Pregnancy test is positive.
- **Twisted ovarian tumor**: Causes sudden pain with vomiting but usually no fever is seen in these patients. Mass is better appreciated. Uterus is normal in size.
- **Ruptured ovarian cyst**: Though acute pain is present but there is no pyrexia and no vaginal discharge.
- **Septic abortion**: Mimics clinical features of PID. History of amenorrhea is significant.
- **Degenerated fibroids**: Clinical findings like fixity and tenderness are similar if it is adherent to the pelvic organs.
- **Pelvic endometriosis**—clinical features of endometriosis are related to the menstrual cycle.
- **Urinary tract infection**—often features of dysuria and increased urinary frequency are present.

Making a Diagnosis of PID

Making a definitive diagnosis of PID is not simple because of following reasons (Box 12.3):

Clinical Features

Some women with PID are symptomatic while others could be asymptomatic. PID clinical features lack sensitivity and specificity (the positive predictive value of a clinical diagnosis is 65–90% compared to laparoscopic diagnosis).[7-9]

Investigations

It is helpful in making a diagnosis of PID when gonorrhea and chlamydia are tested positive in the lower genital tract. However, a negative test in lower genital tract does not exclude PID. Also elevated ESR and/or C-reactive protein (CRP) support a diagnosis of PID but are non-specific.[10] The absence of endocervical or vaginal pus cells has a good negative predictive value (95%) for a diagnosis of PID but their presence is non-specific (poor positive predictive value—17%).[11]

TREATMENT

The antibiotic regimens are the main stay of PID treatment. Antibiotics should provide empiric, broad-spectrum coverage of likely pathogens including *Neisseria gonorrhoeae*, *Chlamydia trachomatis*, Gram-negative facultative bacteria, aerobes, anaerobes, and streptococci commonly present in upper genital tract in women with PID.

Sexual partners of women with PID should be traced, evaluated, and treated for urethral infection with chlamydia or gonorrhea.

It is important to understand that delaying treatment increases the risk of long-term sequelae, which include pelvic pain, ectopic pregnancy, and infertility.[12]

Because there is a lack of definitive diagnostic criteria and the risk of long-term consequences, Royal College of Obstetricians and Gynaecologists (RCOG)[13] and British Association for Sexual Health and HIV[14] recommend a low threshold for empiric antibiotic treatment of PID.

Patients should be advised to avoid unprotected intercourse until they, and their partner(s), have completed treatment and follow-up. Future use of barrier contraception significantly reduces the risk of PID.

Removal of the IUD should be considered and may be associated with better short-term clinical outcomes. The decision to remove the IUD needs to be balanced against the risk of pregnancy in those who have had otherwise unprotected intercourse in the preceding 7 days. Hormonal emergency contraception may be appropriate for some women in this situation.[14]

Acute PID

Mild

These patients are treated on outpatient basis with the combination of antibiotics. It is convenient for the patients and save time and money.

Moderate to Severe

These patients treated in the hospital. Hospitalization is required to perform investigations and gives time to diagnose the disease.

The indications for the hospitalization in PID are as following:

- When diagnosis is uncertain.
- Pelvic abscess or mass is suspected.
- Clinical disease is severe.
- Temperature ≥38° C.
- Compliance with an outpatient regimen is doubtful.
- The need of surgical intervention.

The indications for discharging inpatients (hospitalized) in PID are as following:[15]

- When fever has totally settled (<99.5°C for more than 24 hours).
- Total leukocyte count has become normal.
- Rebound tenderness is absent.
- Repeat examination shows marked amelioration of pelvic organ tenderness.

SECTION 1 General Gynecology

Inpatients Treatment Plans
1. Rest: In PID women are weak and they require bed rest till they feel stable.
2. Medical management with antibiotics, analgesics, and intravenous fluids.
3. Minimal invasive surgery.
4. Major surgery.

Medical Management
Intravenous Fluids
Required to correct dehydration because of vomiting and fluid loss and electrolyte imbalance. Nasogastric (Ryle's) tube aspiration is required in case of peritonitis and intestinal distention.

Analgesics
Antispasmodics and NSAID group to relieve the patient from pain.

Antibiotics (Boxes 12.4 and 12.5)
The antibiotic therapy should be instituted without waiting for culture and sensitivity reports, since a wait may worsen the situation. In most cases of PID the polymicrobial factors are responsible including aerobes and anaerobes. So it is wise to administer a combination of antibiotics to get the quick response of therapy and to prevent the permanent damage to the tubes. Initially intravenous route is employed and once patient becomes stable oral therapy should be provided. Timely and appropriate change in antibiotics is required if therapy fails or culture and sensitivity report demands.

Treatment of PID
Metronidazole improves coverage for anaerobic bacteria, which are of importance in patients with severe PID. But metronidazole may be discontinued in patients with mild or moderate PID who are unable to tolerate it.

Ofloxacin should be avoided in patients who are at high risk of gonococcal PID because of increasing quinolone resistance. Quinolones should also be avoided as first line empirical treatment for PID in areas where >5% of PID is caused by quinolone resistant *Neisseria gonorrhoeae*. Levofloxacin is the L isomer of Ofloxacin and has the advantage of once daily dosing (500 mg OD for 14 days). It may be used as a more convenient alternative to ofloxacin.

Treatment of Sexual Partners
Current and recent male partner(s) of women with PID should be contacted and offered health advice and screening for gonorrhea and chlamydia.

Tracing of contacts within a six month period of onset of symptoms is recommended. Gonorrhea or chlamydia diagnosed in the male partner should be treated concurrently with the index patient. Broad-spectrum empirical therapy should also be offered to male partners, e.g. azithromycin 1 g single dose because all cases of PID are not associated with gonorrhea or chlamydia.

If screening for gonorrhea is not available additional specific antibiotics effective against *Neisseria gonorrhoeae* should be offered, e.g. ceftriaxone 500 mg IM single dose.

Box 12.4: Outpatient regimen.

Recommended intramuscular/oral regimens
- **Ceftriaxone** 250 mg IM in a single dose
PLUS
- **Doxycycline** 100 mg orally twice a day for 14 days
WITH* or WITHOUT
- **Metronidazole** 500 mg orally twice a day for 14 days
OR
- **Cefoxitin** 2 g IM in a single dose and Probenecid. 1 g orally administered concurrently in a single dose
PLUS
- **Doxycycline** 100 mg orally twice a day for 14 days
WITH or WITHOUT
- **Metronidazole** 500 mg orally twice a day for 14 days
OR
- Other parenteral third-generation cephalosporin (e.g. ceftizoxime or cefotaxime)
PLUS
- **Doxycycline** 100 mg orally twice a day for 14 days
WITH* or WITHOUT
- **Metronidazole** 500 mg orally twice a day for 14 days

Box 12.5: In patient regimen.

Parenteral treatment
Recommended parenteral regimens
- **Cefotetan** 2 g IV every 12 hours
PLUS
- **Doxycycline** 100 mg orally or IV every 12 hours
OR
- Cefoxitin 2 g IV every 6 hours
PLUS
- **Doxycycline** 100 mg orally or IV every 12 hours
OR
- Clindamycin 900 mg IV every 8 hours
PLUS
- Gentamicin loading dose IV or IM (2 mg /kg) followed by a maintenance dose (1.5 mg/kg) every 8 hours. Single daily dosing (3–5 mg/kg) can be substituted
Alternative parenteral regimen
- Ampicillin/Sulbactam 3 g IV every 6 hours
PLUS
- Doxycycline 100 mg orally or IV every 12 hours

Sexual Intercourse during the Treatment
Both male and female partners are advised to avoid intercourse until they have completed the antibiotic treatment course.

Follow-up[16]

72 Hours Review
It is recommended that these patients are reviewed at 72 hours, particularly for those with a moderate or severe clinical presentation, and should show a significant improvement in clinical symptoms and signs. If no improvement is observed by 72 hours then further investigation, parenteral antibiotic therapy and surgical intervention should be considered.

2–4 Weeks Review
This review is useful to ensure:
- Adequate clinical response to treatment
- Compliance with oral antibiotics
- Screening and treatment of sexual contacts
- Education of both partners about PID and its sequelae
- Repeat testing for gonorrhea or chlamydia after 2 to 4 weeks in those in whom persisting symptoms
- Tracing of sexual contacts.

Surgical Treatment
Approximately, 75% women with TO abscess will respond to antimicrobial therapy alone. Failure of medical therapy suggests the need for surgical exploration and drainage of the abscess.[17]
- Colpotomy or colpocentesis: To drain pelvic abscess.
- Laparotomy
  - To drain peritoneal pus.
  - To correct intestinal obstruction.
  - In ruptured and twisted TO masses or abscesses.
- Laparoscopy to drain TO abscess indicated when:
  - Size of abscess is less than 10 cm.
  - No response to antibiotic treatment in 42–72 hours.
  - Abscess ruptures.
  - Pyoperitoneum.
- Ultrasound guided abscess aspiration vaginally is less invasive, and may be equally effective.[18,19]

Treatment of Chronic Pelvic Inflammatory Disease
Apart from medical management these patients require surgical intervention as this condition is the end result of acute PID. Surgical treatment depends on the age and parity of the patients, symptoms, and pelvic pathology.

In young patients, conservative surgery like salpingectomy or salpingo-oophorectomy may be required. When extensive damage precludes conservative surgery or when the patient is old and multiparous, abdominal hysterectomy and bilateral salpingo-oophorectomy is needed.

Tuboplasty
In mild and adequately treated women having minimal tubal damage and infertility require corrective surgery of the fallopian tube. Hysteroscopic falloposcopy or laparoscopic salpingoscopy is preferably performed to assess the damage before embarking on surgery. Adhesiolysis may be needed in cases where tube is blocked or anatomy is disturbed due to pelvic adhesions. Fluoroscopic tubal recannulation or hysteroscopic balloonplasty is advised for cornual blocks due to mild intratubal adhesions or cellular debris or plugs.

Uncommon Complications of Chlamydia and Gonorrhea
Both these infections may spread into the abdominal cavity and cause periappendicitis and perihepatitis.

Fitz-Hugh Curtis Syndrome
Pelvic inflammatory disease with perihepatitis has been known as "Fitz-Hugh Curtis syndrome". These women present with right hypochondrial pain and tenderness and hyperpyrexia. This may be confused with cholecystitis. One has to look for other features of PID. If laparoscopy is performed in these patients, fine 'violin string' adhesions are seen between the liver capsule and visceral peritoneum. The optimum treatment for this is to give an antibiotic course for three weeks.

Sexually Acquired Reactive Arthritis (SARA)
This occurs due to dissemination of chlamydia to joints and is seen in less than 1% of PID patients. There is usually an asymmetrical oligoarthritis, affecting large joints of the lower limb.

Reiter's Syndrome
In this condition, Chlamydial arthritis is accompanied by uveitis and a rash that, if florid, may be similar to psoriasis.

Gonococcal Arthritis
Disseminated gonococcal infection occurs rarely and presents as a septic oligoarthritis, usually affecting the small joints of the hand or wrist, with a scanty papular rash.

REFERENCES

1. Soper DE, Brockwell NJ, Dalton HP. Microbial etiology of urban department acute salpingitis: treatment with Ofloxacin. Am J Obstet Gynaecol. 1992;167:653-60.
2. Soper DE, Brockwell NJ, Dalton HP, Johnson D. Observations concerning the microbial etiology of acute salpingitis. Am J Obstet Gynaecol. 1994;170:1008-17.
3. Padubidari V, Daftary SN (Eds). Howkins & Bourne Shaw's Textbook of Gynaecology, 12th edn, New Delhi: BI Churchil Livingstone Pvt Ltd, 2000, pp 106-14 & 351-66.
4. Hillis SD, Joesoef R, Marchbanks PA, Wasserheit JN, Cates W Jr, Westrom L. Delayed care of pelvic inflammatory disease as a risk factor of impaired fertility. Am J Obstet Gynaecol. 1993;168:1503-9.
5. Westrom J. Diagnosis and treatment of salpingitis. J Reprod Med. 1983;28:703-8.
6. Lewis FR, Holcroft JW, Boey J, Dunphy JE. Appendicitis: a critical review of diagnosis and treatment in 1000 cases. Archives of Surgery. 1975;110:677-84.
7. Bevan CD, Johal BJ, Mumtaz G, Ridgway GL, Siddle NC. Clinical, laparoscopic and microbiological findings in acute salpingitis: report on a United Kingdom cohort. British Journal of Obstetrics & Gynaecology. 1995;102(5):407-14.
8. Haggerty CL. Evidence for a role of Mycoplasma genitalium in pelvic inflammatory disease. Current Opinion in Infectious Diseases. 2008;21(1):65-9.
9. Centers for Disease Control. Sexually Transmitted Diseases Treatment Guidelines 2006. MMWR - Morbidity & Mortality Weekly Report 2006;55(RR-11):56-60.
10. Miettinen AK, Heinonen PK, Laippala P, Paavonen J. Test performance of erythrocyte sedimentation rate and C- reactive protein in assessing the severity of acute pelvic inflammatory disease. Am J Obstet Gynecol. 1993;169(5):1143-49.
11. Yudin MH, Hillier SL, Wiesenfeld HC, Krohn MA, Amortegui AA, Sweet RL. Vaginal polymorphonuclear leukocytes and bacterial vaginosis as markers for histologic endometritis among women without symptoms of pelvic inflammatory disease. American Journal of Obstetrics and Gynecology. 2003;188(2):318-23.
12. Hillis SD, Joesoef R, Marchbanks PA, et al. Delayed care of pelvic inflammatory disease as a risk factor for impaired fertility. Am J Obstet Gynecol. 1993;168(5):1503-9.
13. RCOG Green Top Guidelines (2009) – Management of Acute Pelvic Inflammatory Disease (www.rcog.org.uk).
14. National Guideline for the Management of Pelvic Inflammatory Disease 2011 (updated June 2011) Clinical Effectiveness Group British Association for Sexual Health and HIV, http://www.bashh.org/documents/3572.
15. Soper DE. Pelvic inflammatory disease. Infect Dis Clin North Am. 1994;8:821-40.
16. Centers for Disease Control. Sexually Transmitted Diseases Treatment Guidelines 2015. MMWR - Morbidity & Mortality Weekly Report 2015;64(3):78-81.
17. Reed SD, Landers DV, Sweet RL. Antibiotic treatment of tubo-ovarian abscesses: comparison of broad spectrum beta lactum agents versus clindamycin-containing regimens. Am J Obstet Gynaecol. 1991;164:1556-62.
18. Aboulghar MA, Mansour RT, Serour GI. Ultrasonographically guided transvaginal aspiration of tubo-ovarian abscesses and pyosalpinges: an optional treatment for acute pelvic inflammatory disease. Am J Obstet Gynecol. 1995;172(5):1501-3.
19. Corsi PJ, Johnson SC, Gonik B, Hendrix SL, McNeeley SG, Jr, Diamond MP. Transvaginal ultrasound-guided aspiration of pelvic abscesses. Infectious Disease in Obstetrics and Gynecology. 1999;7(5):216-21.

CHAPTER 13

Sexually Transmitted Infections
(Formerly Known as Sexually Transmitted Diseases)

Siya Sharan Sharma, Sucheta Jindal

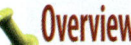

Overview
- STI's are two varieties—curable and difficult to cure.
- Common STI's are ulcerative and non-ulcerative.
- Symptoms vary from urethritis to cervicitis endometritis and tubo-ovarian masses.
- Curable STI's have specific infections.
- Difficulty to cure STI's have specific infection but efficacy is being analyzed.

INTRODUCTION

The female genital tract is vulnerable to acquire infection from the external environment because of its anatomical location. The defense mechanisms are so protective that the organisms are not allowed access to the genital tract despite its anatomical vulnerability.

DEFENSE MECHANISM OF FEMALE GENITAL TRACT (BOX 13.1)

Variations in the Efficiency of Defense Mechanisms

With Age

During Childhood and Menopause
The defenses are imperfect during childhood and after the menopause when:
- The vagina has thin and vulnerable epithelium, its content of glycogen and Doderlein bacilli is low, and its pH approaches 7 or the acidity is reduced.
- The endometrium is also poorly developed or atrophied at these ages, respectively, and does not undergo cyclical shedding.

With Menstruation
- During menstruation, the cervical plug is absent and vaginal acidity is lowered by the alkaline menstrual discharge.

Box 13.1: Defense mechanism of female genital tract.

Defense mechanisms
- Vulva:
  - Closure of the introitus by apposition of the labia protects entry of organisms
  - Secretion of the apocrine glands which is rich in undecylenic acid is fungicidal
- Vagina:
  - Closure by apposition of its anterior and posterior walls
  - Well-developed and mature stratified squamous epithelium
  - Vaginal acidity: The normal vaginal pH is lower than 4.5 being acidic, which is maintained by the production of lactic acid from epithelial glycogen by the lactobacilli
  - Vaginal flora: Doderlein's bacillus (lactobacillus) is normally predominant and it is this which by its lactic acid production, keep other organisms in check and maintains vaginal acidity. Vaginal defense is directly proportional to the relative number of bacilli
- Cervix: Functional closure of the cervix is effected by mucus which is also said to be bacteriolytic
- Uterus: Periodic shedding of surface endometrium during menstruation tends to eliminate any infection which may try to gain a hold
- Infection may ascend to the uterus and tubes at this time.

During Puerperium
In adult women the genital tract defenses are weakened during and immediately after abortion or labor because:
- There is raw placental site
- There are often breaks in the epithelial lining of the cervix and the vagina

- The tissues are bruised and devitalized
- The vulva, vagina, and cervix are wide open
- The discharge of liquor and lochia are alkaline so reduced vaginal acidity
- Degenerating blood clots and fragments of decidua offer a nidus for infections
- Patients' general resistance is lowered by pregnancy and possibly by anemia and malnutrition.

SEXUALLY TRANSMITTED INFECTIONS

Introduction

The incidence of sexually transmitted infections (STIs) is increasing due to high promiscuity and multiple sex partners. Sexually transmitted diseases being common in all parts of the globe require a clear understanding of etiology, clinical features, and treatment. The appropriate treatment is the key to the success in relieving the patients of their chronic and irritating symptoms and signs. Timely intervention in the disease processes will reduce the long-term adverse effects on the genital tract system and on the psychology of the women.

STIs are responsible for infertility—due to blocked tubes and pelvic adhesions, ectopic gestation, and precancer of cervix and vulva. Transplacental and perinatal transmission of infection can cause abortion, intrauterine fetal death, fetal anomalies, and neonatal diseases like ophthalmia.

Traditionally, only few infections such as gonorrhea, syphilis, human papillomavirus (HPV), and chancroid, were considered STIs. In recent times some more diseases have been associated with sexual transmission (Flowchart 13.1). These include Trichomoniasis, Candidiasis, Herpes genitalis, Chlamydial infection, Genital warts, HIV, and hepatitis A and B. Coitus triggers a few infections such as Candidiasis although it colonise in vagina normally. It is evident that STIs are caused by bacteria, viruses, fungi, and parasites (Table 13.1).

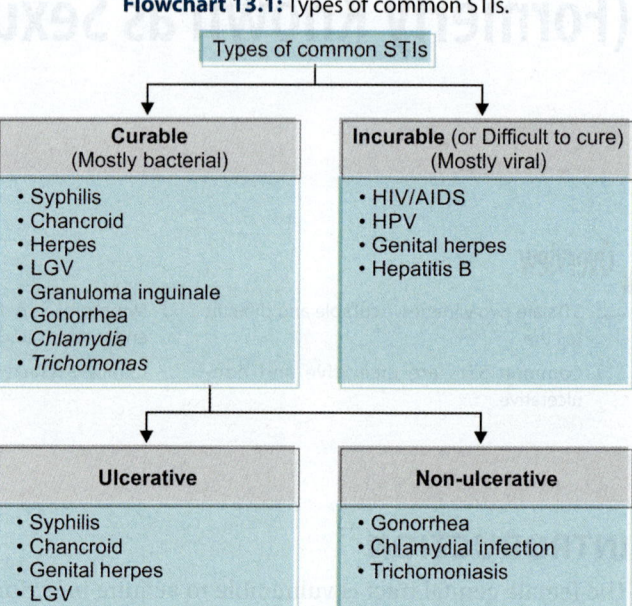

Flowchart 13.1: Types of common STIs.

(LGV: lymphogranuloma venereum; HPV: human papillomavirus; HIV, human immunodeficiency virus; AIDS: acquired immunodeficiency syndrome)

Table 13.1: Summary of STIs—Organisms, mode of transmission and sequelae.

Name of disease	Causative organism	Mode of transmission	Sequelae
• **Bacterial**			
– Gonorrhea	Neisseria gonorrhoeae	STI	Urethritis, epididymitis, cervicitis, salpingitis, endometritis, disseminated
– Chlamydial infection	Chlamydia trachomatis	STI	same as above and Reiter's syndrome
– Syphilis	Treponema pallidum	STI	Vulval ulcers, lymphadenopathy, tabes dorsalis, aortic aneurysm
• **Viral**			
– AIDS	HIV	STI, contaminated needles, transfusion of infected blood and blood products, mother to fetus	Multisystem infections Kaposi's sarcoma Death
– Herpes	HSV	STI	Genital herpes Neonatal herpes Aseptic meningitis
– Condyloma accuminata	HPV	STI	CIN, cancer cervix, penile cancer
• **Protozoa**			
– Trichomoniasis	Trichomonas vaginalis	STI	Vaginitis, vulvitis
• **Fungal**			
– Candidiasis	Candida albicans	Contact, non-STI	Vaginitis, vulvitis

(STI: sexually transmitted infection; HPV: human papillomavirus; AIDS: acquired immunodeficiency syndrome; HSV: herpes simplex virus; HIV: human immunodeficiency; CIN: cervical intraepithelial neoplasia)

CHLAMYDIAL INFECTION

Chlamydia is the commonest bacterial sexually transmitted infection. About 10% of women of childbearing age are infected.[1]

Women under 25 years of age are more prone to develop this infection.[2] Unfortunately many patients, approximately 70–80% women are asymptomatic though they have infection. Risk factors include new and multiple sexual partners and irregular use of barrier condoms.

Organism

Chlamydia trachomatis is small, Gram-negative and an obligate intracellular parasite bacterium. Commonly it causes genital infections but some strains are responsible for trachoma, conjunctivitis, and lymphogranuloma venereum (LGV).

Pathology

The infectious particle (the elementary body) infects columnar epithelial cells in genital tract. They gain entry to the cell by binding to the specific surface receptors. These appear as intracytoplasmic inclusion bodies. These reproduces inside the host cells by binary fission. After a 48 hours life cycle elementary bodies are released from cell surface. Heavily infected cell die but it is the inflammatory response to infection that contribute most to damaging the epithelial surface.

Route of Spread

Sexual intercourse is primary route. Although conjunctival and nasopharyngeal infections can be present without coexisting genital tract infection.[3]

Clinical Features

Chlamydia trachomatis causes cervicitis and pelvic inflammatory disease. Risk of PID increases with each recurrence of Chlamydia infection.[4] It is present in cervix often without symptoms. *Chlamydia trachomatis* infect only the glandular epithelium and are responsible for mucopurulent endocervicitis producing purulent endocervical discharge (mucopus), generally yellow or green in color. Edema, erythema, and friability of glandular epithelium are present specially when glandular epithelium is visible in cases of cervical ectropion. Touching the ectropion with a cotton swab can assess the friability or easily induce bleeding. Dysuria and frequency of micturition are the urinary symptoms of chlamydial infection. Infection may spread upwards to the tubes, causing chronic salpingitis, pelvic inflammatory disease (PID), and consequent infertility.

Chlamydia: Clinical Features

- Lower abdominal pain
- Purulent vaginal discharge
- Mucopurulent cervicitis and/or contact bleeding
- Post-coital or intermenstrual bleeding
- Dysuria.

Chlamydia Infection: Possible Complications

- PID
- Peri-hepatitis (Fitz-Hugh-Curtis syndrome)
- Reiter's syndrome—conjunctivitis, arthritis
- Neonatal conjunctivitis and pneumonia.

Up to two-third of male partners of chlamydia-positive women show positive chlamydia test.[5,6]

In pregnancy, this infection may cause miscarriage (abortion), preterm labor and intrauterine growth restriction (IUGR). During the delivery, ophthalmia neonatorum may be caused by chlamydia derived from maternal cervix.

Investigations[7]

Nucleic Acid Amplification Tests

Nucleic acid amplification tests (NAATs) show superior sensitivity and high specificity in the diagnosis of *C. trachomatis* over enzyme immunoassays (EIAs), point of care tests (POCTs) or DNA probe technology. NAATs have a positive predictive value (PPV) over 90% and detect all known variants, making it test of choice for urethral, cervical, lower vaginal and first catch urine specimens.[8] NAAT detect both viable and non-viable organisms.

Culture and Inoculation

It is 60–80% sensitive and 100% specific. After cleaning ectocervix of its secretions with a swab, a small cotton swab is placed into the endocervical canal and the cervical mucus is extracted. It must be cultured by inoculation in suitable cells, in which inclusion bodies develop and can be recognized after staining.

Serological Tests

- Antigen detection: Immunofluorescent and enzyme-linked immunosorbent assay (ELISA, sensitivity 40–70% only) tests are used to detect specific antigens.
- Antibody detection: Micro-immunofluorescence is used to detect serum antibodies.

Detection of DNA

To detect DNA of chlamydia, polymerase chain reaction (PCR) and ligase chain reaction (LCR) are much more sensitive than all the above mentioned tests. They are non-invasive methods.

Repeat Testing
UK's National Chlamydia Screening Programme (NCSP) for England recommended that persons under the age of 25 years treated for chlamydia should be offered a repeat test for chlamydia three months after the completion of treatment.[9]

Specimen
In women, appropriate specimen can be endocervical swab, lower vaginal swab or first catch urine. However, first catch urine samples may be less sensitive than endocervical or self taken lower vaginal swabs for the detection of *C. trachomatis*. A urethral swab is used if urethral symptoms persistent and tests from other sites are negative or in women who have undergone a hysterectomy.

Treatment
It is essential to treat the sexual partner(s) together.

Advice: Patient and partner are advised to avoid any kind of sexual intercourse until after completion of antibiotic treatment.

The treatment choices are as following:
1. Doxycycline 100 mg orally, bid for 7 days and for 14 days in case of salpingitis, is the most commonly used and effective drug.
   Or
2. Azithromycin 1 g orally single dose.
   Or
3. Clindamycin 500 mg orally, QID (6 hourly) for two weeks.
   Or
4. Erythromycin 500 mg BID for 14 days.
   Or
5. Ofloxacin 200 mg BID (or 400 mg OD) orally for 7 days
6. In Pregnancy:
   - Erythromycin sterarte, 500 mg 12 hourly for two weeks is the suitable alternative to tetracycline.
   - Azithromycin 1 gm orally single dose is also equally effective, recommended by WHO.
   - Amoxicillin 500 mg three times a day (TID) for 7 days.

GONORRHEA
Introduction
Gonorrhea was described by Hippocrates as 'Strangury' as early as 400 BC. The present name was given in 130–200 AD. This infection may occur at any age but common in reproductive young age when patient is sexually active. It is acquired during coitus. Most women are asymptomatic carriers.

Organism
This infection is caused by *Neisseria gonorrhoeae*. The intracellular Gram-negative cocci are kidney-shaped, seen in pairs (diplococci), with their long axes parallel.

Pathology
Glandular columnar epithelium, such as that of cervix, urethra, Skene gland, Bartholin's gland, or fallopian tube, is easily invaded. The infection spreads along the mucous membranes; thus after infection of the cervix it may ascend to the endometrium and fallopian tubes, causing acute salpingitis. It also ascends in a piggy-back manner attached to the sperms. Squamous epithelium of the adult vagina is resistant to infection by gonococcus, but in children the vaginal epithelium is thinner and less resistant, so vaginitis may develop.

There is intense inflammatory response in the mucosa of involved parts. Abscess may be formed in Skene or Bartholin's glands, and if left untreated may rupture or become chronic in nature.

In salpingitis edema of stroma, swollen and adherent plicae, and exudation of pus in the tubal lumen are present. Chronic infection leads to tubal blockage resulting in infertility. Occasionally pyosalpinx, hydrosalpinx, tubo-ovarian mass, pelvic abscess, or peritonitis may develop.

Incubation Period
The initial symptoms usually are seen 2–7 days after exposure.

Clinical Features in Gonorrhea[10-12]
A patient may harbor gonococci, and transmit the infection, without having any symptoms. About 50% of women have chronic asymptomatic infection.[10]

In young patients it causes vaginitis and vulvitis with clinically evident discharge without the involvement of upper genital tract.

Symptoms
- Infection at the endocervix is frequently asymptomatic (up to 50%).
- Increased or altered vaginal discharge is the most common symptom (up to 50%).
- Lower abdominal pain may be present (up to 25%).
- Urethral infection may cause dysuria (12%), but not frequency.

- Gonorrhea is a rare cause of intermenstrual bleeding or menorrhagia.
- Pharyngeal infection is usually asymptomatic (90%).

Signs
- Mucopurulent endocervical discharge and easily induced endocervical bleeding (50%).
- Pelvic/lower abdominal tenderness (5%).
- Commonly, no abnormal findings are present on examination.

ACUTE GONORRHEA

Symptoms and signs of gonorrhea in women are relatively mild in comparison to men. In acute phase, patients may have involvement of lower or upper genital tract alone or both.

Lower Genital Tract
- **Urethritis and cystitis:** Little micturition discomfort with slight yellowish purulent urethral discharge is present.
- **Bartholinitis and skeinitis:** The Bartholin glands are inflamed and patient complains of tender swelling. If the gland is compressed a bead of pus is seen at its opening on the inner surface of the labia minora. Bartholin's abscess may rupture through the skin or vaginal mucosa.
- **Vaginitis and vulvitis:** Not common but at times patient may have swelling of labia.
- **Cervicitis:** An increased mucopurulent cervical secretion, which is yellowish green in color, is the characteristic. The cervical hyperemia and erosions may be seen.
- **Proctitis:** About one-third of patients may have rectal discharge, discomfort during defecation, and rectal bleeding. It is frequent in women who have anal intercourse.

Upper Genital Tract (Pelvic Inflammation)

Salpingitis may produce severe symptoms of PID, which includes pain abdomen, low backache, dysmenorrhea, and fever. It may cause pyosalpinx, hydrosalpinx, or tubo-ovarian mass.

Chronic Gonorrhea

This is difficult to diagnose since the signs and symptoms cannot be distinguished from those of non-gonococcal genital and pelvic infections. In such situations the past history in patient herself or in her partner is important. The common complaints are backache, vaginal and cervical discharge, bartholinitis, mild chronic urethritis, and proctitis. Patients are chronically ill. Patients may give history of recurrent attacks of backache, low-grade fever, and dyspareunia in cases of salpingitis and pelvic infections. Uterus is retroverted and fixed. Adnexal swelling due to pyosalpinx, hydrosalpinx, or tubo-ovarian mass may be felt.

Investigations[11,13]

Gonorrhea is diagnosed by detecting *Neisseria gonorrhoeae* in culture.

Microscopic Smear Examination

The most likely place to obtain pus or discharge containing the gonococcus is the urethra and the cervical canal. First wipe away gross discharge then urethral and cervical discharge is taken. Gram-staining reveals the presence of an increased number of neutrophils (> 30 high-power fields). The presence of intracellular Gram-negative diplococci, leads to the diagnosis of gonococcal infection.

Culture

A swab is required for the culture since urine is not suitable for culture. The inoculum must be incubated immediately. *Neisseria gonorrhoeae* is a delicate organism so swabs require prompt transport to the laboratory. The gonococcus is grown on blood agar or Thayer–Martin media in an atmosphere of 5–10% carbon dioxide. Culture is not as sensitive as NAATs.

Gonococcal Complement Fixation Test

It is the standard test for the presence of antibody. This test is positive only after some weeks from the onset of infection.

Nucleic Acid Amplification Techniques (NAATs)

Generally more sensitive than culture. Lower volvo-vaginal or endocervical swab is choice of specimen. Urine specimen is not considered optimal specimen due to lower sensitivity. NAATs can also detect chlamydia on the same specimen. Antibiotic sensitivity by culture must be established from all patients with NAAT positive results so as to offer most suitable antibiotic therapy.

Treatment

Screen for other STIs (Chlamydia, HIV, syphilis) should be carried out. Male partner(s) should be traced, investigated and treated as appropriate.

Gonorrhea is treated with one of the following modalities:

Uncomplicated Ano-genital Infection in Adults

Main Option
Ceftriaxone 500 mg as a stat IM injection **plus** Azithromycin 1 g orally stat.

Alternative Option – 1
Cefixime 400 mg orally stat **or** Spectinomycin 2 g IM stat **or** Cefotaxime 500 mg IM stat **plus** Azithromycin 1 g orally stat.

Alternative Option – 2
Quinolones should only be used if sensitive. Ciprofloxacin 500 mg orally stat or Ofloxacin 400 mg orally stat.

Treatment of Complicated Infections

Gonococcal PID[14]
Ceftriaxone 500 mg IM immediately followed by Doxycycline 100 mg orally twice daily plus Metronidazole 400 mg twice daily for 14 days.

Disseminated Gonococcal Infection
Ceftriaxone 1 g IM or IV every 24 hours or Cefotaxime 1 g IV every 8 hours or Ciprofloxacin 500 mg IV every 12 hours or Spectinomycin 2 g IM every 12 hours.

Therapy should continue for 7 days but may be switched 24–48 hours after symptoms improve to one of the following oral option:

Cefixime 400 mg twice daily or Ciprofloxacin 500 mg twice daily or Ofloxacin 400 mg twice daily.

Women with Drug Allergy
Spectinomycin 2 g IM single dose plus Azithromycin 1 g orally single dose or Azithromycin 2 g orally single dose or Ciprofloxacin 500 mg orally single dose if quinolone sensitive.

Surgery
A Bartholin's or other abscesses requires drainage and marsupialization along with antibiotic course.

Follow-Up
Follow-up visit will help to:
- Confirm compliance with treatment.
- Ensure resolution of symptoms.
- Enquire about adverse reactions.
- Take a sexual history to explore the possibility of reinfection.
- Partner tracing.
- Test of cure and this helps to identify emerging resistance and potential failure to treatment indicated by persisting symptoms or signs.[15]

TRICHOMONAS VAGINITIS

Introduction
It is the disease of childbearing period but even the young girls and postmenopausal women are not immune. This infection is sexually transmitted but it can be transmitted due to poor hygiene and by using the infected person's bath towels or clothes. Poor immune resistance and high pH (5-6) of vagina favor this infection as seen during menstruation. It accounts for about 20–30% of cases of vulvovaginitis. About 70% male partners contract the disease after a single exposure to an infected woman and this transmission rate is even higher from male to female.

Organism
Trichomonas vaginitis is caused by the sexually transmitted, flagellated, protozoan parasite, actively motile anaerobic *Trichomonas vaginalis*. It exists only in trophozoite form. It is found in the vagina, urethra and paraurethral glands. In women with this infection, 90% have urethral infection. It is interesting that the isolated urethral infection is seen in less than 5% of cases. In male counterparts Trichomonas infection usually involves the urethra, occasionally organism has been found in the subpreputial sac and penile lesions.

Clinical Features[16,17]
Clinical symptoms and signs range from asymptomatic (10–50%) to mild to severe forms depending on the amount of parasitic load apart from individual's immune resistance.[3] In 10–15% women no obvious signs are noted.

Vaginal discharge can be seen in 70% cases, is greenish-yellow, thin, usually profuse, purulent, malodorous and characteristically frothy (seen only in up to one-third cases). The pH of vaginal secretions is usually higher than five.

Discharge causes intense itching and inflammation of the vulva, which may extend up to the perineum. Patchy erythema and hemorrhagic punctations give the appearance of "Strawberry Cervix" in 2% cases. Strawberry spots may also be seen on vaginal wall.

Urinary symptoms include dysuria and frequency of micturition and a low-grade urethritis may be revealed on examination.

Abdominal pain, low backache and dyspareunia may some times occur.

Pregnancy and Trichomonas vaginalis
In pregnancy, trichomonas vaginitis increases the risk of premature rupture of the membranes and preterm delivery.

Investigations

- **Wet smear under microscope:** Wet smear is prepared by mixing 1-2 drops of vaginal discharge with normal saline on a slide. Motile trichomonads and increased number of leukocytes are visualized under microscopic examination. The sensitivity of this test in detecting the microorganism is 60% and specificity is high.[18] Motile organism is identified from its shape and four flagellae. Its constant motion distinguishes it from pus cells.
- **Culture:** Culture is carried out on high or low vaginal swab. The reliability of culture is up to 96%.[19]
- **Nucleic acid amplification techniques**: NAATs have highest sensitivity for the detection of Trichomonas and are considered 'gold standard' test; with sensitivities of 88-97% and specificities of 98-99%.[20]

Treatment[21]

Both the sexual partners should be treated simultaneously. Both partners are advised to avoid the coitus during the therapy and until after the follow-up. Tests for other STIs should be carried out in both the partners.

Oral antibiotics given in a single dose or a longer course results in cure in >90% of cases. Intravaginal treatment showed cure rates around 50%. Spontaneous cure rate is observed 20-25%.[22] These drugs better are avoided in first trimester of pregnancy.

One of the following options are used to treat *Trichomonas vaginalis*:

First Regimen

- Metronidazole is the drug of choice for the effective treatment of Trichomonas vaginitis. The 95% cure rates achieved with Metronidazole in the dose of 400 mg twice or thrice daily for 7 days. Equally effective cure rates are achieved with single dose therapy with 2 g orally. This is convenient to take and has better patient compliance.
- Secnidazole in a single dose of 1 g is also good alternative.
- Tinidazole 2 g orally in a single dose.

Treatment Options for Non-Responders

Second Regimen

If the initial therapy is not effective, these patients should be treated for 7 more days - Metronidazole in the dose of 400 mg twice or thrice daily for 7 days. Amongst women who failed to respond to a first course of treatment, 40% respond to repeat course of treatment.[23]

Third Regimen[24]

If repeated treatment is not yet effective, the patients should be treated with one of these regimens:

- Metronidazole 2 g single dose daily for 3-5 days.
- Tinidazole 2 g single daily dose for 5-7 days.
- Metronidazole 800 mg three times daily orally for 7 days.

In women who failed to respond to a second regimen, 70% respond to this third regimen.

Fourth Regimen

Tinidazole 1 g twice or three times daily, or 2 g twice daily for 14 days with or without intravaginal Tinidazole 500 mg twice daily for 14 days.

About 90-92% respond to this fourth regimen.[25]

VULVOVAGINAL CANDIDIASIS (MONILIASIS)

This is the commonest infection of the female genital tract, experienced by over 75% women at least once in their life time and about half the women will experience two or more episodes per year.[26]

Organism

Gram-positive fungus *Candida albicans* is responsible for 85-90% of vaginal fungal infections. It grows in acid medium with an abundant supply of carbohydrates. Candida is dimorphic fungi existing as blastopores and mycelia. Blastopores are responsible for transmission and asymptomatic colonization, and mycelia, which result from blastopore germination, enhance colonization and facilitate tissue invasion. The organism is carried in the vagina, under the nails, and on the skin.[27] Non-*albicans* species also causes candidiasis and these may include *C. glabrata, C. tropicalis, C. krusei, C. parapsilosis*, and *Saccharomyces cerevisiae*.

Predisposing Factors

- *Pregnancy:* Pregnancy predisposes to infection because of the increased vaginal acidity and high glycogen content. Also there is qualitative decrease in cell-mediated immunity.
- *Hormonal oral contraceptive pills* also predispose to monilial vaginitis for the same reasons.
- *Antibiotic use*—normally lactobacilli prevent the overgrowth of opportunistic fungi. Antibiotics decrease lactobacilli concentration and thus allowing the overgrowth of fungi.
- *Diabetes mellitus:* Rich supply of glucose and a qualitative decrease in cell-mediated immunity lead to a higher incidence of vulvovaginal candidiasis.
- *Sexual contact* is not important in the transmission of this infection, but the possible trauma caused by the coitus may be sufficient to trigger an attack in a predisposed individual.

Clinical Features

The classical symptoms of vulvovaginal candidiasis consist of vulvar pruritis, and a profuse vaginal discharge that typically resembles cottage cheese or curd, and it smells like yeast. During micturition, inflamed vulvar and vestibular epithelium come in contact to urine causing external dysuria, which is known as "splash" dysuria. Women may also present with associated history of superficial dyspareunia.

Examination reveals erythema and edema of the labia and vulvar skin. Often there is excoriation from scratching. Discrete pustule-papular lesions may also be seen. The whitish discharge is adherent to vaginal walls, which on separation leaves behind the petechial oozing surface. Typically cervix appears normal. The pH of vagina in patients with vulvovaginal candidiasis is usually normal or lowered (<4.5). In child-bearing age about 10–20% women may have *Candida sp. colonization* with no clinical features. Such asymptomatic women do not require treatment.

Investigations

- **Wet smear:** A drop of vaginal discharge is taken on a slide and a drop of 10% KOH is added, mix it and put cover slip. KOH dissolve all the cellular debris. In about 80% patients, either budding yeast forms or mycelia are observed under the microscope.
- **Culture:** Culture of vaginal fluid on Sabouraud's medium can grow the fungi and reveal rounded colonies 1–2 mm in diameter within 48–72 hours. The growth of fungus has yeast-like odor.

Treatment[28]

Patients are advised to maintain strict genital and perineal hygiene, avoid tight synthetic undergarments, and avoid scratching the vulva with finger nails.

- Predisposing factors if present should be treated accordingly.
- Antifungal medication: The symptomatic relief is seen after 2–3 days. The usual duration of therapy is for 7 days but duration can be decreased to 1–3 days by increasing the concentrations of the antifungal agents. Topical use is better since it reduces the side effects.

Azole Group Antifungals[29,30]

In uncomplicated cases with acute vulvovaginal candidiasis topical and oral azole treatments give a clinical and mycological cure rate of over 80%, however nystatin gives better results (90%).

Tropical Azole Group Antifungal

- *Clotrimazole*
    - Vaginal tablets:
        - 100 mg vaginal tablet for seven days
        - 200 mg vaginal tablets for three days
        - 500 mg vaginal tablet for single dose only.
    - Cream
        - 1% cream 5 g vaginal for 7–14 days
        - 10% cream 5 g intravaginally stat.
- *Miconazole*
    - Vaginal tablets:
        - 100 mg vaginal for 7–14 days
        - 200 mg vaginal for 3 days
        - 1.2 g vaginal stat.
    - Cream
        - 2% cream 5 g vaginal for 7 days.
- *Econazole*
    - Vaginal tablets
        - 150 mg for 3 days.
- *Nystatin:* Both preparations contain 100,000 units.
    - Vaginal tablets:
        - 1–2 vaginal for 14 days.
    - Cream
        - 4 g vaginal for 14 days.

Oral Antifungal Agents

- *Fluconazole* is used in a single 150 mg dose. This therapy protocol appears to have equal efficacy like topical application, in the treatment of mild to moderate vulvovaginal candidiasis.[6]
- Itraconazole is used in dose of 200 mg twice only for a day.

CHRONIC VULVOVAGINAL CANDIDIASIS

A small number of women develop chronic or recurrent vulvovaginal candidiasis. These patients experience persistent irritative symptoms of the vulva. Burning replaces itching as the prominent symptom in patients with chronic vulvovaginal candidiasis.

Treatment

The treatment of patients with chronic vulvovaginal candidiasis consists of inducing a remission of chronic symptoms with daily Ketaconazole 400 mg or fluconazole 200 mg until symptoms resolve. Patients should than be maintained on prophylactic doses of these agents (ketaconazole 100 mg/daily, fluconazole 150 mg /weekly) for 6 months.[31]

Vulvovaginal Candidiasis in Complex Situations

Pregnancy

Asymptomatic colonization with *Candida* species is more common (30–40%) and symptomatic candidiasis is more prevalent throughout pregnancy.³² Candid colonization is not associated with IUGR or preterm delivery.

Treatment in Pregnancy

Oral antifungal treatment is not safe and contraindicated. Symptomatic vulvovaginal candidiasis in pregnancy is treated with topical azoles. Longer courses are recommended; a four-day course will cure just over 50% whereas a seven day course cures over 90%.³³

Recurrent Vulvovaginal Candidiasis

Recurrent vulvovaginal candidiasis occurs in about 5% women.³⁴ To make a diagnosis of recurrent vulvovaginal candidiasis there should be at least four episodes of symptomatic vulvovaginal candidiasis in a year with:
- Partial or complete resolution of symptoms between episodes.
- Positive microscopy or culture growth of *Candida albicans* on at least two occasions.

Treatment

Patient Advice

Additional advice includes as following:
- Vulval emollients may give symptomatic relief if vulval dermatitis is present.
- Avoid high-estrogen containing contraceptive pills—Depo-Provera.

Antifungal Treatment

An induction regimen (Fluconazole 15 mg every 72 hours for three doses only) is used for clinical remission, followed by a maintenance regimen (Fluconazole 150 mg every week for six months). This results in disease free period of 6 months in about 90% of women and up to 1 year in 40% cases.³⁵

Follow-up: If symptoms resolve then there is no need of follow up review.

Sexual partner: Male partners are not required to be treated.

GENITAL ULCERATIVE DISEASES (FLOWCHART 13.2)

Herpes Genitalis

Organism

Genital infection is caused by two main types of DNA containing herpes simplex virus (HSV). HSV II is the usual cause of herpes genitalis. HSV I usually causes Herpes labialis but occasionally it may cause herpes genitalis through orogenital contact. This virus enters in the cell by invasion and reproduces itself in large number in the cell resulting into the disruption of the cell.

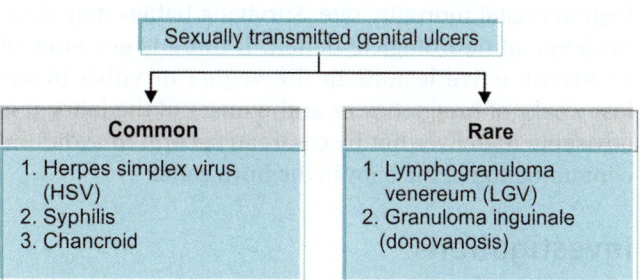

Flowchart 13.2: Sexually transmitted genital ulcers.

Clinical Features

Primary Herpes

First symptom attack, appear in less than 7 days of the sexual contact, incubation period ranges between 3–6 days. In a few infected individual lesions are not noticed but there may be complaints of tingling and burning in genital region.

Lesions

Small and extremely painful vesicles appear on an erythmatous base on clitoris, labia, and vestibule, but they may also occur on the vaginal wall and cervix. These vesicles soon break down to form small painful shallow ulcers, and within few days scab appears over the ulcer. Grouped vesicles mixed with small ulcers are almost pathognomonic of genital herpes. Virus is shed from the lesions until healing is complete in about a fortnight to three weeks. Inguinal lymph nodes are enlarged and tender.

In some women, micturition may be painful. About 30% patients suffer from fever, malaise, and headache.

Recurrent Herpes

Following the primary herpes, virus colonize the neurons in the dorsal root ganglia causing latent infection. In some patients, the virus remains dormant, but in others recurrent attacks occur at irregular intervals. Acute infection occurs intermittently when virus particles are produced and track down the axons to the skin. Although, recurrent attacks may be milder and shorter than the primary attack, they cause much discomfort and misery to both partners. The signs and symptoms last for 7–10 days.

Pregnancy with Herpes

In early pregnancy the primary attack may cause an miscarriage (abortion). During the last weeks of pregnancy the primary attack may be responsible for transplacental spread of the virus to the fetus, where it subsequently may cause damage to the central nervous system with a high neonatal mortality rate. Surviving babies may show evidence of neurological deficit. If there is evidence of recurrent active lesions in the vagina or vulva in the last weeks of pregnancy or at the onset of the labor it is advisable to deliver her by cesarean section to avoid the contamination of the baby in the birth canal.

Investigations

- **Direct smear:** Microscopic examination of smear, from the ulcer shows giant multinucleated cells with characteristic intranuclear inclusion bodies.
- **Culture:** The serum is obtained from the vesicle or a sterile culture swab is rubbed over the ulcer. Culture is most sensitive and specific test; specificity is 100%, sensitivity approaches 100% in the vesicle stage and 89% in the pustular stage and drops to as low as 33% in patients with ulcers.
- **HSV DNA:** DNA detection by polymerase chain reaction (PCR) increases HSV detection rates by 11–71% compared with virus culture.
- **Serology for HSV antibody:** HSV-1 IgG or HSV-2 IgG or both, in a single serum sample represents HSV infection. It is difficult to say whether the infection is recent as IgM detection is unreliable. Serum samples taken a few weeks apart can be used to show seroconversion and, hence, recent primary infection. HSV-2 antibodies are indicative of genital herpes. HSV-1 antibodies do not differentiate between genital and oro-pharyngeal infection.

Treatment[36]

General

- Saline baths relieve the local pain.
- Analgesia.
- Topical anesthetic agents, e.g. 5% lidocaine (lignocaine) ointment.

Antivirals

Oral antiviral drugs are commenced within 5 days of the start of the episode and while new lesions are still forming. These drugs reduce the severity and duration but not the natural disease progressions. Topical agents are less effective than oral agents and there is benefit with combined oral and topical treatment. Intravenous therapy is indicated when there is difficulty in swallowing or in vomiting. There is no evidence for benefit from courses longer than five days except when new lesions are still appearing at this time.

Primary infection of genital herpes should be treated for 5 days only with any one of the following:

1. Aciclovir, 200 mg orally five times daily.
2. Aciclovir 400 mg three times daily.
3. Valaciclovir 500 mg twice daily.
4. Famciclovir 250 mg three times daily.

Recurrent Infection

Recurrent episodes are self-limiting and generally have minor symptoms.

If required management include:

- General advice.
- Supportive treatment.
- Episodic antiviral treatments.
- Suppressive antiviral therapy.

Episodic antivirals include any one of the following for five days:

- Aciclovir 200 mg five times daily.
- Aciclovir 400 mg three times daily for 3–5 days.
- Valaciclovir 500 mg twice daily.
- Famciclovir 125 mg twice daily.

Suppressive Antiviral Therapy

Daily suppressive long-term therapy reduces the frequency of HSV recurrences by at least 75%. Suppressive treatment does not totally eliminate the potential for transmission. Any one of these antivirals can be used:

1. Aciclovir 400 mg twice daily.
2. Aciclovir 200 mg four times daily.
3. Valaciclovir 500 mg once daily.

Follow-up

Patients and their partners should be informed and warned that they are infectious whenever they have any evident lesions. Women should have annual cervical smears for the follow-up since HSV may cause precancerous lesions of the cervix.

HERPES IN PREGNANCY[36,37]

Primary Episode of Genital Herpes in First and Second Trimesters

Women should be referred to a genitourinary physician for appropriate management with oral or intravenous aciclovir in standard doses. Type-specific HSV antibody testing, which can help to differentiate between primary and recurrent infections, should be undertaken if a woman presents with a first episode of genital herpes in the third trimester.

First episode genital herpes has been associated with first trimester miscarriage. There is no conclusive evidence to associate these episodes with fetal developmental abnormality if the pregnancy continues. Such infection is not an indication for termination of pregnancy. An anomaly scan would be sufficient 20–22 weeks gestation.

Daily suppressive aciclovir from 36 weeks gestation may be considered for women who experience a first-episode of genital herpes in order to reduce the likelihood of HSV lesions at term, and the offer of cesarean section delivery. Aciclovir 400 mg TID can be used because of the altered pharmacokinetics of the drug in late pregnancy.

Primary Infection in Third Trimester
Mode of Delivery
Cesarean section should be offered to all women presenting with first episode genital herpes lesions at the time of delivery, or within 6 weeks of the expected date of delivery or onset of labor. However, cesarean section may not be of benefit in reducing transmission for women presenting with ruptured membranes for greater than four hours. In all these cases the pediatricians should be informed.

Vaginal Delivery
If vaginal delivery is unavoidable or where the mother opts for a vaginal birth, prolonged rupture of membranes should be avoided and invasive procedures (fetal blood sampling) should not be used.

Antivirals
Continuous aciclovir in the last 4 weeks of pregnancy reduces the risk of both clinical recurrence at term and delivery by cesarean section. IV aciclovir given to the mother during labor (intrapartum) and subsequently to the neonate may be considered by the pediatricians.

Recurrent Herpes Infection in Pregnancy
Antivirals
Antiviral treatment is rarely indicated for treatment of recurrent episodes of genital herpes during pregnancy. Symptomatic recurrence if any during the third trimester is brief. Aciclovir suppressive treatment from 36 weeks gestation may be considered.

Mode of Delivery
Vaginal delivery is safe if no lesions are present at the time of delivery as cesarean section is not more beneficial in preventing neonatal herpes.

Herpes Genitalis Lesions at the onset of Labor
Cesarean section should be considered for women with recurrent genital herpes lesions at the onset of labor. Recurrent genital herpes at any other time during pregnancy is not an indication for delivery by cesarean section. The risks of vaginal delivery for the fetus are small and must be set against risks to the mother of CS.

SYPHILIS[38]
Organism
It is caused by a spirochete bacterium *Treponema pallidum*, it replicates slowly.

Transmission
This is transmitted from one person to another either by:
- Direct contact with an infectious lesion usually occurring during sexual contact.
- During pregnancy from mother to child.
- Via infected blood products.

Classification
See Flowchart 13.3.

Clinical Presentation
Syphilis presents in three stages of its clinical course.

Primary Syphilis
A minute abrasion of the skin, on contact allows the organism to reach the subcutaneous tissue where they multiply. The incubation period is 9–90 days. The continuous multiplication of the spirochete gives rise to a lesion, which usually ulcerates, and is termed a chancre. The ulcer is the typical of the first stage of syphilis.

Syphilitic Ulcer (Chancre)
Syphilitic ulcer usually is single, painless, circular and indurated, with an eroded base. There is marked edema of the surrounding tissue. It may not be noticed by the patient and will heal spontaneously in 3–10 weeks, leaving a very slight scar. The most common site of the chancre is the cervix but it may occur on the labia.

The chancre first takes the form of a raised papule with an indurated base, and later it breaks down to form a shallow punched out ulcer with well-defined edges and a smooth shiny floor. It exudes a serous discharge, unless secondarily infected when the discharge is more purulent. About a week after the chancre appears, the related lymphatic glands enlarge and in 3–6 weeks, they become rubbery, but remain painless, discrete, and mobile. These glands do not suppurate until septic secondary infection occurs.

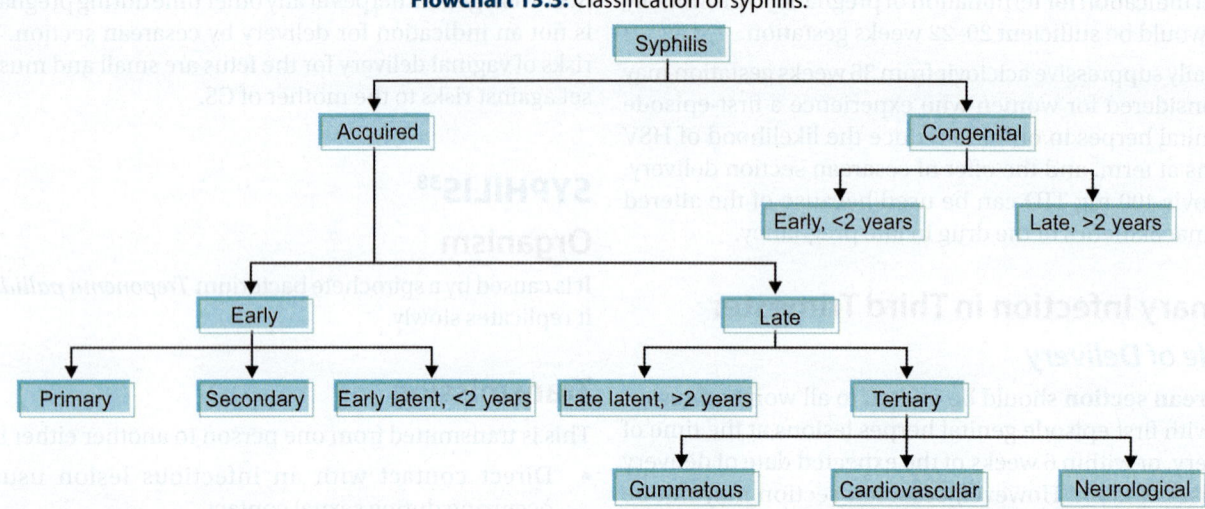

Flowchart 13.3: Classification of syphilis.

A cervical chancre is less friable, has less tendency to bleed on touch, and has the sharp outline of the ulcer than the cervical cancer.

Secondary Syphilis

Skin Rash
After 2 months of the appearance of the chancre the first evidence of dissemination of the spirochetes occurs in the form of a non-irritating extragenital rash, which is usually symmetrical. This is a coppery colored maculopapular rash on the trunk and limbs. It can also appear on the face and forehead (corona veneris). In addition, there may be anemia, slight pyrexia, headache and occasional alopecia. Some patients may develop sore throat and 'mucus patches' within the mouth, which are whitish areas on the inner aspects of the lips, cheek and palate.

Condylomata Lata
Another form of manifestation, which occurs soon after the appearance of the rash, is the formation of the condylomata lata in moist areas like around vulva and anus. They appear as raised plaques, which may be bilaterally symmetrical. They tend to become macerated, and so appear as raised discs with a flat or slightly indented top, which is covered by grayish exudate (Sodden white areas).

Latent Syphilis
Treponema pallidum infection diagnosed on serological testing with no symptoms or signs. Within the first two years of infection this is early latent syphilis and beyond that late latent syphilis.

Tertiary Syphilis (Table 13.2) (Symptomatic Late Syphilis)

Gummata
In the later stage of the disease, perhaps many years after the chancre has healed, lesions occur due to end-arteritis. These lesions are firm elastic tumors and may be seen on skin, mucus surfaces, bones, and viscera, although they are very rare in the female genital organs.

Neurosyphilis
It includes meningovascular disease with focal lesions, tabes dorsalis and general paralysis of insane.

Cardiovascular Lesions
These include aneurysm of the aorta and other large arteries.

Syphilis in Pregnancy
Sometimes the disease is discovered as the result of a routine serological test during an antenatal visit. If the patient becomes pregnant soon after acquiring the syphilis the fetus may die, usually in the second half of pregnancy, and spirochetes may be found in its liver or in the intima of the umbilical cord. If untreated, subsequent pregnancies may proceed nearer to term until a child is born alive with signs of congenital syphilis.

Syphilis may be transmitted transplacentally at any stage of pregnancy. Consequences of syphilis in pregnancy are miscarriage, preterm labor, intrauterine death (stillbirth), polyhydramnios, fetal hydrops, and congenital syphilis.

Table 13.2: Clinical features in late syphilis.

	Duration since infection	Clinical features
Asymptomatic neurosyphilis	Early and/or late	Abnormal CSF; significance is uncertain (Abnormal CSF observed in up to 30% of primary and secondary syphilis) Still abnormal CSF does not become clinically significant in the majority of patients
Meningovascular	2–7 years	Focal arteritis with infarction and meningeal inflammation; Occasional headache, labile emotions, insomnia
Parenchymatous general paresis	10–20 years	Cortical neuronal loss; gradual decline in memory and cognitive functions, labile emotions, personality change, psychosis and dementia. Seizures and hemiparesis are late complications
Tabes dorsalis	15–25 years	Inflammation of spinal dorsal column and nerve roots; lightening pains, areflexia, paresthesia, sensory ataxia, Charcot's joints, optic atrophy, pupillary changes
Cardiovascular	10–30 years	Aortitis—asymptomatic, substernal pain, aortic regurgitation, heart failure, coronary ostial stenosis, angina, aneurysm
Gummatous	1–46 years Average 15	Inflammatory granulomatous destructive lesions can occur in any organ but most commonly affect bone and skin

Investigations

Microscopy

To demonstrate the presence of spirochete the edge of the lesion (primary syphilis) is gently wiped with a swab dipped in normal saline until serum, but not blood, exudes. The serum is transferred to a glass slide and examined under dark ground illumination. Under the oil immersion lens the treponemata appear as mobile white corkscrew-shaped organisms against the dark background. The examination is repeated on three successive days if the initial test is negative.

Serology

Confirmation by serological reaction on the patient's serum is obtained 4–6 weeks after the appearance of the chancre. Serological reactions are strongly suggestive of syphilis but the final diagnosis should never be made only on the basis of one type of test. While the tests are almost completely reliable in the secondary stage, they do not become positive for 4–10 weeks after the infection.

- **Non-specific antigen tests** include non-treponemal rapid plasma reagin (RPR) test, or Venereal Disease Research Laboratory (VDRL) test for antibody.
- **Specific and confirmatory tests** for treponemata: Treponemal enzyme immunoassay (EIA) detects IgG and IgM. Tests include fluorescent treponemal antibody absorption (FTA ABS) test and the *Treponemal pallidum* hemagglutination assay (TPHA). These tests may remain positive for many years, even after the disease has been effectively treated. The best combination for screening is to use the VDRL and TPHA tests. Other tests are *T. pallidum* chemiluminescent assay, *T. pallidum* particle agglutination assay (TPPA), and *T. pallidum* recombinant antigen line immunoassay.

When **primary syphilis** suspected IgM are tested via EIA, which can be detected by the end of second week. IgG can be detected in 4–5 weeks of infection. Specific tests are usually positive in **secondary** and **early latent syphilis**.

Polymerase Chain Reaction

Suitable to use on oral or other lesions where contamination with commensal treponemes is likely to be present. Also polymerase chain reaction (PCR) is helpful in diagnosis by demonstrating *T. pallidum* in tissue samples, vitreous fluid and CSF.

Chest X-ray (CXR)

In late latent syphilis or if there are any signs of aortic disease.

Computed Tomography of the Head

If neurological feature are present.

CF Examination

In presence of neurological or ophthalmic signs or symptoms and when treatment fails.

Management and Treatment of Syphilis

General Advice

- Offer screening for other STIs including HIV to all patients.
- Explain to patient about syphilis, it's long-term implications; reinforce this by written information.

- Advise to avoid sexual activity until the lesions of early syphilis are fully healed or until after the results of the first follow-up serology are known.

Management in Pregnancy

A multidisciplinary team (MDT) approach is essential to manage these women and this includes Obstetric, Midwifery and Pediatric teams along with genitourinary Medicine team. Fetal medicine units are able to manage these pregnancies by serial ultrasound to evaluate fetal involvement including non-immune hydrops or hepatosplenomegaly. Fetal monitoring for fetal distress in the early stages of therapy is recommended after 26 weeks gestation.

Recommended Regimens

A treponemicidal level of antimicrobial must be achieved in serum, and in the CSF in cases of neurosyphilis. In following each regimens any one drug can be selected with first choice for the first drug if suitable and not contraindicated.

Incubating Syphilis or Epidemiological Treatment

- Benzathine penicillin G 2.4 MU IM single dose.
- Doxycycline 100 mg oral bd for 14 days.
- Azithromycin 1 g oral stat.

Early Syphilis (Primary, Secondary and Early Latent)

1. Benzathine penicillin G 2.4 MU IM single dose.
2. Procaine penicillin G 600,000 units IM daily for 10 days.

Early Syphilis: Alternative Regimens

1. Doxycycline 100 mg oral bd for 14 days.
2. Azithromycin 2 g oral stat; or Azithromycin 500 mg oral daily for 10 days.
3. Erythromycin 500 mg oral qds for 14 days.
4. Ceftriaxone 500 mg IM daily for 10 days (only if no anaphylaxis to penicillin).
5. Amoxycillin 500 mg oral qds plus Probenecid 500 mg qds for 14 days.

Late Latent, Cardiovascular and Gummatous Syphilis

1. Benzathine penicillin 2.4 MU IM weekly for two weeks (three doses).
2. Procaine penicillin 600,000 units IM od for 17 days.

Alternative Regimens for Late Syphilis

1. Doxycycline 100 mg oral bd for 28 days.
2. Amoxycillin 2 g oral tds plus probenecid 500 mg qds for 28 days.

Neurosyphilis including Neurological/Ophthalmic Involvement in Early Syphilis

1. Procaine penicillin 1.8–2.4 MU IM od plus probenecid 500 mg oral qds for 17 days.
2. Benzyl penicillin 18–24 MU daily, given as 3–4 MU every four hours for 17 days.

Alternative Regimens for Neurosyphilis

1. Doxycycline 200 mg oral bd for 28 days.
2. Amoxycillin 2 g oral tds plus probenecid 500 mg oral qds for 28 days.
3. Ceftriaxone 2 g IM (with lidocaine as diluent) or IV (with water for injections as diluent, Not lidocaine for IV route) for 10–14 days.

Early Syphilis in Pregnancy

1. Benzathine penicillin G 2.4 MU IM single dose in the first and second trimesters.
   When maternal treatment is initiated in the third trimester, a second dose of benzathine penicillin G 2.4 MU IM should be given after one week (day 8).
2. Procaine penicillin G 600,000 unit IM daily for 10 days.

Alternative Regimens in Early Syphilis in Pregnancy

1. Amoxycillin 500 mg oral qds plus probenecid 500 mg oral qds for 14 days.
2. Ceftriaxone 500 mg IM daily for 10 days.
3. Erythromycin 500 mg oral qds for 14 days or Azithromycin 500 mg oral daily for 10 days plus evaluation and treatment of neonates at birth with penicillin.

Late Syphilis in Pregnancy

Manage as in non-pregnant patients but without the use of doxycycline.

Follow-up in Syphilis

- **Early syphilis:** Minimum clinical and serological (VDRL or RPR) follow-up should be at months 1, 2, 3, 6 and 12, then six monthly until VDRL/RPR negative or serofast.
- **Late syphilis:** Minimum serological follow-up is three monthly until serofast.
- **Re-infection and relapse:** A sustained two bottle dilution (i.e. four-fold) or greater increase in the VDRL or RPR titre suggests re-infection or treatment failure. Reinfection or relapse should be retreated preferably with supervised treatment schedules to ensure compliance, and sexual partners should be screened and treated.

- **Treatment failure:** It is characterized by four-fold or greater increase in non-treponemal test titre, recurrence of signs or symptoms, and re-infection is excluded. CSF examination and re-treatment is indicated and same is also considered for patients whose non-treponemal test titres do not decrease four-fold within 6–12 months of therapy.

  Such patients are treated with benzathine penicillin G 2.4 MU (million units) IM, three doses each at weekly intervals, if CSF examinations are normal.
- Specific treponemal tests may remain positive for life following effective treatment.
- If the patient remains asymptomatic and the VDRL/RPR is negative or serofast at 1 year, the patient may be discharged.

CHANCROID[39]

Organism

This condition, commonly known as soft sore, is caused by sexually transmitted infection with *Haemophilus ducreyi* (Ducrey's bacillus). It is Gram-negative facultative anaerobic cocco-bacillus (bacilli). The incidence of chancroid has now decreased markedly throughout the world and even in African countries where it used to be common and currently the incidence is 1–4%.

Clinical Features

The incubation period is 3–5 days. Small shallow ulcers occur on the vulva and vagina. The ulcers are multiple and painful, and may be surrounded by a zone of hyperemia. They are irregular in outline with undermined edges. Their bases are covered with greenish slough, which is contagious.

The lymphatic glands in groin become enlarged and known as "Bubo". They are tender, soft, and fluctuating in some, thus differing with syphilis, in which the glands are discrete, firm and painless. Frequently the suppuration of these lymph glands is observed, as secondary infection with pyogenic organisms is common.

The sore tend to heal spontaneously if kept clean, but if secondary pyogenic infection occurs there may be considerable destruction of tissue and consequent scarring.

Chancroid is distinguished from primary syphilis by the short incubation period, the multiplicity of lesions, and the inguinal lymph nodes' characteristics.

Investigations

- DNA detection by PCR.
- **Gram staining:** It is Gram-negative bacilli, arranged like fish in a streak of mucus.
- **Culture:** Bacilli can be cultured on a medium. Material is obtained from the ulcer base, or the undermined edges of the ulcer, or from pus aspirated from the bubo.
- **Ito test:** *H. ducreyi* vaccine, 0.3 mL is injected intradermally, and appearance of an area of erythema 8 mm across at 24 hours is considered positive.
- The Centers for Disease Control and Prevention in the USA have proposed that a "probable diagnosis", for both clinical and surveillance purposes be made if the patient has one or more painful genital ulcers, and (a) no evidence of *T. pallidum* infection by dark field examination of ulcer exudate or by a serologic test for syphilis performed at least 7 days after onset of ulcers, and (b) the clinical presentation, appearance of the genital ulcers and regional lymphadenopathy, if present, is typical for chancroid and a test for HSV performed on the ulcer exudate is negative.[40]

Treatment

Three to seven days after initiation of therapy the gradual resolution of the genital ulcer is seen and completely heals within 2 weeks unless it is large.

General Advice

Patient is advised to avoid sexual intercourse until she and her partner have completed treatment and follow-up.

Regimens to Treat Chancroid

One of the following drug can be used in preferential order.

- Azithromycin 1 g orally in a single dose.
- Ceftriaxone 250 mg IM in a single dose.
- Ciprofloxacin 500 mg orally in a single dose.
- Ciprofloxacin 500 mg orally bd for 3 days.
- Erythromycin base 500 mg orally qds for 7 days.

LYMPHOGRANULOMA VENEREUM[41]

Lymphogranuloma venereum is caused by a sexually transmitted strain of *Chlamydia trachomatis*, which belongs to lymphogranuloma-psittacosis group. The incubation period is 7–21 days. From the point of entry, the agent is disseminated via the bloodstream and lymphatics to result in a chronic inflammatory disease.

Clinical Features

The earliest genital lesion is a vesicopustular eruption, which becomes a painless shallow ulcer, which gradually deepens and extends. The inguinal bubo is a hard cutaneous induration, reddish-blue in color and it is seen unilaterally in up to two-third of women or bilaterally, in about 10–30 days after inoculation. The enlarged inguinal nodes may break down to form multiple sinuses. One lymph node or more including the entire chain may be involved, which can become matted.

Groove Sign
This is observed when both inguinal and femoral lymph nodes are involved and are separated by the inguinal ligament. It is pathognomonic of LGV and seen in 15–20% of affected women.

The destruction of lymph nodes may result in genital lymphedema (elephantiasis) with persistent suppuration and pyoderma.

Secondary infections of these ulcers may cause severe pain. Systemic symptoms such as fever, headache, arthralgia, chills and abdominal cramps are seen in the later part of the disease. Ulcers eventually heal, leaving irregular scars, and characteristic 'windows' in the labia minora where the tissue has been destroyed. As the edema and subsequent ulceration cause fibrosis, the urethra may also be destroyed; and the involvement of rectum causes stenosis, sometimes with a rectovaginal fistula. After some years epithelioma may develop in the involved skin.

LGV proctitis can present as rectal pain, anorectal bleeding, mucoid and/or hemopurulent rectal discharge, tenesmus, and constipation.

Investigations
Chlamydia is intracellular organisms so samples should aim to contain cellular material, which is obtained from ulcer base exudate and aspiration of involved enlarged or fluctuant lymph nodes or buboes.

- **Nucleic acid amplification tchniques (NAATs):** NAATs detect LGV-associated *C. trachomatis* DNA/RNA by polymerase chain reaction (PCR), strand displacement amplification (SDA) or transcription mediated amplification (TMA). Detection of LGV DNA confirms the diagnosis.
- **Chlamydia serology:** These tests include complement fixation test, single L-type immunofluorescence test, the micro-immunofluorescence test (micro-IF) and the anti-MOMP IgA assay.
- **Frei's test:** Antigen (0.1 mL) is inoculated intradermally on forearm. In positive response there is inflammatory nodule at the site of test in 2 days, it may reach to maximum size of 7 mm in 4–5 days. This test is positive in 2–6 weeks after the infection and remains positive for several years.
- **Culture:** Culture on cycloheximide-treated McCoy cells of material from suspected LGV lesions has a sensitivity of 75–85% at best, and less for bubo aspirates.
- **Detection of inclusion bodies** in the smear from urethra and vaginal ulcer.

Treatment
One of the following treatment option should be chosen:

Option 1 for 21 days: Doxycycline 100 mg oral bd daily or Tetracycline 2 g oral daily or Minocycline 300 mg oral loading dose followed by 200 mg oral bd daily.

Option 2 for 21 days: Erythromycin 500 mg oral qds daily or Azithromycin 1 g oral weekly for 21 days.

- Surgical treatment may be required if the urethra is destroyed or there is a rectal stricture.

GRANULOMA INGUINALE[42]

Organism
It is caused by Donovania granulomatis (*Klebsiella granulomatis*) and is sexually transmitted.

Clinical Features
This is a chronic ulcerative granulomatous disease that develops in vulva, perineum and inguinal region. The incubation period is 8–12 weeks.

The disease begins as discrete papules, which break down to form painful ulcers, with a meat-red granular zone with clean sharp edges. Ulceration may extend over the vulva, perineum and groins, and the vaginal epithelium or rectal mucosa may be involved.

The ulcer may develop into chronic ulcer with satellite lesions, enlarged lymph nodes with superadded infection resulting in an inguinal swelling (bubo). This bubo may show redness, ulceration, or formation of granulation tissue. A chronic inflammatory exudate comprising lymphocytes, giant cells and histiocytes exude from these buboes. Healing is followed by dense fibrosis, and there may be extensive swelling of the vulva (pseudoelephantiasis). Epithelioma may occur in the damaged skin.

Investigations
Demonstration of Donovan bodies in cellular material or biopsy from lesions confirms the diagnosis. Donovan bodies are characteristically located within large (20–90 µm) histiocytes, pleomorphic in appearance 1 – 2 × 0.5 – 0.7 µm, visible in bipolar densities with a capsule, and stain Gram-negative.

- **Gram-staining:** Smear from the ulcer shows gram negative bipolar rods within leucocytes (these are Donovan bodies).
- **Biopsy:** The diagnosis is made by discovery of Donovan bodies in a biopsy. It may show granulation tissue infiltrated by plasma cells and large macrophages with rod shaped cytoplasmic inclusion bodies (Mikulicz cells).
- **Culture:** Culture of the causative organism, *Klebsiella granulomatis*, in human peripheral blood monocytes.

Treatment
Any one drug is suitable and the duration of treatment should be until lesions have healed at least for three weeks.

1. Azithromycin 1 g oral weekly or 500 mg oral.
2. Ceftriaxone 1 g IM IV daily.
3. Co-trimoxazole 160/800 mg oral bd.
4. Doxycycline 100 mg oral bd.
5. Erythromycin 500 mg oral qds.

Surgery
Residual fibrosis at the sites of lesions may require surgical treatment.

GENITAL WARTS (TABLE 13.3) (CONDYLOMA ACUMINATA)[43]

Organism
Genital warts are caused by human papilloma virus (HPV) infection. Amongst the various types of HPV, the non-oncogenic HPV types 6 and 11 are usually responsible for genital warts. Occasionally, HPV types 16 and 18, which cause cervical precancer, may also cause genital warts. It is advised to screen all the patients with past and present HPV warts for cervical cytology.

Clinical Features
The incubation period is three months. The warts tend to occur in areas most directly affected by coitus, namely the posterior fourchette and lateral areas on the vulva. Less frequently, warts can be found throughout the vulva, in the vagina, and on the cervix. Minor trauma associated with coitus can cause breaks in vulvar skin, allowing direct contact between the viral particles from an infected male and the breached skin of female sexual partner. Infection may be latent or may cause viral particles to replicate and produce a wart. On dry areas of skin the warts are usually flat and small, although on warm moist areas they may be much larger. Exophytic genital warts are highly contagious; more than 75% of sexual partners develop this manifestation of HPV infection when exposed.

Extragenital lesions may be seen on the oral cavity, larynx, conjunctivae, and nasal cavity.

Treatment
The aim of treatment is removal of warts since it is not possible to eradicate the viral infection. Treatment is most successful when warts are small and that have been present for less than 1 year. Selection of specific treatment regimen depends on the anatomic site, size, and number of warts, as well as expense, efficacy, convenience, and potential adverse effects. Recurrences more often result from reactivation of sub-clinical infection.

Specific Treatment
These are not suitable in pregnancy.

- **Podophyllin**: Consists of the local application of 10–25% podophyllin in spirit. This should be washed away 4–6 hours after the application to prevent local skin ulceration. This therapy may need to be repeated several times before the warts disappear. If this therapy fails to remove the warts, cutting diathermy, cryotherapy, laser therapy, or interferon can be used.
- **Podophyllotoxin**: It is a purified extract of podophyllin (0.5% solution or 0.15% cream) and is used for 4–5 weeks. Treatment cycles consist of twice daily application for 3 days, followed by 4 days rest for 4–5 cycles.
- **Trichloroacetic acid**: 80–90% solution is used for weekly application. It results in cellular necrosis. An intense burning sensation may be experienced for 5–10 minutes after application.
- **5-Fluorouracil**: It is a DNA anti-metabolite. A 5% cream used.
- **Interferons**: Interferons alfa, beta, and gamma are used as cream and as intralesional or systemic injection.
- **Imiquimod**: Imiquimod is an immune response modifier. It is used as a 5% cream, applied to lesions three times weekly and washed off 6–10 hours later, for up to 16 weeks.

Table 13.3: Comparative clinical presentations of genital ulcers suggestive of specific diagnosis.

Ulcer	Syphilis	HSV	Chancroid	LGV	GI
Number	Single	Multiple and grouped	One to three	Single	Multiple and discrete
Appearance	Circular, shallow, well-defined edges	Small and shallow with grouped vesicles	Small, shallow, irregular outline, undermined, greenish slough	Shallow, gradually deepens,	Beefy-red granular, clean sharp margins
Pain and tenderness	Painless	Painful	Painful	Painless	Painful
Lymphadenopathy	Rubbery, discrete, painless, mobile	Enlarged, tender	Tender, soft, fluctuating	Tender, hard, form sinuses over skin	Tender, hard, form sinuses over skin

(HSV: herpes simplex virus; LGV: lymphogranuloma venereum; GI: granuloma inguinale)

REFERENCES

1. LaMontagne DS, Fenton KA, Randall S, Anderson S, Carter P. The National Chlamydia Screening Steering Group. Establishing the National Chlamydia Screening Programme in England: results from the first full year of screening. Sex Transm Infect. 2004;80(5):335-41.
2. McKay L, Clery H, Carrick-Anderson K, Hollis S, Scott G. Genital Chlamydia trachomatis infection in a subgroup of young men in the UK. Lancet. 2003;361(9371):1792.
3. Postema EJ, Remeijer L, van der Meijden WI. Epidemiology of genital chlamydial infections in patients with chlamydial conjunctivitis: a retrospective study. Genitourinary Medicine. 1996;72(3):203-5.
4. Westrom LV. Sexually transmitted diseases and infertility. Sexually Transmitted Diseases. 1994;21(2 Suppl):S32-S37.
5. Clad A, Prillwitz J, Hintz KC, Mendel R, Flecken U, Schulte-Monting J, et al. Discordant prevalence of Chlamydia trachomatis in asymptomatic couples screened using urine ligase chain reaction. European Journal of Clinical Microbiology & Infectious Diseases. 2001;20(5):324-8.
6. Khan AM. The prevalence of chlamydia, gonorrhea, and Trichomonas in Sexual Partnerships: implications for partner notification and treatment. Sexually Transmitted Diseases. 2005;32(4):260-4.
7. Chlamydia trachomatis UK Testing Guidelines - http://www.bashh.org/documents/3352.pdf.
8. Watson EJ, Templeton A, Russell I, Paavonen J, Mardh P-A, Stary A, et al. The accuracy and efficiency of screening tests for Chlamydia trachomatis: a systematic review. J Med Microbiol. 2002;51:1021-31.
9. The British Association of Sexual Health and HIV (BASHH)'s National Chlamydia Screening Programme (NSCP) for England, www.bashh.org.
10. Barlow D, Phillips I. Gonorrhoea in women: diagnostic, clinical and laboratory aspects. Lancet. 1978;i:761-4.
11. Bignell C, FitzGerald M; UK national guideline for the management of gonorrhoea in adults, 2011; International Journal of STD & AIDS. 2011;22:541-7. (www.bashh.org).
12. Lewis DA, Bond M, Butt KD, et al. A one-year survey of gonococcal infection seen in the genitourinary medicine department of a London district general hospital. Int J STD AIDS. 1999;10:588-94.
13. United Kingdom National Guideline for Gonorrhoea Testing 2012, Clinical Effectiveness Group, British Association of Sexual Health and HIV. (http://www.bashh.org/documents/4490.pdf)
14. UK National Guideline for the Management of Pelvic Inflammatory Disease 2011, Clinical Effectiveness Group, British Association for Sexual Health and HIV. http://www.bashh.org/documents/3572.pdf.
15. Chisholm S, Mouton J, Lewis D, et al. Cephalosporin MIC creep among gonococci: time for a pharmacodynamics rethink? J Antimicrob Chemother. 2010;65:2141-18.
16. Wolner-Hanssen P, Kreiger JN, Stevens CE, et al. Clinical manifestations of vaginal trichomoniasis. JAMA. 1989;264:571-6.
17. Hollman D, Coupey SM, Fox AS, Herold BC. Screening for Trichomonas vaginalis in high-risk adolescent females with a new transcription-mediated nucleic acid amplification test (NAAT): associations with ethnicity, symptoms, and prior and current STIs. J Pediatr Adolesc Gynecol. 2010;23:312-6.
18. Nye MB, Schwebke JR, Body BA. Comparison of APTIMA Trichomonas vaginalis transcription-mediated amplification to wet mount microscopy, culture, and polymerase chain reaction for diagnosis of trichomoniasis in men and women. American Journal of Obstetrics and Gynecology. 2009, 200:188.e181-188.e187.
19. Huppert JS, et al. Use of an immunochromatographic assay for rapid detection of Trichomonas vaginalis in vaginal specimens. Journal of Clinical Microbiology. 2005;43:684-7.
20. Schwebke JR, Hobbs MM, Taylor SN, Sena AC, Catania MG, Weinbaum BS, et al. Molecular testing for Trichomonas vaginalis in women: results from a prospective U.S. clinical trial. J Clin Microbiol. 2011;49(12):4106-11.
21. United Kingdom National Guideline on the Management of Trichomonas vaginalis 2014, Clinical Effectiveness Group, British Association for Sexual Health and HIV (BASHH). http://www.bashh.org/documents/UK national guideline on the management of TV 2014.pdf).
22. Forna F, Gülmezoglu AM. Interventions for treating trichomoniasis in women. Cochrane Database of Systematic Reviews 2003, Issue 2. Art. No.: CD000218. DOI: 10.1002/14651858.CD000218.
23. Das S, Huengsberg M, Shahmanesh M. Treatment failure of vaginal trichomoniasis in clinical practice. Int J STD AIDS. 2005;16:284-6.
24. Centers for Disease Control and Prevention. Sexually transmitted diseases treatment guidelines. MMWR 2010;59:1-116. http://www.cdc.gov/std/treatment/2010/vaginal-discharge.htm#a2.
25. Mammen-Tobin A, Wilson JD. Management of metronidazole-resistant Trichomonas vaginalis – a new approach. Intl J STD & AIDS. 2005;16:488-90.
26. Hurley R. Recurrent Candida infection. Clin Obstet Gynaecol. 1981;8:208-13.
27. Sobel JD. Vulvovaginal candidiasis. In: Pastorek J, (Ed). Obstetric and Gynaecologic Infectious Disease. New York: Raven Press, 1994:523-36.
28. United Kingdom National Guideline on the Management of Vulvovaginal Candidiasis (2007); Clinical Effectiveness Group, .British Association of Sexual Health and HIV; http://www.bashh.org/documents/1798.pdf.
29. Watson MC, Grimshaw JM, Bond CM, Mollison J, Ludbrook A. Oral versus intra-vaginal imidazole and triazole anti-fungal agents for the treatment of uncomplicated vulvovaginal candidiasis (thrush): a systematic review. BJOG: an International Journal of Obstetrics & Gynaecology. 2002;109(1):85-95.
30. Watson MC, Grimshaw JM, Bond CM, Mollison J, Ludbrook A. Oral versus intra-vaginal imidazole and triazole anti-fungal treatment of uncomplicated vulvovaginal candidiasis (thrush).

[update of Cochrane Database Syst Rev. 2001;(1):CD002845; 11279767.]. [Review] [37 refs]. Cochrane Database of Systematic Reviews 2001;(4):CD002845.

31. Sobel JD. Management of recurrent vulvovaginal candidiasis with intermittent ketoconazole prophylaxis. Obstet Gynaecol. 1985;65:435-60

32. Bauters T, Dhont M, Temmerman M, I, Nelis H. Prevalence of vulvovaginal candidiasis and susceptibility to fluconazole in women. American Journal of Obstetrics and Gynecology. 2002;187(3):569-74.

33. Young GL, Jewell D. Topical treatment for vaginal candidiasis (thrush) in pregnancy. [update of Cochrane Database Syst Rev. 2000;(2):CD000225; 10796183.]. Cochrane Database of Systematic Reviews 2001;(4):CD000225.

34. Nyirjesy P. Chronic vulvovaginal candidiasis. Am Fam Physician. 2001;63(4):697-702.

35. Sobel J, Wiesenfeld H, Martens M, Danna P, Hooton T, Rompalo A, et al. Maintenance fluconazole therapy for recurrent vulvovaginal candidiasis. The New England Journal of Medicine. 2004;351(9):876-83.

36. National Guideline for the Management of Genital Herpes 2007, Clinical Effectiveness Group, British Association for Sexual Health and HIV. http://www.bashh.org/documents/115/115.pdf.

37. Management of genital herpes in pregnancy, Green-top Guideline No. 30, RCOG.https://www.rcog.org.uk/globalassets/documents/guidelines/gt30genitalherpes2007.pdf.

38. UK National Guidelines on the Management of Syphilis 2008, http://www.bashh.org/documents/1879.pdf.

39. UK National Guideline for the Management of Chancroid 2014. Clinical Effectiveness Group, British Association for Sexual Health and HIV (BASHH) http://www.bashh.org/documents/Chancroid%202014%20.pdf.

40. Centers for Disease Control and Prevention. Sexually transmitted diseases treatment guidelines, 2010. MMWR 2010; 59(RR-12).

41. UK National Guideline for the management of lymphogranuloma venereum: Clinical Effectiveness Group, the British Association for Sexual Health and HIV (CEG/BASHH). John White, Nigel O'Farrell and David Daniels *Int J STD AIDS* 2013 24: 593. http://std.sagepub.com/content/24/8/593.

42. United Kingdom national guideline for the management of Donovanosis (Granuloma inguinale) 2011. Clinical Effectiveness Group, British Association for Sexual Health and HIV. http://www.bashh.org/documents/3194.pdf

43. United Kingdom National Guideline on the Management of Ano- genital Warts, 2007. Clinical Effectiveness Group, British Association for Sexual Health and HIV. http://www.bashh.org/documents/86/86.pdf.

CHAPTER 14

Human Immunodeficiency Virus in Women (Including in Pregnancy)

Siya Sharan Sharma, Sucheta Jindal

Overview

- HIV retrovirus characteristically process reverse transcriptase and enzyme which enables RNA virus to make a copy of itself when into host cell DNA replicates further and destroys the host cell.
- Absolute number of CD4 T helper lymphocyte is reduced.
- Prevention of mother to child transmission has to be reduced.
- Importance of viral load to be considered.

EPIDEMIOLOGY

The World Health Organization estimates that around 34 million people in the world are living with human immunodeficiency virus (HIV). The virus is particularly widespread in sub-Saharan African countries.

The adult HIV prevalence in India is declining from estimated level of 0.41% in 2000 through 0.36% in 2006 to 0.32% in 2008 to 0.31% in 2009 with further reduction to 0.27% in 2013. This decreasing trend is also evident in HIV prevalence among the young population of 15–24 years. The estimated number of new annual HIV infections has declined by more than 50% over the past decade in Indian subcontinent.

In 1981, acquired immune deficiency syndrome (AIDS) was first noticed as a clinical entity in men suffering from an unusual outbreak of pneumonia due to *Pnemocystitis carinii*. They were found to have fatal opportunistic infection, which arose due to defective cell-mediated immunity caused by retrovirus HIV. In 1986, HIV epidemic was seen amongst sex workers in the Southern part of India. To control the spread of virus, HIV screening centers were set up along with the provisions of health education.

With the help from United Nations and World Health Organization, the Government of India set-up an organization in 1992 called National AIDS Control Organization (NACO) to oversee the policies, prevention and control programs relating to HIV and AIDS. As a part of the second phase of the programs of NACO, in 1999 the steps were taken to reduce the Mother-To-Child Transmission (MTCT).[1-3]

PATHOPHYSIOLOGY

Human immunodeficiency virus is a retrovirus comprised of single stranded RNA. It is different from other retrovirus because it characteristically possesses reverse transcriptase, an enzyme which enables the RNA virus to make a copy of itself; this copy can be inserted into the host cell DNA where it replicates further and destroys the host cell. HIV in particular targets cells, which have a CD4 protein on their surface, such as CD4+ T-helper lymphocytes. These cells are required for cell-mediated immunity. The absolute number of CD4+ T-helper lymphocytes is reduced and there is abnormal T-cell function with reduced immunity resulting in the opportunistic infections. Autoimmune phenomenon, such as thrombocytopenia also sets in the HIV infection.

Long-term HIV infection leads to AIDS. The continuous HIV virus replication causes the depletion of CD4+ T-helper lymphocytes, which results in the rising state of immune activation and increase in the proinflammatory markers like cytokines. Although new T cells are continuously produced by the thymus to replace the ones lost, the regenerative capacity of the thymus is slowly destroyed by direct infection of its thymocytes by HIV. Eventually, the minimal number of CD4+ T cells necessary to maintain a sufficient immune response is lost, leading to AIDS.

Transmission of HIV (Tables 14.1 and 14.2)

The HIV has been isolated from semen, plasma, tears, saliva, cerebrospinal fluid, urine, breast milk and cervical mucus. Amongst all the bodily fluids, semen, pre-ejaculate secretions, vaginal and cervical secretions, rectal secretions have been shown to transmit infection. Hence, HIV transmission occurs after unprotected vaginal or anal intercourse.

Among the other etiological factors, intravenous drug abuse, sharing injecting equipments and infected blood or blood products are the important risk factors for HIV in women.

HIV can be passed on by receiving blood transfusions or other blood-related products from someone living with HIV, or donations of semen (artificial insemination), skin grafts and organ transplants.

Mothers can transmit HIV infection to their babies during pregnancy, labor and breastfeeding.

The risk of transmission is increased by genital ulcerative disease, such as herpes, syphilis, and chancroid. There is probably an increased risk of transmission of infection when the patient is viremic soon after infection or during the later stages of disease.

Myths about HIV

HIV infection is not transmitted by household or close physical nonsexual contact, swimming pools, by sharing cups, cooking utensils or toilets, or by breathing the same air as an infected person.

Table 14.1: Sources of HIV transmission (%).

• Sexual intercourse	75
– Vaginal	60
– Anal	15
• Transfusion of blood and blood products	5
• IV drugs	4
• Needle pricks	<0.4
• Perinatal (MTCT)	10
• Others	6

Table 14.2: MTCT transmission (%).

• Antepartum	25
• Intrapartum	65
• Breastfeeding	10

CLINICAL PROGRESSION OF HIV

In HIV infection, clinical disease spectrum spreads from an asymptomatic state to fully blown AIDS, progression being variable in individuals. Time taken from contract of HIV infection to AIDS ranges from a few months to more than 12 years, median time being considered is 10 years.

Once HIV infection is contracted, symptoms develop in 70–85% infected patients and AIDS is seen in 55–60% patients within 12 years. Terminal period of illness is relatively short lasting for 1–2 years only. Survival following AIDS is approximately 18 months but may be prolonged if health services are provided adequately.

A febrile illness appears soon after the infection due to viremia. At this stage a person is seronegative but infective. After 6–8 weeks he/she becomes seropositive and may remain asymptomatic for many years. The illness may occur in form of pneumonia, weight loss, and CNS symptoms. Some persons pass through first stage with fever and throat infection like a bad cold. They can then be without symptoms for a time period. For some period before the final diagnosis can be made, the person might suffer from symptoms of infection. They are grouped into what is called ARC (AIDS-related complex). The manifestations of disease vary widely in the world. Different sign and symptoms may be predominant in different areas. For example, "slim disease" stressing the weight loss is most common in Africa, while pneumonia is common in USA and Tuberculosis may be more common in India.

Women with HIV infection, due to reduced immunity, are more prone to other infections as Tuberculosis, bacterial pneumonia, *Pnemocystitis carinii* pneumonia, toxoplasma, CMV, and malignancies, such as Kaposi's sarcoma, which is rare in women. The efficacy of antimicrobial therapy against STDs and other infections is decreased due to reduced immunity.

Schematic representation of HIV disease progression can be seen in Flowchart 14.1.

DIAGNOSIS

HIV is best diagnosed by HIV antibody detection tests.[4,5]

- **Screening test**: Enzyme-linked immunosorbent assay (ELISA)
- **Confirmatory test:** Western Blot

Enzyme-linked immunosorbent assay was the first screening test used which has high sensitivity of 99.7% and specificity of 98.5% with some false positive results. Hence, not all positive or inconclusive HIV ELISA tests mean that the person is infected by HIV. A confirmation test, Western Blot remains the standard method for diagnosing HIV infection which has very low, i.e. 1 in 2,50,000 chance of false positive test.

SECTION 1 General Gynecology

Flowchart 14.1: Schematic representation of HIV disease progression, including symptoms that may occur at each stage of HIV infection.

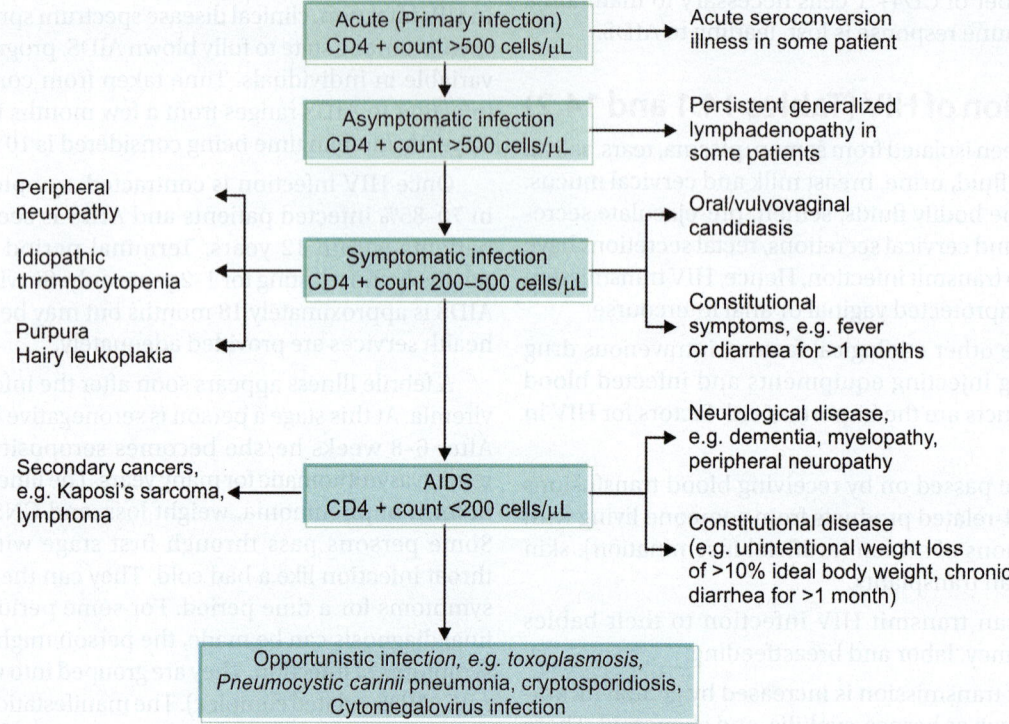

Rapid antibody test or a point-of-care test is a qualitative immunoassay, which can also be used as a screening tool, but its positive predictive value has not been yet evaluated.

Indicator of Immunosuppression

The CD4+ T lymphocyte count is the best laboratory indicator of clinical progression, and management strategies for HIV infection are based on CD4+ count.

A normal CD4+ count range from 500 cells/mm^3 to 1000 cells/mm^3. Patients with CD4+ count from 200–500 cells/mm^3 are more likely to develop HIV-related symptoms and to require medical intervention. Patients with CD4+ counts <200 cells/mm^3 are at increased risk for developing opportunistic infections.

PREVENTION OF SPREAD

- Health education of the population is the major preventive strategy. Everyone including high-risk individual, such as homosexual and bisexual men and women and intravenous drug users, must be made aware of the risks associated by having multiple sexual partners and in failure to use barrier contraceptive precautions.
- Blood donors need to be screened worldwide.
- Semen to be used for artificial insemination should be stored frozen for 3 months until it is established that the donor is not infected.
- Organ donors also need to be screened.

Some social strategies which might be considered for HIV prevention include the following:
- Sex education
- Needle-exchange programs
- Safe injection sites
- Safe sex
- Serosorting
- Sexual abstinence
- Immigration regulation.

GYNECOLOGICAL PROBLEMS DUE TO HIV

- **Infections**: Vaginal candidiasis is common and difficult to treat. Pelvic inflammatory disease (PID), herpes, and human papillomavirus infection (HPV) infections are also frequent in these patients. The prompt diagnosis and aggressive treatment should be employed.
- **Menstrual problems**: Menorrhagia may be due to thrombocytopenia associated with HIV infection. Premature menopause may be observed in these patients.
- **Malignancy screening**: Women with HIV infection have a greater risk of cervical intraepithelial neoplasia (CIN) specially in immunosuppressed individuals. Premalignant lesions may also occur in the vagina and vulva. These women need 6 monthly Pap smears and colposcopy should be employed to avoid the missing of lesions by only cytology.

CLINICAL ASSESSMENT AFTER INITIAL DIAGNOSIS[6-8]

History
- Symptom enquiry (physical, psychological)
- Sexual health
- Partner, status disclosed, safer sex
- Conception issues
- Past and current medical [including tuberculosis (TB) and TB contacts]
- Psychiatric history
- Vaccination history
- Children
- Lifetime travel history, smoking, alcohol, drug-using history
- Animal contact
- GP contact/disclosure.

Physical Examination
- General, skin, oropharynx, lymph nodes, heart, lungs, abdominal (hepatosplenomegaly), anogenital, musculoskeletal and neurological system including cognitive function, dilated fundoscopy (if CD4 T-cell count <50 cells/mm^3)
- Weight, height, BMI, blood pressure, waist circumference.

Investigations
- CD4 T-cell count (absolute and percentage)
- HIV-1 plasma viral load (repeat to confirm baseline within 1–3 months)
- HIV-1 drug-resistance test and HIV-1 subtype determination
- Biochemistry: Creatinine, estimated glomerular filtration rate (eGFR), liver function tests (LFTs), bone profile
- Hematology: Full blood count (FBC)
- Urinalysis: Dipstick for blood, protein and glucose
- Urine protein/creatinine ratio
- Metabolic assessment: Lipid profile [total cholesterol, high-density lipoprotein (HDL) cholesterol, total/HDL cholesterol, triglycerides], glucose
- Syphilis serology
- Hepatitis A virus immunoglobulin (IgG)
- Hepatitis B virus surface antigen (HBsAg), anticore total antibody (anti-HBc), antisurface antibody (anti-HBs)
- Hepatitis C virus antibody (followed by hepatitis C virus RNA testing if antibody positive and confirmation of antibody-positive status if RNA negative)
- Toxoplasma IgG antibody (if CD4 T-cell count <200 cells/mm^3)
- Measles IgG antibody
- Varicella IgG antibody
- Rubella IgG antibody in women of child-bearing age
- Stool for ova/cysts/parasites (if from, or spent >1 month in, tropics)
- Schistosoma serology (if >1 month spent in sub-Saharan Africa)
- Sexual health screen
- Cervical cytology.

Systemic Assessment
- Cardiovascular Disease (CVD) risk
- Fracture risk (if aged >50 years)
- Bone mineral density (BMD) (if aged >65 years)

Treatment with Combined Antiretroviral Therapy (cART) (Table 14.3)

All women must be given the opportunity to be involved in making decisions about their treatment. The primary aim of ART is the prevention of the mortality and morbidity associated with chronic HIV infection at low cost of drug toxicity. Treatment should improve the physical and psychological well-being of people living with HIV infection. The effectiveness and tolerability of ART has improved significantly over the last 15 years.

In primary HIV infection—commence cART in the following:
- Neurological involvement
- Any AIDS-defining illness
- Confirmed CD4 cell count <350 cells/mm^3.

In chronic HIV Infection—Commence cART in the following:
- CD4 cell count is <350 cells/mm^3
- HIV-related comorbidity, including HIV-associated nephropathy (HIVAN), idiopathic thrombocytopenic

Table 14.3: Summary recommendations for choice of ART.

	Preferred	Alternative
NRTI backbone	Tenofovir and emtricitabine	Rilpivirine‡
Third agent	Atazanavir/ritonavir	Abacavir and lamivudine*‡
	Darunavir/ritonavir	Lopinavir/ritonavir
	Efavirenz	Fosamprenavir/ritonavir
	Raltegravir	Nevirapine†
	Elvitegravir/cobicistat	

*Abacavir is contraindicated if HLA-B*57:01 positive
†Nevirapine is contraindicated if baseline CD4 cell count is greater than 250/400 cells/mm^3
‡Use recommended only if baseline VL <1,00,000 copies/mL: rilpivirine as a third agent, abacavir and lamivudine as NRTI backbone.

purpura, symptomatic HIV-associated neurocognitive (NC) disorders irrespective of CD4 cell count
- Coinfection with hepatitis B virus (HBV) if the CD4 cell count is <500 cells/mm³
- Coinfection with hepatitis C virus (HCV) if the CD4 cell count is <500 cells/mm³
- AIDS diagnosis [e.g. Kaposi sarcoma (KS)] irrespective of CD4 cell count
- Non-AIDS defining malignancies requiring immunosuppressive radiotherapy or chemotherapy
- Coinfection with HBV if the CD4 cell count is >500 cells/mm³ and treatment of hepatitis B is indicated.

Start cART containing two nucleoside reverse transcriptase inhibitor (NRTIs) plus one of the following: a ritonavir-boosted protease inhibitor (PI/r), a non-nucleoside reverse transcriptase inhibitor (NNRTI) or an integrase inhibitor (INI).

Factors, such as potential side effects, comorbidities, drug interactions, patient preference and dosing convenience need to be considered in selecting cART in individual women.

Following approach could be adopted in order to ascertain the adherence to cART:
- A 'no-blame' approach is important to facilitate open and honest discussion
- A patient's motivation to start and continue with prescribed medication is influenced by the way in which they judge their personal need for medication (necessity beliefs), relative to their concerns about potential adverse effects
- Delayed uptake and nonadherence are associated with doubts about personal need for cART and concerns about taking it
- Interventions to support adherence should be individualized to address specific relevant perceptual and practical barriers. A three-step 'perceptions and practicalities approach' may be helpful:
  - Identify and address any doubts about personal need for cART
  - Identify and address specific concerns about taking cART
  - Identify and address practical barriers to adherence.
- Because evidence is inconclusive, only use interventions to overcome practical problems, if there is a specific need
- Interventions might include:
  - Suggesting patients to record their medicine-taking
  - Encouraging patients to monitor their results
  - Simplifying the dosing regimen
  - Using a multicompartment medicines system.
- If side effects are a problem:
  - Discuss benefits and long-term effects and options for dealing with side effects
  - Consider adjusting the dosage, switching to another combination or other strategies, such as changing the dose timing or formulation.
- Patients' experience of taking cART and their needs for adherence support may change over time
- Patients' knowledge, understanding and concerns about medicines and the benefits they perceive should be reviewed regularly at agreed intervals.

PREVENTION OF MOTHER-TO-CHILD TRANSMISSION

Provider-initiated testing and counseling for pregnant women and linkage to prevention and care is recommended to promote the mother's health and prevent new pediatric infections.

In the pre-cART era, HIV-positive women were advised to avoid getting pregnant because of high-risk of mother-to-cilld (MTCT). Despite the lack of licence for the use of cART in pregnancy, the global consensus is that the benefits of using cART outweigh the risks of not using it during the pregnancy. Zidovudine has a licence to be used in pregnancy but in the cART era, the evidence for the efficacy of using zidovudine is poor although its use in combination with cART is beneficial if the HIV viral load is >1000/mL. Also, the combination of latest evidence and research has changed the picture completely and the following steps are recommended in the HIV-positive pregnant women in order to achieve MTCT to 0%:

1. Women conceiving on an effective cART with or without zidovudine should continue their drug regimen. Exceptions are:
   - Protease inhibitor (PI) monotherapy should be intensified to include (depending on tolerability, resistance and prior antiretroviral history) one or more agents that cross the placenta.
   - The combination of stavudine and didanosine should not be prescribed in pregnancy.
2. Women requiring cART for their own health should commence treatment as soon as possible during pregnancy.
3. No routine dose alterations are recommended for ARVs during pregnancy if used at adult licensed doses.
4. Women who do not require cART for themselves should still have commenced ART by 24th week of pregnancy.
5. Zidovudine plus lamivudine, tenofovir plus emtricitabine or abacavir plus lamivudine are acceptable nucleoside backbones.
6. Protease inhibitors can be used to boost cART.
7. Zidovudine monotherapy can be used in women planning a cesarean section who have a baseline VL of <10,000 HIV RNA copies/mL and a CD4 of >350 cells/mm³.

8. If the baseline VL is >30,000 HIV RNA copies/mL, commence cART in early second trimester and if the baseline VL is >100,000 HIV RNA copies/mL, commence cART in first trimester.
9. A woman who presents after 28 weeks should commence cART without delay.
10. If the viral load is unknown or >1,00,000 HIV RNA copies/mL, a three or four drug regimen that includes raltegravir is suggested in late presenting woman with no treatment.
11. An untreated woman presenting in labor at term should be given a stat dose of nevirapine and commence fixed-dose zidovudine with lamivudine and raltegravir. Intravenous zidovudine (Loading dose of 2 mg/kg IV over one hour, then 1mg/kg/hour till delivery) is infused for the duration of labor and delivery.
12. Untreated women with a CD4 cell count ≥350 cells/mm^3 and a viral load of <50 HIV RNA copies/mL can be treated with zidovudine monotherapy or with cART (including abacavir/lamivudine/zidovudine) and can aim for a vaginal delivery.
13. One CD4 cell count must be done at the point of contact as a baseline and another one at 36 weeks at least.
14. HIV viral load should be performed 2–4 weeks after commencing cART, at least once every trimester, at 36 weeks and at delivery.
15. Liver function tests should be performed as per routine initiation of cART and then at each antenatal visit.
16. Routine fetal ultrasound imaging and combined screening test for trisomy 21 should be performed regardless of maternal HIV status.
17. External cephalic version (ECV) can be performed in women with HIV.
18. For women with a plasma viral load of <50 HIV RNA copies/mL at 36 weeks, and in the absence of obstetric contraindications, a planned vaginal delivery is recommended.
19. For women with a plasma viral load of 50–399 HIV RNA copies/mL at 36 weeks, planned cesarean delivery at 38–39 weeks should be considered.
20. For women with a plasma viral load of >400 HIV RNA copies/mL at 36 weeks, planned cesarean delivery at 38–39 weeks is recommended.
21. Vaginal birth after cesarean section (VBAC) should be offered to women with a viral load <50 HIV RNA copies/mL.
22. In all cases of term prelabor, spontaneous rupture of the membranes (ROM) delivery should be expedited.
23. In all cases of 34–37 weeks prelabor spontaneous ROM delivery should be expedited and intrapartum group B streptococcus prophylaxis should be given.
24. In all cases of <34 weeks prelabor spontaneous ROM, mode and timing of delivery should be planned after multidisciplinary discussions, intramuscular steroids should be administered for fetal lung maturity and virological control should be optimized.
25. All mothers known to be HIV positive, regardless of antiretroviral therapy, and infant pre-exposure prophylaxis, should be advised to exclusively formula feed from birth.
26. If a mother who is on cART and with undetectable viral load chooses to breast feed, intensive support and monitoring by monthly viral loads is recommended for both (mother and baby).

REFERENCES

1. Overview of HIV and AIDS in India. Retrieved from http://www.avert.org/aidsindia.htm.
2. Appay V, Sauce D. Immune activation and inflammation in HIV-1 infection: causes and consequences. J Pathol. 2008;214(2):231-41.
3. Morgan DC, Mayanja MB, Whitworth JA. Progression to symptomatic disease in people infected with HIV-1 in rural Uganda: prospective cohort study. BMJ. 2000;324(7331):193-196.
4. UNAIDS/WHO policy statement on HIV Testing (PDF), accessed 5 October 2006.
5. Chou R, Huffman LH, Fu R, Smits AK, Korthuis PT. Screening for HIV: a review of the evidence for the US Preventive Services Task Force. Ann Intern Med. 2005;143(1):55-73.
6. British HIV Association. HIV Medicine. 2012;13:1-44.
7. British HIV Association. HIV Medicine. 2014;15(Suppl. 1):1-85.
8. British HIV Association. HIV Medicine. 2014;15(Suppl. 4):1-77.

CHAPTER 15

Benign Lesions of the Genital Tract

K Jayakrishnan, P Manjula

Overview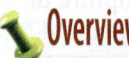

- Benign lesions of the vulva are lichen sclerosis, squamous cell hyperplasia (formerly hyperplastic dystrophy) and other dermatomes.
- Condyloma acuminata are the most common lesions in the vagina. Vaginal cysts are rare because there are no glands in the mucous layer. The common cysts are Gartner's cyst and inclusion cyst.
- The squamous epithelium of the ectocervix is replaced by columnar epithelium which is continuous with the lining of endocervix. Various forms of erosions are present. Ectropion is because of the bilateral tears of the cervix exposing the endocervix. Polyps are the other benign lesions of the cervix.
- Uterine fibroids are the commonest benign tumors, which arise from the smooth muscle cells and termed correctly as leiomyoma.
- These are cysts, which form in the ovary during normal ovarian cycles. Because of the easy availability of the ultrasound, this is often found incidentally. They are mostly seen in young women. The common cysts are follicular cysts and corpus luteum cysts.
- Neoplasms of the ovary can occur from the epithelium, stroma or the germ cells.

INTRODUCTION

This Chapter will be confined to discussion of the benign lesions of the female genital tract. The emphasis is on the common and important lesions of vulva, vagina, uterus and ovaries. The intention is to provide a sound and thorough framework upon which the advanced knowledge is built.

BENIGN LESIONS OF VULVA

Benign gynecological conditions can present with a variety of symptoms like pruritus, pain, dyspareunia, discharge, ulceration and pigmentation. However, some vulval lesions are asymptomatic and are noted during gynecological examination.

Classification

Benign lesions of the vulva are classified, according to The International Society of Gynecological Pathologists as:

- Lichen sclerosis
- Squamous cell hyperplasia (formerly hyperplastic dystrophy)
- Other dermatomes.

A systematic approach with appropriate treatment and reassurance of benign pathology should alleviate the symptoms.

Lichen Sclerosis

This is a common condition found in elderly women complaining of itching in the vulval area. It is sometimes seen in children and less commonly in young women. The etiology remains unknown, but may be associated with autoimmune disorders. It is hormone dependent as it is influenced by testosterone. The lesions are seen to improve following local application of testosterone. Lichen sclerosis may be due to infection commonly spirochetal; as these organisms may be found in histological sections of LS. About 4% women with lichen sclerosis develop invasive carcinoma of vulva. Vulval intraepithelial neoplasia and lichen sclerosis can coexist in the same patient. The affected skin looks thin white and crinkled. The contour of the vulva disappears and labial adhesions form.

The diagnosis can be made clinically but a biopsy is performed whenever possible. If the patient is asymptomatic, no treatment is needed. Mild itching may be relieved by aqueous cream or 1% hydrocortisone ointment, applied three times daily for 6 weeks. For severe pruritus, application of a potent corticosteroid such as betamethasone, fluocinolone or clobetasol for 8-12 weeks is required. Thereafter, frequency of application can be reduced to once or twice a week. Hormonal creams like 2% testosterone ointment applied 2-3 times per day for 6 weeks and then reduced 1-2 times a week produced reversal of labial fusion and clitoral adhesions. There is no place for vulvectomy in view of high morbidity and recurrence rate.

Squamous Cell Hyperplasia

Squamous cell hyperplasia is diagnosed when there is histological evidence of hyperplasia with out any other clinical features to account for the lesion. The lesion is mainly confined to labia majora, minora and introitus.

Histology
The characteristic histological features include elongation of rete pegs, hyperkeratosis and dermal inflammation.

Clinical Features
Pruritus vulvae is the main complaint. If cracks develop, secondary infection may result, the margins are well-defined. Histology is mandatory. Atypia is present in 8-10% of cases. If atypia is present, the chances of malignancy is very high.

Treatment
Hydrocortisone cream 2% can be effectively applied locally. If atypia is present considering the risk of development of malignancy, simple vulvectomy may be advised, especially in cases of severe atypia and in cases where regular follow-up is unlikely.

Other Dermatoses

Many of these lesions will have manifestations elsewhere. They are diagnosed by history, examination and in few cases biopsy may be needed. This includes lichen simplex chronicus, lichen planus, psoriasis, allergic dermatitis and intertrigo.

- *Lichen simplex chronicus*: The lesions are dry, thick and scaly and is treated with mild topical corticosteroids.
- *Lichen planus*: The lesions are purple white papules with a shiny surface, often asymptomatic and self-limiting. Histology is diagnostic, treated by topical steroids.
- *Psoriasis*: May occur on vulva, lesion is erythematous with sharp outline and silvery scaling surface, treated with a strong long topical steroid.
- *Allergic dermatitis*: Occurs as an allergic response to various irritants. Usually, presents with vulval itching, present clinically as a diffuse erythema and edema.
- *Intertrigo*: Lesions are red, moist and susceptible to secondary infection.

Vulval ulcers: The causes of benign vulval ulcers are:
- Aphthous ulcers
- Behcet's disease
- Lipschutz ulcers
- Crohn's disease
- Herpes genitalis
- Primary syphilis
- Lymphogranuloma venereum
- Chancroid
- Donovanosis
- Tuberculosis.

Disorders of Pigmentation

- Melanosis vulvae (lentigo) is the commonest pigmented lesion on the vulva, producing light brown, multiple macules which are asymptomatic and diagnosed by excision biopsy
- Benign nevi
- Vitiligo.

BENIGN TUMORS OF VULVA

Majority of the benign tumors of vulva are of epidermal origin. Less commonly, they arise from epidermal appendages, mesoderm or from greater or lesser vestibular glands. Other vulval swellings may be due to cyst of the canal of Nuck, mesonephric duct (Gartner's), hydrocolpos, hematocolpos and vulva endometriosis.

Cystic Lesions

- Epidermoid and sebaceous cysts are treated by excision. Mucinous cysts may arise from the minor vestibular glands
- Mesonephric cysts are found on the labia majora
- Cysts of the canal of Nuck are found on the anterior part of the vulva
- *Bartholin's cysts*: These cysts arise from the ducts of Bartholin's gland, which lies in the subcutaneous tissue below the lower third of labia majora. This is a retention cyst, occurs when the duct becomes blocked, forming a tense cyst which when infected, forms a painful abscess. It is treated by incision and marsupialization of the abscess and antibiotic therapy.

Nonepithelial Tumors

Lipomas and fibromas are the commonest benign tumors of the vulva arising from the mesoderm. Other less common tumors are leiomyoma, neurofibroma, lymphangioma, hemangioma.

Epithelial Tumors
- Squamous papilloma and 'skin tags' are common benign tumors
- *Basal cell papilloma (seborrheic keratosis/wart):* It is a benign proliferation of the epidermis. It is a raised pigmented lesion with a 'stuck-on' appearance. No treatment is required
- *Keratoacanthoma*: It is a nodular lesion developing into ulceration, resolves spontaneously. As it resembles squamous carcinoma, excision biopsy is done for histological study
- *Angiokeratoma*: It is a form of hemangioma, seen as a vascular or pigmented lesion on the labia majora
- *Condyloma acuminata*: These are small papules sometimes sessile, often polypoidal, caused by human papilloma virus type 6/11. Majority can be treated by application of 80% trichloroacetic acid. Podophyllin is less effective and more toxic. If lesions are large and widespread, removal by diathermy or CO_2 laser is performed.
- *Condyloma lata* are sessile papules which become highly infectious when they ulcerate.

Ectopic Tissue
- Breast lesions may be found on the vulva and presents as a firm mobile vulval mass during pregnancy
- *Endometriosis:* It may be found on the vulva after implantation in a surgical wound, e.g. episiotomy.

BENIGN LESIONS OF THE VAGINA
- Benign tumors of the vagina are uncommon. Condyloma acuminata are the most common lesions with frond-like surface. Biopsy is confirmative
- *Endometriotic* deposits of vagina are most common in an episiotomy wound
- *Vaginal cysts* are rare because there are no glands in the mucous layer. The common cysts are Gartner's cyst and inclusion cyst
- *Gartner's cyst*: It is a simple mesonephric cyst, seen high up near the fornices and anterolateral walls of vagina. The cyst is lined by low columnar cells and secretes mucinous material. They are usually asymptomatic and treated by marsupialization in symptomatic patients. Marsupialization is safer and effective than excision
- *Inclusion cysts* arise from vaginal epithelium, buried under the mucosa during healing from trauma mainly following childbirth. They are lined by stratified squamous epithelium and treated by excision.

BENIGN LESIONS OF THE CERVIX
- *Cervical erosion*: The squamous epithelium of the ectocervix is replaced by columnar epithelium which is continuous with the lining of endocervix. Various forms of erosions are described.
  - *Congenital erosion*: It is due to the maternal estrogenic effect on the newborn. It is self-limiting. It may reappear at or soon after puberty under the influence of estrogen
  - *Acquired erosion*: It occurs following chronic cervicitis, the squamous epithelium of ectocervix is replaced by columnar epithelium
  - *Hormonal or papillary erosion*: During pregnancy and in oral contraceptive pill users, the hyperplasia of end cervical epithelium causes papillary type of cervical erosion which is estrogen dependent. This usually returns back to normal within three months of delivery or withdrawal of pill. The patient may be asymptomatic or may present with profuse mucoid discharge.

  It is seen as a raised reddened smooth glistening area around the external OS with well-defined margins and the inner margin continuous with the end cervical lining.

  Symptomatic patients are treated with local application of antiseptics and antibiotics to the cervix, diathermy cauterization, cryosurgery, conization or laser therapy.
- *Ectropion*: It is the eversion of endocervical canal, exposing the lining mucosa. It is caused by cervical lacerations. It is usually accompanied by chronic cervicitis and produces mucopurulent discharge. Treated by excision of scar tissue and suturing the edges of the torn cervix.
- *Cervical polyps*: They include mucous myomatous and fibroadenomatous polyps. Mucous polyps arise from mucous membrane of cervical canal and are frequently associated with chronic inflammatory disease of cervix. It forms a small red vascular pedunculated swelling which bleeds on touch, being attached to mucous membrane of the cervical canal (Figs. 15.1A and B). It causes increased vaginal discharge, irregular and postcoital bleeding. Avulsion of the polyp is the treatment.

BENIGN TUMORS OF UTERUS
Uterine fibroids are the commonest benign tumors, which arise from the smooth muscle cells and termed correctly as leiomyoma.

Incidence: At least 20% of women of reproductive age group have fibroids.

CHAPTER 15 Benign Lesions of the Genital Tract

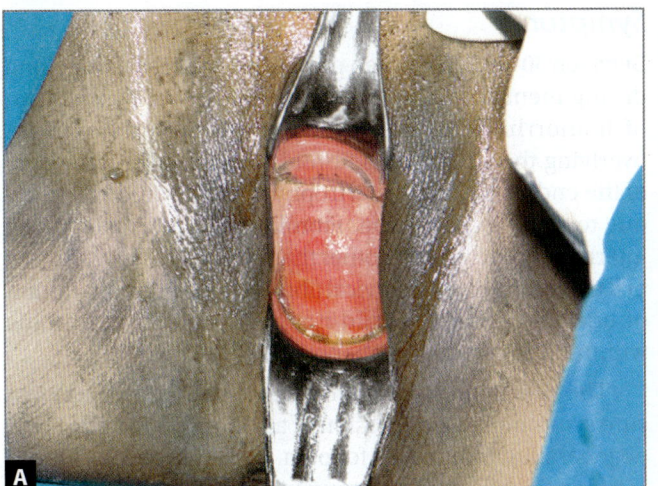
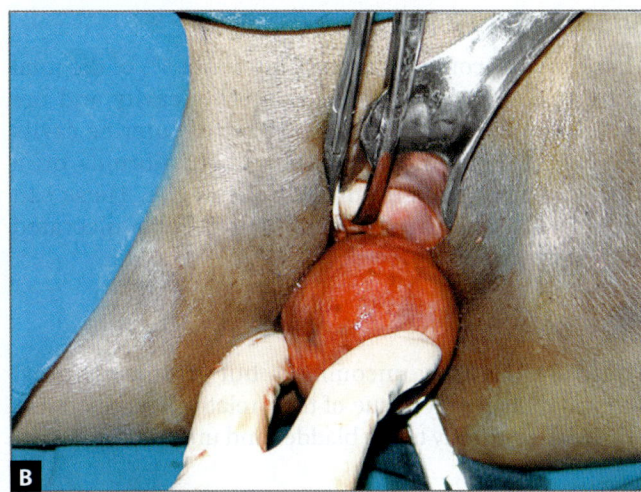

Figs. 15.1A and B: Cervical polyps.

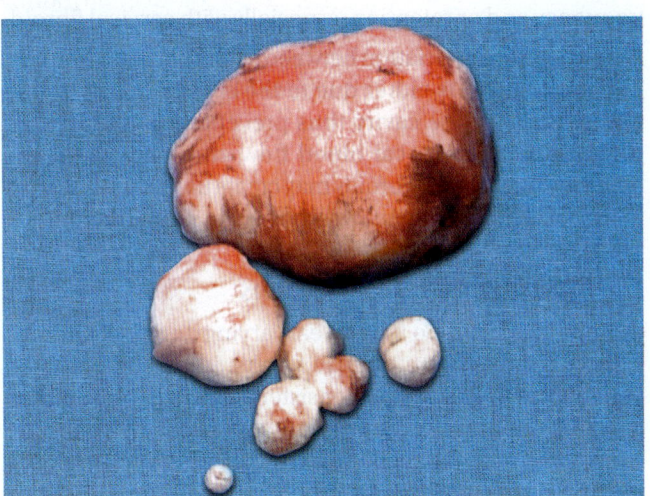

Fig. 15.2: Multiple fibroids.

Etiology: It is unknown, estrogen dependent, common in nulliparous and undergoes atrophy after menopause.

Pathology: Fibroids are firm, round tumors, become soft and cystic when degenerative changes occur, may be single or multiple, usually arising from body of uterus and less commonly from cervix (Fig. 15.2). They can be intramural, submucous, subserous of intraligamentary.

Fibroids undergo various degenerative changes like hyaline, cystic calcific and red degeneration. Rarely, sarcomatous degeneration may occur.

Signs and Symptoms

Most of them are asymptomatic. Usually, they present with abdominal swelling and menstrual irregularities, menorrhagia being common.

Pain may be due to congestive dysmenorrhea, red degeneration or torsion of pedunculated fibroid.

They may cause infertility by causing distortion of uterus or mechanical obstruction of fallopian tube.

Classification and Pathophysiology

Macroscopically, fibroids are round and firm in consistency with a characteristic whorled appearance on cross-section. They may be single or multiple with varying sites and sizes. Four clinical subgroups which are intramural, subserosal, submucosal and cervical are described below.

Intramural

They lie within the uterine wall separated from the adjacent normal myometrium by a thin layer of connective tissue, which forms the false capsule. Small nutrient arteries penetrate this capsule. Large intramural fibroids enlarge and distort the uterine cavity.

Subserosal

These project outward from the uterine surface and are covered with peritoneum. As growth is not restricted by surrounding myometrium, they may attain a very large size. These fibroid can become pedunculated. Subserosal fibroid arising from the lateral wall may lie in between the layers of broad ligament and can displace the ureters laterally. These broad ligament fibroids (otherwise called false broad-ligament fibroid) are different from true broad-ligament fibroid which have no attachment to uterine wall, but have their origin in smooth muscle fibers within the broad ligament.

Submucous Fibroid

These are less common comprising about 5% of the total fibroids. They project into the uterine cavity and are covered by endometrium and distort the uterine cavity (Fig. 15.3). Pedunculated submucous fibroids on a long stalk may prolapse through the cervix. These can produce intermenstrual bleeding or become ulcerated and infected.

Cervical Fibroids

These are relatively uncommon, but give rise to great surgical difficulty by virtue of their relative inaccessibility and close proximity to the bladder and ureters.

Microscopic Appearance

Microscopically, fibroids are composed of smooth muscle cell bundles, arranged in whorl-like patterns (Fig. 15.4) admixed with variable amount of connective tissue. The center of the fibroid is relatively poor in blood supply. Hence, they can undergo degenerative changes. Hyaline degeneration results in a homogeneous consistency and may become cystic. Fatty change or calcification also can happen. Red degeneration happens almost exclusively in pregnancy. The symptoms are pain and tenderness and may present as an acute abdomen. Fibroid in this condition is reddish and with a peculiar fishy smell. Sarcomatous changes can occur very rarely.

Etiology

The etiology is unknown. The growth of the fibroid is dependent on ovarian hormones. Fibroids are unknown before menarche and it will regress after menopause.

Symptoms

Between 30–50% of women present with excessive bleeding during menstruation. It can lead to anemia. Mechanism of hemorrhage is due to ulceration of endometrium overlying the submucous fibroids, increased surface area of the endometrium, hypertrophy of the myometrium and due to venous congestion. Fibroids will not usually cause intermenstrual bleeding other than when there is ulceration or it is a submucous or cervical fibroid. Hence, any disruption of normal cyclicity should not be attributed to fibroids without first excluding other causes.

The next major symptom is pelvic pain and other pressure symptoms. Acute torsion of a pedunculated fibroid or degeneration is the cause for pain. If the submucous fibroid is trying to get expelled through the cervix, it will produce pain. Rarely, this can cause inversion of uterus. Large fibroids can produce bladder symptoms such as increased frequency and or retention, especially with cervical fibroid.

There is an association between subfertility and fibroids. The mechanism is either due to the cornual block or due to distortion of the cavity thus preventing implantation. Alterations in the local blood flow and increase in the binding of steroids to fibroids may create unfavorable factors in the local environment, which prevent implantation.

Diagnosis and Investigations

General examination may reveal varying degree of anemia. If the fibroid is more than 14 weeks, it may be palpated per abdomen. It is firm in consistency, with a well-defined margin. Bimanual examination shows the uterus to be enlarged. It may be regular or irregular enlargement. The uterus is not felt separate from the swelling and cervix moves with the movement of the swelling. In a subserous

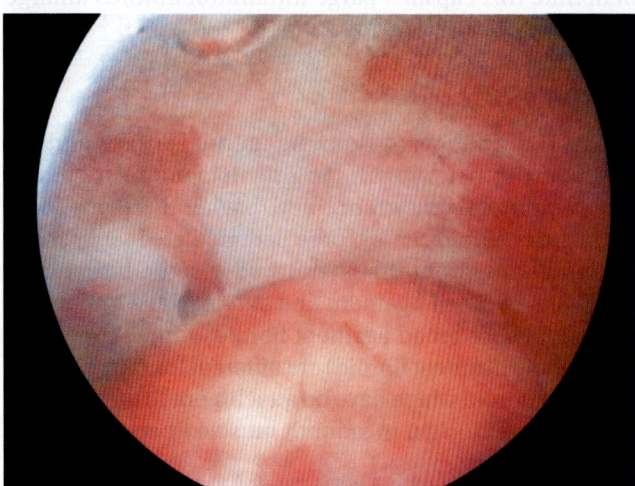

Fig. 15.3: Submucous fibroid (hysteroscopy).

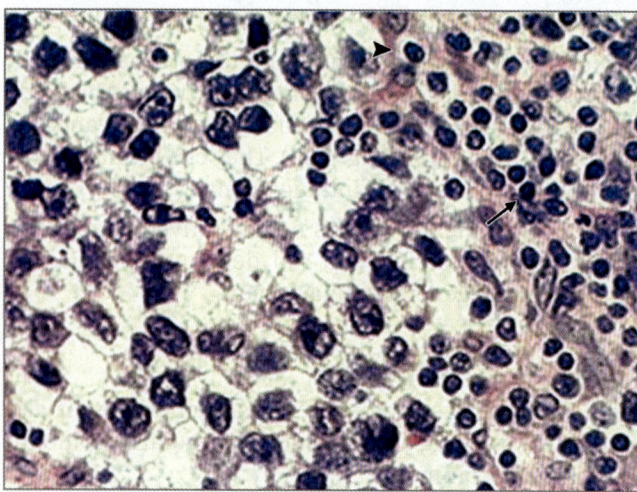

Fig. 15.4: Microscopic appearance of fibroids.

fibroid it may feel separate from the uterus, especially if it is pedunculated.

Ultrasound will confirm the diagnosis.

- A fibroma is seen as well-defined rounded tumor, hypoechoic with cystic spaces if degeneration has occurred. Ultrasound cannot differentiate a pedunculated subserous fibroid from a solid ovarian tumor.
- Magnetic resonance imaging is highly accurate in depicting number, size and location of fibroids. But it is costly, not widely available and rarely necessary.
- *Hysterosalpingography:* It identifies a submucous myoma and checks the patency of fallopian tubes in infertility.
- *Hysteroscopy*: Direct visualization through hysteroscopy will diagnose a submucous myoma and at the same time enables its excision.
- Laparoscopy is of value in diagnosing coincidental endometriosis, pelvic adhesions or other tubal pathology. It differentiates between pedunculated fibroid and ovarian neoplasm and enables removal of fibroids.

Differential Diagnosis

These are pregnancy, full bladder, adenomyosis, chocolate cysts, ovarian pathology or tubo-ovarian mass, hematometra, bicornuate uterus.

Treatment Methods

Recent advances in medical and surgical methods of treatment have increased the potential range of therapeutic options for women with fibroids. While surgery remains the treatment of choice for most symptomatic women, alternatives may be appropriate in some situations.

Expectant Management

Fibroids are frequently asymptomatic and therefore, active treatment is unnecessary. The risk of sarcomatous change is 1 in 1,000, making prophylactic removal of fibroid unjustified. Annual pelvic examination for assessing the growth of the fibroid supplemented with ultrasound is enough to manage these cases. Fibroids do not carry any long-term detrimental effects and spontaneous regression after menopause may be anticipated.

Hysterectomy

This is the definitive treatment for symptomatic fibroids, who do not wish to preserve reproductive function. In asymptomatic women with large fibroids and rapid increase in size, hysterectomy is justified.

Abdominal hysterectomy with ovarian conservation is the procedure of choice where fibroids are very large.

Vaginal Hysterectomy

Preoperative treatment with GnRH analogues can shrink the fibroids and make vaginal hysterectomy possible.

Due consideration is given to factors like women's wish to preserve reproductive function. Conservative surgical management of myomectomy, i.e. removal of fibroids, is done in those desiring to conserve the uterus. In most cases, total abdominal hysterectomy will be the procedure of choice.

Myomectomy

Is the removal, individual fibroids, current surgical techniques are largely attributed to Victor Bonney. Enucleation of intramural fibroid from their false capsule can be rapid and simple but sometimes, technical difficulties, major hemorrhage and greater postoperative morbidity and mortality than hysterectomy are seen.

Principle of Myomectomy

- It is restricted to women who have not completed childbearing age
- When fibroids are solitary or few in number
- To minimize postoperative adhesions, hemostasis should be achieved from incision sites as many fibroids as possible should be removed through single incision
- Avoid opening of uterine cavity to prevent intrauterine adhesions
- Careful obliteration of large cavities left by enucleation of fibroids is very important. Bonney described "hood" method of closure of the cavity left after enucleation of large single posterior fibroid. Suturing the redundant flap of serosal covered myometrium over the fundus and low down on to the anterior wall to avoid adhesion formation
- Use of Bonney's myomectomy clamp placed across the lower uterus to occlude the uterine artery or use of rubber tourniquet placed around the uterus through incision in broad ligament at the level of lower uterine segment. Such methods are unsuitable for large cervical or broad ligament fibroids
- Local injection of vasopressin into fibroids
- Preoperative treatment with GnRH analogues to reduce vascularity of uterus and size of the fibroids.

Endoscopic Surgical Methods

Hysteroscopy

- Most submucous fibroids protruding through cervix can be removed vaginally with ligation of the pedicle
- Submucous fibroids can be diagnosed and at the same time removed through hysteroscopy which is gaining

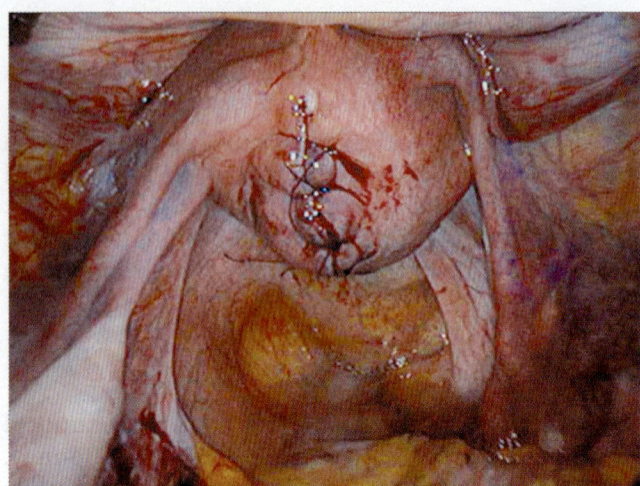

Fig. 15.5: Laparoscopic myomectomy.

popularity. Prior shrinkage with GnRHa for large fibroids enables removal. Postoperative bleeding can be controlled by tamponade with the balloon of a Foley catheter.

Laparoscopic myomectomy (Fig. 15.5) is gaining popularity over abdominal myomectomy in recent times: If the fibroid is very large, in order to reduce the bleeding in these cases preoperative treatment with GnRH analogue is recommended.

The fibroids are morcellated or removed by colpotomy.

Medical Management

Two main objectives of medical management are relief of symptoms and reduction in the size of fibroids. But do not cause complete regression of the tumor. There is a greater role for medical therapy both for symptomatic treatment and fibroids and as adjuncts to surgery. For this reason, medical management has got its own limitations.

- *Progestogens*: Progestogens are widely used in the management of DUB but are not effective in reducing the size and bleeding with fibroids
- *Androgenic steroids*—such as danazol or gestrinone are useful in reducing menstrual blood loss by virtue of their direct effect on the endometrium and negative feedback inhibition of pituitary gonadotropin release. A small reduction in the size of fibroids has been reported, with relief of menstrual symptoms. Due to androgenic properties and side effects they are unsuitable for long-term use. It is used only for short-term waiting for the operation or to raise the hemoglobin level before operation
- *Prostoglandin synthetase inhibitors*: These may be used in relieving the pelvic pain in women with fibroid. Are ineffective in treating menorrhagia
- *Antifibrinolytics*: Useful agent for menorrhagia, reduces blood loss by 50%
- *Estrogen-progestogen combination*: Modest reduction of blood loss is seen, but can cause enlargement of fibroids. They can be given with GnRH analogues to reduce vasomotor side effects and bone loss caused by GnRHa
- *GnRH agonists*: These agents significantly reduce the size of uterine fibroids, relieves pressure symptoms and menorrhagia by their sustained pituitary down regulation, and resultant ovarian suppression. It causes amenorrhea and at the same time causes vasomotor symptoms and vaginal dryness. Uterine volume shrinks by 35% after 3 months of administration and 50% after 6 months with little further change thereafter. Once treatment is stopped, rapid growth to their preoperative size is seen. Therefore, their use is confined to short-term use as adjuncts to surgery to reduce vascularity and size of fibroids and relief of severe menorrhagia. This treatment is advocated in medically unfit women, obese women and in those known to have severe pelvic adhesions, where surgery is not safe option.

GnRHa play a valuable role in the management of uterine fibroids but they will not replace the role played by surgery.

- *GnRH antagonist*: They directly inhibit the action of GnRH on pituitary gland resulting in immediate suppression and rapid shrinkage of fibroid
- *Antiprogesterones*: RU 486, mifepristone cause shrinkage of fibroid and amenorrhea. Exciting new approach to medical treatment of fibroids.

While hysterectomy gives the best results in terms of symptomatic cure, this will be inappropriate in a woman wishing to preserve reproductive potential.

UTERINE POLYPS

Uterine polyps are common and usually benign. They are found in the body of the uterus and in the endocervix.

Polyps cause menorrhagia, intermenstural and post-menopausal bleeding. They are treated by removal using sponge forceps and curettage or hysteroscopically.

BENIGN TUMORS OF OVARY (TABLE 15.1)

The ovary gives rise to a wide variety of tumors than any other organ in the body, ranging from epithelial, connective tissue, germinal, embryonal cell and hormone secreting tumors. Commonest are the epithelial tumors, forming 80% of all ovarian tumors. Of these, 80% ovarian tumors are benign and 20% are malignant, many of which may

CHAPTER 15 Benign Lesions of the Genital Tract

Table 15.1: Difference between benign and malignant ovarian tumors.

	Benign	Malignant
Age	Mostly reproductive age	Menopausal, adolescent, young adults
Symptoms	Not associated with pain	Associated with pain
Bleeding	Seen with functional ovarian tumors	Postmenopausal bleeding
Side of the tumor	Unilateral or bilateral	Bilateral

Table 15.2: Difference between cystic and solid ovarian tumors.

	Cystic (solid—fibroma, Brenner, theca cell)	Solid
Consistency	Smooth	Nodular
Surface mobility	Mobile	Fixed
POD	Free	Nodular, hard, fixed
Size	Less than 10 cm	More than 10 cm
Septation	Less than 3 mm	Multiple septation more than 3 mm
Ascites	Absent (except in Brenner or fibroma)	Present
CA 125	Below 35 unit/mL	More than 35

be asymptomatic. Benign small cysts of the ovary are asymptomatic and often disappear spontaneously.

Benign ovarian tumors can be broadly classified into functional or physiological and pathological cysts.

Physiological Cysts (Table 15.2)

These are cysts, which form in the ovary during normal ovarian cycles. Because of the easy availability of the ultrasound, this is often found incidentally. They are mostly seen in young women. The common cysts are follicular cysts and corpus luteum cysts.

The features of the functional cysts are:
- They are rarely complicated in appearance
- They are related to hormonal changes
- Usually, they do not exceed more than 5 cm in diameter
- They are mostly unilocular and contain clear fluid.

Follicular Cyst

This is lined by granulosa cells, and is the commonest benign cyst. This results from nonruptured dominant follicle and can achieve a diameter of up to 10 cm. It can persist for several menstrual cycles. Small cysts may resolve and intervention is required in the form of ultrasound-guided aspiration, laparoscopy or laparotomy if symptoms develop or if the cyst do not resolve after 8–12 weeks. Combined steroidal contraceptive can be prescribed for a short duration to suppress cyst formation.

Corpus Luteal Cyst

This is less common than follicular cysts. This is mainly due to the overactivity of corpus luteum. It can be associated with pregnancy and usually disappears around 12 weeks. The cyst can enlarge and continue producing progesterone and the menstrual period can get delayed. One complication is cyst rupture that produces intraperitoneal bleeding and acute abdomen. With a delayed period and intraperitoneal bleed, this can mimic a ruptured ectopic pregnancy. If features of acute abdomen appear, laparoscopy or laparotomy may be needed to arrest bleeding and to enucleate the cyst.

Pathological Cysts or Benign Ovarian Neoplasms

WHO classification of ovarian tumors (major groups):
- Common epithelial tumors
  - Serous tumors
  - Endometrioid tumors
  - Clear cell (mesonephroid tumors)
  - Brenner tumors
  - Mixed epithelial tumors
  - Undifferentiated carcinoma
  - Unclassified epithelial tumors.
- Sex-cord (gonadal stromal) tumors
  - Granulosa-stromal cell tumors, theca cell tumors
  - Androblastomas: Sertoli-Leydig cell tumors
  - Gynandroblastomas
  - Unclassified.
- Lipid (lipoid) cell tumors
- Germ cell tumors:
  - Dysgerminoma
  - Endodermal sinus tumor
  - Embryonal carcinoma
  - Polyembryoma
  - Choriocarcinoma
  - Teratoma
  - Mixed forms.
- Gonadoblastoma:
  - Pure
  - Mixed with dysgerminoma or other germ cell tumors.
- Soft tissue tumors not specific to ovary
- Unclassified tumors
- Secondary (metastatic) tumors
- Tumor-like conditions.

It is important to establish whether the ovarian tumor is benign or malignant before operation.

Benign Germ Cell Tumors

This is the commonest ovarian tumor seen in women less than 30 years of age, accounting for 15–20% of all ovarian tumors, 95% are benign cystic teratomas, also called demoids.

- *Mature teratomas:* These are rare tumors and contain mature tissues with minimal cystic areas. Immature teratomas are malignant and this should be identified and proper therapy instituted
- *Dermoid:* This is the common benign germ cell tumor, accounting for 5–10% of all cystic tumors of the ovary. It is usually unilocular and contains sebaceous material and hair. It is lined by squamous epithelium with hair follicles, sebaceous glands, teeth, bone, cartilage, etc. being found in the cyst wall. It is bilateral in 12–15% of cases and occurs in any age. These cysts are usually heavy because of the presence of bone and cartilage and is prone to torsion. This can rupture and slow leak of the contents can produce chemical peritonitis
- Malignant change is seen in 1.7% of cases.

Benign Epithelial Tumors

The majority of ovarian tumors, both benign and malignant are epithelial in origin, forming 80% of all ovarian tumors.

- *Serous cystadenoma*: These are the most common benign tumor, occur in 3rd to 5th decades of life. They are bilateral in 50% of cases. Usually, they are unilocular with papillary projections into the cavity. The cavity is lined by cuboidal or columnar cells which may have cilia. The cyst contains thin serous fluid (Fig. 15.6)
- *Mucinous cystadenoma* constitutes 25% of the ovarian tumors, are usually unilateral, large and multiloculated (Fig. 15.7), and occur between 30–60 years of age. The cyst wall consists of mucin secreting columnar cells and contains thick gelatinous mucinous material. If the cyst ruptures, it may cause pseudomyxoma peritonei
- *Endometrioid cystadenoma*: Benign endometrioid cysts are difficult to differentiate from endometriotic cysts and most of these are malignant
- *Brenner tumor*: These account for 1–2% of all ovarian tumors. They are rare, solid fibroepithelial tumors and consists of nests of transitional epithelium in a dense fibrous stroma. They are unilateral, small to moderate size, essentially benign and seen around menopause. Most of them are benign and less than 2 cm in size
- *Clear cell tumor (Mesonephroid tumor)*: These arise from serosal cells and are rarely benign. Typical clear or 'Hobnail' cells are seen on histological sections.

Benign Sex Cord Stromal Tumors

These constitute only 6% of ovarian tumors. They originate from sex cords of the embryonic gonad before differentiation into male or female or from stroma of the ovary and are also known as mesenchymoma. These may occur at any age and produce hormones.

Feminizing Functional Mesenchymomas

- *Granulosa cell tumors*: These are composed of cells resembling the granulosa cells of the Graafian follicle, secretes estrogens and most of these are malignant. These tumors can produce precocious puberty if they occur before puberty, cystic glandular hyperplasia of endometrium in adult and postmenopausal bleeding

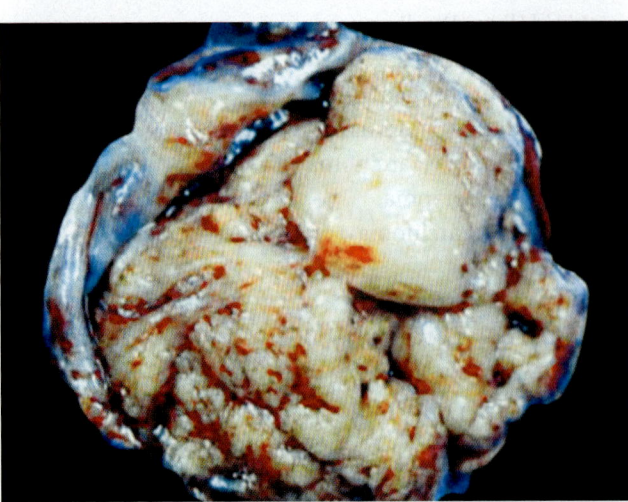

Fig. 15.6: Papillary serous cyst.

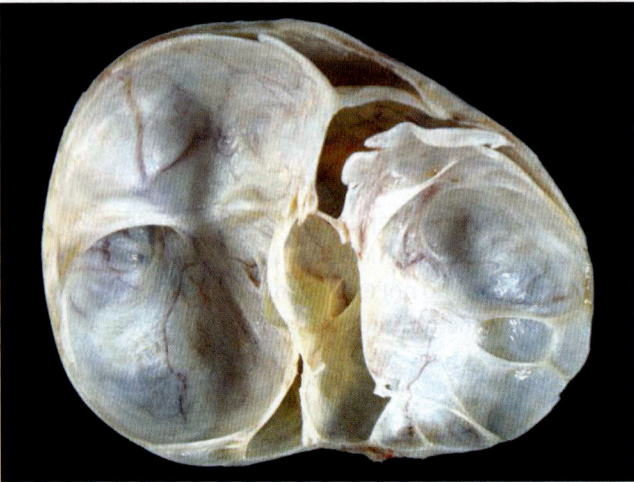

Fig. 15.7: Mucinous cystadenoma with multiple septae.

- *Theca cell tumors*: Almost all are benign and unilateral and seen after menopause. They consist of spindle-shaped cells with fat-laden polyhedral cells, are estrogenic and cause postmenopausal bleeding.

Virilizing Mesenchymoma
- *Sertoli-Leydig tumors*: These are usually of low-grade malignant potential. Many produce androgens and thus produce virilizing features; they are usually small and bilateral
- *Arrhenoblastoma*: Secrete androgens and cause defeminization followed by masculinization
- *Adrenal cortical tumors*: Composed of cells resembling large clear cells of adrenal cortex
- *Hilus cell tumors* are rare and arise from ovarian hilum cells. It consists of Reinke crystals.

Gynandroblastoma combines characteristics of granulosa cell tumors and arrhenoblastoma.

Tumors Arising from the Connective Tissue of the Ovary

Ovarian fibroma is the most common benign connective tissue tumors of the ovary and occurs frequently around 50 years of age. They are firm mobile smooth cysts with glistening capsule and consist of network of spindle-shaped cells. Ascites and pleural effusion may occur with fibroma and is known as Meigs' syndrome in 1% of cases.

Clinical Features

Benign ovarian cysts though grow to large size, rarely give rise to symptoms. Presentations of benign tumors are as follows:
- Asymptomatic
- Pain
- Abdominal swelling
- Pressure effects

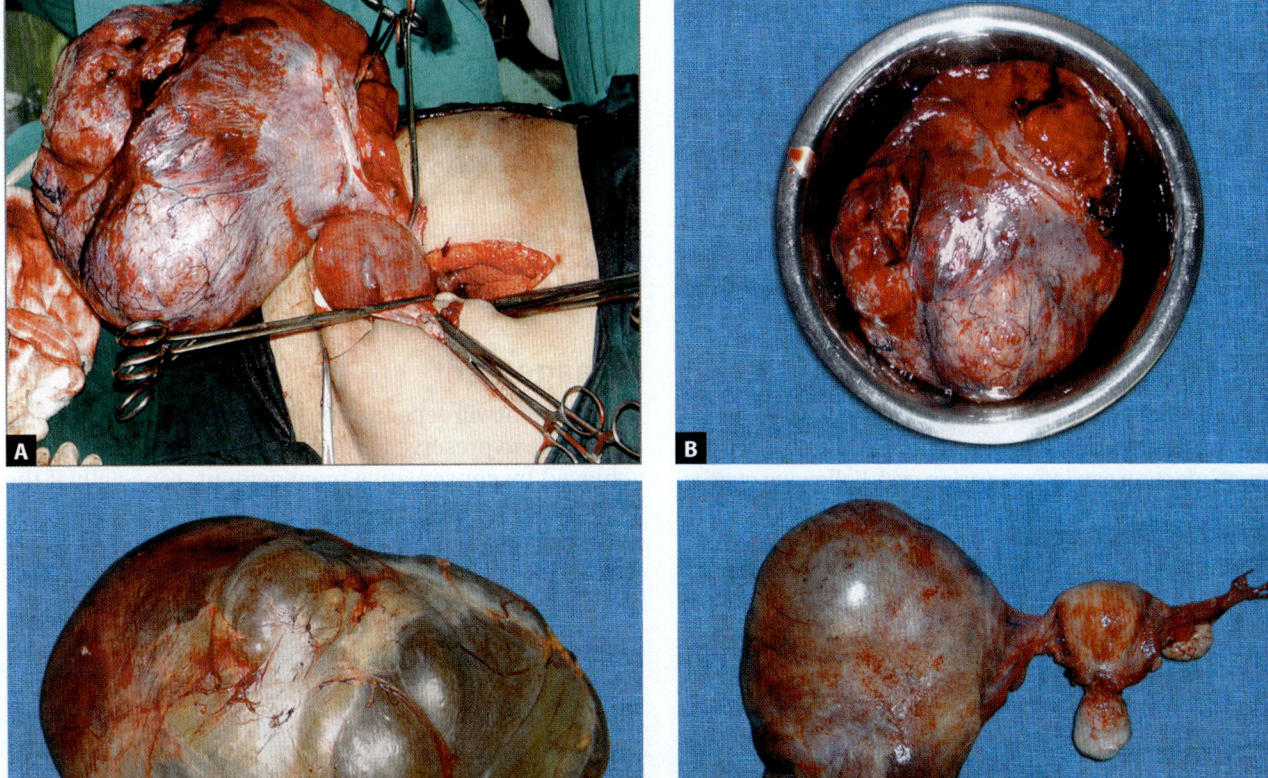

Figs. 15.8A to D: Gross specimens of ovarian tumor.

- Menstrual disturbance
- Hormonal effect.

Many tumors are found incidentally. Some gross specimens of ovarian tumors are presented in Figures 15.8A to D. Ovarian tumors can undergo torsion, rupture, hemorrhage and infection producing acute abdomen. The patient may come with a visible enlargement of abdomen, especially in mucinous tumors. Pressure from the tumor can produce bowel or bladder symptoms. In extreme cases, it can produce edema of the legs, varicose veins and hemorrhoids. Menstrual disturbance is associated with hormone-secreting tumors.

Differential Diagnosis
- Full bladder
- Pregnancy
- Ectopic gestation
- Appendicitis
- Pelvic inflammatory disease
- Fibroids.

Complications of Ovarian Tumors
- *Axial rotation or torsion:* Torsion of an ovarian cyst is a common complication, occurs in about 12%, commonly seen in cysts of about 10 cm diameter. As the result of rotation, ovarian arteries and veins in the pedicle becomes occluded, the tumor becomes congested, interstitial hemorrhage in the wall of the tumor and into the loculi (Figs. 15.9 and 15.10). The increased tension causes severe abdominal pain and signs of peritoneal irritation
- *Infection:* Infection of ovarian tumor is rare, most cases follow acute salpingitis, when the cyst becomes infected by direct spread. During puerperium, ascending genital tract infection can infect ovarian cyst. Following ovarian torsion, adhesion forms between tumor and intestine and thereby the ovarian cyst becomes directly infected. Sebaceous material in dermoid cyst also causes infection in the tumor
- *Rupture of ovarian cyst:* This may be traumatic or spontaneous. When mucinous cystadenoma ruptures, mucinous material is discharged into the peritoneal cavity which rarely leads to development of pseudomyxoma of the peritoneum. Here, the peritoneal cavity is filled with mucinous material adherent to omentum and intestines which cannot be removed completely at operation
- *Hemorrhage:* Follows rupture of ovarian cyst
- *Malignancy.*

Investigations
The patient presenting to the casualty ward may require emergency surgery. Pelvic examination will show an adnexal mass and the uterus is felt separate from the mass. The mass is usually mobile. Abdominal examination may show the swelling if it is large enough. Ultrasound can demonstrate the presence of ovarian mass with reasonable sensitivity and fair specificity. Chest X-ray is taken to rule out secondaries. Intravenous urogram to rule out pressure effects is also advised in relevant situations. A raised CA 125 is strongly suggestive of malignancy. CT scan and magnetic resonance imaging (MRI) aids in diagnosis of ovarian tumors as well as other tumor markers like cancer antigen (CA 125), carcinoembryonic antigen (CEA), alpha-fetoprotein (AFP) and β human chorionic gonadotropin (β hCG).

Management
Management will depend upon the severity of the symptoms and desire to preserve fertility. In older women nothing is achieved by conservative management, especially if the

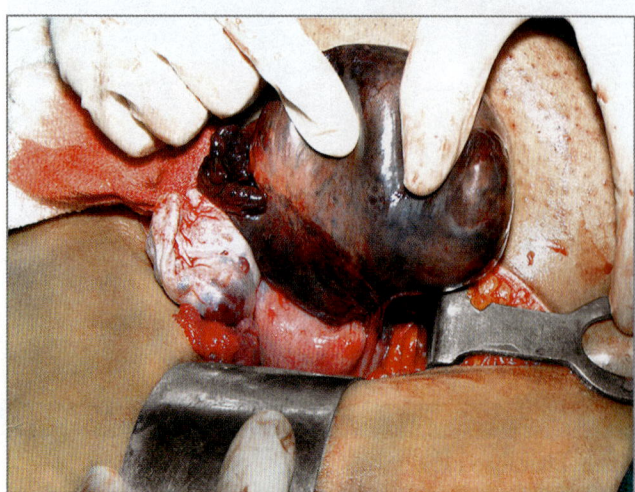

Fig. 15.9: Torsion of the ovarian tumor.

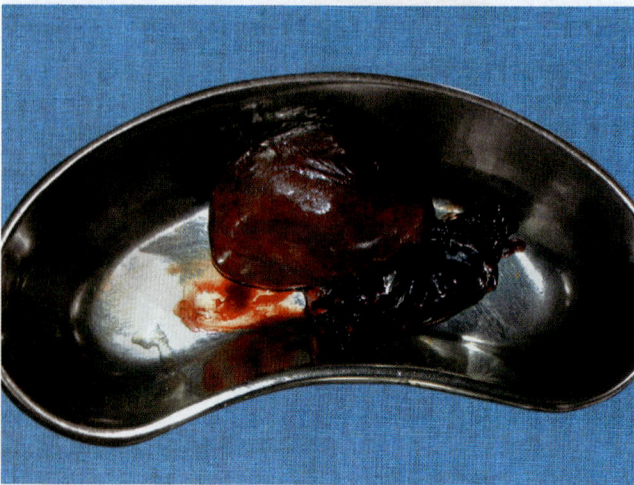

Fig. 15.10: Gross specimen of the ovarian tumor showing hemorrhage of congestion.

CHAPTER 15 Benign Lesions of the Genital Tract

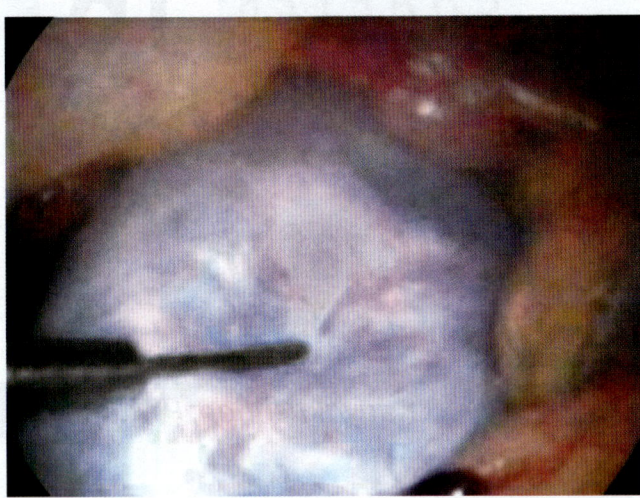

Fig. 15.11: Laparoscopic appearance of benign ovarian cyst.

tumors are more than 5 cm. Surgery is advised. In younger women if the cysts are above 10 cm, they are unlikely to disappear spontaneously. Laparoscopy (Fig. 15.11) or laparotomy is indicated. Patients with symptoms obviously require treatment.

The treatment comprises of:

- Abdominal hysterectomy and bilateral salpingo-oophorectomy
- Unilateral ovariotomy
- Ovarian cystectomy
- Laparoscopy cystectomy-ovariotomy
- Laparoscopy/ultrasound guided aspiration of the cyst.

Surgery

In perimenopausal women, total hysterectomy with bilateral salpingo-oophorectomy is done, even if the tumor is benign or unilateral.

In young women, conservation of healthy ovary is desirable. Ovarian cystectomy or enucleation is done, leaving behind normal ovarian tissue. If not possible, ovariotomy, i.e. removal of the whole diseased ovary is done, either laparoscopically or by laparotomy. Laparoscopy permits quick recovery and has low morbidity without an abdominal scar. It is a recent minimal invasive surgery in vogue per small cysts. Cyst is first aspirated followed by dissection of cyst. No further follow-up is required in benign tumors unless the histopathology reveals unsuspected cancer when further treatment depends on type of the tumor staging, etc.

In pregnancy, the tumor can undergo torsion and surgery is advised irrespective of gestational age, if they present with symptoms. In asymptomatic patients, it is advisable to wait until 14–16 weeks are completed when chances of torsion are greater and chances of miscarriage will be less.

BIBLIOGRAPHY

1. Aharoni A, Reiter A, Golan D, Paltiely Y, Sharf M. Patterns of growth of uterine leiomyomas during pregnancy. A prospective longitudinal study. British Journal of Obstetrics and Gynecology. 1988;95:510-13.
2. Buttram VC, Reiter RC. Uterine leiomyomata: aetiology, symptomatology and management. Fertility and Sterility. 1981;36:433-45.
3. Campbell S, Bhan V, Royston P, Whitehead MI, Collins WP. Transabdominal ultrasound screening for early ovarian cancer. British Medical Journal. 1989;299:1363-67.
4. Friedrich EG. Vulvar disease. 2nd edition. Philadelphia: Saunders; 1983.
5. Nezhat C, Winer WK, Nezhat F. Laparoscopic removal of dermoid cysts. Obstetrics and Gynecology. 1989;73:278-81.
6. Novak ER, Woodruff JD. Myoma and other benign tumors of the uterus. In: Novak's gynecological and obstetric pathology. 8th edition. Philadelphia WB Saunders; 1979;260-79.
7. Ridley CM. The vulva. Churchill Livingstone: Edinburgh; 1988.
8. West CP, Lumsden MA. Fibroids and menorrhagia. Bailliere's Clinical Obstetrics and Gynaecology. 1989;2:689-709.

CHAPTER 16

Contraception and Sterilization

K Jayakrishnan, P Manjula

Overview

- There are natural, temporary and permanent methods.
- The Pearl index is defined as the number of failures per 100 woman-years of exposure (HWY).
- Combined oral contraceptives are made of synthetic estrogen and progesterone. Ethinylestradiol (EE) and the mestranol are the synthetic estrogens, ethinylestradiol being more potent. There are three groups of progesterone currently used in OC pills.
- The newest pill contains drosperonone which is a progesterone with both antiandrogenic and mineralocorticoid activity.
- Emergency contraception is a form of contraception that women can use to prevent pregnancy after unprotected intercourse such as when act occurs without contraception or contraception fails. Two types of emergency contraception are available; emergency contraceptive pills (ECPs) and emergency copper bearing intrauterine device insertion.
- IUDs are effective method of reversible long-term contraception. They do not affect lactation, do not interfere with intercourse and they do not have systemic side effects (except for hormone containing devices).
- Sterilization provides permanent contraception for women who do not want any more children, done by laparotomy or laparoscopy.

The need for limiting population by virtue of limiting family size is a global emergency. Many women die each year from complications of pregnancy, childbirth and induced abortions. Effective contraception can reduce maternal morbidity, mortality as well as population explosion and its consequences. Therefore, contraceptive advice is a component of good preventive health care. The clinician's approach is a key.

DEFINITION

A method or system which prevents pregnancy.

An ideal contraceptive agent should be safe, effective, convenient, independent of coitus, initiated by single simple procedure, reversible, cheap, socially and culturally acceptable and requiring no or minimal medical supervision. But such a method does not exist. So, all the available methods are offered, to be chosen by the individual to meet their needs.

Efficacy of Contraception

Contraceptive efficacy[1] is assessed by measuring the number of unplanned pregnancies that occur during a specified period of exposure while using a contraceptive method. Pearl index and Life-table analysis are the two methods used to measure contraceptive efficacy.

Pearl Index

The Pearl index created by Raymond Pearl in 1933, is defined as the number of failures per 100 woman-years of exposure (HWY).

Pregnancy rate per HWY

$$\frac{\text{Total accidental pregnancies} \times 12 \times 100}{\text{Total months of exposure to unintended pregnancies}}$$

Life-Table analysis calculates a failure rate for each month of use. A cumulative failure rate can then compare methods for any specified length of exposure.

Contraceptive failure—do occur for many reasons. Thus "method effectiveness" and "use effectiveness" have been used to designate efficacy with correct and incorrect use of a method (Table 16.1).

The likelihood of pregnancies is usually reported in two ways.[2]

- Effectiveness when used correctly and consistently (perfect use)
- Effectiveness as commonly used that is the typical or average likelihood of pregnancy, whether or not method is used correctly and consistently (typical use).

Revised WHO Eligibility Criteria

World Health Organization (WHO) has published the medical eligibility criteria[3] to classify health conditions into four categories for initiation and continuation of each contraceptive, taking into account the health risk and benefits of using such method for a woman with given conditions:

Category 1: *Always usable, No restriction on use.*
Category 2: *Broadly usable, advantages overweigh risks.*
Category 3: *Use with caution, risks out weigh advantages.*
Category 4: *Do not use, has unacceptable health risk.*

Contraception and litigation: The best way to avoid litigation is good patient communication, keeping good records, good history taking and documentation which is vital.

Documentation should include discussing risks and benefits of all methods with patient, a plan for follow-up and all interactions made with the patient.

CLASSIFICATION OF CONTRACEPTIVE AGENTS

Reversible (Temporary)

Traditional
- Natural family planning method (periodic abstinence)
- Withdrawal method (coitus interruptus)
- Postcoital douche
- Lactational amenorrhea method.

Barrier
- Physical:
  - Male condom
  - Female
    - Diaphragm
    - Cervical cap
    - Condom
- Chemical: Spermicidal agents

Table 16.1: Failure rates in first year of use.[4]

Method	Typical use	Perfect use
No method	85	
Spermicides	29	18
Withdrawal	27	4
Periodic abstinence	25	
Calendar		9
Ovulation method		3
Symptothermal		2
Diaphragm	16	6
Condom—female, male	2115	52
Combined pill and mini pill	8	0.3
Combined hormonal patch	8	0.3
Combined hormonal ring	6	0.3
DMPA (Depo-Provera)	3	0.3
Combined injectable (Lunelle)	3	0.05
IUD Copper TMirena (LNG IUS)	0.80.1	0.60.1
LNG implants (Norplant, Norplant-2/Jadelle)	0.05	0.05
Female sterilization	0.5	0.5
Male sterilization	0.15	0.10

Hormonal Contraceptives
- Combined oral contraceptives
- Progesterone only pills
- Injectable contraceptives
- Hormonal implants
- Vaginal rings
- Transdermal patches
- Intrauterine systems.

Intrauterine Devices
Emergency Contraception
Permanent: Male and female sterilization.

TRADITIONAL METHODS

Natural Family Planning Method (Periodic Abstinence and Withdrawl)

The natural family planning method requires observation of naturally occurring symptoms and signs of fertile phase of the menstrual cycle and to avoid coitus during that period. Accurate prediction or indication of ovulation is essential for the success of this method. Ovulation is variable, even in women who menstruate regularly. This method take into account the viability of sperm in the female genital tract (2–7 days) and lifespan of ovum (1–3 days).

The period of maximal fertility begins 5 days before the day of ovulation and ends on the day after ovulation.

Implantation occurs 6–12 days after ovulation.

Couples using natural family planning method may use one technique or a combination of techniques to identify the beginning and end of woman's fertile period.

1. The rhythm or calendar method
2. Basal body temperature method (BBT)
3. The cervical mucus method (Billings method)
4. The symptothermal method
5. The standard days method (SDM)
6. Hormone monitoring[5]

Calendar Method

The woman should record the length of 6 cycles. The beginning of fertile period is obtained by subtracting 18 days from the length of the shortest cycle, and the end of the fertile period by subtracting 11 days from the length of the longest cycle.

Basal Body Temperature Method

Basal body temperature (BBT) is more reliable compared to calendar method. The evidence of ovulation is obtained by recording basal body temperature. The BBT is recorded with any thermometer before getting out of bed. After ovulation the body temperature rises by about 0.2–0.4°C (0.4–0.8°F) in response to the increasing levels of progesterone. The abstinence is practiced until the night of 3rd day of shift in temperature.

The Cervical Mucus Method

This method is based on change in quantity and consistency of cervical mucus during various phases of menstrual cycle. The cervical mucus becomes thin, watery and stretchable starting from few days before and until just after ovulation, it is thick and opaque at other times. The abstinence is observed when the mucus becomes moist and sticky till 4th day after the last day of sticky, wet mucus. This method cannot be used by women with abnormal vaginal discharge. It requires a lengthy period of abstinence. This is also called Billings method, the Creighton Model Fertility Care System or the two day method.

Symptothermal Method

This method combines BBT and mucus method. Abstinence begins when the mucus becomes sticky and moist till the night of either the 3rd day of a temperature shift or the 4th after the last day of sticky mucus whichever is later. Efficacy is slightly better though the method is more complicated.

The Standard Days Method (SDM)

Standard days method (SDM) is simple calendar based method in which the users are counseled to abstain from unprotected intercourse from day 8 through day19 of the 26–32-day cycle to avoid pregnancy. It is simple as there are no symptothermal observations involved.

Hormone Monitoring[5] (Persona)

Urinary concentrations of estrone-3-glucuronide and luteinizing hormone can be detected with disposable test sticks and hand held monitor (The Persona Monitor). The monitor indicates fertile days by displaying a red light after the insertion of the stick into urine.

Natural family planning methods can be used safely throughout reproductive years if couples are satisfied with the method. It has no side effects, does not require any medical supervision or follow-up. It is available regardless of the economic status and does not use unnatural substance which may be harmful. It also avoids religious prohibition. But this method cannot be used by women with irregular menses. It demands long period of abstinence and commitment of both the partners. Long period of abstinence can be overcome by using a barrier method during the fertile period. Failure rate is high; 20 per 100 women. But with consistent use, failure rate can be reduced. It is 9 per 100 women for calendar method, 1 per 100 for BBT method and 3 per 100 for cervical mucus method if used consistently.

Coitus Interruptus (Withdrawal)

Coitus interruptus is one of the oldest contraceptive methods. Withdrawal of the penis before ejaculation results in deposition of the semen outside the female genital tract. Failure rate is high (18 per 100 users in first year; WHO 1994).

Postcoital Douche

Vaginal douching with water, vinegar or the other commercial solutions immediately after coitus may flush the semen out of the vagina. The method is unreliable and failure rate is high (20–41 per HWY).

Lactational Amenorrhea Method

Lactation plays a very important role in spacing pregnancies. It depends on the intensity and the frequency of suckling and to the extent to which the supplementary food is added to infant diet. Amenorrheic women who exclusively breastfeed at regular intervals including at night, during the first 6 months have contraceptive benefit. The chance of ovulation increases with menstruation or after 6 months.

Mechanism of Action

Elevated prolactin acts at both central and ovarian level to produce anovulation and amenorrhea. Suckling results in high prolactin levels which inhibits the pulsatile secretion of gonadotropin releasing hormone (GnRH) leading to lower luteinizing hormone (LH) and follicle-stimulating hormone (FSH) levels which inhibits follicular growth and estrogen secretion. Prolactin appears to affect granulosa cell function in vitro by inhibiting the synthesis of progesterone.

Failure rate is 0.5–2 per 100 women.

BARRIER METHODS

Risks and Benefits

Provide Protection against STDs and PID

Barrier methods can be physical (mechanical) barriers or chemical spermicidal agents, used either alone or in combination. They can be used by either males or females. Mechanical barriers prevent entry of sperms into cervical canal. They also provide protection against sexually transmitted diseases (STDs) and pelvic inflammatory disease (PID).

Male Condoms

Condoms are made of either latex, polyurethane or silicone rubber, used as a cover for the penis and prevent the deposition of the semen in the vagina. The condom is simple and inexpensive contraceptive without any side effects except for occasional allergic reactions. It is proven to prevent HIV, and other sexually transmitted infections. Most condoms are made of latex that is 0.3–0.8 mm thick, which is impermeable to both sperms and most bacterial and viral organisms that cause STIs and HIV infection.

The condom must be placed on the erect penis before it touches the genitalia of the partner. After the intercourse, the condom should be held at the base of the penis as the still erect penis is withdrawn. If there is doubt of spill or leakage, a spermicidal agent should be quickly inserted into the vagina and emergency contraception should be used. *Failure rate* is 2% for perfect use and 15% with typical use.

Reasons for Failure

- An error in the technique such as applying the condom after some semen has escaped into vagina, or spill as a result of failure to withdraw the penis when it is erect.
- Breakage of condom
- Manufacturing defect.

Disadvantages

- Natural rubber causes an allergic reaction in approximately 3% of users
- Condoms are alleged to reduce penile glans sensitivity and may reduce sexual satisfaction of male partner
- It is coitus dependent
- Has high failure rate.

Vaginal Diaphragms

The diaphragm acts as a mechanical barrier between the vagina and the cervical canal (Fig. 16.1). They are circular rings ranging from 50–105 mm in diameter, designed to fit the vagina and cover the cervix. Most women use sizes between 65 and 80 mm.

The diaphragm which fits properly should be selected for successful use. This can be done either by a physician or a trained paramedical person by a pelvic examination. The diaphragm should be inserted into the vagina as far as it will go, the leading edge is behind the symphysis, and no longer than 6 hours prior to sexual intercourse. A contraceptive jelly or cream should be placed on the cervical side of the diaphragm before insertion. This also serves as a lubricant for insertion. The diaphragm should be left in place for at least 6 hours, no more than 24 hours after coitus as there is a chance of infection.

Advantages

- Safe, no major side effects
- Low cost, durable and with proper care can last for several years
- Reduces the incidence of STIs, PID.

Disadvantages

- Intercourse dependent
- Medical supervision is required initially to assess the size and to teach the technique

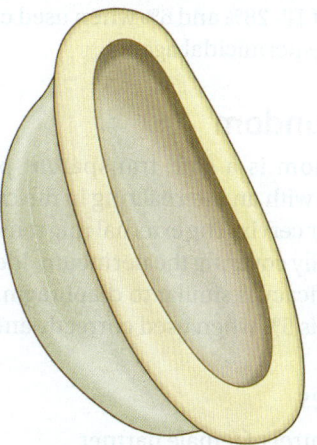

Fig. 16.1: Diaphragm.

- Weight loss or gain, vaginal delivery, presence of cystocele, rectocele require reassessment of size
- High failure rate.

Side Effects
- Occasionally causes vaginal irritation due to latex rubber or the spermicidal agent used (<1%)
- Urinary symptoms are common
- Rarely causes toxic shock syndrome.

Failure rates for diaphragm users vary from 2–23% per year.

The Cervical Cap

The cervical cap is a small latex cup with a firm flexible rim. It is 32–38 mm long and fits snugly over the cervix. It is held in place by suction. Caps should be fitted by a trained clinician and woman must be able to identify the cervix, and then slide the cap into the vagina, up to the posterior wall and onto cervix. The cap should be fitted with spermicide on its dome at least 20 minutes prior to intercourse. It should remain in place for 8 hours in order to ensure that no motile sperms are left in the vagina.

Advantages Over Diaphragm
- It can be used by women with vaginal wall or pelvic relaxation
- It can be left in place for longer time up to 48 hours.

Disadvantages
- Cannot fit adequately if the cervix is too long, too short, inflamed or in cases of acute anteversion or retroversion
- It is difficult to feel the cervix and place the cup onto the cervix
- Dislodgement of cap from cervix is more frequent
- Less protection against STIs.

Vaginal diaphragms and cervical caps have typical failure rates of 18–28% and 6% when used consistently and properly with spermicidal agents.

Female Condom

Female condom is a soft, transparent pouch made of polyurethane with an internal ring in the closed end of the pouch to cover cervix. The external ring remains outside the vagina, partially covering the perineum. Ideally should not be reused. Efficacy is similar to diaphragm. Typical failure rate is 21%, it is 5% when used correctly and consistently.

Advantages
- Under control of female partner
- Offers some protection against STIs.

Disadvantages
- High cost and bulkiness
- More cumbersome than condoms
- Relatively high rates of slippage.

Spermicidal Preparations

Spermicidal agents are chemicals which in addition to being toxic to sperms, act as mechanical barrier to entry of sperm into the cervical canal. Jellies, creams, gels, suppositories and soluble films are used as vehicles for chemical agents that inactivate sperms in the vagina. The spermicidal agents currently used are nonoxynol-9, octoxynol-9, benzalkonium chloride and menfegol. Spermicides may be used alone or in combination with diaphragm, cervical cap or condom. It should be applied 10–30 minutes prior to intercourse for adequate dispersion throughout the vagina and failure may result if dispersion is not allowed to occur. Typical failure rate is 21%.

Advantages
Inexpensive, widely available and simple to use.

Disadvantages
- High failure rate
- Causes allergy in 1–5% of cases
- Spermicide users also alter vaginal flora promoting the colonization of *E.coli* and *Staphylococcus saprophyticus*. Therefore, women are susceptible to urinary tract infection
- Vaginal and cervical mucosal damage caused by non-oxynol-9 may have an adverse impact on transmission of HIV.

The contraceptive sponge is a sustained-release system for a spermicide "Today" sponge is a small polyurethane sponge containing 1 g of nonoxynol-9. It can be worn for 24 hours. This is less effective than diaphragm. It was thought to be associated with toxic shock syndrome.

Side effects associated with the sponge include allergic reactions, vaginal dryness or itching.

HORMONAL CONTRACEPTIVES

Combined Oral Contraceptive Pills

Combined oral contraceptives (COCs) are made of synthetic estrogen and progesterone. Ethinylestradiol (EE) and the mestranol are the synthetic estrogens, ethinylestradiol being more potent. There are three groups of progesterone currently used in OC pills.

- First generation contain 50 μg or more of ethinyl-estradiol: Norethisterone group: norethisterone, norethisterone acetate, ethynodiol diacetate and lynestrenol

- Second generation contain levonorgestrel, norgestimate, and other members of the norethindrone family and 20, 30, or 35 µg ethinylestradiol.
- Third generation contain desogestrel or gestodene with 20, 25, or 30 µg of ethinylestradiol.
- Fourth generation: The newest pill contains drospirenone which is a progesterone with both antiandrogenic and mineralocorticoid activity, dienogest or nomegestrol acetate.

Monophasic pills contain same dose of estrogen and progesterone in all active pills.
- *High dose pills* contain 50 µg of EE.
- *Low dose pills* contain 20–35 µg of EE.

Multiphasic pills: The dose of estrogen and progesterone is different in different phases to simulate physiological levels of hormone. Side effects like breakthrough bleeding and amenorrhea are less. The carbohydrate and lipid metabolism are less affected.

There are two types:
- Biphasic (not commonly used because of high failure rates)
- Triphasic pills: It contain 30 µg of EE and 50 µg of LNG per day for first 6 days, 75 µg of LNG for next 5 days and 125 µg of LNG for last 10 days.

Mechanism of Action
- Inhibition of ovulation by inhibiting gonadotropin secretion via an effect on both pituitary and hypothalamus. Estrogen suppresses the development of ovarian follicles, progesterone primarily suppresses LH
- Progesterone produces a decidualized endometrium with atrophic glands which is not receptive for implantation of fertilized egg
- Progesterone makes cervical mucus thick and impermeable to sperms
- Progesterone may also influence on secretion and peristalsis of the fallopian tube and provide additional contraceptive effect.

Failure rate with perfect use is 0.3 per 100 women and with typical use 6 to 8 per 100 women in first year.

Systemic and Metabolic Effects
Cardiovascular system pharmacological estrogens increase the production of clotting factors. Progesterones have no significant impact. Oral contraceptives increase the risk of venous thromboembolism by 3 to 4 fold.[6] Smoking and hypertension add on to risks for arterial thrombosis and stroke.

Carbohydrate metabolism oral contraceptive use does not produce an increase in diabetes mellitus. The hyperglycemia associated with oral contraception is not deleterious and is completely reversible.

Liver: Estrogen influences the synthesis of hepatic DNA and RNA, hepatic cell enzymes, serum enzymes formed in the liver and plasma proteins. The active transport of biliary components is impaired by estrogen and some progesterones.

The risk of cancer:[7] The use of oral contraceptives protects against endometrial carcinoma, epithelial ovarian carcinoma, colorectal cancer and salivary gland carcinoma. Oral contraceptive use increases the risk of dysplasia and carcinoma in situ of uterine cervix, hepatic adenomas and long-term use is associated with slightly increased risk of molar pregnancy and melanoma.

Oral contraceptives have protective effect on benign breast disease, but increased risk of premenopausal breast cancer.

Infections: Oral contraceptives provide protection against pelvic inflammatory disease by making cervical mucus thick, thus preventing the movement of pathogens into uterus and tubes. It also protects against bacterial vaginosis and trichomoniasis. OC use may increase the risk of candidiasis, lower genital chlamydia and urinary tract infections.

Noncontraceptive Beneficial Effects
- Regular cycles with less flow and less dysmenorrhea
- Reduces the incidence of iron deficiency anemia
- Useful in blood dyscrasias and dysfunctional bleeding.

Reduces the incidence of
- Mittelschmerz
- Endometriosis
- Acne
- Hirsutism
- Premenstrual syndrome
- Menstrual porphyria.

Protects against
- Osteoporosis
- Benign breast diseases
- Endometrial carcinoma
- Ovarian cyst
- Ovarian cancer
- Pelvic inflammatory disease, therefore against ectopic pregnancy.

Causes less
- Rheumatoid arthritis
- Fibroids
- Ectopic pregnancy.

Side Effects
Minor problems account for 40% of discontinuation:[8]
- Nausea is seen in 10% of users, declines after several months of use

- Intermenstrual bleeding is experienced in 10–20% of users in first few months of use
- Oligomenorrhea, amenorrhea (reversible)
- Weight gain and fluid retention
- Breast tenderness
- Headache
- Mood changes and loss of libido.

Major Problems

Increased risk of:
- Venous thromboembolism and stroke
- Myocardial infarction
- Cervical intraepithelial neoplasia (CIN), carcinoma cervix
- Breast cancer and liver adenoma.

Absolute Contraindications[9]

- Thrombophlebitis, past history of thromboembolic disorders or with history of a first degree relative with thrombosis
- Acute viral hepatitis, cirrhosis, benign or malignant liver tumors
- Undiagnosed abnormal vaginal bleeding
- Known or suspected breast cancer
- Hypertension with >160 systolic and >100 diastolic or with vascular disease
- Smokers of >35 years age, >15 cigarettes per day
- Diabetes for >20 years or with severe vascular disease or with severe nephropathy or retinopathy
- Breastfeeding <6 weeks postpartum
- Migraine >35 years of age or migraine with aura or focal neurological deficits
- History of coronary heart disase or cerebrovascular disease.

COCs can be Used by Women

- Uncomplicated diabetes of less than 35 years of age, who do not smoke
- Well-controlled hypertension, history of preeclampsia
- Obese women
- Seizure disorders
- Benign breast disease
- Uncomplicated valvular heart disease.

Drug Interactions

Certain antiepileptic drugs (barbiturates, carbamazepine, phenytoin, primidone) and antimicrobials (rifampicin and griseofulvin) may reduce contraceptive efficacy of OCPs.

Pill Taking

A family and personal history with particular attention paid to cardiovascular risk factors, such as thromboembolism and blood pressure recording is sufficient before prescribing oral contraceptive pills.[10]

Effective contraception is achieved during the first cycle of pill use, provided pills are started no later than the 5th day of the cycle and no pills are missed. Starting the pill on the first day of the menses ensures immediate protection. Quick-Start method[11] encourages women to take the pill at first visit and to continue daily pill taking regardless of the menstrual cycle day, to avoid pregnancy while waiting for the next menses, especially in patients with irregular cycles. But additional protection is required in the first week of use. After termination of pregnancy of less than 12 weeks, OC can be started immediately. It is better to wait for 2 weeks after 2nd trimester termination or after premature delivery to avoid the risk of thrombosis. If lactating women choose COCs, they should start 6 months after child birth as it has been demonstrated to diminish the quantity and quality of milk.

One pill to be taken daily at bed time for 21 days, stopped and restarted after a gap of 7 days irrespective of onset or stoppage of menstruation during this pill-free interval. If the packet contains 28 tablets, the last 7 tablets are placebos, the pills from the next packet should be started the very next day after a pack of tablets is finished.

Extended cycle combined contraceptive pills:[12] To avoid the inconvenience of monthly withdrawal bleeding, there are regimens containing active pills for 3 months or 6 months followed by placebo for 1 week, thus reducing the cycle to 4 or 2 per year.

Missed Pills

If a woman misses 1 pill, she should take that pill as soon as she remembers and take the next pill as usual. No backup method is needed. If she misses 2 pills in first 2 weeks, she should take 2 pills on each day for next 2 days with the backup for the next 7 days. The backup method should be used for 7 days. If the lady forgets 2 pills in the 3rd week or misses more than 2 pills at any time in any case she should continue taking pills of that packet.

In women who became pregnant while taking COCs or inadvertent use during cycle of conception, there was no increased risk of major malformations, congenital heart defects or limb defects in the fetuses.[13]

Reproduction after Discontinuation of COCs

Combined oral contraceptives users had a low monthly percentage of conceptions for the first 3 months. 90% conceive within 24 months after stopping the pills.

PROGESTERONE ONLY PILLS (MINI PILLS)

Mini pills are estrogen free oral contraceptive pills made from very low dose of synthetic progesterone (25% of that in combined pills) in order to eliminate the side effects attributable to estrogen component of conventional pills. Progestin-only mini pill provides a modest boost to milk production, protects against the bone loss associated with lactation. They do not increase the risk of venous thrombosis. They can be started immediately after the delivery.

Preparations
- Levonorgestrel: 0.030 mg
- Norethindrone: 0.350 mg
- Norgestrel: 0.075 mg
- Lynestrenol: 0.5 mg
- Ethynodial diacetate: 0.5 mg
- Desogestrel: 0.075 mg.

Mechanism of Action
- Makes cervical mucus thick and impermeable
- Endometrium is made hostile for implantation
- Gonadotropins are not consistently suppressed; ovulation is inhibited only in 50–60% of patients.

There are no significant effects on carbohydrate and lipid metabolism. Coagulation factors remain unchanged.

Efficacy: Failure rates are slightly more than COCs 1.1–1.9 per HWY in the first year; typical failure rate is 3–10 per 100 women.

Pill should be started on the first day of menses. Mini pill must be taken everyday at the same time of the day, continuously without any break. If there is more than 3 hours delay in taking a pill, a backup method should be used for next 48 hours.

Indications
- Mini pill[14] is a good choice for breastfeeding woman as it has no adverse effect on lactation and has slight positive impact
- Women over the age of 40. Fecundity decreases as age advances, therefore slightly high failure rate of mini pill may not result in pregnancy. The risk of arterial and venous thrombosis is more at this age if estrogen is added
- In any situation where estrogen is contraindicated such as diabetes with vascular disease, uncontrolled hypertension, smoking and SLE
- For those who cannot tolerate minor complaints of COCs like gastrointestinal upset, headaches and diminished libido.

Disadvantages
- Irregular menstrual bleeding is common. 10% of patients may have spotting and amenorrhea
- Levonorgestrel pills may be associated with acne
- Ectopic pregnancy is not prevented as effectively as intrauterine pregnancy
- Strict adherence to daily pill taking at the same time is required and overall effectiveness is less than that of combined pills.

TRANSDERMAL PATCH

Transdermal patch is a small (20 cm²), thin adhesive square which is applied tropically. It releases 150 µg of norelgestromin (progesterone) and 20 µg of ethinylestradiol daily into circulation. It is pharmacologically similar to COCs. The patch can be applied to the upper arm, lower abdomen, or buttocks, once in every week for 3 weeks in a month.

VAGINAL RING

The vaginal ring is a flexible, single sized ring which releases 15 µg of ethinylestradiol and 120 µg of etonogestrel per day. Hormones are absorbed through the vaginal epithelium and suppress ovulation. The insertion and removal is easy. The ring is inserted by the patient on the first day of menses and worn for 3 weeks and then removed to allow withdrawal bleeding. The new ring is inserted after one week. Efficacy is maintained if the ring is replaced within 3 hours. Failure rate is 1.18/HWY.

INJECTABLE CONTRACEPTION

The injectable contraceptives contain synthetic hormones that are administered by deep intramuscular injection. Two types of injectable contraceptives are available: progesterone only and combined injectables that contain both estrogen and progesterone. Depot medroxyprogesterone acetate (DMPA) and Norethisterone enanthate (NET-EN) are the progestin only injectables; cyclofem and mesigyna are the combined injectables available.

DMPA (Depot-provera) contains 150 mg of medroxyprogesterone acetate that protects pregnancy for at least 3 months. Norethisterone enanthate 200 mg is used as an 8 weekly injection.

Monthly injectables like 25 mg medroxyprogesterone acetate plus 5 mg estradiol cypionate and 50 mg norethindrone plus 5 mg estradiol valerate.

Newer formulation allows self-administration of a subcutaneous dose of 104 mg of medroxyprogesterone acetate every 3 months.

Mechanism of Action

Thickening of cervical mucus and alteration of the endometrium and high level of the progestin blocks the LH surge, and therefore ovulation does not occur.

To ensure effective contraception, the first injection should be taken within the first 5 days of menstruation before a dominant follicle emerges, or a backup method is required for 2 weeks. The injection is given deeply into muscle by the Z-track technique, and the area should not be massaged.

Efficacy: 0.3 pregnancies per 100 when injections are regularly taken, typical failure rate is 3% in first year.

Advantages
- Not associated with compliance problems
- Not related to the coital event
- Very effective
- Free from side effects of estrogen, therefore can be prescribed to women with congenital heart disease, sickle cell anemia, previous history of thromboembolism and women over the age of 35 years
- Increases the quantity of milk in nursing mothers
- Improvement in seizure control can be achieved probably due to sedative action of progestins.

Disadvantages
- **Irregular menstrual bleeding:** Up to 25% of women discontinue in the first year because of irregular bleeding. The bleeding and spotting decrease progressively and after 5 years 80% of users become amenorrheic with DMPA.
- **Women may have minor symptoms like:**
  - Breast tenderness
  - Weight gain, headache, dizziness and fatigue
  - Depression.
- **Bone density:**[15] Modest reduction in bone mineral density (BMD) was observed in women using DMPA. Loss of BMD occurs only while using DMPA and is reversible after stopping. In adolescents DMPA slows the accumulation of bone mass.
- **Effects on future fertility:** DMPA usually causes delay in conception after stopping the use. The delay is about 9 months after the last injection. 90% conceive within 18 months. However, amenorrhea which persists 12 months after the last injection needs to be investigated.

Beneficial Effects
- Reduced risk of endometrial cancer and ovarian cancer
- Reduced bleeding, therefore, reduced anemia
- Reduced risk of pelvic inflammatory disease, endometriosis, fibroid and ectopic pregnancies
- Prevents sickling and development of abnormal shaped red blood cells. Therefore, best choice for patients with sickle cell anemia.

Combined Injectable Contraceptives

Cyclofem (Lunelle, Cyclo-provera) contains 25 mg of DMPA and 5 mg estradiol cypionate and mesigyna contains norethindrone enanthate 50 mg with estradiol valerate 5 mg. Both are administered monthly as deep intramuscular injection and are rapidly reversible.

CONTRACEPTIVE IMPLANTS

Contraceptive implants[16] consist of hormone filled capsules that are inserted under the skin. Norplant system consists of six thin, flexible capsules made of silicone (Fig. 16.2). Each capsule is 2.4 mm in diameter and 34 mm in length and contains 36 mg of levonorgestrel. Contraceptive action lasts for 8 years; it is approved for 5 years. Norplant-2 (Jedelle) is two rod system, action lasts for 5 years. Implanon and uniplant are single rod systems 4 cm long and 2 mm in diameter. Implanon contains 68 mg of 3- keto-desogestrel (Etonorgestrel), and lasts for 3 years. Uniplant contains 38 mg of nomogestrel acetate and lasts for one year.

Biodegradable implants deliver sustained levels of progestin from a vehicle that dissolves in body system. It eliminates the need for surgical removal. Capranor is a single capsule, biodegradable levonorgestrel releasing subdermal implant. Anulle is a biodegradable norethindrone pellet that is injected subdermally.

Mechanism of action of implants is same as progesterone only pills.

Efficacy: 0.05 to 0.1 pregnancies per women in first year, it is 1.6 per 100 over 5 years.

Advantages
- Safe, highly effective and continuous method of contraception
- Rapidly reversible
- Not related to coitus
- No estrogenic side effects

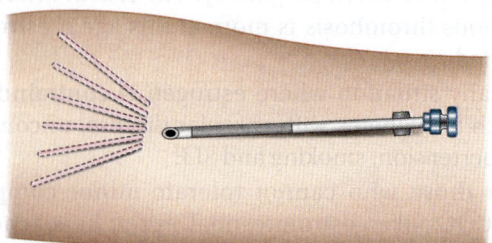

Fig. 16.2: Norplant rods.

- No suppression of lactation
- Return of fertility within few weeks.

Disadvantages
- Pain, reaction and infection at the site of insertion
- Needs surgical procedure for insertion and removal and special training is required
- Irregular menstrual bleeding in up to 80% of users especially in first year of use
- Expensive
- Do not protect against sexually transmitted infection (STI).

EMERGENCY CONTRACEPTION (POSTCOITAL CONTRACEPTION)

Emergency contraception is a form of contraception that women can use to prevent pregnancy after unprotected intercourse such as when act occurs without contraception or contraception fails. Two types of emergency contraception are available; emergency contraceptive pills (ECPs) and emergency copper bearing intrauterine device insertion. ECPs can be used up to 72 hours after an unprotected intercourse; intrauterine device can be inserted up to 5 days.

Methods

Levonorgestrel alone is the method of choice, initiated as soon after exposure as possible, no later than 120 hours.

Progesterone only, 2 dose regimen: Levonorgestrel (LNG) 0.75 mg, two doses taken 12 hours apart, prevents about 85% of expected pregnancy.

Progesterone only, one dose regimen:[17] single 1.5 mg of LNG can substitute for two 0.75 mg doses.

Yuzpe regimen: 100 mg ethinylestradiol + 5 mg LNG; 2 tablets taken immediately followed by another 2 tablets 12 hours later.

Mechanism of Action

Acts by preventing or delaying ovulation, preventing fertilization and local effect on endometrium.

Other Methods: Progesterone Receptor Modulators

Mefipristone (RU 486): A single dose of 600 mg can be used. It is an antiprogestogen. It causes sloughing and shedding of decidua and prevents implantation.

Ulipristal acetate has similar biologic effect as mifepristone, given as a single oral dose of 30 mg.

Centchroman: Two tablets of 60 mg are taken twice in 24 hours, within 24 hours of intercourse. It prevents implantation in 99% of cases.

Prostaglandins have luteolytic effect on ovary, increase the tubal motility and prevent implantation. Vaginal suppository administered following unprotected intercourse can prevent pregnancy.

A 3 week follow-up visit should be scheduled to assess the result, and to counsel for regular contraception. ECPs are intended for occasional emergency use, other method should be used consistently to provide more effective ongoing contraceptive protection.

Intrauterine device is an effective method if inserted within 5 days of unprotected intercourse, prevents pregnancy in 99% of cases. Advantage is that, it can be used as ongoing contraception. But not suitable for women who have multiple sexual partners and rape victims because of high-risk of STIs. IUDs act by causing giant cell and lymphocytic infiltration and enzymatic and other cellular changes in the endometrium. It can directly damage the blastocyst.

INTRAUTERINE DEVICES

Intrauterine devices (IUDs) are small flexible devices that prevent pregnancy when inserted into uterus through vagina. IUDs are an effective method of reversible long-term contraception. They do not affect lactation, do not interfere with intercourse and they do not have systemic side effects (except for hormone containing devices).

Types of Intrauterine Devices

Various types of intrauterine devices are shown in Figure 16.3.

Unmedicated or Inert IUDs
- The Lippes loop is made of plastic (polyethylene), double S-shaped device impregnated with barium sulfate
- Safe T-coil is a flexible stainless steel ring.

These inert devices can be left in place for several years. They are associated with increased incidence of menorrhagia, dysmenorrhea and pelvic inflammatory disease, therefore, are rarely used nowadays.

Copper-Containing IUDs

They are smaller compared to inert devices. Therefore, cause less pain and bleeding. The first copper IUDs (with failure rate of 2 per 100 women) contain copper wire of surface area 200 to 250 mm wrapped round the vertical stem of polypropylene frame.

- Copper T 200—contains copper of 200 mm^2 surface area and effective for 4 years
- Copper 7—effective for 3 years
- Multiload 250—effective for 3 years.

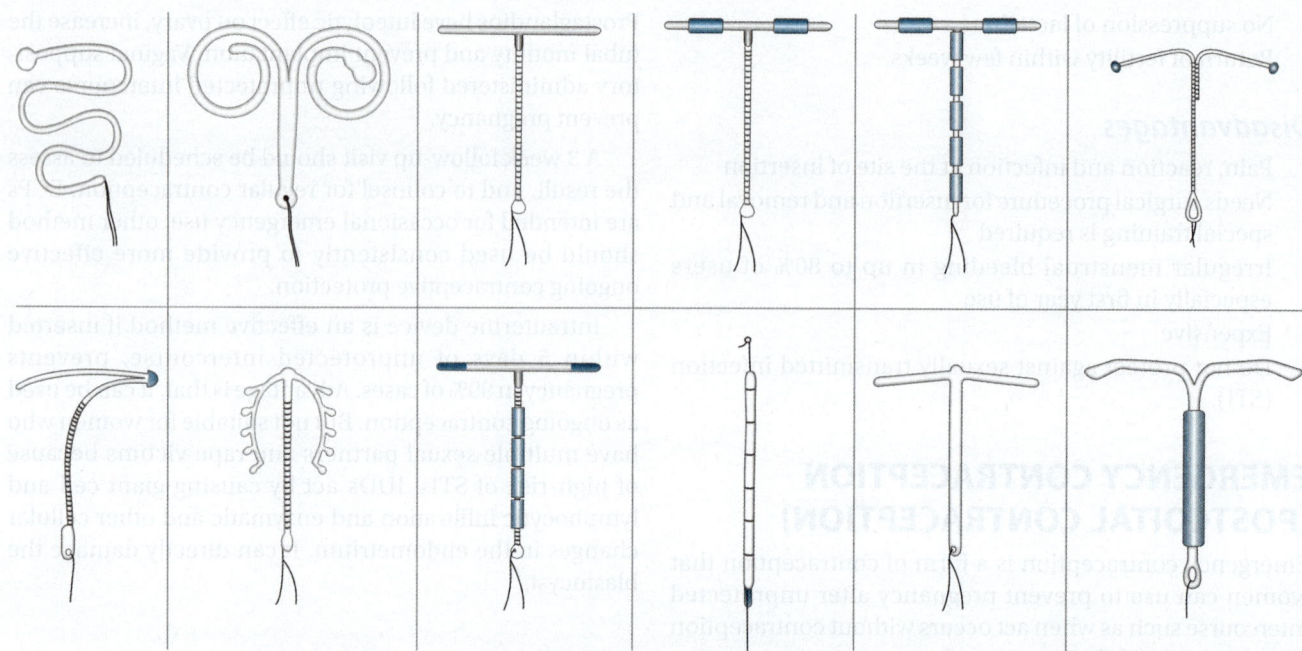

Fig. 16.3: Intrauterine devices.

The modern copper IUDs contain more copper increasing the efficacy (0.6 to 0.8 pregnancies per year) and the lifespan.
- Copper T 380 A—is a T-shaped device holding 380 mm^2 of exposed surface area of copper, efficacy lasts for 10 years
- Nova T—contains 200 mm of copper, effective for 5 years
- Multiload 375—has 375 mm^2 of copper wire around its stem, effective for 5 years.

Others
- Copper T 380 Ag which is identical to the Cu T 380 A, but in addition to copper, stem has a silver core to prevent fragmentation and extend the lifespan of copper
- The Cu T 380 slimline has 300 mm^2 of copper sleeves flushed at the ends of the arms to facilitate easier loading and insertion
- The Cu SAFE – 300 IUD has 300 mm^2 of copper in its vertical arm and a transverse arm with sharply bent ends that are adapted to the uterine cavity and help hold this device at fundus. It is made from a more flexible plastic and is smaller in size, therefore is associated with less bleeding and pain
- Frameless IUD, the flexi Gard consists of 6 copper sleeves (330 mm^2) strung on a surgical nylon thread that is knotted at the end. The knot is pushed into the myometrium during insertion. The incidence of bleeding and pain is less, but has higher failure rate.

Hormone Releasing Intrauterine Devices (Intrauterine Systems)

Progestasert
A T-shaped IUD, the vertical stem contains 38 mg progesterone which is released at a rate of 65 µg per day. It needs to be replaced yearly. It has failure rate of 1.3–1.6 per 100 women.

The LNG-IUS 20 (Mirena)
This T-shaped device has a collar attached to the vertical arm, which contains 52 mg levonorgestrel. LNG is released at a rate of 20 µg/day in vivo. The LNG–IUD is effective up to 10 years, the failure rates 0.1 per HWY. It reduces menstrual blood loss and pelvic infection rates.

Mechanism of Action
Mechanism by which IUDs prevent conception is not clear.
- Foreign body effect—causes cellular and biochemical reaction in the endometrial fluid, and also sterile inflammatory response causing mobilization of leukocytes. These are spermicidal and prevent implantation
- Provoke uterine contractility, increase tubal peristalsis so that fertilized egg is propelled down more rapidly from fallopian tube before endometrium is ready for implantation
- Copper-containing devices cause increase in uterine and tubal fluid containing copper ions, enzymes, pro-

staglandins and macrophages which impair sperm function and fertilization
- Progesterones cause decidualization of endometrium, alters characteristics of cervical mucus which becomes thick.

Contraindications: Absolute

- Current, recent or recurrent pelvic inflammatory disease and pelvic tuberculosis
- Abnormal uterine anatomy incompatible with IUD insertion—bicornuate uterus, submucus fibroid
- Undiagnosed abnormal vaginal bleeding
- Genital tract malignancies
- Wilson disease
- Immunocompromised conditions like patients suffering from AIDS.

Relative Contraindications

- Nulliparity
- History of pelvic inflammatory disease
- Multiple sexual partners
- Patients with heavy menstrual flow
- Moderate to severe dysmenorrhea
- Iron deficiency anemia
- Women with bleeding disorders or who are on anticoagulants
- Valvular heart disease (should receive prophylactic antibiotics at insertion and removal)
- Uncontrolled diabetes (women with well-controlled diabetes can use IUDs)

- Mucopurulent discharge at cervix (can be inserted after treating the infection).

Suitable candidates for intrauterine device are parous women in a mutually monogamous relationship who do not have history of PID, and have normal menstrual periods.

Timing

- Within 10 days of beginning of menstruation.
    - Insertion is easier as
        - Cervical canal is patulous
        - Endometrial cavity is more distensible
        - The uterine contractions which may expel the device are less
        - The woman in unlikely to be pregnant.
    - Within 4–8 weeks after delivery. The risk of infection, perforation and expulsion are more with immediate postpartum insertion.
- An IUD can be inserted immediately after a first trimester termination of pregnancy, but after a second trimester termination it is recommended to wait for the involution to occur.

But the device can be inserted any time during a menstrual period if pregnancy is ruled out either by history or by a sensitive pregnancy test.

Technique of Insertion (Fig. 16.4)

A pelvic examination is done to rule out conditions that contraindicate IUD insertion and to note the position

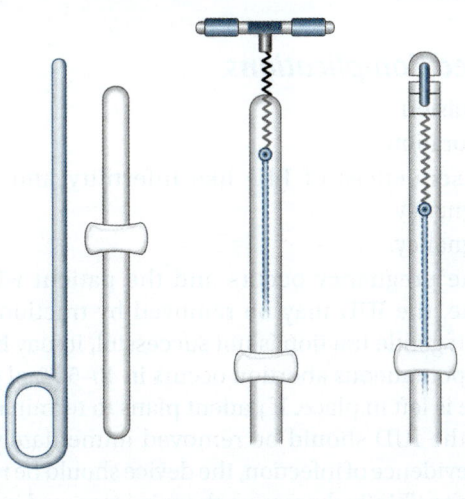
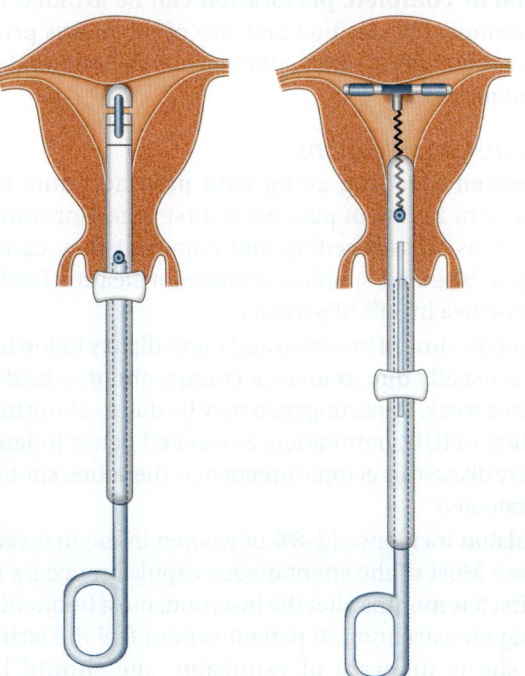

Fig. 16.4: Cu T 380 A: insertion technique.

and the size of the uterus. The length of uterine cavity is measured with a uterine sound. The stop on the tube is adjusted to the length of uterine cavity. The transverse arm of the device and that of the stop should be at the same plane so that the device gets released in the coronal plane at the fundus. The insertion tube, along with the plunger is advanced into the uterine cavity till the stop is at the external os. The inserter is withdrawn over the plunger (withdrawal technique) and the device will get released into uterine cavity, the tips of T will rest in the cornual region. The strings (thread) are trimmed. They allow the patient to feel them and facilitate removal.

Prophylactic antibiotics such as doxycyclin 200 mg or azithromycin 500 mg orally one hour prior to insertion are not recommended routinely,[18] however, it should be given for women who get the device replaced.

Follow-up

A one month follow-up after the next menstruation is recommended to visualize the strings and to discuss about the minor problems. Patient should be advised to feel the strings periodically.

Complications

At the Time of Insertion

- **Pain**—can be reduced by giving an anti-inflammatory drug one hour prior to insertion and by giving paracervical block during insertion
- Occasional **syncopal attack** due to cervical dilatation or endometrial insertion
- **Partial or complete perforation** can be avoided by ascertaining the position and size of the uterus prior to insertion and to strict adherence to recommended techniques.

Immediate Complications

- **Increased bleeding along with pain** accounts for removal in 2–10% of patients in first year. Hormonal IUDs cause less bleeding and pain, but they cause irregular bleeding, spotting, oligomenorrhea and finally amenorrhea in 50% of patients
- **Pain** at the time of insertion and immediately following that is usually due to uterine cramps and it subsides within a week. Persisting pain may be due to abnormal position of IUD, perforation, associated pelvic inflammatory disease or ectopic pregnancy, therefore, should be evaluated
- **Expulsion** incidence (2–8% of women in the first year of use): Most of the spontaneous expulsion occurs in the first few months after the insertion, most frequently during menstruation. If patient cannot feel the string and she is unaware of expulsion, she should be examined to visualize the string. The reasons for the missing threads can be:
  - Expulsion
  - Thread may have been drawn back
  - The tail may have separated from the device and expelled unnoticed
  - The device may have perforated the uterine wall or passed into peritoneal cavity
  - Patient may have conceived and thread might have moved up as uterine cavity enlarges.

A real time ultrasound is the best method to locate the lost IUD. If the device is not visualized with ultrasonography or if the facility is not available, a plain X-ray of abdomen and pelvis will identify as IUDs are radiopaque. Insertion of another IUD should be done if prior ultrasound is not done, to find the exact location of the device. If the device is in the uterine cavity, it can be removed by grasping with a forceps or Shirodkar's hook under ultrasound guidance or hysteroscopically. If the IUD is perforating the myometrium, it should be removed using operative laparoscopy under general anesthesia. Copper in the abdominal cavity can lead to adhesion formation; therefore, it may require laparotomy for retrieval.

- **Pelvic infection:** IUD related bacterial infection is due to contamination of endometrial cavity at the time of insertion. The risk of infection is 6 times higher during the 20 days after the insertion. If there is evidence of endometritis and salpingitis, treatment must be instituted and device should be removed. Infection with *Actinomyces israelii* has been reported in association with IUDs.

Delayed Complications

- Expulsion
- Perforation
- Consequences of PID like infertility and ectopic pregnancy
- Pregnancy.

If the pregnancy occurs and the patient wishes to continue, the IUD may be removed by traction on the thread. If gentle traction is not successful, it may be left in place. Spontaneous abortion occurs in 40–50% of patients if device is left in place. If patient plans to terminate pregnancy, the IUD should be removed immediately. But if there is evidence of infection, the device should be removed after the antibiotic therapy as there is increased incidence of septic shock.

There is no evidence that, exposure of fetus to medicated IUDs is associated with increased risks of congenital anomalies. But the incidence of preterm labor and delivery is increased when an IUD is left in place during pregnancy.

The use of an IUD, other than progestasert, offers some protection against ectopic pregnancy. But when an IUD user becomes pregnant, it is more likely to be ectopic than in women using oral contraceptives.

Efficacy of IUDs: The actual use failure rate in the first year is approximately 3% with 10% expulsion ratend a 15% rate of removal, mainly for bleeding and pain.

IUD Removal

Removal of an IUD is done by grasping the thread with forceps and exerting firm traction. If an IUD is embedded, it can be removed either under ultrasound guidance or hysteroscopically. Fertility returns after removal of an IUD, at a normal rate.

Beneficial Effects of IUDs

- IUD use has been associated with decreased risk of endometrial cancer.
  Protection against PID, endometrial hyperplasia and polyps associated with postmenopausal estrogen therapy or tamoxifen treatment.
- Levonorgestrel IUS[19] is used for the treatment of:
  - Idiopathic menorrhagia
  - Menorrhagia and pain secondary to small fibroids, endometriosis, adenomyosis and endometrial hyperplasia.

SURGICAL STERILIZATION

Female Sterilization

Sterilization provides permanent contraception for women who do not want any more children. During the procedure, the fallopian tubes are occluded in such a way as to prevent sperm from reaching the ovum. Sterilization protects women from unwanted pregnancies. It saves them from common problems of temporary methods like compliance, inconvenience, disposal problems, privacy, partner compliance and harmful side effects.

Sterilization can be accomplished by:
- Laparotomy
- Laparoscopy
- Vaginal approach
- Transcervically.

Minilaparotomy

In this method, tubal ligation is done through a small suprapubic incision, usually 2 to 4 cm in length.

Puerperal Ligation (Postpartum Sterilization)

Puerperal sterilization is done within 7 days of childbirth. Procedure is technically easy because, uterus remains abdominal organ; therefore, it is easy to find fallopian tubes. Tubal ligation can be combined with cesarean section.

Interval Sterilization

It is done 6 weeks after delivery or at any time in a non-pregnant woman. Ideally, the procedure should be done within 7 to 10 days of onset of menstruation before ovulation occurs.

Postabortal Sterilization

Tubal ligation can be done immediately following evacuation of uterus for induced or incomplete abortion.

Procedure

The operation can be performed under local anesthesia with sedation or under general anesthesia. The abdomen is opened; the fallopian tubes are identified by their fimbrial ends and caught with an atraumatic forceps. Several techniques have been described to perform tubal ligation.

Pomeroy technique: The tube is held with a Babcock forceps about 4 cm lateral to the uterine cornu at an avascular space of the mesosalpinx and pulled up to form a loop (Fig. 16.5). The base of the loop is tied, keeping about 2 cm of tube above the base with chromic catgut Number 0, needle passing through the mesosalpinx. The loop is cut and about 1.5 cm of the tube is removed. *Failure rate* is 1 in 300 to 400.

Irving technique: The tube is doubly ligated with chromic catgut Number 0, about 2.5 cm from cornu and then cut (Fig. 16.6). The medial end of the tube is buried into a tunnel made on the posterior uterine wall. The distal end is buried in the mesosalpinx. *Failure rate* is less than 1 in 1,000 cases.

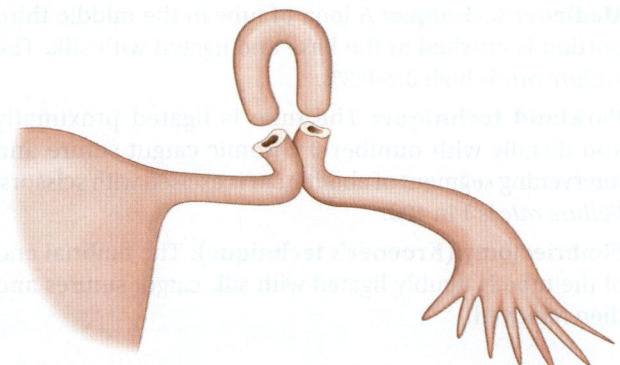

Fig. 16.5: Pomeroy technique.

SECTION 1 General Gynecology

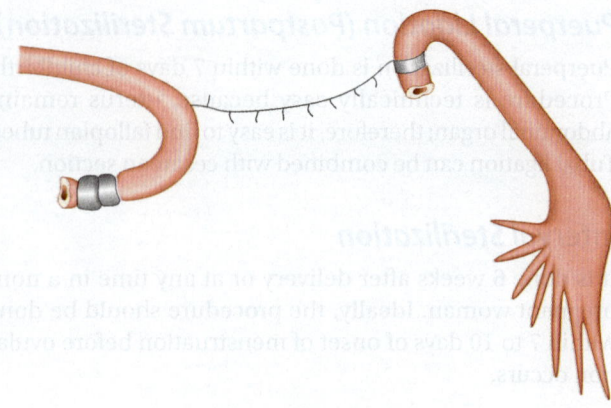

Fig. 16.6: Irving technique.

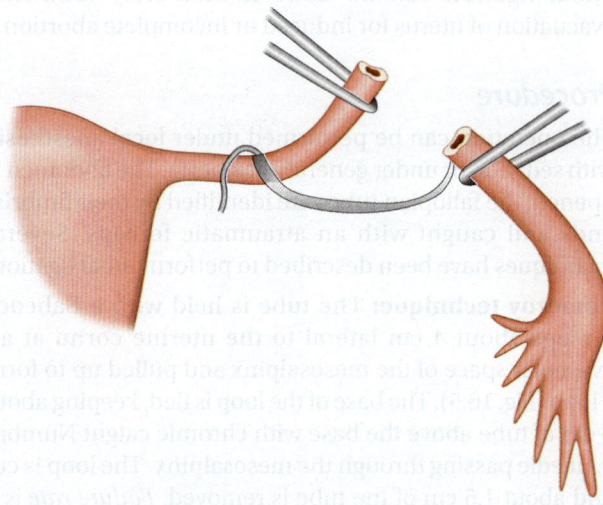

Fig. 16.7: Uchida technique.

Uchida technique: The tubal serosa is separated from the muscularis. About 5 cm of the tube is cut after separating the mesosalpinx and tying both the ends separately (Fig. 16.7). The medial end of the tube is buried in the mesosalpinx, lateral end remains outside the mesosalpinx.

Madlener technique: A loop of tube in the middle third portion is crushed at the base and ligated with silk. The *Failure rate* is high 0.2–0.3%.

Parkland technique: The tube is ligated proximally and distally with number 0 chromic catgut suture and intervening segment of about 2 cm is excised with scissors. *Failure rate* is 1 in 400.

Fimbriectomy (Kroener's technique): The fimbrial end of the tube is doubly ligated with silk/catgut sutures and then removed.

Complications of Minilaparotomy
- Injury to bladder or intestines
- Injury to tube or mesosalphyngeal vessels leading to hematosalpinx
- Wound hematoma, infection or dehiscence
- Rarely pelvic infection and peritonitis
- Incisional hernia
- Bowel and bladder fistulae if damage is not recognized and repaired immediately.

Contraindications
No contraindications are permanent, but the procedure is delayed or patient is referred to higher center if woman has conditions that either increase anesthetic or surgical risk.

Advantages
- Safe, effective, easy method and can be performed by a junior doctor
- Does not need special training, or expensive equipments
- Complications are minor. Many can be avoided and can be tackled easily
- Can be performed soon after delivery, after termination of pregnancy.

Disadvantages
- Higher chance of wound and pelvic infections
- Bigger incision is required
- Postoperative pain is more severe and lasts longer
- Longer convalescent period.

Laparoscopic Sterilization
Laparoscopic sterilization can be done by following methods:
- Occlusion with silastic rings
- Occlusion with clips.
- Occlusion or transaction or resection either with unipolar or bipolar electrocoagulation.

Silastic (Falope or Yoon) rings are nonreactive silastic rubber bands (Fig. 16.8). The outer diameter is 3.6 mm and inner diameter is 1 mm and thickness is 2.2 mm. Rings are loaded onto a special applicator, tube is grasped about 3 cm from the uterus, and band is pushed over the knuckle of the tube. Failure rate of the procedure is 1 per 100 women.

Hulka-Clemens spring clips (consists of two plastic jaws made of Lexan) and Filshie clips (made of titanium lined with silicone rubber) are available. The clips are applied at 90° angle to include some mesosalpinx at the proximal part of the isthmus of a stretched fallopian tube (Figs. 16.9 and 16.10). These destroy 3–4 mm of the tube. It has a *Failure rate* of 0.2 per 100 women years.

Procedure
The procedure is ideally done under general anesthesia, but can be done under local anesthesia with sedation. Initially, a pneumoperitoneum is created to displace the intestines

CHAPTER 16 Contraception and Sterilization

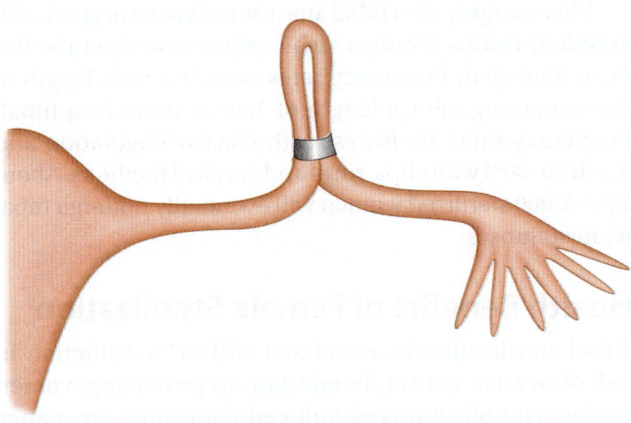

Fig. 16.8: Falope ring.

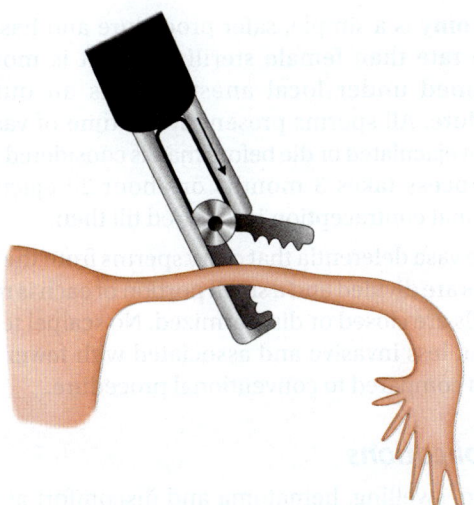

Fig. 16.9: Hulka-Clemens spring clip.

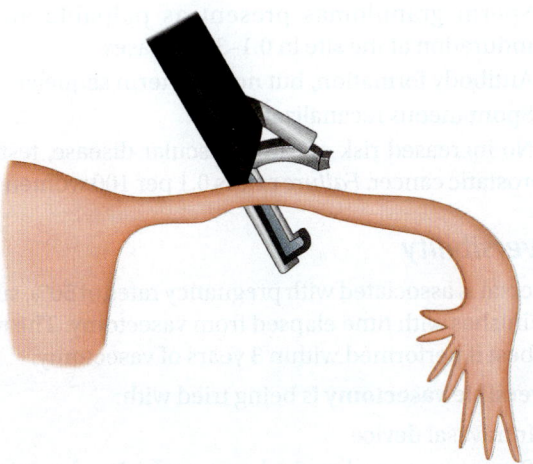

Fig. 16.10: Filshie clip.

away by inserting a Verres needle into abdomen through a small incision at the lower margin of the umbilicus. Trendelenburg position facilitates displacement of bowel. The laparoscope is introduced and the pelvic organs are inspected carefully, the fallopian tubes are identified and occluded by one of the above mentioned techniques.

Complications

- Abdominal wall emphysema
- Bleeding from inferior epigastric vessel, mesosalpingeal vessel and rarely great vessels
- Bladder and intestinal injury
- Uterine perforation
- Air embolism
- Cardiorespiratory embarrassment.

Contraindications

- A patient with cardiac or respiratory disease who cannot tolerate pneumoperitoneum and Trendelenburg position
- Previous abdominal surgery which may lead to intestinal perforation if adhesions were present
- Puerperal uterus or any other big abdominal masses
- Diaphragmatic or umbilical hernia.

Advantages

- Laparoscopy permits direct visualization and manipulation of the abdominal and pelvic organs with minimal abdominal disruption
- Small incision
- Minimal discomfort postoperatively
- Shorter convalescence
- Better choice for fixed, immobile uterus
- Success after reversal procedure is more except for electrocoagulation
- Simultaneous diagnosis of other pathological conditions is possible.

Disadvantages

- Complications are rare, but when occurs, they are usually serious and life-threatening
- Special expensive equipment and special training is required
- Not suitable for postpartum patients.

Vaginal Approach

Vaginal approach is associated with higher rates of infection and occasional pelvic abscess; they are technically difficult and occasionally laparotomy in needed to complete the procedure.

Transcervical Approach

Many methods have been described including instillation of sclerosing agents (quinacrine, erythromycin) or tissue adhesives (Femcept), electrocoagulation, thermal occlusion, cryosurgery, laser and mechanical occlusive devices (Essure, Adiana). These techniques can be performed either blindly or with hysteroscopic guidance. They destroy the interstitial portion of the tube or mechanically obstruct the tubal lumen.

Advantages
- No scar
- Less pain, recovery is faster
- Complications are less
- Suitable for obese patients and patients who have medical conditions that contraindicate laparotomy or laparoscopy.

Disadvantages
- Delay in sterility as the devices used to take time to occlude the tube completely
- The need for a test to document tubal block like hysterosalpingography
- Special equipment (hysteroscope) and special training is required.

Long-term Complications of Sterilization Procedures

- **Failure:** Failure rate is highest for spring clip application, after that in decreasing order for bipolar cautery, interval sterilization, silicone rings, unipolar coagulation and postpartum sterilization
- **Ectopic pregnancy:** One-third of the pregnancies following sterilization are ectopic. They are more likely to occur 3 or more years after sterilization
- **Regret:** Some women regret the decision of permanent method. Risk factors include young age at the time of sterilization, low parity, unstable relationship, change in family structure or illness/death of child
- **Post-tubal sterilization syndrome** includes abnormal menstrual bleeding, dysmenorrhea and premenstrual distress. The cumulative evidence provides little or no support to the existence of such syndrome.

Reversal of Sterilization

The sterilization must be considered as irreversible and permanent procedure. The success rate for reversal of sterilization is usually less than 50%, however, with some procedures like clips, it may be 75%. It is least with electrocoagulation and fimbriectomy. The incidence of ectopic pregnancy is high following reversal surgery.

Microsurgery with tubal anastomosis is associated with excellent results if only a small segment of the tube has been damaged. Pregnancy rates correlate with length of the remaining tube, a length of 4cm or more is optimal. Pregnancy rates are lowest with electrocoagulation and reach 70–80% with clips, rings and surgical methods. About 2 per 1,000 sterilized women will eventually undergo tubal reanastomoses.

Health Benefits of Female Sterilization

Tubal sterilization is associated with 67% reduction in risk of ovarian cancer, in addition to protecting women against complications of induced abortions, pregnancy and delivery.

Male Sterilization

Vasectomy is a simple, safer procedure and has a lower failure rate than female sterilization. It is more often performed under local anesthesia as an outpatient procedure. All sperms present at the time of vasectomy must be ejaculated or die before man is considered infertile. The process takes 3 months or about 20 ejaculations. Additional contraception is required till then.

The vasa deferentia that carry sperms from the testicles to penis are divided and a small portion of each is removed, the ends are closed or diathermized. No scalpel technique is faster, less invasive and associated with fewer complications compared to conventional procedure.

Complications
- Pain, swelling, hematoma and discomfort at the site. These complications are less with no scalpel technique
- Infection usually is mild
- Hypersensitivity reaction to local anesthetic agents and anaphylaxis are rare
- Sperm granulomas present as palpable areas of induration at the site in 0.1–3% of cases
- Antibody formation, but no long-term sequelae
- Spontaneous recanalization.

No increased risk of cardiovascular disease, testicular or prostatic cancer. *Failure rate* is 0.1 per 100 women years.

Reversibility

Reversal is associated with pregnancy rates of 50%, success diminishes with time elapsed from vasectomy. The results are best if performed within 3 years of vasectomy.

Reversible vasectomy is being tried with:
- Intravasal device
- Percutaneous chemical vas occlusion by injecting a mixture of carbolic acid and n-butyl alpha-cyanoacrylate directly into vas lumen are under study.

NEWER METHODS

Male Hormonal Method

Hormonal suppression of spermatogenesis by exogenously administered androgen and progestin to inhibit the hypothalamic-pituitary axis. The following are under trial:

- Weekly injections of testosterone enanthate
- Transdermal patch, implants of testosterone
- Adding depot medroxyprogesterone to testosterone.

Immunocontraception

Research on contraceptive vaccines has focused on sperm antigen, zona pellucida and human chorionic gonadotropin antigens.

Genetic Research

Blocking the function of genes that control the release of eggs, sperm development, sperm motility and sperm-egg fusion may help in preventing conception.

HIV and Contraception[20]

The only method, which helps protect against pregnancy and STIs, including HIV, is condom. But it is better to use another method for contraception as condoms have higher failure rates. Women who are infected with HIV or suffering from AIDS or those who are on antiretroviral treatment (ARV) can use:

- Combined oral contraceptive pill
- Progesterone only pills
- Injectable hormonal contraceptives
- Subdermal implants.

ARV drugs may reduce the effectiveness of these hormones; condoms provide additional protection in such situation.

Intrauterine device can be used by women who are at risk of HIV infection or who are infected with HIV, but **not** if they have AIDS.

Vaginal diaphragms, cervical caps and spermicides are not recommended.

Adolescent Girls

They have less information about contraceptives, consequences of unprotected intercourse such as risk of sexually transmitted diseases, teenage pregnancy, induced abortions and their impact on future fertility. They are usually less compliant. Combined oral contraceptives are the best options if used regularly and consistently. It is better if condoms are also used to protect against STIs. Emergency contraceptives play an important role as adolescents are more likely to forget pills and they are more likely to have infrequent, unplanned coitus. Implants are usually not preferred by teenagers as they cause minor problems like irregular menses, weight gain and acne. DMPA may cause reduced bone mineral density. Diaphragms and spermicidal agents are not ideal for adolescents.

Contraception for Women more than 35 and Perimenopausal Women

Childbearing is associated with greater risk for both the mother and fetus after the age of 35. The fecundity and frequency of intercourse usually reduces as age advances. Therefore, methods with higher failure rates can be used. Aging is accompanied by medical conditions that may restrict the use of certain contraceptives (Table 16.2).

Options available are:

- Permanent sterilization
- Intrauterine device till menopause
- Subdermal implants and injectables
- Progesterone only pills
- Barrier methods
- Combined oral contraceptive pills if woman is not a smoker and has no other medical contraindications
- Emergency contraception.

Women who use temporary methods are advised to continue contraception for one year following their last menstrual period if aged 50 years or more, or for 2 years if aged 50 years or less.

Table 16.2: Medical conditions and method of choice.

Conditions	Preferred method	May be used	Not to be used
Lactating mothers	• LAM • POPs • DMPA • Copper IUDs • Barrier methods		COCs till 6 months
Diabetes	• DMPA • IUDs • POPs • Other methods	COCs if uncomplicated	COCs, DMPA if diabetes for 20 years or more or if vascular disease
Migraine	• All other methods	COCs if no focal neurological deficits or other risk factors for stroke	COCs if migraine with aura, focal neurological deficits, or other risk factors

(LAM: lactational amenorrhea method; POPs: progestin only pills; DMPA: depot medroxyprogesterone; IUDs: intrauterine device; COCs: combined oral contraceptives)

REFERENCES

1. Trussel J, Hatcher RA, Cates Jr W, Stewrat FH. A guide to interpreting contraceptive efficacy studies. Obstet Gynecol. 1990;76:558.
2. Hatcher RA, Rinehart W, Blackburn R, Geller JS, Shelton JD. The essentials of contraceptive technology. Baltimore: John Hopkins University School of Public Health, Population Information Program, 1997.
3. WHO. Medical eligibility criteria for contraceptive use. Geneva: WHO; 2004.
4. Selected Practice Recommendations. Department of Reproductive Health and Research, Family and Community Health, WHO, Geneva. 2nd edition. 2004.
5. Speroff I, Darney PD. A clinical guide for contraception. 3rd edition. Philadelphia, US: Lippincott Williams & Wilkins; 2001.
6. Shulman LP. Oral contraceptives risks. Obstetrics and Gynecology Clinics of North America. 2000;27:695-704.
7. Family planning. A global hand book for providers. Baltimore and Geneva: CCP and WHO; 2007.
8. Burkman R. Contraception and family planning. Current diagnosis and treatment. Obstetrics and Gynecology. 10 edition. A Lange Medical Book, McGraw-Hill, 2006.
9. Scott A, Glasier A. Evidence based contraceptive choices: Best Practice and Research. Clinical Obstetrics and Gynaecology. 2006;20:665-80.
10. Hannaford PC, Webb AMC. Evidence guided prescribing of combined oral contraceptives: Consensus statement. Contraception. 1996;54:125.
11. Westhoff C, Kerns J, Morroni C, et al. Quick start: a novel oral contraception initiation method. Contraception. 2002;66:141-5.
12. Steinauer J, Autry AM. Extended cycle combined hormonal contraception. Obstetrics Gynecology Clinics of North America. 2007;34:43-55.
13. Bracken MB. Oral contraception and congenital malformation in offspring: a review and meta-analysis of the prospective studies. Obstet Gynecol. 1990;76:552.
14. Chaudhari SK. Practice of fertility control. 6th edition. India: Elsevier Publication; 2004.
15. Gbolade B, Ellis S, Murby B, Randall S, Kirkman R. Bone density in long term users of depot medroxyprogesterone acetate. Br J Obstet Gynaecol.1998;105:790.
16. L Mascarenhas, J Newton. Contraceptive implants. In: Stud J (Ed). Progress in Obstetrics & Gynecology. Churchill Livingstone;1996;12:279-92.
17. Von Hertzen H. Low dose mifepristone and two regimens of levonorgestrel for emergency contraception: a WHO multicentric randomized trial, for the WHO research group on postovulatory methods of fertility regulation (WHO, Geneva, et al.). Lancet. 2002; 360:1803-10.
18. Grims DA, Schulz FK. Antibiotic prophylaxis for intrauterine contraceptive device insertion. Cochrane database of systematic reviews. 1999, issue 3.
19. Hockey J, Verma V, Panay N. The wider role of intrauterine progestogens. In: Studd J (Ed). Progress in Obstetrics and Gynecology. 2005;16:389-409.
20. Population reports, Series L-15, Family Planning Choices for Women with HIV. John Hopkins School of Public Health; 2007.

CHAPTER 17

Psychosexual Problems and Sexual Dysfunction

Claudine Domoney

Overview

- Prevalence of sexual problems in primary care is high with 22% of men and 40% of women having a diagnosis of sexual dysfunction, although this was poorly recognized or documented – only 3–4% had an entry in their medical notes.

- *Sexual pain disorders* include dyspareunia, defined as persistent or recurrent genital pain associated with sexual intercourse. This may be physical and/or psychological, i.e. psychosomatic in origin.

- Management of sexual difficulties will always be tailored to the individual and/or couple as with any intervention.

INTRODUCTION

Sexual health is a state of physical, emotional, mental and social well-being in relation to sexuality; it is not merely the absence of disease, dysfunction or infirmity. The World Health Organization declared this as long ago as 1978 and stated that "sexual health requires a positive and respectful approach to sexuality and sexual relationships, as well as the possibility of having pleasurable and safe sexual experiences, free of coercion, discrimination and violence".[1] For this to be achieved and maintained, the sexual rights of all persons must be respected, protected and fulfilled. As society changes, the status of women gradually changes, in turn. Health professionals aim to embrace a holistic approach to health care, which includes understanding sexual behavior and its impact on quality of life. In tandem, the academic pursuit of 'sexology' has followed an increase in sexual expression for many women and an individual expectation to achieve sexual satisfaction. Both women and men are more likely to seek solutions to their sexual difficulties, although they may present with (occasionally) unrecognized somatization of these problems. The inseparability of mind and body with respect to sexuality allows a plethora of symptomatology. This is turn offers the clinician the challenge of interpretation and individual management planning in order to fulfill the patient's known or unknown wishes. This Chapter hopes to introduce key aspects of sexual dysfunction, focusing on the female, and an approach to managing individual patients. Patients may expect health professionals to have some training in sexual medicine, but in practice the majority feel poorly equipped to deal with these problems.

Female Sexuality

To try to encapsulate female sexuality as a series of physiological reactions will always disappoint but knowledge of the workings of the female sexual cycle will help understand some difficulties and the complex inter-relationship of multifactorial features. Although, true also of male sexuality, a more physical model as demonstrated by Masters and Johnson in the 1950s,[2] can aid and direct treatment for some; although psychosexual factors will always play a key part in any sexual difficulties. It is important to understand that it is universal to have a psychological reaction to malfunction whether it be physical or psychological. Basson et al. have expanded the female sexuality models developed over the latter 20th century to include the importance of intimacy and sexual stimuli on the innate sexual drive or 'hunger' (Fig. 17.1).[3]

This contrasts to the linear human sexual response model of Masters and Johnson more in keeping with male sexuality, with an inbuilt sexual drive, i.e. libido and desire to be involved in sexual behavior that causes excitement and arousal. Orgasm is achieved if the physical mechanisms

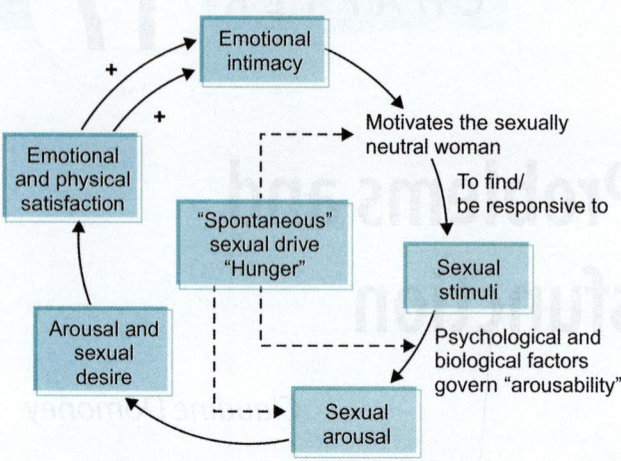

Fig. 17.1: Basson model of female sexuality.

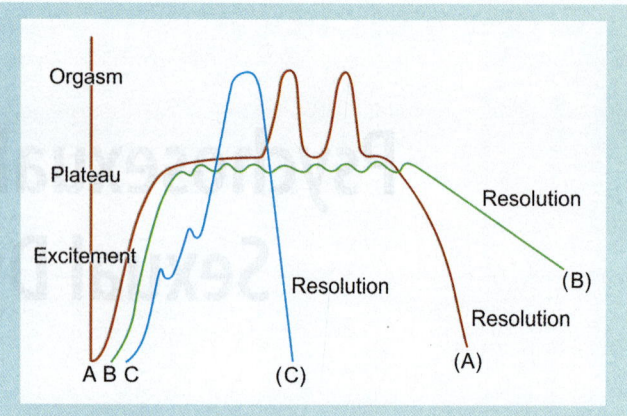

Fig. 17.2: Masters and Johnson model of human sexuality.

are intact and psychologically there are no hurdles. Their model also incorporated those without orgasm and with multiple orgasmic potential (Fig. 17.2).

Studies of female sexuality indicate that an inbuilt sexual drive to be involved in sexual activity does not need to be present for satisfactory relationships to be maintained. Women seek sexual activity for many different reasons, including the strong need to be intimate. The content of sexual activity therefore *may* be less goal driven than that of men. Therefore, it is important to understand the other features influencing the individual woman's ability to be sexual in order to explain why she may be experiencing difficulties. These may be well-hidden in a wide variety of physical symptoms commonly presenting to the gynecologist. Sexuality may be modulated by many factors and normal features of life, including life events, reproductive events, health, relationships and cultural factors. Overall, female sexuality is a complex interplay of physiological, psychological and cultural factors.

PRESENTATION OF SEXUAL DIFFICULTIES

Sexual difficulties are common in both men and women. Whether these are circumstantial and temporary will determine their effect on an individual and couple's functioning. The often cited paper of Laumann et al. reported a sexual dysfunction rate of 43% in women and 31% in men from a North American population.[4] However, the definition of female sexual dysfunction (FSD) was arguably not what a clinician would call a clinical problem, i.e. a persistent and bothersome to the individual. The International Consensus conference panel modified the framework of the International Classification of Diseases-10 and DSM-V (Diagnostic and Statistical Manual of Mental Disorders of the American Psychiatric Association) to categorize clinical sexual disorders and thereby improve diagnosis and treatment. For men, the advances in physical treatments have greatly fuelled interest in their sexual disorders but perhaps at the cost of the psychosexual factors. The early hopes that medications would follow to treat female desire and arousal problems have largely been unrealized. Yet, the financial support and interest has fired interest overall in management of FSD. Hormonal treatments are more commonly suggested although also have perhaps suffered from the general decrease in hormone replacement therapy since the publication of the Women's Health Initiative (WHI) study in 2002.[5]

British studies have indicated that prevalence of sexual problems in primary care is high with 22% of men and 40% of women having a diagnosis of sexual dysfunction, although this was poorly recognized or documented—only 3–4% had an entry in their medical notes.[6] This is reflected in gynecology clinics where presentation can be covert or overt (Table 17.1). There is frequently a psychosexual element to any gynecological complaint. Referrals from primary care may include diagnoses of vaginismus, superficial dyspareunia, lack of libido yet exploration of chronic pelvic pain, vulval pain disorders may frequently mask primary sexual disorders. Difficult consultations are often covert presentations of FSD (Table 17.2). The patient and /or the doctor may subconsciously collude in avoiding identifying the problem. Women complaining of perimenopausal or urogynecological symptoms are thankful for the opportunity to discuss their sex lives. It may however, be recognized that the primary problem is in fact their relationship, that will generally be outside the remit of the gynecologist. Rather than be viewed as the older woman whose sexual being is all in the past, to be reassured that the possibilities of future satisfactory relationships are there for the taking of a few simple measures can be very important at this often tumultuous time.

The concept of the 'calling card' is important. Those women in whom one appears not to be able to diagnose their

CHAPTER 17 Psychosexual Problems and Sexual Dysfunction

Table 17.1: Common presentations of sexual problems in the gynecology clinic.

Overt presentation	Covert presentation
Loss of libido	Pelvic pain
Loss of sensation	Prolpase symptoms
Nonconsummation	Vulval pain
Vaginismus	Vaginismus
Coital urinary leak	Difficulty with smear taking
Vaginal dryness	Requests for labial reduction
Dyspareunia	Dyspareunia

Table 17.2: Communication difficulties between patient and clinician.

Patient difficulty	Clinician difficulty
Embarrassment	Embarrassment
Shame	Other health factors more important
Expectation, e.g. older or life event	Lack of time
Poor knowledge of interventions	Lack of training
Poor general health	Lack of shared language
Physician issue, e.g. gender, age	Poor recognition of somatization. Perceived lack of treatment
Perceived lack of confidentiality	

problem or determine what they want from your service, those who mention a sexual difficulty with their hand on the door as they leave the consultation room (allowing both patient and doctor room to 'flee' as necessary), those who indicate that they may be 'too old' to expect any different, are reflecting their ambivalence and testing you as a clinician. These women often warrant further exploration of their sexual difficulties or an offer of referral to a different practitioner as this may be the first time she has been able to broach the subject. You may be the first clinician to have touched upon an area that she may not have consciously thought about. The frequent feeling of being overwhelmed or out of one's depth may reflect the feelings of the patient herself. The reaction of both clinician and patient is to often ignore rather than confront these feelings. Offering a diagnostic laparoscopy for a 'case' of pelvic pain when the clinical suspicion of physical pathology is low may miss an important opportunity to explore other psychosomatic, if not psychosexual disorders. The financial and human expense of missing these diagnoses is enormous.

Categorization of Female Sexual Disorders

- Sexual desire disorders
- Hypoactive sexual desire disorder (HSDD)
  - Sexual aversion disorder
- Sexual arousal disorders
- Orgasmic disorder
- Sexual pain disorder
  - Dyspareunia
  - Vaginismus
  - Noncoital sexual pain disorders.

DEFINITIONS OF SEXUAL DISORDERS IN WOMEN

Desire Disorders

Hypoactive sexual desire disorder (HSDD) is the persistent or recurrent deficiency or absence of sexual desire or sexual fantasies or thoughts, and/or the desire for or receptivity to sexual activity which causes distress. The emphasis on causing distress and focus on sexual thoughts allows the flexibility of definition to include those who are not in a relationship or have lost their relationships secondary to their HSDD. Sexual aversion disorder is the persistence of phobic aversion to and avoidance of sexual activity which causes personal distress.

Sexual arousal disorder is defined as the persistent or recurrent inability to attain or maintain sexual excitement causing personal distress, which may be described as subjective feelings and/or lack of physical changes.

Orgasmic Disorder

This is defined as the persistence or recurrent difficulty or absence of achieving orgasm following sufficient stimulation and arousal. It may follow from both desire or arousal disorders or be truly independent.

Sexual pain disorders include dyspareunia, defined as persistent or recurrent genital pain associated with sexual intercourse. This may be physical and/or psychological, i.e. psychosomatic in origin. It is important not to dismiss this as nonorganic pain without sufficient exploration which may not always require physical invasive investigations. Vaginismus has been described by the International Consensus Group as recurrent or persistent involuntary spasm of the pelvic musculature that interferes with intercourse. However, it may be situational, i.e. with only certain partners or just at speculum examination. This should be more often interpreted as a sign not a pelvic symptom or considered alone a diagnosis. If a woman complains of vaginismus, explore what this means to her. Where did she find this diagnosis? As so often with sexual issues, we all use different language, be it to describe difficulties or our anatomy. Basic language can allow misinterpretation and often proves difficult with patients in whom their native language is different to that of their health professional. This works both ways. Never assume we understand what the patient means! Let her explain the meaning in her words and feelings.

The patient is the expert. The doctor often needs to assume a position of ignorance to interpret the patient's symptoms and feelings. This is difficult when we are trained to be the expert and ask closed questions to streamline care down preplanned pathways. Particularly with respect to sexual difficulties, all circumstances and individuals are unique. Just as expectations and frequency of intercourse are individual to a particular woman or couple, so are the difficulties that ensue.

Noncoital sexual pain disorders are genital pain disorders induced by nonsexual stimulation, most commonly vulval pain disorders.

The prevalence of these disorders is varied depending on the population and age group. They can vary from 16–75% with desire disorder, 12–64% with arousal, 16–48% with orgasm and 7–68% with sexual pain; with considerable overlap.

MANAGEMENT

Questions

The most basic questions that should be incorporated into a basic general gynecological consultation regarding sexual function should be as follows:

- Do you have a partner? Are you in a sexual relationship?
- Do you have any difficulties? Do you have pain during intercourse?
- Are these difficulties a problem for you?

The words used should be tailored to the patient and the situation. Following her lead, or not as she prefers, answers to such questions are likely to reveal the most useful information. If there are no difficulties that the patient wishes to discuss, her sexual life will remain private. Only those who offer further discussion should be tackled at this time. However, further into a consultation, if there appear to be related issues, these topics can be approached again, but with great caution. Any previous suggestion that a woman did not want to discuss her sexual life needs to be addressed sensitively. Inquisitiveness without a therapeutic benefit can be interpreted as inappropriate. Also, be careful about making assumptions regarding sexual orientation.

Use of Questionnaires

Questionnaires can be extremely useful as they introduce the subject of sex to those who find it uncomfortable, both clinician and patient. It indicates that clinicians are interested in sexual history, which frequently patients feel is not the case or there is no treatment that the doctor can offer. However many questionnaires are unwieldy tools designed by psychologists and for some people may be intrusive. There are those with up to 35 'items' or questions so far many practical purposes, short form questionnaires have been validated for clinical use. These may not be as useful for research but can be beneficial for introducing the subject and screening for sexual problems in a clinical setting. They may also be useful to monitor the sexual effects of a new intervention in a population rather than for individuals. Questionnaires can be generic or disease or condition specific. An example of a disease specific questionnaire is the Prolapse and Incontinence Sexual Questionnaire (PISQ) which comes in a long and short form-12.[7,8] Generic questionnaires such as the Female Sexual Function Index (FSFI) are well-accepted by most patients and can be downloaded from the Internet, including analysis instructions.[9] There are strengths and weaknesses of every questionnaire and it is important to know in what population they have been validated. Some are not sensitive enough to deal with difficulties in those that are not sexually active. This can have clinical implications depending on why they are not active—secondary to their own difficulties, health or disease status, their partner's or personal preference.

Sexual History

A sexual history may be a combination of a medical and psychiatric history. During specific sexual therapy, it is necessary to gain details of an individual sexual biography to place the current sexual difficulties in context. In a more general setting, it is important to know medical details including medical conditions, psychiatric disorders, surgical history, current symptoms particularly those of a gynecological nature or psychological problems, medications, drug and alcohol use. A social history including details of relationships (do not assume there is only one), housing, who lives at home, work and general relationships will 'set the scene.' Sexual expectations and previous experiences may be explored during the 'sexual biography' and should be addressed. Family history and details of first sexual experiences or sexual awareness, how sex education and family attitudes to sexual matters as well as the body in general are frequently revealing. The limitations of clinician or sexual therapist must be recognized—in general the aim is not to be a relationship counsellor. Sexual difficulties that are a symptom not a cause of marital breakdown may be best dealt with by a relationship counsellor. When ascertaining the specific problem, determine what is the patient specifically complaining of as patients frequently use broad terms rather than be specific. Complaints of loss of libido may mean loss of desire, loss of arousal and/or loss of orgasmic potential to the patient.

Many patients may resist psychosexual exploration until the mind-body link is explained. There is always a psychological reaction to a physical illness, and in the arena

CHAPTER 17 Psychosexual Problems and Sexual Dysfunction

of sexuality, physical problems can be accentuated by the psychological consequences. The reverse somatization of psychological problems into sexual and physical problems is a very powerful sequence of processes. This in part explains the resistance for change in those who refuse to acknowledge a psychological component. Patients presenting with non-consummation may have deep seated issues that have been suppressed. Non-consummation may in these circumstances be protective and an examination under anesthesia (EUA) will not cure these difficulties. Physical examination must obviously exclude physical abnormalities, although vaginismus and adductor spasm may prevent full examination. An ultrasound scan may exclude congenital malformations of the genital tract if there is any degree of concern but this would be an indication for an EUA.

INVESTIGATIONS

In the vast majority of women, few investigations are required. Baseline tests that may be considered are:

- Follicle stimulating hormone (FSH)
- Luteinizing hormone (LH)
- Estradiol (E_2)
- Androgen profile
  - Testosterone
  - Sex hormone binding globulin (SHBG)
  - Free androgen index (FAI)—calculated from total testosterone and SHBG (Normal range 0.4–0.8 ng/L)

$$FAI = \frac{TT \text{ (in mmol/L)}}{SHBG \text{ (in mmol/L)}} \times 100 \text{ (ng/L)}$$

- Prolactin
- Blood sugar

See Tables 17.3 and 17.4 for pre- and postmenopausal androgens. Table 17.5 provides mean hormone levels in women.

However, it is pertinent to remember that during the perimenopause, hormone levels are frequently of little clinical value as they may be rapidly fluctuating and therefore are only a snapshot in time. They may be of benefit in those who have iatrogenic premature or early menopause (below 40 and 45 years respectively).

Table 17.3: Premenopausal androgen distribution.

	Ovarian secretion	Adrenal secretion	Peripheral conversion
Testosterone	25%	25%	50%
Androstenedione	40%	50%	10%
DHEA	10%	60%	30%
DHEA-S	90%	10%	

(DHEA-S: dehydroepiandrosterone-sulfate)

Table 17.4: Postmenopausal androgen distribution.

	Ovarian secretion	Adrenal secretion	Peripheral conversion
Testosterone	50%	10%	40%
Androstenedione	20%	70%	10%
DHEA	10%	60%	30%
DHEA-S		90%	10%

Table 17.5: Mean hormone levels in women (pg/mL).

Hormone	Reproductive age	Natural menopause	Surgical menopause
Estradiol	100–150	10–15	10
Testosterone	400	290	110
FSH	<10	>30 (×2, 6 weeks apart)	>30
LH	<6	>10	>10

(FSH: follicle-stimulating hormone; LH: luteinizing hormone)

Hormone levels can also be useful for those who have been prescribed estrogen and/or androgen therapy but appear to be having no therapeutic effect. It is important to measure SHBG as this will alter the free levels of other sex steroids. Only 1 to 2% of testosterone is free in the circulation: 66% is bound to SHBG, 31% to albumin (which is also bioavailable). Peripheral conversion occurs in adipose and muscle tissue. Therefore, women with a higher body mass index have higher circulating sex steroid levels and therefore higher risk of hormone dependant tumors such as endometrial and breast cancers. Androgens fall by 50% after the menopause but are more dramatically lowered after bilateral oophorectomy, therefore causing significant symptoms in those who are already menopausal. SHBG is altered by other interventions and may impact on free circulating androgens and therefore female sexual response. Most importantly in a gynecological context, HRT and the combined oral contraceptive pill (COCP) increase SHBG and therefore reduce free testosterone. Some progestogens within the COCP also impact negatively on mood.

TREATMENT

Management of sexual difficulties will always be tailored to the individual and/or couple as with any intervention. However, there is frequently a pressure to treat the couple. On many levels this may be alienating—a woman presenting to a gynecologist is frequently asking for help for herself. She may not have a partner, not have discussed or revealed her difficulties to her partner and have features of her past life she does not wish to disclose. Different therapists work

Table 17.6: Interventions used in sexual medicine.

Psychosexual	Pharmacological	Physical
Brief psychodynamic therapy	Estradiol—systemic or topical	Physiotherapy—pelvic floor exercises +/– biofeedback
Psychotherapy	Testosterone—implant/gel/patch/oral	Vaginal trainers/dilators
Sex education	Tibolone	Lubricants
Couple therapy	Analgesics	Clitoral stimulators
Sensate focus	Antidepressants	Visual sexual aids
Cognitive behavioral therapy	Gabapentin	Physical sexual aids, e.g. vibrators
Psychoanalysis	?DHEA	'Bibliotherapy'
	Sildenafil	
	Local anesthetics	

in different ways and many prefer to work with couples. Gynecologists have a responsibility to their patient, the woman, and therefore, it is reasonable to deal with her individual problems. She may have a problem with intimate examinations or cervical smear taking that then unravels sexual difficulties. Fantasies (or less often reality) regarding anatomy or surgery may be disclosed to a gynecologist. If the patient brings their partner then it is appropriate to see them together although the dynamic of the consultation is different. It may reveal much information about their sexual functioning and this can be explored in a 'safe' environment.

There are three main approaches to treatment (Table 17.6). A combination is most common amongst sex therapists but a gynecologist has the advantage of prescribing ability in addition to the revelations of 'the moment of truth'—the genital examination. They also have recourse to surgery, although with greater recognition of psychosexual problems, this may be less often required.

- Psychosexual
- Pharmacological
- Physical.

Pharmacological Interventions

Patient and physician are drawn to the 'magic pill' or quick fix of a pharmacological intervention. If there is a hormonal deficiency or need for analgesics or antidepressants for pain disorders, other subconscious or learned behaviors need to be corrected for normal sexual functioning to return. For the vast majority of women, drug interventions will not be the first treatment choice. Perimenopausal women and those who have an iatrogenic menopause may be the exceptions. There has been much discussion in the medical and lay press regarding the medicalization of female sexual function. Female sexual dysfunction (FSD) has been used as a definition loosely. Whether the condition is determined by the impact a pharmacological intervention may have and therefore the revenue it may generate is arguable.

Estrogen replacement therapy may improve ability to be aroused and genital tissue response. Testosterone may be linked to sexual drive and ability to achieve orgasm. Studies have currently determined that adequate estrogen replacement is given to sex hormone deficient women before androgen replacement. Testosterone implants have been the mainstay of androgen replacement for women for decades. Oral androgen is produced for men and has a higher risk of hepatic derangement. Testosterone gels for men have been used by women at a fraction of the dose. There are currently no licensed testosterone products available for women in the UK. Ongoing studies will assess the use of testosterone without estrogen and in those women with a diagnosis of HSDD without oophorectomy. At present, testosterone is used pre- and postmenopausally off license but care must be taken that psychosexual issues are not being ignored in the face of a pharmacological intervention. Tibolone is a synthetic sex steroid with estrogenic, progestogenic and androgenic effects. It has been shown to have a positive effect on some sexual symptoms in a few studies. Topical estrogen cream or pessaries may be sufficient for estrogen deficient women with vaginal dryness and dyspareunia, although adequate arousal during intercourse should be enquired after. Breastfeeding women who are estrogen deficient may need topical estrogens as this often contributes to the trauma of post-childbirth perineal injury. Topical estrogens can be used long-term in postmenopausal women if one of the weaker preparations that do not stimulate the endometrium is chosen. For those who cannot or will not use hormonal therapy, vaginal moisturizers such as Replens MD can be used.

Dihydroepiandrostenedione (DHEA) is a nonlicensed prohormone that has been suggested to have a beneficial effect on female sexual drive, arousal and orgasmic potential but the data are not conclusive at present.

With the remarkable effect sildenafil has had on male erectile difficulties worldwide, there were high hopes for sildenafil in women. 5-phosphodiesterase inhibitors have limited value for FSD but some works have indicated that it may have a role in female sexual arousal disorder. As this is unconfirmed it is not recommended for off license treatment at present.

Pain disorders may require more specific treatment. Generic pain treatment can include use of amitriptyline, gabapentin and local anesthetic injections or nerve/ganglion blocks. Steroid and anesthetic injections for point tenderness have a role, particularly post-surgery or post-childbirth. Others are advocating the use of botulinum toxin for levator spasm and vaginismus. The previous reservations regarding physical interventions for somatized deep distress which protect the individual must be considered. Anesthetic gels suitable for genital skin can be useful to decrease sensitivity, especially in women with vulval pain syndrome.

Physical Interventions

There are a wide range of physical interventions, many of which will be available to the gynecologist. The use of vaginal trainers or dilators is popular but often it is more appropriate to try to encourage self-exploration with fingers (patient's own or partner's) and looking with mirrors. Encouragement of tampon use can familiarize women with their genitals and vagina, and empower the woman to 'own' her vagina. It can aid dispelling of long held fantasies, such as the vagina 'with teeth', with a 'bone' inside or the 'dark tunnel'. Physiotherapists are involved with exercises to facilitate pelvic floor muscle relaxation in those with vaginismus. Pelvic floor dysfunction involving urinary and bowel function in addition to pelvic organ prolapse, can have a fundamental effect on sexual function. Surgical approaches to these sexual problems often have limited success, and further accentuate the role of those trained in sexual medicine. Clinicians who have awareness of or additional training in sexual medicine may improve overall functioning and success of their surgical interventions by acknowledging sexual issues.

Women in couples and single women may want advice regarding sexual aids. This is very individual but with greater access for many, either directly or via the internet, visual erotic stimuli and aids can be suitable for some. Clitoral stimulators are discrete devices that are for external use, but more women are exploring the use of vibrators. They may be cheaper to buy than medical devices such as the vaginal dilators. There has been some concern that vibrators can desensitize genital tissue but for the vast majority, the sexual experience with an aid does not replace that within a relationship. 'Bibliotherapy' is often used by therapists to introduce discussion of some subjects that individuals may find uncomfortable.

Although, the use of sex education can cross over with therapy, basic information is frequently sought by patients (Box 17.1). Written material and models are useful to have to hand in addition to internet access (although hospitals may block access to some sites!) when demonstrating to patients. Again, it is important to be aware of the patient who devolves responsibility to the 'expert' doctor and wants to be taught how to have sex or experience feelings.

It is always better to remind couples or women about the use of lubricants. The commonly used water based lubricants are not generally useful for those with difficulties. They can help in penetration but thereafter become sticky. Silicone or oil-based lubricants are less cloying but their compatibility with condoms must be checked. Vegetable oils may be readily available but not especially 'sexy'.

Psychosexual Medicine

There are many varying approaches to managing sexual problems. All involve recognition of the powerful effect of the mind on the body which is so marked in sexual matters. Therapists will offer treatment options based on their particular training. Many will have cognitive behavioral techniques targeted at sexual problems. These involve techniques such as sensate focus (Fig. 17.3) and

Box 17.1: Features of sex education for the adult with sexual difficulties.

- Anatomy
- Physiological changes at differing stages of life
- Surgical changes
- Sexual development
- Contraception
- Fertility
- Sexual behavior variations and norms
- Sexual orientation
- Sexuality changes in life
- Effect of ill health and medications on sexuality

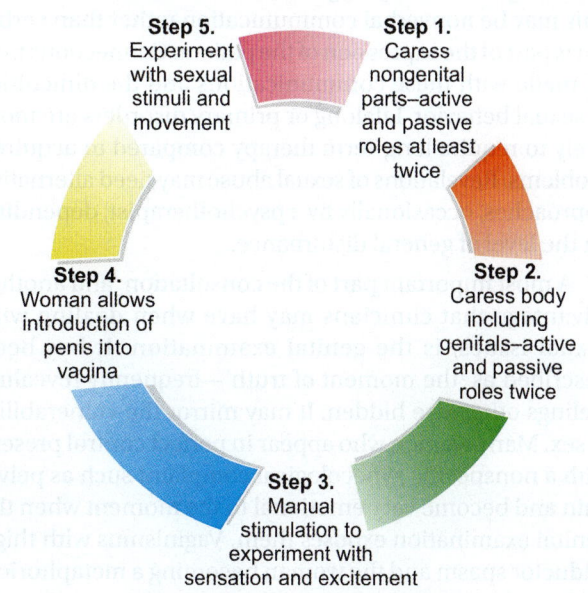

Fig. 17.3: Sensate focus program.

desensitization using dilators/trainers. Other therapists will use alternative psychological approaches, some more psychodynamic than others. It is rare that long-term psychoanalytic therapy will be necessary for most sexual difficulties, although there may be a place for those with other longstanding issues, which sexual problems are a reflection thereof. Behavioral therapists may work with individuals or couples. Many prefer to work with couples as the problem may be between two partners. Those involved in women's health care may discover sexual problems not necessarily when they are involved in a relationship and it may be important to deal with these as they present. The mainstay of gynecologists trained in psychosexual medicine is one that is based on analysis of the doctor-patient relationship reflecting the dynamics of the patient's sexual problems. The basic tenets of the psychosexual consultation are:

- Listen
- Observe
- Feel
- Think
- Interpret

The patient is central to the process—she is the 'expert'—the therapist aims to help reveal the causative and maintaining factors; understanding then facilitating change and hopefully improvement. The empathic consultation may enable the exposure of subconscious feelings and fantasies, as a reflection of the physical symptoms and sexual problems. Psychosexual medicine uses consultation, counseling and psychodynamic skills in addition to the psychosomatic examination to manage these difficulties. Consultations should always be sensitive to the patient's mood although observations can be made reflecting the anxiety/aggression/defensiveness, etc. felt. This may be nonverbal communication rather than verbal but is part of the expression of the patient. Connections may be made with these communications and the difficulties in sexual behavior. Lifelong or primary disorders are more likely to require long-term therapy compared to acquired problems. Revelations of sexual abuse may need alternative approaches, occasionally by a psychotherapist, depending on the level of general disturbance.

A most important part of the consultation, and another advantage that clinicians may have when dealing with sexual issues, is the genital examination. It has been described as 'the moment of truth'—frequently revealing feelings otherwise hidden. It may mirror the vulnerability of sex. Many women who appear in perfect control present with a nonspecific gynecological complaint such as pelvic pain and become very emotional to the moment when the genital examination exposes them. Vaginismus with thigh adductor spasm and the woman becoming a metaphorical 'little girl', trying to escape up the couch may reveal much about her sexual feelings. The woman disconnected from her examination may also be 'disconnected' from sex, not able to feel or therefore react with desire or arousal. She may have had many investigations—all the more reinforcing a perception that her genitals do not belong to her. The woman with persistent discharge who tells the clinician what an awful job they have, is reflecting her disgust with her genital tract. Is her discharge physiological? Requests for labial reduction are becoming more common—are they a response to the trend of increased shaving and therefore, exposure to adult female vulva rather than the physiologically exposed prepubescent vulva or an individual reaction to their 'abnormal' genitalia? The vagina that is too small that bleeds or splits with any penetration, the vagina that is blocked and cannot tolerate anything inside, or the vagina that is sharp and will damage any penis put inside. All these are common fantasies that need understanding before the genitals can become a pleasurable place.

Active listening and observing is what is valuable in these consultations to try to facilitate an exposure of features that may never have been explored before in a safe environment. A patient coming to an understanding of his problem facilitates his acceptance and then ability to deal with it. The 'patient cures herself with the help of the doctor. The doctor is the agent of cure, but does not prescribe the cure'. The behavioral and physical doctoring can occur in addition but is not the main tenet of treatment. An important role of the gynecologist is to assess other physical disease (Table 17.7) in conjunction with recognition of somatized symptoms.

Silence can be therapeutic and time for thought. The patients can be invited to interpret their feelings at that time

Table 17.7: Physical illness and prescribed medications related to sexual problems (men and women).

Condition	Medications
Vascular disease—hypertension, atherosclerosis	Antidepressants
Dyslipidemias	Antihypertensives
Diabetes	Antipsychotics
Chronic disease	Mood stabilizers
Depression	Diuretics
Anxiety	Anticonvulsants
Pelvic floor dysfunction—incontinence (fecal and urinary), prolapse	GnRH analogues
Pelvic surgery	H2 anatagonists
Radiotherapy	Antihistamines
Pelvic adhesions	Combined contraceptive pill
Endometriosis	Mirena IUS
Hormonal	Cyproterone
Addiction	Synthetic progestogens

by the doctor as necessary. The doctor repeatedly asking questions needs to think whether this is a reflection of the effort, the patient's partner needs to input to get a response.

PARTNERS

Within gynecology, women present individually with their symptoms. If they have been referred with a specific sexual difficulty, they may bring their partners. Yet, in the majority, they present alone. As discussed previously, presentation may be overt or covert, planned or incidental. Revelations not spoken of for years can be unearthed during consultations. The fear of opening Pandora's box is what deters many physicians from asking questions. Yet the mere sharing of these memories with contemporary sequelae can be therapeutic.

It appears that women are protective of their partner's sexual difficulties, with development of secondary problems when their male partners develop erectile or ejaculatory disorders, particularly in the older age group. Yet, as the patterns of sexual behavior change, this may alter. It is apparent that there is a significant increase in sexually transmitted infections in those over the age of 50. The use of condoms is low, i.e. less than 10% in this group and the rates of chlamydia, gonorrhea, herpes simplex and warts are rising. The popularity of phosphodiesterase inhibitors has increased the expectations of some who may have abandoned all hopes previously. Yet, their female partners may feel pressure to accept penetrative sex that is no longer as easy, with the effects of genital atrophy secondary to estrogen deficiency and pelvic floor dysfunction with incontinence and/or prolapse.

The most common male sexual problem is erectile dysfunction (ED) but desire and ejaculatory problems are also commonly reported. It is important that the patient's description of impotence is clarified as it can be very generic and nonspecific to laymen. ED increases with age and a careful medical and sexual history may elicit a predominantly organic problem. Although, difficult to elicit, a situational ED is different from a partner who has lost his early morning erections—the latter much more likely to indicate organic disease. Routine tests recommended are serum glucose, lipids and early morning testosterone. There is some concerns that new onset erectile difficulty may predate the onset of cardiovascular disease. Therefore, the evaluation of men with sexual dysfunction requires blood pressure, pulse, weight, genital and prostate examination. Although, ED and, to a certain extent, premature ejaculation, are compatible with pharmacological treatment, it is important to assess the psychosexual aspects of these difficulties for the couple. Physical treatment options for men with sexual problems are outlined in Table 17.8.

Table 17.8: Physical treatment options for men with sexual dysfunction.

Phosphodiesterase inhibitors	
Sildenafil (Viagra)	Improves ED in 60–70%, acts in 20–60 minutes, lasts up to 8 hours
Tadalafil (Cialis)	May be useful for premature ejaculation, half-life 17 hours. May be useful for psychogenic ED
Vardenafil (Levitra)	Duration of action 8 hours
Apomorphine	Dopamine agonist, sublingual, rapid onset, shorter duration, less efficacious 50–60%.
Androgens	For men with hypogonadism NB PSA measurements
Intracavernous prostaglandin	Alprostadil, most common, papaverine and phentolamine occasionally used
Intraurethral prostaglandin pellets	Alprostadil (less effective than intracavernosal)
Vacuum devices	Cost, require dexterity
Penile implants	Good success and patient satisfaction, but failure has serious implications
Surgery	Appropriate for condition but rarely valuable

PHASES OF LIFE

Sexuality develops throughout childhood. During the 20th century, many have superimposed theories of sexual development onto the development of the child. Freud suggested sexual dysfunction was symptomatic of adverse childhood experiences leading to disorders of maturation and personality. The normal phases of sexual maturation as a child were disturbed reflecting abnormal child-parent relationships and therefore the model for future intimate relationships. The power of the unconscious could only be addressed through long-term psychoanalysis or psychotherapy. The immature woman could not progress from the less satisfactory or immature clitoral orgasm to that of the mature woman and her vaginal orgasm. It has more recently become apparent that only 20% of women achieve orgasm with vaginal penetration alone and 30% with vaginal and concurrent clitoral stimulation.

Adolescence

Adolescence is a time of massive hormonal upheaval, peer group pressure and evolving self-realization. Prior education with respect to genital function, menstrual cycles, sexual behavior, contraception and functional relationships are significant throughout this period as well as there exposure to family attitudes.

Reproductive Years

Sexual function is inextricably linked with reproductive function despite the ability to control fertility and infection in the modern age. There is not scope in this Chapter to cover these areas in great depth but those commonly encountered are mentioned for discussion.

Sexually Transmitted Diseases

Education to prevent sexually transmitted disease and treatment seeks to prevent long-term psychological consequences as well as physical. The circumstances under which an infection is introduced, its consequences and the approach to treatment has a bearing on future sexual behavior. Clinicians in genitourinary clinics try to minimize adverse future behavior, in the form of both high-risk taking sexual behavior and normalizing sexuality in general. The specter of HIV temporarily altered sexual behavior in some societies but in many is returning to higher rates of unprotected intercourse. Advertising strategies for sex education reflect the standards and expectations of the younger age groups but may not target all communities as required.

Infertility

Sexual function in couples with sub- and infertility are of such significance that most fertility clinics will employ counselors often with experience in psychosexual work. It is not uncommon to encounter couples who are not having penetrative intercourse, either consciously or not. The demands of performing to specific menstrual cycle dates and maintaining celibacy at other times takes its toll on most couples. Sex becomes goal-orientated and the spontaneity may disappear. The financial, physical and psychological impact of fertility alters the relationship between the couple, and for some raise questions regarding their motivation and wishes at odds with their previous desires.

Termination of Pregnancy

At the other end of the spectrum, control of fertility by termination of pregnancy is repeatedly cited in women recounting their sexual biography: the relationships that change with unresolved issues after a pregnancy; the vagina as a tomb for a pregnancy unwanted or miscarried, that cannot be entered lightly any longer has been expressed in different versions by many women. This may often be years after the event, when another precipitating life event brings it to the fore.

Childbirth

Pregnancy and childbirth herald major changes for a couple, embarking with their first child to a different role in society. Their primary role as partner and lover changes to include mother/parent. For some pregnancy increases orgasmic potential, theoretically via an increase

Table 17.9: Management of postnatal sexual problems.

Condition	Intervention
Superficial dyspareunia—scar tenderness, skin bridge	Fentons procedure
Spot tenderness	Perineal injections
Superficial dyspareunia—estrogen deficiency and genital atrophy	Topical estrogen cream Lubricants—not water-based
Poor pelvic floor tone/vaginismus	Physiotherapy
Lack of sensation/libido/orgasm	Psychosexual counseling
Postnatal depression	Support, antidepressants
Post-traumatic stress disorder	Support, SSRIs

in oxytocin receptors, but changes may be secondary to other psychological and behavioral effects such as bonding and protection. Childbirth itself will alter sexual health but there is no good evidence to suggest that vaginal delivery decreases postnatal sexual health compared with cesarean section, despite claims to justify the increasing cesarean section rate. Episiotomy, however, does increase the persistence of superficial dyspareunia. In one study, women who breastfed their babies were significantly less interested in sex than bottle-fed babies, irrespective of tiredness or depression, although this was not maintained long-term. It also revealed that 7–13% of women expressed a need for help, but 25% had not sought it.[10] Overall sexual problems were common. Changes and dissatisfaction are common but many factors can contribute to this. Mind and body doctorine is fundamental in these circumstances. Debriefing is commonly a feature of perineal clinics for postpartum injuries and although not evidence-based at present, should be incorporated as far as possible into routine postnatal care. Advice regarding sexual function is also reassuring for the pregnant and postnatal, even if they feel it is the 'last thing on their mind'. Great care should be taken when deciding on operative intervention in those with dyspareunia, especially if they plan to have more children and are estrogen deficient. Topical estrogen cream can safely be used in breastfeeding women (Table 17.9).

Colposcopy

Many procedures are experienced very differently by patients when compared to health care professionals' perceptions. These include smear taking, speculum examination and colposcopy. Examinations may allow the patient to reveal their difficulties but clinicians may miss the opportunity to discuss them in their haste to 'console' the patient. Care must be taken to make these procedures as minimally traumatic as possible as the potential to impact on sexual functioning is marked. The potential of a diagnosis of human papillomavirus (HPV) to cause distress due to its STD nature, be it almost ubiquitous, must be recognized. Careful explanation of all aspects of colposcopy care and screening are paramount to circumvent adverse effects.

Menopause and Aging

There have been a number of studies exploring sexual activity and dysfunction in perimenopausal and aging women. Overall, there is a reduction in activity with age but this correlates with partner status—both those with partners and those whose partners have sexual problems. One study reported 32% of women over 60 years were active but 56% of married women.[11] There is some evidence that cessation of activity is more likely to be linked to the male partner. In Australian menopausal women aged, between 45 and 55 years, increased rates of FSD from 44 to 88% was seen from the early to late menopause.[12] Other works from this group seem to indicate that sexual responsivity is related to aging but libido, frequency of intercourse and dyspareunia are associated with estrogen deficiency. Simple measures can improve the physical sequelae of hormone deficiency and aging; such as topical estrogen, nonhormonal vaginal remoisturisers and lubricants in addition to consideration of surgery for those with symptomatic prolapse and stress incontinence. Correction of other health concerns should be complemented by a psychosexual approach.

Cancer

Aside from the physical effects of surgery, chemotherapy and radiation therapy, the impact of a cancer diagnosis on the patient is enormous. In addition, the role of partner as carer and provider of comfort may not sit well with the sexual partner. Understanding the individual feelings as experienced by the patient and their partner is key. One patient was worried that a hormone dependent cancer had recurred, as she perceived a high sex drive that she attributed to high hormone levels and increasing tumor size. Having made this connection herself she rapidly lost her libido, only to rediscover it once she had aired her anxieties.

Sexual Abuse

The possibility of sexual abuse or unwanted sexual experiences should be explored. The lifetime risk of sexual assault for women worldwide is 1 in 4 to 6 and (in the UK 1 in 20) with a worldwide risk for men of 1 in 10. Only one in 5 adult rapes are reported to the police with a much lower number being pursued through the legal system. In children, it is estimated at most 1 in 20 to 50 as yet is known to supervising authorities. Most presentation will be 'historical'. What constitutes sexual trauma will vary with individuals and is dependant on circumstances and support systems, such as the reaction of a family awareness of child sexual abuse, or within the context of physical abuse. In others, over exposure to nudity and sexuality in some may constitute abuse. Changes to the British Sexual Offences Act in 2003, responds to the changes in accessibility of children and vulnerable adults via the Internet, e.g. grooming and deems them prosecutable sexual offences and terms any penile penetration of vagina, anus or mouth as rape, rather than sexual assault.

Role of the Internet

The internet offers access to help, support and education in addition to misinformation and resources available in privacy. It provides an opportunity to find partners with its negative and positive consequences. But it has afforded easy access to hard core pornography and sexual alliances that may hinder relationships. The diversion of sexual energy may be a scapegoat for underlying difficulties.

CONCLUSION

Sexual function is a basic and important part of female well-being. Recognition of sexual problems as presented to the gynecologist is mandatory. All professionals involved in women's health should have basic training and some understanding of these issues. They should feel able to initiate consultations dealing with sexual difficulties and determine those who need referral and the ability to start first line interventions, including hormone therapy. Psychosexual medicine, as a branch of psychosomatic medicine pertaining to sexual problems, is a major part of the work of gynecologists and obstetricians.

REFERENCES

1. Declaration of Alma-Ata. International Conference of Primary Health Care, Alma-Ata, USSR, 1978. http://www.who.int/hpr/archive/docs/almaata.html
2. Masters WH, Johnson VE. Human sexual response. Boston: Little Brown, 1966.
3. Basson R, Berman J, Burnett A, Derogatis L, Ferguson D, Fourcroy J, et al. Report of the international consensus development conference on female sexual dysfunction: definitions and classifications. Urology. 2000; 163: 888-93.

4. Laumann E, Paik A, Rosen R. Sexual dysfunction in the United States: prevalence and predictors JAMA. 1999; 281: 537-44.
5. Writing Group for the Women's Health Initiative Investigators. Risks and benefits of estrogen plus progestin in healthy postmenopausal women. Principal results for the Women's Health Initiative Randomized controlled trial. JAMA. 2002;288: 321-33.
6. Nazareth I, Boynton P, King M. Problems with sexual function in people attending London general practitioners:cross sectional study. BMJ. 2003;327:423-6.
7. Rogers RG, Rockwood TH, Constantine ML, Thakar R, Kammerer-Doak DN, Pauls RN. A new measure of sexual function in women with pelvic floor disorders (PFD): the Pelvic Organ Prolapse/Incontinence Sexual Questionnaire, IUGA-Revised (PISQ-IR). Int Urogynecol J. 2013;24(7): 1091-103.
8. Rogers RG, Coates KW, Kammerer-Doak D, Khalsa S, Qualls C. A short form of the Pelvic Organ Prolapse/Urinary Incontinence Sexual Questionnaire (PISQ-12) Int Urogynecol J Pelvic Floor Dysfunct. 2003;14:164-8.
9. Rosen R, Brown C, Heiman J, Leiblum S, Meston C, Shabsigh R. The Female Sexual Function Index (FSFI): a multidimensional self-report instrument for the assessment of female sexual function. J Sex Marital Ther. 2000;26(2):191-208.
10. Glazener CM. Sexual function after childbirth: women's experiences, persistent morbidity and lack of professional recognition. Br J Obstet Gynaecol. 1997;104(3):330-5.
11. Diokno AC, Brown MB, Herzog AR. Sexual function in the elderly. Arch Intern Med. 1990;150:197-200.
12. Dennerstein L, Alexander JL, Kotz K. The menopause and sexual functioning: a review of the population-based studies. Annu Rev Sex Res. 2003;14:64-82.

CHAPTER 18

Pelvic Organ Prolapse

Pralhad Kushtagi

Overview

- Prolapse is commonly classified on the basis of anatomical structure that is protruded or prolapsed; namely, uterine prolapse, cystocele (for bladder descent), urethrocele (for descent of urethra), enterocele (for small bowel), rectocele (for protrusion of rectum), etc.
- All pelvic prolapse conditions and urethral hypermobility result from pelvic floor relaxation.
- The type of prolapse caused due to damage level I supports with be different from that caused due to damage of level II supports. Defects in the support provided by level II vaginal supports (pubocervical and rectovaginal fasciae) result in cystocele and rectocele, and loss of the upper suspensory fibers of the paracolpium and parametrium (level I) is responsible for the development of vaginal vault and uterine prolapse.
- Since pelvic support defects are frequently associated with specific alteration in bowel or bladder, or sexual function, both the evaluation and management of poor support and abnormal visceral function are important in developing a treatment plan and assessing therapeutic outcome.
- The modalities of treatment include follow-up, surgical repair, or use of a vaginal pessary. Prolapse has been treated by surgery, the nature of which depends on degree and type of prolapse, patient's general health status and the need for preservation of menstrual, reproductive or coital function. The goal of surgery should be to relieve the patient of her symptoms by repairing each aspect of abnormal pelvic support in a durable and long-lasting manner.
- Pelvic organ prolapse is not due to single etiology. Normal support of the pelvic organs depends on a combination of fascial and muscular support. The specific type of prolapse that exists in an individual corresponds with specific defects in the anatomic structures responsible for normal support. Hence, surgical management needs to be individualized.

DEFINITION AND INCIDENCE

A prolapse is a downward or forward displacement of one of the pelvic organs from its normal location. Traditionally, prolapse is referred to displacement of the bladder, the uterus, or the rectum. It will be author's endeavor to address the problem of pelvic organ prolapse excluding true rectal prolapse, in this chapter.

Of the common gynecological complaints one comes across in clinical practice, the problems related to pelvic support disorders are common. The true incidence of pelvic organ prolapse is unknown as many women with clinically severe prolapse are largely asymptomatic, and many with mild degrees of prolapse may have severe pelvic floor symptoms. The development of effective operations to alleviate pelvic organ prolapse (to be specific, the uterus and vaginal prolapse) was one of the key factors that led to the establishment of gynecologic surgery as a separate specialty.[1]

CLASSIFICATION

Pelvic organ prolapse can be classified etiologically into: (1) congenital (neonatal)—which is a rare event found at birth in some neonates and disappears soon, unless it is associated with spinal cord defects; (2) acquired—(a) can be caused by childbirth or any kind of injury; and (b) nulliparous—where childbirth injury to the supports is not the cause.[2]

Prolapse is commonly classified on the basis of anatomical site and structure that is protruded or prolapsed, namely, (1) anterior vaginal wall with descent of bladder (cystocele) and/or urethra (urethrocele); (2) central or the descent of cuff with uterus (uterine descent or prolapse) or vault in patients with hysterectomy (vault prolapse); (3) posterior vaginal wall with protrusion of small bowel (enterocele) and/or rectum (rectocele).

These descriptive terms have been in use since time immemorial, but they tend to prejudge the true nature of

SECTION 1 General Gynecology

Table 18.1: Classification of pelvic (genital) organ prolapse.

	Etiological classification	

	1. Congenital
	2. Acquired
	    a. due to child birth injuries
	    b. not due to child birth injuries	

Anatomical classification	**Structure**	**Type of prolapse**
1. Anterior vaginal wall	Posterior aspect of bladder urethra	Cystocele Urethrocele
2. Central or cuff	Uterus Vaginal vault	Uterine prolapse Vault prolapse
3. Posterior vaginal wall	Small bowel Anterior rectal wall	Enterocele Rectocele

Table 18.2: Shaw's degrees of uterine descent[1].

Degrees	Descriptions
1°	Cervix below ischial spines
2°	Cervix up to the introitus
3°	Cervix outside introitus*
4° (Procidentia)	All of the uterus outside the introitus*

*Some workers combine 4° with 3° prolapse

Table 18.3: Baden–Walker Halfway system for grading each site of pelvic relaxation.

Grade 0: Normal position for each respective site
Grade 1: Descent halfway to the hymen
Grade 2: Descent to the hymen
Grade 3: Descent halfway past the hymen
Grade 4: Maximum possible descent for each site

Notes for using the grading system:
1. Prolapse is graded at each site (cystocele, uterine prolapse, vault prolapse, rectocele, enterocele) with patient straining maximally. The upright position may also be used.
2. When choosing between 2 grades, choose the higher grade.

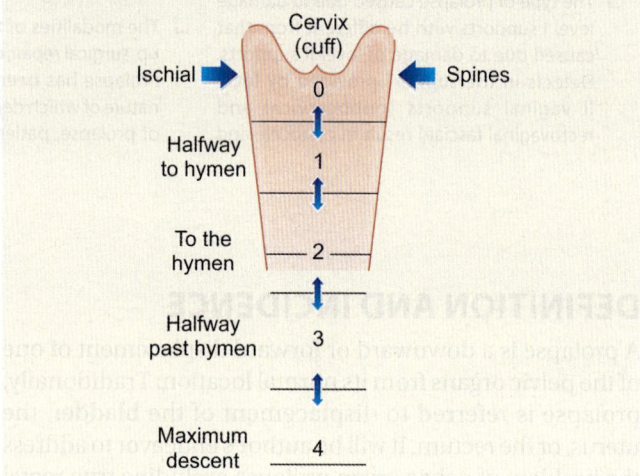

Source: Baden and Walker.[2]

any prolapse by focusing attention on bladder, rectum, or uterus rather than on the specific defects that are responsible for alteration in vaginal support (Table 18.1).

Normally, the cervix or vaginal cuff is supported at or above the level of ischial spines. Pelvic organ prolapse, particularly the prolapse of uterus is usually graded on a scale of 0–4, the grade increasing with increasing severity of prolapse, with 0 referring to no prolapse and 4 referring to descent of uterus with its fundus outside the level of (procidentia) introitus (Table 18.2).

Since introitus is an ill-defined and imprecise term, hymen is preferred as landmark to evaluate prolapse, even though plane of hymen is somewhat variable depending on the degree of levator ani dysfunction.[3] In the latter system of evaluation, consideration is given to anterior and posterior vaginal wall descents (Table 18.3 and Fig. 18.1). It consists of four grades: Grade 0—no prolapse, grade 1—halfway to hymen, grade 2—to hymen, grade 3—halfway past hymen, grade 4 –maximum descent.

However, International Continence Society has adopted a site-specific descriptive system, pelvic organ prolapse quantification (POPQ) system, that takes hymen as a fixed point of reference and measurements are taken from that point on the anterior and posterior vaginal walls and to the vaginal apex. In addition, the genital hiatus, width of perineal body and total vaginal length are measured and recorded on a grid form (Fig. 18.1).[3] This system is complex. It ensures uniform, reliable, and site specific descriptions of pelvic organ prolapse, provides a standardized measurement system to allow for more accurate assessments of postoperative outcome.

ETIOLOGY

The etiology of pelvic floor disorders is more likely to be multifactorial. All pelvic prolapse conditions and urethral hypermobility result from pelvic floor relaxation.

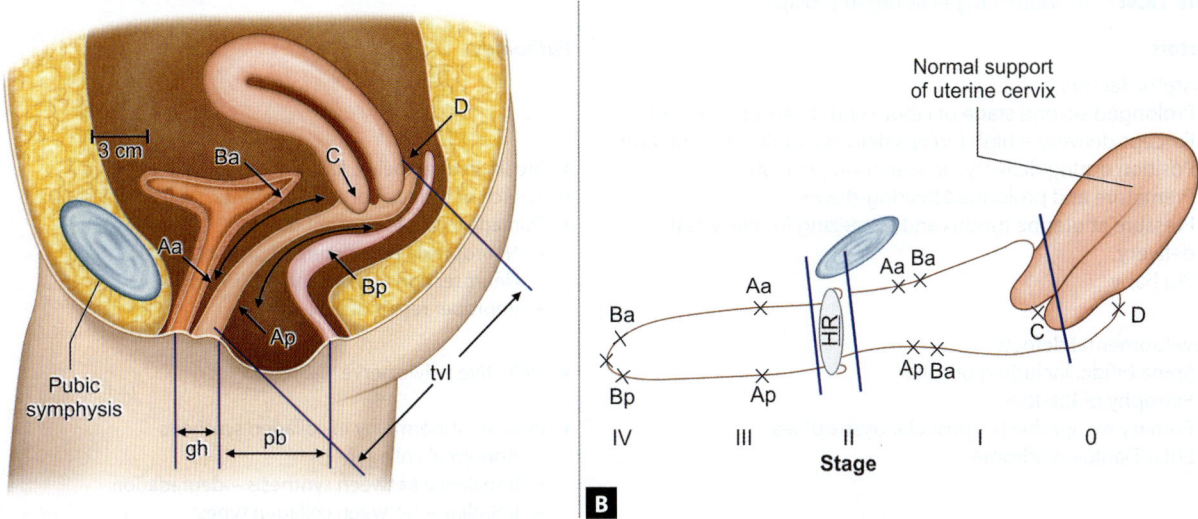

Figs. 18.1A and B: Pelvic organ prolapse quantification system (A) Points and measurements: Six sites (Aa, Ba, C, D, Bp and Ap), genital hiatus (gh), perineal body (pb), and total vaginal length (tvl) used for pelvic organ support quantification. (b) POPQ ordinal staging system: The maximal descent observed for each of the three compartments (anterior, apical, and posterior) is graded with reference to the hymenal remnant (HR). Stage 1 occurs when the leading edge of that segment is more than 1 cm above the HR; stage 2 when the leading edge is within 1 cm (above or below) of HR; stage 3 when the leading edge is more than 1 cm below the HR; and stage 4 when there is essentially complete eversion of that compartment.
(*Source:* Bump RC, Mattiasson A, Bo K, Brubaker LP, DeLancey JO, Klarskov P, etal. The standardization of terminology of female pelvic organ prolapse and pelvic floor dysfunction. Am J Obstet Gynecol. 1996; 175:10-17)

The etiopathology is often attributed to childbirth injury. Prolonged labor and high forceps delivery, particularly if prolonged traction is required, have always been reasonably blamed as etiological factors in the development of genital prolapse. Considerable stresses imposed on the pelvic floor if delivery is conducted in 'squatting' position might increase the risk of subsequent prolapse.[4] 'Bearing down' before full cervical dilatation puts a tremendous strain on the uterine supports and contributes to an increased risk of prolapse. Fundal pressure used to be a recommended method of placental delivery, but it could lead to gross stretching of the uterine ligaments and has now been abandoned in favor of patience, maternal effort and judicious controlled cord traction. Neuromuscular damage to the pelvic floor is associated with development of pelvic organ prolapse.[5] The function of the levator ani muscle can be compromised in two ways: First, there can be direct injury to the muscle resulting in mechanical destruction to the entire muscle. Second, damage to the nerve supply of the muscles could lead to their inability to contract, even though they themselves remain intact. The direct nerve supply from the sacral plexus to the levator ani is placed under great stretch during parturition resulting in transient neuropraxia and repeated childbirth could further injure such patients and ultimately produce symptoms of prolapse and incontinence as the muscular supports are progressively damaged. A prolonged second stage and high fetal weight seem to cause most neural damage.[6]

However, previous pregnancy is not a required precondition for prolapse, because it can occur in nulliparous women, especially when the cervix is congenitally elongated. Women with congenital defects like overt sacral abnormalities such as spina bifida, or those with defects of pelvic floor muscles as in exstrophy of the bladder or those with primary myopathies, such as muscular dystrophy, have a striking propensity to develop uterine prolapse, often before pregnancy and at remarkably early age. Syndromes such as Ehler-Danlos syndrome characterized by fascial and connective tissue weakness have significantly higher prevalence of genital prolapse.

An underlying abnormality of connective tissue in pelvic floor ligaments and fascia is also believed to be the cause of pelvic support disorders. This may be due to an intrinsic abnormality of collagen synthesis (e.g. abnormal collagen, imbalance between synthesis and degradation, imbalance between collagen types) that leads to pelvic support disorders regardless of outside stressors. A second mechanism might be mildly abnormal fascia and ligaments that can withstand normal pressures, but with excessive strain (e.g. high parity, chronic straining, or loss of pelvic floor contraction) develop genitourinary prolapse. In these individuals, the abnormality might be errors in repair of damaged ligaments and fascia, or lack of remodeling in mature collagen.[7]

The tendency to prolapse is more likely to manifest itself after the menopause, when the ovarian steroidogenesis

Table 18.4: Contributors to pelvic organ prolapse.

Factors	Pathology

Obstetric factors
• Prolonged second stage of labor - with bearing-down efforts
• Forceps delivery—high forceps delivery, prolonged traction
• Position during delivery - in squatting position
• Premature and prolonged bearing-down
• Pressure at uterine fundus and squeezing for placental delivery
• Big baby
	• Breaks in deep pelvic fascia
	• Stretch of the supporting ligaments
	• Damage to the levator ani due to:
	  – Neuropraxia by pressure of presenting part
	  – Neurosection at tears and episiotomy
	  – Improper repair of tear

Developmental defects
• Spina bifida, including occulta
• Extrophy of bladder
• Primary myopathies—muscular dystrophies
• Ehler Danlos syndrome
	• Defective pelvic nerve
	• Intrinsic abnormality in collagen synthesis
	  – Abnormal collagen
	  – Imbalance between synthesis—degradation
	  – Imbalance between collagen types

Precipitators • High parity—frequent childbirths • Chronic cough • Chronic constipation • Menopause	• Repeated damage and less recovery time • Increased abdominal pressure • Decreased estrogen support and muscle mass
Prior hysterectomy	• Inadequate suspension of vault after surgery • Insufficient obliteration of rectouterine *cul-de-sac*

ceases. Although, inherent tissue weakness and childbearing are among the most common causes of vaginal prolapse conditions, an additional cause is a prior hysterectomy. If the vaginal vault is not sufficiently resuspended and the cul-de-sac is not obliterated, vault prolapse and/or enterocele are common sequelae.

The greatest forces that affect the pelvic floor come from increases in abdominal pressure and the weight of the abdominal organs in a woman with some weakness induced by child birth trauma or inherent connective tissue weakness or aging and menopausal hypoestrogenism. Chronic intra-abdominal pressure from pulmonary disease or work involving lifting heavy weights, chronic straining during bowel movements, ovarian tumor, ascites, and fibroid uterus contribute to aggravation of the prolapse condition (Table 18.4).

ANATOMY OF THE PELVIC FLOOR

Understanding of the anatomy of structural components that support uterus and pelvic floor is essential to understand the problems of the pelvic floor and in planning surgical correction.

The top layer of the pelvic floor is created by the endopelvic fascia, which attaches the pelvic organs especially the vagina and uterus to the pelvic walls, thereby suspending the pelvic organs. Support of the pelvic organs is provided by a group of muscles referred to as the levator ani.

Viscero-fascial Layer

The fascial layer of the pelvic floor is a combination of the pelvic viscera and endopelvic fascia. Hence, it is referred to as viscero-fascial layer. On each side of the pelvis, the endopelvic fascia attaches the uterus and vagina to the pelvic wall. It forms a continuous sheet-like mesentery. It runs continuously from uterine artery at its cephalic margin to the point at which the vagina fuses with the levator ani muscle below. The part that attaches to the uterus is called the parametrium, and that which attaches to the vagina, the paracolpium.

The parametria are made up of the cardinal (transverse cervical) and uterosacral ligaments, which are two different parts of a single mass of tissue. Opposite the external cervical os, the sheet of tissue that attaches the genital tract to the pelvic wall arbitrarily changes name from the parametrium to the paracolpium. These supportive tissues contain prominent blood vessels, nerves, and fibrous connective tissue. Paracolpium can be considered as mesenteries that supply the genital tract bilaterally. The paracolpium attaches to the upper two-thirds of vagina.

DeLancey divided this vaginal support into three levels (Fig. 18.2).[8]

- **Level I:** It is the proximal vaginal support. It consists of the cardinal and uterosacral ligaments attachment to the cervix and upper vagina. Damage to level I support results in uterovaginal prolapse, posthysterectomy vaginal prolapse, and enterocele. The primary

CHAPTER 18 Pelvic Organ Prolapse

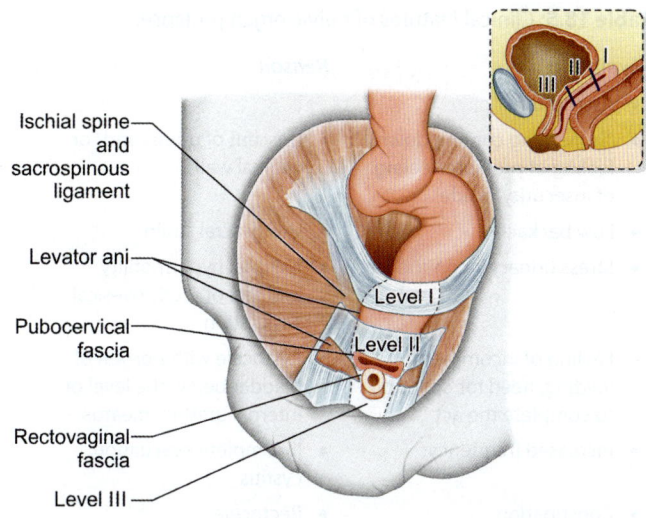

Fig. 18.2: DeLancey's levels of vaginal support.
(*Source:* DeLancey JOL. Anatomy and biomechanics of genital prolapse. Clin Obstet Gynecol. 1993; 36: 897-909.)

load-bearing elements are the uterosacral ligaments and, to a lesser extent, the cardinal ligaments. It may be noted that prolapse occurs only after 85% of the integrity of the paracolpium is severed.

- **Level II**: It is a midvaginal support. It is due to lateral attachment of the fascia to the pelvic sidewalls. This portion attaches laterally to the arcus tendineus fascia pelvis, the arcus tendineus fasciae rectovaginalis and also to the medial border of levator ani muscles. This attachment stretches the vagina transversely between the bladder and rectum and has functional significance. Damage at this level results in paravaginal and pararectal defects. The structural layer that supports the bladder (pubocervical fascia) is composed of anterior vaginal wall and its attachment through the endopelvic fascia to the pelvic wall. The suburethral endopelvic fascia is better developed than that in the area of bladder. It therefore is designed to provide better support for the vesical neck. Loss of this normal support at the vesical neck is one of the factors responsible for stress urinary incontinence.
- **Level III**: The constituents are perineal body, superficial and deep perineal muscles, and fibromuscular connective tissue. In distal vagina, the vaginal wall is directly attached to surrounding structures without any intervening paracolpium. The support is attributed to fusion to the urogenital diaphragm anteriorly and to the proximal perineum posteriorly. Damage at these sites results in urinary incontinence anteriorly and in perineal body deficits posteriorly. Cystocele and rectocele are central defects in the pubocervical and rectovaginal septum.

Levator Ani Muscles

The levator ani consists of two portions: the pubovisceral muscle and the iliococcygeus muscle.[9,10] The pubovisceral muscle is a thick U-shaped muscle whose ends arise from the pubic bones on either side of the midline and passes behind the rectum, forming a sling-like arrangement. It has several components. The pubococcygeus is the most cephalic portion of the levator ani and passes from the pubic bones to insert on the inner surface of the coccyx. This portion does not contribute substantially to supporting the pelvic organs. The puborectalis portion of the pubovisceralis passes beside the vagina, and lateral vaginal walls are attached to it. The muscle then continues dorsally where some fibers penetrate the rectum between internal and external sphincter, while others pass behind the anorectal junction. Laterally, the iliococcygeus arises from the fibrous band on the pelvic wall (arcus tendineus levator ani) and forms a relatively horizontal sheet that spans the opening within the pelvis and forms a shelf on which the organs may rest.

The opening in the levator ani muscle, through which urethra and vagina pass is the urogenital hiatus. The normal baseline activity of the levator ani muscle keeps the hiatus closed and thereby the lumen of vagina, urethra and rectum. This eliminates any opening in the pelvic floor through which prolapse could occur and forms a shelf on which the pelvic organs are supported.

The interaction between the pelvic floor muscles and the supportive ligaments is critical to support of pelvic organs. As long as the levator ani muscles function normally, the pelvic floor is closed and the ligaments and fascia are under no tension. The fasciae stabilize the organs in their position above the levator ani muscles. When the pelvic floor muscles relax or are damaged, the pelvic floor opens and the vagina lies between the high abdominal pressure and low atmospheric pressure. Although the ligaments can sustain the organs in place for short periods of time, if the pelvic floor muscles do not close the urogenital hiatus, then the connective tissue will become damaged and eventually fail to hold the vagina in place. This situation is likened to a ship in its berth, floating on the water attached by rope on either side to a dock—where the water supports ship's weight and the moorings simply keep the ship from straying away.[11]

SECONDARY ANATOMICAL CHANGES

Uterus gets retroverted before prolapsing through the vagina. The prolapse leads to further kinking of its blood supply especially the venous drainage and results in congestion. The chronic congestion of the cervix will be responsible for the bulky cervices seen in menopausal women with prolapse.

Box 18.1: Prolapse uterus: Secondary changes.

- Retroversion
- Hypertrophied cervix
- Decubitus ulcer
- Keratinization of vaginal skin
- Elongation of supravaginal cervix
- Obstructive uropathy—hydroureter, hydronephrosis

The venous congestion over a period of time leads to decreased oxygenated blood in the most dependent portions of the cervix. Decubitus ulceration is the result of such tissue hypoxia. It is a trophic ulceration and heals on reposition of the uterus into the vagina, which restores venous drainage and improves availability of oxygenated blood.

In a patient with prolapse the vaginal skin shows areas of keratinization and pigmentation due to exposure and friction. It also loses rugosities from stretching.

As is already indicated, childbirth injury usually affects integrity of pelvic floor. In such patients, traction from below by the weight of the uterus on damaged levator ani and paracolpos, while the strain imposed by pull of parametrium (cardinal and uterosacral ligaments) to keep the cervix and uterus in position, result in stretching and elongation of softened, congested supravaginal portion of cervix.

Anterior vaginal wall prolapse and the resultant descent of posterior bladder wall near trigone cause stretching of the ureteric openings. It may also result in cystoureteric reflux of urine. The effect of these is hydroureter and hydronephrosis in a case of long-standing prolapse of severe degree (Box 18.1).

SYMPTOMS

It is a common clinical experience that the degree of prolapse bears little relationship to the presenting symptoms; someone with a severe prolapse, say procidentia, may have few symptoms, whereas others with a small anterior wall descent may complain vociferously.

Symptomatic prolapse may manifest in several different ways (Table 18.5). Majority of the patients referred to hospital with genital prolapse complain of 'something coming down'. There may be only a feeling of pressure or insecurity 'inside'.

Low backache may be one of the symptoms due to strain on the periosteal attachment of uterosacral ligaments caused by downward pull of uterine descent. The patient fails to pin point the site of pain. It is felt more at the end of days' work and is relieved after taking rest lying down.

Table 18.5: Clinical features of pelvic organ prolapse.

Symptom	Reason
• Asymptomatic	
• 'Something coming down'/ feeling of pressure/feeling of insecurity 'inside'	• Descent of uterus and/ or vaginal walls
• Low backache	• Uterosacral strain
• Stress urinary incontinence	• Urethral hypermotility and loss of urethrovesical angulation
• Feeling of incomplete voiding; need for 'splinting' to complete the act	• Cystocele with portion of bladder below the level of internal urethral meatus
• Increased frequency	• Incomplete evacuation; cystitis
• Constipation	• Rectocele
• Dyspareunia	• Protruding prolapsed tissues in vagina; dry vagina
• Dissatisfaction at sex	• Lax vagina
• Vaginal discharge	• Cervix congestion
• Vaginal bleeding/ blood stained vaginal discharge	• Decubitus ulceration

Anterior vaginal wall prolapse leads to urethral hypermobility, loss of urethrovesical angulation and direct transmission of increased abdominal pressure to urethra through bladder, which in turn often (but not necessarily) results in stress urinary incontinence. A larger prolapse, prolapsing posterior bladder wall through anterior vaginal wall coming out below the urethra, can produce symptoms of voiding difficulty. Such patients may have feeling of incomplete voiding and require digital pressure on the prolapsed vaginal wall for completion of the act. They may also have frequency and urgency of micturition due to cystitis.

Protrusion of the posterior vaginal wall by rectum can cause symptoms of inefficient rectal emptying, often described by the patient as constipation, necessitating splinting of the posterior vagina to reduce the pocket of trapped stool.

A sexually active woman may complain of dyspareunia or obstruction to the penetration because of tissues protruding outside the introitus. Lax vagina and introitus could be the reason for decreasing sexual pleasure or there may be diminished frequency of sexual intercourse because of anxiety on the part of her partner.

Congested and hypertrophied cervix by itself or the secondary infection may be the cause for discharge per vagina. The patient with decubitus ulcer on cervix will present with blood stained discharge.

CLINICAL EVALUATION[12]

Since, pelvic support defects are frequently associated with specific alteration in bowel or bladder, or sexual function, both the evaluation and management of poor support and abnormal visceral function are important in developing a treatment plan and assessing therapeutic outcome.

There are no universally agreed-upon definitions either for normal pelvic support or for pelvic support defects.

The patient is examined in the dorsal lithotomy position with moderate amount of urine in the bladder to help evaluate stress incontinence. Pelvic support is assessed when the patient is straining maximally as each individual site is identified. Envision an imaginary line, the midvaginal axis extending from the mid-portion of the hymen to the hollow of the sacrum. During maximal strain in women with normal support, the urethra, bladder, cul-de-sac, and rectum will not cross the midvaginal axis. Support defects may occur at any or all of these sites.

Using any of the classification of grading the prolapse or pelvic organ descent (see Classification above), the urethra, bladder, cervix or vaginal cuff, cul-de-sac, and rectum are described as grade 0 to 4. If the patient is not straining effectively, the prolapse may not be apparent. If one is unable to make prolapse protrude when patient is in lithotomy position, repeat examination may be necessitated while she is standing and straining.

Urethra

Urethral support defects are generally associated with paraurethral loss of support. When the patient having urethral hypermobility strains, the urethra rotates posteriorly, and its junction with the bladder straightens. The meatus rotates anteriorly. The paraurethral support defect can be confirmed by using an open ring forceps (sponge holding forceps) in a position lateral to the urethra to provide support paraurethrally as the patient bears down. As lateral support is applied, one should look to see if there is any correction in the rotational descent. The cotton swab stick (Q-tip; Fig. 18.2) test objectively quantifies the degree of mobility. When an individual is straining, the urethra usually does not rotate more than 30° from the horizontal plane, but some continent multiparas may have loss of urethral support with no stress incontinence.

Bladder

Support defects involving the anterior vaginal wall may occur in the midline, laterally or paravaginally, superiorly, or in any combination of these sites. Defects can be identified clinically by evaluating each individual area.

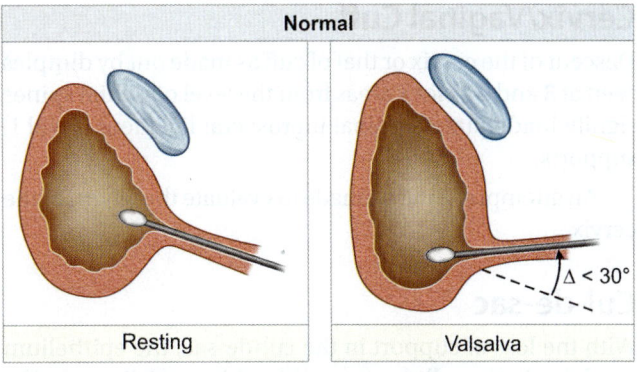

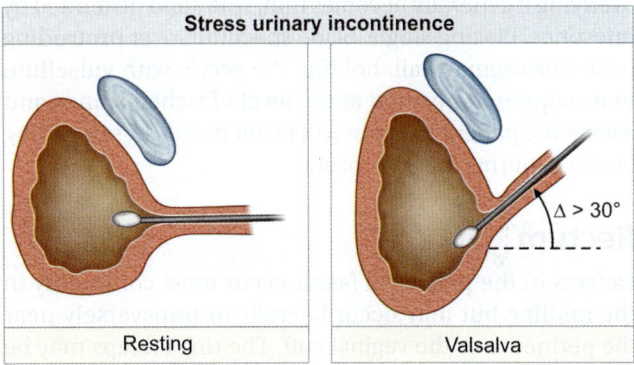

Fig. 18.2: Diagrammatic presentation of Q-tip test showing mobility of urethrovesical angle in continent and the patient with stress urinary incontinence.

Anterior vaginal wall is retracted using the ring (sponge holding) forceps and is directed along the anterior vaginal wall towards ischial spines and the forceps is opened such that the ring ends point towards the lateral vaginal walls. This makes the lateral aspects of the anterior vagina and pubocervical fascia to return to their normal point of attachment along the arcus tendineus fasciae pelvis. The patient is asked to strain maximally; if there are no evidences of anterior defects, she has lateral or paravaginal loss of support. If, when she strains, there is some improvement in anterior support, but she continues to have a midline bulge through the open arms of the forceps, she also has a midline defect in pubocervical fascia. The forceps may be closed, turned sideways and used to support the base of the bladder centrally. When the patient strains and if she has no midline descent, the support defect is central or midline.

Superior loss of support is characterized by several clinical clues. When the patient strains, if the anterior vaginal epithelium appears thin and, with loss of rugae from the vaginal cuff along the base of the bladder, and the anterior vaginal wall is longer than the posterior vagina, the patient is likely to have superior loss of support of her pubocervical fascia. Superior defects are usually associated with midline defects.

Cervix/Vaginal Cuff

Descent of the cervix or that of cuff as made out by dimples seen at 3 and 9 o'clock areas from the level of ischial spines signify inadequate cardinal uterosacral ligament (level I) supports.

An attempt should be made to evaluate the length of the cervix.

Cul-de-sac

With the loss of support in the cul-de-sac, the epithelium overlying it generally becomes thin, shiny and distended by intestines. Placing single-blade speculum over protruding posterior vaginal wall, holding the cervix with vulsellum in its supposed position at the level of ischial spines and asking the patient to strain will result in cul-de-sac gliding over it confirms the enterocele.

Rectum

Defects in the perirectal fascia occur most commonly in the midline but may occur laterally or transversely near the perineum or the vaginal cuff. The ring forceps may be placed posteriorly and laterally in an effort to reduce the posterior defect. If there continues to be a bulge between the open arms of the forceps, the defect is midline. The forceps may be closed and used to support the midline. The defect is considered to be present laterally, if there is bulge on the sides of the forceps when the patient strains.

Perineum

The distance between the anal orifice and posterior fourchette should be noted. With a finger in the rectum and the thumb pressing against the perineum, the thickness of the perineum can be felt.

Loss of support at cul-de-sac and at perineal body is best identified intraoperatively. A full general and abdominal examination is necessary. It is necessary to exclude chronic chest problems, gross obesity and abdominal masses. Bimanual vaginoabdominal palpation should always be carried out to exclude pelvic masses such as ovarian cysts or fibroids.

DIFFERENTIAL DIAGNOSIS

Diagnosis of prolapse should not pose a problem, but the correct identification of site-specific defect in the pelvic floor will do.

Descent of anterior vaginal wall along with portions of bladder or hypermobile urethra may at times have to be differentiated from vulval cyst/tumor, Gartner's duct cyst, or urethral diverticuli.

Table 18.6: Differential diagnosis of vaginal mass pelvic organ prolapse.

• Anterior vaginal wall	– Vulvar cyst/tumor – Gartner's duct cyst – Urethral diverticuli
• Central mass at vault	– Congenital elongation of cervix – Cervical/fibroid polyp – Chronic inversion of uterus – Rectal prolapse

Congenital elongation of cervix, cervical/fibroid polyp, or chronic inversion of uterus will be the conditions to be considered while diagnosing uterine descent or vault prolapse.

Rarely, the patient complains of vaginal prolapse, but in fact, she will be suffering from true rectal prolapse (Table 18.6).

TREATMENT OF PELVIC ORGAN PROLAPSE

The modalities of treatment include follow-up, surgical repair, or use of a vaginal pessary.

Expectant Management

Prolapse may be discovered during a routine gynecological examination. Such patient may or may not have symptoms due to pelvic support defect. One should keep in mind the axiom of medicine that "the asymptomatic patient cannot be made to feel better by medical or surgical therapy". The patient should be informed of the physical examination finding and the problems that could make her relaxation worse over time. The importance of buttock squeezing exercises in improving perineal muscle tone should be emphasized,[4] and in some vaginal cones of increasing weight[13] are prescribed for use in vagina for the same purpose. Pelvic floor muscle strengthening exercises as referred as Kegel exercises entail voluntary contraction of the levator ani muscle as if one is holding back the urine midstream and should be performed several times during the day. Efficacy of these exercises can be increased by placing weighted cones in the vagina. Advantage of this advice is that woman learns to consciously contract muscles before and during increases in abdominal pressure and regular muscle strength training may help to build the muscle volume. It is to be remembered that pelvic muscle exercises are virtually never harmful, but they are not likely to correct the problem if there is neuromuscular damage as the underlying pathology. In postmenopausal women use of estrogens as replacement therapy may help strengthen the supports and alleviate trivial symptoms. Periodic examinations while on follow-up will provide comparisons regarding the status of pelvic support defect, changes in patient's physical condition or symptoms.

Surgical Management

Traditionally, prolapse has been treated by surgery, the nature of which depends on degree and type of prolapse, patient's general health status and the need for preservation of menstrual, reproductive or coital function. The goal of surgery should be to relieve the patient of her symptoms by repairing each aspect of abnormal pelvic support in a durable and long-lasting manner. Many different surgeries are used to repair prolapse and pelvic support defects (Table 18.7). There is lack of evidence base for many treatments for genital prolapse. Most reports are observational and outcome measures employed are subjective and clinician based with absence of well-documented clinical trials. A detailed description of the various operations for managing pelvic support defects is beyond the scope of this chapter; however, a few general remarks are in order.

Before undertaking surgery attention should be given to treatment of decubitus ulcer if present. The reduction of the prolapse into the vagina and to keep it reduced will be the mainstay of its management. Repositioning helps to improve the venous drainage, arterial blood supply and relief from the congestion. Use of lubricated tampon with povidone iodine and glycerine will hasten this process by adsorbing the edema fluid from congested cervix. Such daily repositioning-dressing will initiate epithelialization and healing of the ulcer in a week's time. If no signs of healing are seen over a week's time, it is a good practice to take a wedge biopsy to rule out carcinoma.

Removal of the uterus is not the surgery for prolapse. The corrective surgery for prolapse is the repair of support tissues of uterus and vagina. The surgical approach for each patient needs to be tailored to the specific symptoms, objective physical findings, and tests of visceral function. Most patients with prolapse have defects in more than one location, so attention should be paid to correcting all defects during the same operation. Hence, several procedures are combined. Operations for prolapse are generally, but not always, carried out through the vaginal rather than

Table 18.7: Common surgical procedures for the treatment of pelvic organ prolapse.

Clinical condition	Surgical procedures
Cystocele	• Cystocele repair (Figs. 18.4A to D) • Anterior colporrhaphy • Paravaginal repair
Urethrocele	• Urethroplasty (urethral plication)
Uterine prolapse	• Hysterectomy with suspension of vagina with ligaments (transverse cervical/uterosacral) (Figs. 18.4 and 18.5) • Amputation of ectocervix and plication of transverse cervical ligament • Colpocleisis
Vaginal vault prolapse	• Uterosacral/sacrospinous fixation • Abdominal sacral colpopexy • Colpocleisis
Enterocele	• Vaginal enterocele repair • McCall culdoplasty • Abdominal enterocele repair (Halban/ Moschcowitz procedures)
Rectocele	• Posterior colporrhaphy (Fig.18.5C) • Rectovaginal fascia defect repair
Deficient perineum	• Perineorrhaphy

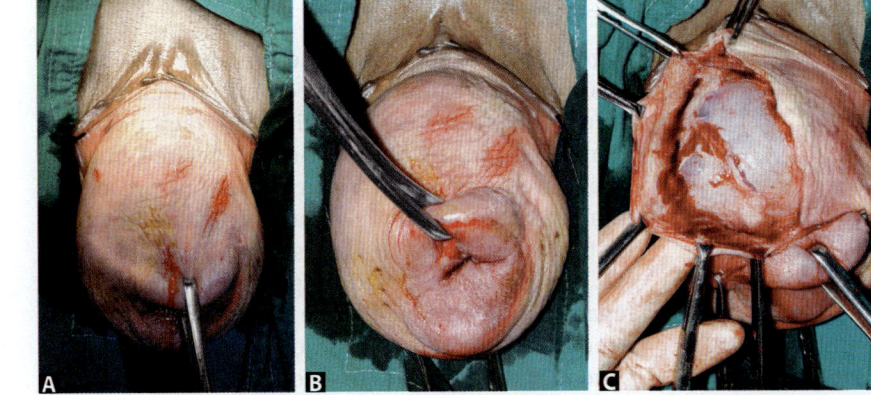
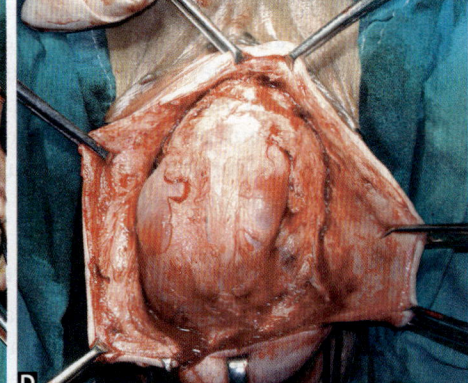

Figs. 18.4A to D: (A) Genital prolapse with cystocele; (B) Cervix held; (C) Incision over the vaginal epithelium overlying the cystocele; (D) Dissection of the underlying fascia until the defect in pubocervical fascia is visualized.

SECTION 1 General Gynecology

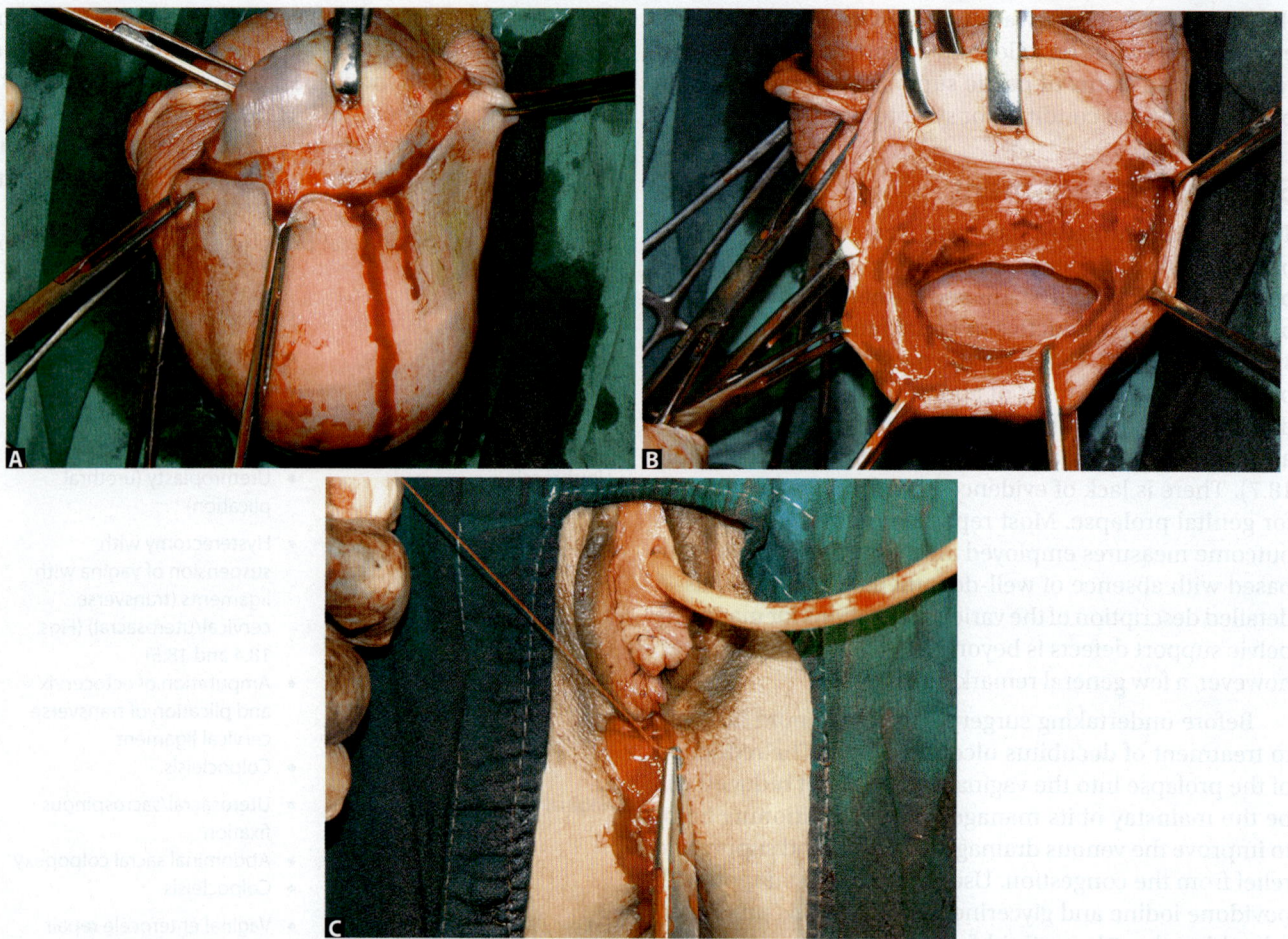

Figs. 18.5A to C: (A) Rectocele seen posteriorly and the vaginal epithelium overlying it is incised; (B) Opening the pouch of Douglas; (C) Perineorrhaphy—subcutaneous approximation in progress.

through the abdominal route. Some conditions, such as stress urinary incontinence, are most reliably handled by an abdominal operation.

The generation next vaginal prolapse repairs are mesh or graft augmented repairs. They allow pelvic organ prolapse to be repaired in a minimally invasive manner with a short procedure time and rapid postoperative recovery. For the repair of anterior vaginal wall prolapse, mesh with two fixing arms (Perigee) will be used and transobturator approach is followed. For the treatment of posterior vaginal wall prolapse and vault prolapse, tension free mesh or graft augmentation with four arms (Apogee) is used through the posterior vaginal and perineal approach.

Repair of Anterior Vaginal Wall Defects

Patients with a central defect are best treated by anterior colporrhaphy, which reapproximates the pubocervical fascia in the midline under the bladder neck. Lateral defects require a different approach in which the vaginal attachments to the pelvic sidewall are reconstituted. These defects are commonly corrected either with a paravaginal repair via the abdominal or vaginal approach where endopelvic fascia is reattached to the arcus tendineus fasciae pelvis,[14] or with a 4-corner bladder neck suspension.[15]

Operations for Uterovaginal Prolapse (Table 18.8)

- *Vaginal hysterectomy:* Uterine prolapse is generally treated with vaginal hysterectomy, which may be accomplished by several different techniques. It is preferred in a woman who has desired number of children and is not particular about preserving menstrual function. The advantage of vaginal hysterectomy is that it allows other vaginal surgery (viz. anterior and posterior colporrhaphy or enterocele repair) to be performed at the same time, without the need for a separate incision or for repositioning the patient. At the time of hysterectomy for prolapse, special attention should be paid to closing the cul-de-sac using a McCall culdoplasty and to reattaching the endopelvic

Table 18.8: Choice of surgery for uterovaginal prolapse according to patient characteristics and requirements.

Surgery → ↓ Variables	Ward Mayo (PFR + Vaginal) hysterectomy	Manchester (Fothergill) repair	Modified Manchester (Shirodkar) repair	Utero-cervicopexy	Sling procedures	Lefort colpocleisis
Menstrual function	NR	R	R	R	R	NR
Reproductive function	NR	±	R	R	R	NR
Sexual function	±	R	R	R	R	NR
Age (years)	any; >40	<40	<40	30-40	< 20-30	>70
Comorbidity						++

(R: Required; NR: Not required; ±: irrespective of the variable; ++: Present and significant; PFR: pelvic floor repair)

fascia and the uterosacral ligaments to the vaginal cuff to provide additional support.[16]

- *Manchester/Fothergill repair:* An alternative to hysterectomy for patients with uterine prolapse who wish to retain the uterus is the Manchester operation. In this operation, the bladder is dissected off the cervix and cervix is amputated. The cardinal ligaments are sewn to the anterior of cervical stump. Anterior colporrhaphy and colpoperineorrhaphy form the essential components of the repair. If desired, vaginal tubectomy can be done along with.
- *Shirodkar's modification of Manchester repair:* In a patient desirous of retaining childbearing function where amputation of cervix could compromise fertility, Shirodkar's modified Manchester repair may be a better option. In this operation, uterosacral ligaments are divided close to their attachment to cervix; the stumps are brought in front of the cervix, crossed and stitched to the cervix. High closure of the peritoneum of the pouch of Douglas is carried out. The cervix is not amputated. As in Manchester repair, anterior colporrhaphy and posterior colpoperineorrhaphy remain the other essential steps.
- *Utero/cevicopexy and sling operations:* Occasionally, marked uterine prolapse may develop in a young nulliparous patient due to inherent weakness of suspensory supports. The basic principle behind these operations is to fortify the supporting ligamentary structures. Abdominal round ligament (Gilliam) uterine suspension with uterosacral plication and culdoplasty may be helpful.[17] There have been efforts to use ribbons of rectus sheath brought out retroperitoneally between leaves of broad ligaments to be attached to isthmus of uterus. As a modification, some surgeons have used mersilene/nylon tapes instead, to be attached between uterus and external oblique aponeurosis.[18] A fascial strap or mersilene/nylon tape can also be interposed between the cervix and the sacrum.[19] Another attempt is to fix the mersilene tape to isthmus posteriorly and bringing the free ends out retroperitoneally to emerge laterally through anterior oblique abdominis for anchoring to anterior superior iliac spines on either side.[20] There is anecdotal evidence of success in such patients using sacrospinous ligament fixation or retroperitonial abdominal uterosacropexy, suturing mesh or fascia to the uterosacral ligaments and then to the anterior longitudinal ligament of the sacrum. There is little information available regarding long-term follow-up of such patients.
- *LeFort repair:* This is reserved for the very elderly menopausal women who are poor medical risks. It should not be advised to a sexually active woman. In this operation, rectangular flaps of the vagina from anterior and posterior walls are excised, the raw areas apposed with absorbable sutures. The repair converts vagina into a double barrel where uterus will be held above by the midline adhesions.

Operations for Vault Prolapse

Among the most challenging cases are those involving complete eversion of the vagina in patients who have had a previous hysterectomy. This condition virtually always requires surgical correction because of the large size of the prolapse, its propensity to increase over time because of increase in intra-abdominal pressure, and the rate of danger of vaginal evisceration if it is not treated.

- *Colpectomy and colpocleisis:* For some patients, particularly elderly women who are not sexually active and who lead a sedentary lifestyle, surgically removing the vagina and closing off the space can manage the condition.
- *Colpopexy:* Another procedure is required for younger women and women who wish to retain sexual function. For these women, the condition can be managed transvaginally or transabdominally. With the transvaginal approach, vaginal eversion is corrected by suturing one side of the vaginal apex (usually the right side) to the sacrospinous ligament with one or

two sutures—a transvaginal sacrospinous colpopexy.[21] In the transabdominal approach, the vaginal apex is suspended from the anterior longitudinal ligament along the sacrum using a graft of fascia or artificial mesh that is sutured to the vagina and to the sacrum and is placed retroperitoneally—a transabdominal sacral colpopexy.[22] Both the operations are highly successful in resuspending the vaginal apex.

Repair of Posterior Vaginal Wall Defect

Repair of posterior vaginal wall prolapse for rectocele and enterocele is performed vaginally using posterior colporrhaphy. In a rectocele repair, the posterior vagina is opened, the rectum is dissected away from the pararectal fascia, and the levator ani muscles are plicated over the rectum in the midline, after which the vaginal epithelium is closed. It is important to note that a rectocele is a defect of the vaginal supporting tissue and not a defect of the rectum. An enterocele is a peritoneal hernia over the rectum, often seen as a second bump higher up in the vaginal canal on examination. The peritoneal sac should be carefully identified, opened, and closed with several purse-string sutures of permanent material; the sac should be excised, and the vagina should be closed once more over the defect. If the perineal body is noted to be deficient and the patient has a gaping introitus, this deficit may be repaired by a perineorrhaphy or a perineoplasty, in which the vaginal fourchette is opened and the base of the levator ani muscle is pulled together in the midline, providing renewed support for the lateral vagina at its outlet. The latter step (perineorrhaphy) is better avoided in the sexually active woman for the fear of causing dyspareunia, unless gaping introitus and related sexual dissatisfaction are the symptoms.

CONSERVATIVE MANAGEMENT

Conservative management of prolapse usually involves fitting the patient with a pessary (Figs. 18.6A and B).[23] It should be emphasized that pessary will not cure prolapse but relieves the symptoms by stretching the urogenital hiatus. The patient who is using a pessary should have a well estrogenized vagina. For women who are past menopause, it is preferable to use intravaginal estrogen cream 4 to 6 weeks before the pessary is inserted, because this makes the pessary more comfortable to wear and dramatically increases compliance and promotes long-term use. Pessaries are advised not only to test as to whether the low backache or urinary stress incontinence is due to prolapse condition, but also as an interim therapy to avoid and/or postpone surgery in early pregnancy, puerperium, patients unfit for surgery with limited life expectancy, or while awaiting surgery. Postmenopausal women should be given hormone replacement therapy, or alternatively, they should use intravaginal estrogen cream on a regular basis.

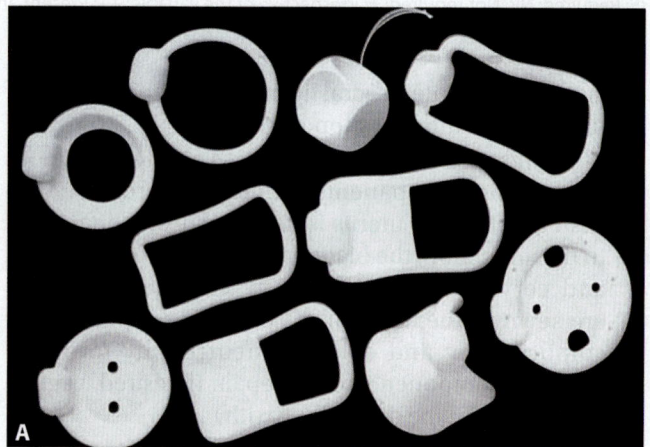

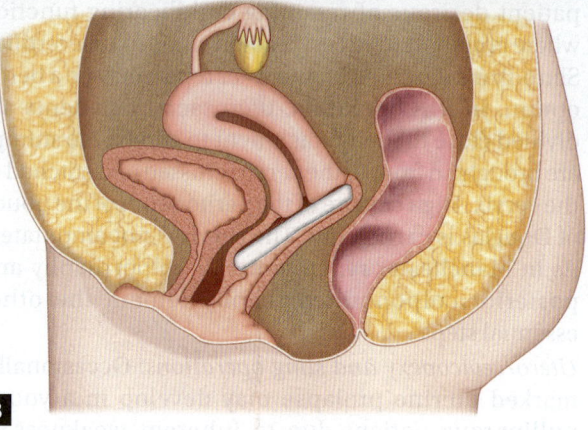

Figs. 18.6A and B: (A) Some of the pessaries used to treat various degrees of prolapse; (B) A line diagram showing a pessary in place after repositioning of prolapsed uterus.
Source: http://www.physio-pedia.com/citerine prolapse

REFERENCES

1. Howkins and Bourne Show's Textbook of Gynecology. In: Padubidri VG, Daftary SN (Eds). 16th edition, RELX India Private Limited, New Delhi; 2011;p.353
2. Baden W, Walker T. Surgical repair of vaginal defects. Philadelphia: JB Lippincott, 1993;9-24.
3. Bump RC, Mattiasson A, Bø K, Brubaker LP, DeLancey JOL, Klarskov P, et al. The standardization of terminology of female organ prolapse and pelvic floor dysfunction. Am J Obstet Gynecol. 1996;175:10-17.

4. Milton PJD. Uterovaginal prolapse. Progress in obstetrics and Gynaecology. 1989;7:319-30.
5. Smith ARB, Hosker GL, Warrel DW. The role of partial denervation of the pelvic floor in the aetiology of genitourinary prolapse and stress incontinence: a neurophysiological study. Br J Obstet Gynaecol. 1989;96:24-28.
6. Allen RE, Hosker GL, Smith ARB, Warrell DW. Pelvic floor damage and childbirth: A neurophysiological study. Br J Obstet Gynaecol. 1990;97:770-79.
7. Norton PA. Pelvic floor disorders: The role of fascia and ligaments. Clin Obstet Gynecol. 1993;36:926-38.
8. DeLancey JO. Anatomy and biomechanics of genital prolapse. Clin Obstet Gynecol. 1993; 36: 897-909.
9. Lawson JO. Pelvic anatomy, I. Pelvic floor muscles. Ann R Coll Surg Engl. 1974;54:244-52.
10. Lawson JO. Pelvic anatomy, II. Anal canal and associated sphincters. Ann R Coll Surg Engl. 1974; 54:288-300.
11. Paramore RH. The uterus as a floating organ. In the Statistics of the Female Pelvic Viscera. London: HK Lewis & Co; 1918;1:12-15.
12. Shull BL. Clinical evaluation of women with pelvic support defects. Clin Obstet Gynecol. 1993;36:939-51.
13. Plevnik S. New methods for testing and strengthening the pelvic floor muscles. In: Proceedings of the 15th Annual Meeting of the International Continence Society, London; 1985: 267.
14. Shull BL, Benn SJ, Kuehl TJ. Surgical management of prolapse of the anterior vaginal segment: an analysis of support defects of morbidity and anatomic outcome. Am J Obstet Gynecol. 1994; 171:1421-39.
15. Raz S, Klutke CG, Golomb J. Four-corner bladder and urethral suspension for moderate cystocele. J Urol. 1989;142:712-15.
16. McCall M. Posterior culdoplasty: surgical correction of enterocele during vaginal hysterectomy; a preliminary report. Obstet Gynecol. 1957;10:595-602.
17. Gilliam DT. Round-ligament ventrosuspension of the uterus : a new method. Am J Obstet. 1900;41:299.
18. Purandare VN, Patel K, Aryan R. Operative treatment for genital prolapse in young woman. J Obst Gynae India. 1966;16:53-56.
19. Shirodkar VN. The problem of prolapse. In: Contribution to Obstetrics and Gynaecology. London: Churchill Livingstone, 1960;16.
20. Khanna SD. A new sling operation for nulliparous prolapse. Proceedings 19th All India Obst Gynae Congress, New Delhi, 1972.
21. Morley GW, DeLancey JOL. Sacrospinous ligament fixation for eversion of the vagina. Am J Obstet Gynecol. 1988;158:872-81.
22. Addison WA, Livengood CH, Sutton GP, Parker RT. Abdominal sacral colpopexy with Mersilene mesh in the retroperitoneal position in the management of posthysterectomy vaginal vault prolapse and enterocele. Am J Obstet Gynecol. 1985;153: 140-6.
23. Streicher LF. Uterine prolapse and pelvic relaxation. www.mygyne.info/uternine prolapse. http://www.physio pedia.com/images|8|86|Pessaries. JPg cascessed 21 march 2017.

CHAPTER 19

Urinary and Fecal Incontinence (Including Fistulae)

Deeksha Pandey

Overview

- Involuntary loss of urine or stool is known as incontinence.
- Urinary and fecal incontinence along with pelvic organ prolapse (POP), are interconnected problems, owing to the same anatomical (pelvic floor), physiological (innervation), and etiological (child birth injuries) background.
- Most important factor for the development of incontinence in women is injury to pelvic floor sustained during vaginal delivery.
- One in three women over age 45 and every second women over age 65 have urinary incontinence.
- The first and foremost investigation to be done in any kind of urinary incontinence is urine microscopy, as cystitis can mimic any of the types of urinary incontinence.
- Lifestyle modification, bladder training and Kegel's exercises are the first line treatment for urge and stress urinary incontinence (SUI).
- Midurethral sling or tension-free vaginal tape (TVT) is becoming increasingly popular operation for SUI due to its minimally invasive nature, ease of use, and good long-term efficacy.
- Though the etiopathogenesis of fecal incontinence is multifactorial, in women child birth related injuries play major role. Occult obstetric anal sphincter injuries (OASIS) have been found to be notoriously associated with anal incontinence.
- In developing countries, the most common cause of genital fistulae is obstetric injuries.
- Most commonly seen genital fistula is vesico-vaginal fistula (VVF).

BACKGROUND

Involuntary loss of urine or stool is known as incontinence. Incontinence can be a major health and social concern for women, across all age groups.

Urinary and fecal incontinence along with pelvic organ prolapse (POP), are interconnected problems, owing to the same anatomical (pelvic floor), physiological (innervation), and etiological (child birth injuries) background. Pelvic floor dysfunction can affect micturition, defecation and sexual activity. Evolutionary modifications like adaptation to upright position, walking on two limbs and delivering fetuses with larger head diameters; has made the support of the pelvic floor vulnerable, therefore predisposing women to POP and incontinence. This Chapter mainly concentrates on urinary and fecal incontinence. Pelvic organ prolapse has been separately discussed elsewhere.

Because of the similar anatomic, physiologic and etiological consideration; these have been described in detail before proceeding onto the specifications of urinary/fecal incontinence.

Anatomy

Pelvic floor is a supporting system for the pelvic organs (bladder, uterus and rectum). It includes all muscles, ligaments and connective tissue that fill the pelvic cavity. Pelvic organs are maintained in their normal anatomic position due to this support system comprised of the levator ani muscles, the endopelvic fascia and its lateral condensation (arcus tendinous fascia pelvis), the uterosacral ligaments and the perineal body (Fig. 19.1).

Neural Control/Physiology

The lower urinary tract and bowel are innervated by: (A) Autonomic nervous system (Sympathetic and Parasympathetic), (B) Somatic nervous system.

Sympathetic system primarily controls storage while parasympathetic facilitates emptying. Somatic nervous system plays only a peripheral role through its innervation of the pelvic floor and external sphincters (Fig. 19.2).

CHAPTER 19: Urinary and Fecal Incontinence (Including Fistulae)

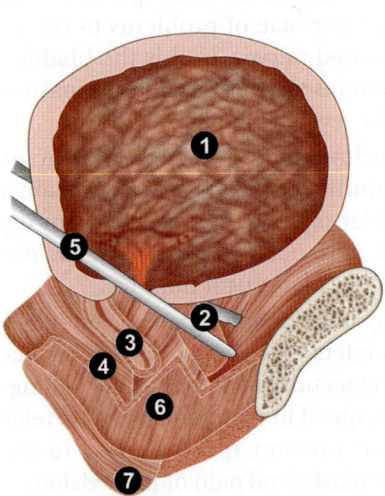

Fig. 19.1: Anatomy of pelvic floor support system for bladder, rectum and uterus. 1. Urinary bladder, 2. Urethra, 3. Vagina, 4. Rectum, 5. Anal sphincter, 6. Levator ani, 7. External anal sphincter.

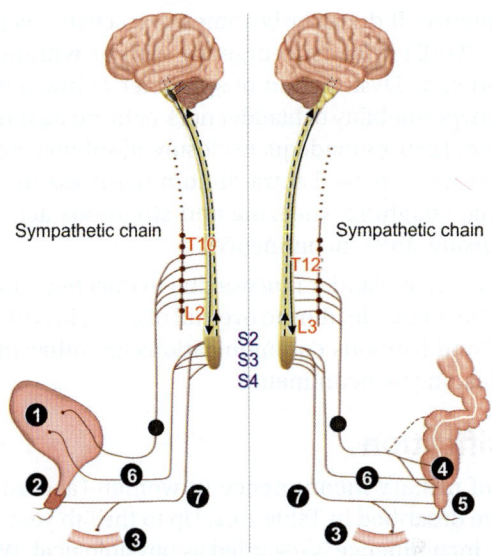

Fig. 19.2: Neural control of lower urinary tract and bowel. 1. Bladder, 2. External urethral sphincter, 3. Perineum, 4. Rectum, 5. External anal sphincter, 6. Pelvic splanchnic nerve, 7. Pudendal nerve.

Autonomic Nervous System (Sympathetic and Parasympathetic)

Storage and emptying of urine and feces is an interplay of sympathetic and parasympathetic nervous system.

- Sympathetic system arises from thoracolumbar spinal cord (T11–L2/L3). Through its neurotransmitter (norepinephrine) it acts on two types of receptors: α-receptors located in urethra, bladder neck and internal anal sphincter; β-receptors located in bladder and anus. Thus stimulation of α-receptors promotes closure, whereas α-receptor blockers have the oppo- effect. Stimulation of β-receptors decreases tone of bladder and rectum.
- Parasympathetic system originates in the sacral spinal cord (S2–S4) and gives rise to pelvic splanchnic nerves. Pelvic splanchnic nerves on either side arise from the ventral rami of the S2–S4. These nerves regulate the emptying of the urinary bladder, control opening and closing of the internal urethral sphincter, influence motility in the rectum and also control sexual functions.

Somatic Nervous System (Pudendal Nerve)

Pudendal nerve is the main nerve of the perineum. This nerve is composed of three roots derived from the ventral rami of the S2–S4. It has both sensory and motor components. It carries sensation from the external genitalia and the skin around of the perineum. It provides motor supply to various pelvic muscles, including external urethral sphincter and external anal sphincter.

ETIOLOGY AND RISK FACTORS

Most important factor for the development of incontinence in women is injury to pelvic floor, sustained during vaginal delivery. Women are prone to develop incontinence usually after they have given birth to at least one child vaginally. Vaginal delivery has been identified as a single most important risk factor for developing stress urinary incontinence. The problem sometimes is occult which gets revealed or aggravated after menopause, due to hypoestrogenism. With increasing life expectancy and thus increasing elderly population, the occult injuries caused in childbirth are being revealed in higher proportion of women with menopause and advancing age.

URINARY INCONTINENCE

Definition

Involuntary loss of urine is called urinary incontinence.

Prevalence

One in three women over age 45 and every second women over age 65 have urinary incontinence.

Pathophysiology

The lower urinary tract basically has two functions: (1) storage (urinary bladder) and (2) emptying (urethra). Storage in the bladder depends on relaxing power of detrusor (bladder muscle) and integrity of sphincter at the bladder neck. Dysfunction of these two can lead to incontinence. If detrusor becomes overactive (overactive bladder/OAB) it leads to urgency with or without urge incontinence. Dysfunction of sphincter at bladder neck (due to hypermobility of bladder neck or intrinsic sphincter deficiency) causes inadequate closure of sphincter during episodes of increased intra-abdominal pressure (as in laughing, coughing, sneezing and strenuous activities), thus causing stress incontinence.

Irritation of bladder mucosa due to infection, obstruction of the urethra leading to overfull bladder, loss of neural control and fistulous communications are other mechanisms leading to incontinence.

Classification

Types of urinary incontinence in women (according to ICS)[1] are described in Table 19.1. Up to the 5th year of life, urinary incontinence is regarded as physiological. Women are prone to develop urinary incontinence after child birth or menopause.

- *Stress urinary incontinence (SUI):* SUI is defined as involuntary leakage of urine upon effort, exertion, sneezing, coughing or laughing (these are the activities that cause increase in the intra-abdominal pressure).
- *Urge incontinence:* Urge incontinence is the involuntary leakage of urine accompanied by or immediately preceded by urgency. Urgency is the sudden compelling desire to pass urine that is difficult to defer. Usually urge incontinence is a result of detrusor over-activity, so it is also associated with symptoms of frequency and nocturia.
- *Mixed incontinence:* When a woman complains of both stress as well as urge urinary incontinence, this is referred to as mixed incontinence.
- *Others:* This includes neurogenic incontinence, overflow incontinence, functional incontinence, transient incontinence and extraurethral causes of incontinence.

  – Neurogenic incontinence (neurogenic bladder): In this condition the neurogenic control to bladder is lost because of problems of brain, spinal cord or related nerves. In this the bladder can have of symptoms of either flaccidity or spasticity depending on the level of damage.
  – Overflow incontinence is characterized by the involuntary release of urine from an over full bladder, often in the absence of any urge to urinate. This may occur due to outflow obstruction or paralysis of detrusor muscles.
  – Functional incontinence is seen in elderly women. This refers to leakage of urine that occurs because of factors unrelated to normal voiding mechanism. This type of incontinence may be related to factors which prevent quick access to the toilet like musculoskeletal pain or poor vision.
  – Transient urinary incontinence is a kind of easily reversible incontinence, which included causes which can be memorized by the mnemonic DIAPPERS (Delirium, Infection, Atrophic urethritis, Pharmacological causes, Psychological causes, Excessive urine production, Restricted mobility, Stool impaction).[2]
  – Extraurethral incontinence includes those causes wherein urine loss occurs through abnormal openings, either because of congenital defects (ectopic ureter, bladder extrophy) or trauma causing fistulous opening (described in detail in the next section).

History

Age

Urinary incontinence is usually a problem of women during reproductive years and beyond. SUI is more commonly seen in younger women while urge incontinence occurs more frequently in older women.

Table 19.1: Types of urinary incontinence.

Type of incontinence	Definition/symptom
• Stress urinary incontinence (SUI)	Involuntary urine loss during episodes of increased abdominal pressure (as in coughing, sneezing, laughing, physical exertion/exercise)
• Urge incontinence (UI)	Involuntary urine loss with sudden sensation of urgency to void
• Mixed incontinence (MI)	SUI + UI
• Others:	
– Neurogenic	• Neurogenic control to bladder is lost
– Overflow	• Outflow obstruction/detrusor paralysis
– Functional	• in elderly with normal voiding
– Transient	• DIAPPERS (mnemonic for causes)
– Extra-urethral	
♦ Fistula	• Acquired (trauma-obstetric/surgical)
♦ Abnormal opening	• Congenital (ectopic ureter, bladder extrophy)

CHAPTER 19 Urinary and Fecal Incontinence (Including Fistulae)

Parity and Mode of Delivery
Pelvic floor trauma caused by vaginal births predisposes woman to SUI. Repeated vaginal births weaken the pelvic floor.

Symptom Details
The most troubling symptom should be ascertained in terms of whether it is predominantly stress, urge, frequency or nocturia.

Specific questions to find out the type of urinary incontinence include:
- Is it a continuous leak or episodic incontinence? (continuous leak denotes fistula)
- Is it associated with frequency and/or dysuria? (more likely to be because of infection)
- If it is episodic: What causes incontinence? Cough, laugh, sneeze, physical exertion, no cause (to find out SUI)
- Is it associated with urgent desire to void immediately? (Urgency/urge incontinence)
- Do you feel the sensation to void? (If no-overflow incontinence)

The other important questions to be asked are: how often does she leak urine, how much urine is lost every time, what provokes it, what improves/worsens the problem and whether she has tried any form of treatment for her problem till now?

Medical History
Some neurological, musculoskeletal or systemic problems (like diabetes) might cause incontinence or may have an indirect relation (with the medications or by predisposition to urinary infection). Chronic cough might be an aggravating factor.

Surgical History
Surgery for prolapse is known to predispose de novo SUI in many women. History of previous pelvic or spinal cord surgeries might also have an association.

Physical Examination

Weight/BMI
Obesity might be an aggravating factor.

General Condition
Physical and mental impairment points to functional causes of urinary incontinence.

Abdominal Examination
Full bladder (if palpable) points towards overflow incontinence. Ascites and abdominal masses (including fibroid uterus) rarely can be associated with incontinence.

Local Examination
Excoriation of surrounding skin and urinary smell from garments helps to assess the severity of the problem. Patients complaining of urinary incontinence should be examined with full bladder. Demonstrable spurt of urine on coughing should be documented.

Speculum Examination
Cystocele if present to be noted. Atrophic vaginitis to be looked for. Fistulous opening to be demarcated in cases of suspected vesicovaginal or ureterovaginal fistulae.

Vaginal Examination
Vaginal examination should be done to rule out pelvic mass.

Special Tests
These tests are not required always. These were meant specifically for SUI: For objective demonstration (stress test), for classifying (Q-tip test), and for forecasting the treatment outcome (Bonney's and Marshall tests).

Stress test: It is done for those women who present with complaint of SUI but routine examination fails to demonstrate it. The patient is asked to empty her bladder. She is then catheterized to note the residual volume of urine. This collected urine can be tested for presence of infection (by dipstick test or laboratory examination). Then the bladder is filled with saline with all aseptic precaution. Patient is now asked to cough or strain. Objective evidence of leakage of urine is noted.

Q-tip test: A cotton tipped swab stick is lubricated with local anesthetic jelly and then placed in urethra. This swab stick will be parallel to the floor. Patient is now asked to strain or cough. Normally, this stick will move 10° to 15° above the horizontal. In cases of SUI this angle can be 20° to 70° thus indicating hypermobility of the bladder neck. This test was popular when SUI was classified as due to hypermobility of bladder neck or intrinsic sphincter deficiency. However with better understanding of the pathology and the treatment modalities this classification has lost its value in cases of uncomplicated SUI, thus outdating the test.

Bonney's and Marshall tests: This test was used to forecast the outcome of surgical treatment in cases of SUI. In Bonney's test, examiner places two fingers in the vagina, to elevate the bladder neck, at the urethrovesical junction on either side of urethra. Absence of leakage now on asking patient to cough predicts positive outcome for surgical treatment. Likewise in Marshall test in place of fingers an open Allis clamp is used, prior to which vaginal mucosa of that area is infiltrated with local anesthetic.

Investigations

1. **Urine microscopy:** The first and foremost investigation to be done in any kind of urinary incontinence is urine microscopy, as cystitis can mimic any of the types of urinary incontinence. Simple rule is to first treat urinary infection and to reassess.
2. **Ultrasound:** An ultrasonographic examination of the pelvis should be performed to rule out secondary causes of incontinence or associated pelvic pathologies. Hydroureteronephrosis should also be ruled out.
3. **Urodynamic studies:** Urodynamics is the dynamic study of the lower urinary tract to evaluate storage and evacuation of urine. Studies have shown a poor correlation between symptoms and urodynamic diagnosis in cases of female urinary incontinence. Thus, it is not indicated for straightforward cases of urinary incontinence in women.[3] It is indicated where patients symptoms are not correlating with examination findings, mixed urinary incontinence, failed surgical treatment or in case of recurrence.[4]
4. **Cystoscopy:** Cystoscopy is visualization of bladder with the help of an endoscope. This test is also not routinely used for evaluation of incontinence in women. It is recommended in patients with complicated urinary incontinence, suspected vesicovaginal fistula, extraurethral incontinence, recurrent bladder infections or suspected tumor/stone in the bladder.

Treatment

Having established the diagnosis, treatment depends upon the type of urinary incontinence.

Stress urinary incontinence

Following are the management options for SUI.

1. **Dietary and lifestyle modification:** Weight reduction is usually of help in overweight or obese women. Simple dietary advice, like cutting down on food and beverages like coffee, tea, colas and chocolates, should be offered. Caffeine can overload the bladder, aggravating SUI symptom.
2. **Pelvic floor muscle training (PFMT) or Kegel's excercises:** This is often used as the first line of management in SUI.[5]
3. **Electrical and magnetic stimulation:** This option is for those who are not able to contract their pelvic floor muscles effectively. Electrical stimulation of these muscles can be achieved by placing electrodes in vaginal or anal canal. Magnetic stimulation of pelvic floor muscles is done extracorporally.
4. **Mechanical devices:** Vaginal inserts including incontinence pessaries or tampons can be used. These act by compressing the bladder neck and urethra, thus decreasing urine loss during episodes of increased intra-abdominal pressure. Urethral inserts are directly inserted in the urethra to prevent leakage. However, all these devices are temporary methods.
5. **Drugs:** There is no Food and Drug Administration (FDA) approved drug to be used for managing SUI. In clinical practice however, antidepressant drug—duloxetine has been used with some objective benefit.[6]
6. **Surgery:** Surgery offers high cure rates and is considered by many to be first-line therapy for uncomplicated SUI in women. Though more than 200 procedures have been described in literature for managing SUI, only few are used in present clinical practice. Burch colposuspension and midurethral synthetic slings are the most popular. The latter has become the more common operation for SUI due to its minimally invasive nature, ease of use, and good long-term efficacy. These midurethral slings are also known as tension-free vaginal tape (TVT) procedures as in these procedures the tape is not fixed to any point rather it remains as a dynamic sling. This dynamicity gives the advantage of urethral occlusion only during the episodes of increased intra-abdominal pressure. Midurethral slings or TVT are classified into two major groups based on the surgical approach: Retropubic approach (ofter referred as TVT) and transobturator approach (often referred as TVT-O or TOT) (Figs. 19.3A and B). Transobturator approach is more popular approach mainly because of lower risk of injuries nearby structures. The tape in this procedure can be inserted below the midurethra either by inside-out or outside-in approach (Figs. 19.4A and B).
7. **Bulking agent:** Injection of a bulking agent at the bladder neck is a minimally invasive method usually reserved for those where all other options have failed or for those who are very high-risk candidates for undergoing surgery. Procedure involves injection of autologous fat, collagen, or carbon beads are injected through a needle placed transurethrally or periurethrally, under urethroscopic guidance.
8. **Artificial urinary sphincter:** This is one of the options where all other methods have failed to make the woman continent. In this device, an inflated cuff keeps the bladder neck closed. Whenever the woman desires to empty her bladder she can do this by deflating the cuff with the help of a control pump which is placed at the labia.
9. **Stem cells:** Stem cell therapy for SUI is still at experimental level. However, the future looks promising.

CHAPTER 19 Urinary and Fecal Incontinence (Including Fistulae)

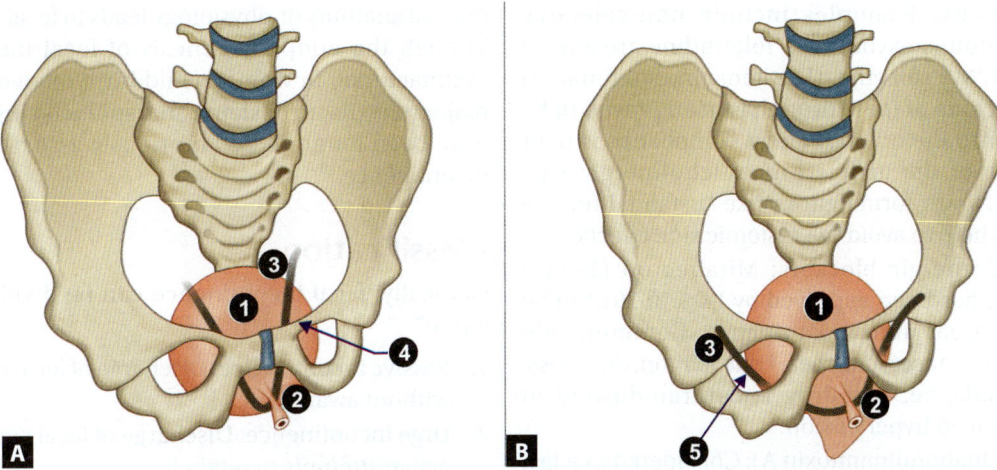

Figs. 19.3A and B: Tension-free vaginal tape for SUI: (A) Retropubic approach. (B) Obturator approach. 1. Urinary bladder, 2. Urethra, 3. Polypropylene mesh, 4. Retropubic space, 5. Obturator fossa.

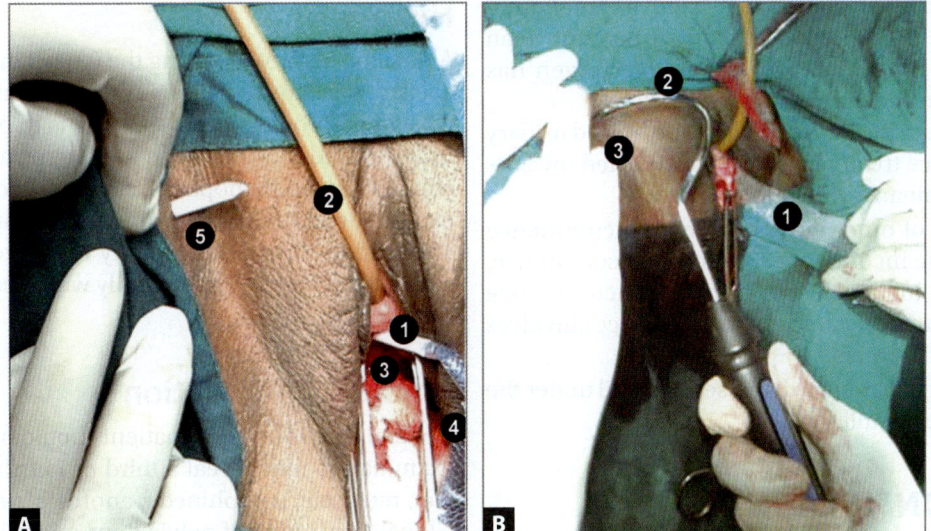

Figs. 19.4A and B: Tension-free vaginal tape (TVT-O) can be inserted in two ways: (A) Inside-out approach: 1. Helical passer attached to the polypropylene mesh, 2. Urethral catheter in, 3. Anterior vaginal wall, 4. Polypropylene mesh/tape, 5. Exit point below the insertion of adductor longus. (B) Outside-in approach: 1. Polypropylene mesh/tape, 2. Helical passer, 3. Entry point.

Urge incontinence

1. **Behavioral therapy:** This should be the first line treatment for urge incontinence. This includes bladder training and PFMT. Contrary to the traditional thinking that PFMT is beneficial only for SUI, it shows very good results for urge incontinence too. It has been demonstrated that properly performed PFMT is more effective than drug therapy in this type of incontinence.[7]
2. **Lifestyle modification:** Patients have to be educated that the symptoms of urge are basically due to overactivity of bladder musculature. So, avoiding certain food substances that either overload the bladder (coffee, tea, colas and alcohol) or are bladder irritants (cigarettes and spicy food items) should be avoided. Minimizing fluid intake especially during bed time might also provide some symptomatic relief.
3. **Neuromodulation:** These techniques include small devices which stimulate nerves that share a common nerve root with nerves supplying the bladder. Posterior tibial nerve stimulator is the most widely used device and it is a office-based procedure. In addition, there are some devices which need a surgical intervention for implantation. These include sacral nerve, paraurethral and pudendal nerve stimulators.
4. **Drug therapy:** Following three groups of drugs can be used to treat urge incontinence.
   - Anticholinergics: This group of drugs block M2/M3 receptors in the bladder, and thus reduce detrusor

overactivity. Examples include non-selective (fesotarodine, oxybutanin, tolterodine, trospium) and M1/M2 selective (Darifenacin, Solifenacin) agents. None of these drugs has been proved to be superior to the others. Patient compliance is poor because of the distressing anticholinergic side effects. Newer formulations like sustained release patches help to avoid the systemic side effects.

- Beta adrenergic blockers: Mirabegron (Beta 3 blocker) has been approved by FDA in 2012 to be used to treat urge incontinence. Common side effects are nausea, diarrhea, constipation, dizziness, and headache. The drug is contraindicated in uncontrolled hypertension.
- Botox (Onabotulinumtoxin A): Considered as a last resort, botox is injected in the detrusor muscle to cause paralysis. Injections need to be repeated in 3 to 6 months.

Warning: Estrogen sometimes used to treat urge incontinence in menopausal women has not been approved by FDA. Moreover systemic estrogen has been shown to worsen the symptoms.[6, 8]

- Mixed urinary incontinence: In case of mixed urinary incontinence treatment should be directed towards the predominant symptom.
- Treatment of other types of urinary incontinence (neurogenic incontinence, overflow incontinence, functional incontinence, transient incontinence and extraurethral causes of incontinence) involves managing the cause.

Note: Urinary fistula has been discussed in detail under the heading of Genital Fistulae.

FECAL INCONTINENCE

Definition
Fecal incontinence is inability to control solid or liquid stool. Anal incontinence is a wider terminology used to describe inability to control gas and mucus in addition to the inability to control stool. However, the two terms are often used interchangeably.

Prevalence
Fecal incontinence may affect individuals of all age groups. However, its prevalence is disproportionately higher in women and elderly. Prevalence of fecal incontinence ranges from 1 to 7.4% in healthy population, whereas in elderly and institutionalized individuals it is reported to be as high as 25%.[9]

Pathophysiology
Fecal continence is maintained by anatomical and functional integrity of anorectal unit. Thus, disruption of normal anatomy or physiology leads to fecal incontinence. Though the etiopathogenesis of fecal incontinence is multifactorial, in women child birth related injuries play major role. Occult obstetric anal sphincter injuries (OASIS) have been found to be notoriously associated with anal incontinence.[10]

Classification
Clinically, fecal incontinence can be divided into three types:[9]

1. Passive incontinence: Discharge of fecal material or gas without awareness.
2. Urge incontinence: Discharge of fecal contents despite active attempts to retain it.
3. Fecal seepage: Leakage of stool following otherwise normal evacuation.

History
A detailed history exploring the type of incontinence to be elicited. Affection to the quality of life should be ascertained. Onset and progression of symptoms to be noted down in order to find out the cause and aggravating factors (e.g. child birth and menopause/aging respectively). Systemic causes (neurological, diabetes, etc.) should be ruled out. Medication should be carefully reviewed. History of any surgical intervention specifically with a perineal approach should be asked for.

Physical Examination
General condition of the patient should be assessed. Local examination may reveal a third or fourth degree perineal tear, rectocele, lax sphincter, anorectal prolapse or fistula. Global weakening of pelvic floor might be evident in the form of associated urogenital prolapse or demonstrable SUI.

Investigations
Following investigations are of help in finding out the cause and severity of the problem before planning the management:

- Proctosigmoidoscopy: To visualize the lumen under magnification and obtain biopsies from abnormal areas.
- Anorectal manometry: To measure the anorectal pressures during rest and squeeze.
- Endoanal ultrasonography: To detect the anatomical integrity of anal sphincter.

Treatment
Treatment of fecal incontinence basically depends on the underlying cause.

- Surgical: Surgical intervention is required in case of perineal tear, anal prolapse or fistula.
- Physiotherapy should be tried in cases of OASIS presenting with fecal incontinence.
- Medical: In refractory cases or where the cause cannot be identified drugs like loperamide and codein may be tried, as they increase the resting tone of anal sphincter.
- Other options: Management of refractory cases may include sacral nerve stimulation or percutaneous tibial nerve stimulation. Fecal diversion or an artificial bowel sphincter may be considered when all else has failed.[11]

GENITAL FISTULAE

Definition

Genital fistula is an abnormal communication between a woman's vagina/uterus and bladder/rectum, through which her urine or feces continually leak.

Etiology

In developing countries, the vast majority of these fistulae are still obstetric in origin. However, the incidence is also in rise owing to the increasing incidence of cesarean deliveries. Unrecognized trauma during pelvic surgeries is another cause of genital fistulae.

Obstetric causes: Prolonged neglected obstructed labor leads to ischemic damage of vagina and bladder. This later leads to necrosis of ischemic tissues and fistula formation. Difficult instrumental delivery (in particular with forceps) might also cause injury to bladder and urethra. There is a chance of bladder injury during cesarean delivery especially in cases of repeat cesarean where the bladder is densely adherent to the lower uterine segment.

Surgical causes: Difficult pelvic surgery usually in presence of dense adhesions, distorted anatomy or malignancy predisposes surrounding tissues and organs for injury. These include bladder, ureteric and intestinal injuries. These injuries if detected in time peroperatively can be managed with the help of specialists. However, if these remain unrecognized, later on might present with fistulous openings into the genital tract.

Malignancy: Malignancy of the pelvic organs may result in fistula formation either as a part of disease process or as a complication of treatment (radiotherapy or surgery).

Classification

Based on the type of discharge genital fistulae can be divided into urinary or fecal fistulae (Table 19.2 and Fig. 19.5).

Among all these fistulae vesicovaginal is the most commonly encountered one. This is discussed in detail.

Table 19.2: Types of genital fistulae.

Urinary fistulae	Fecal fistulae
- Ureterovaginal	- Rectovaginal
- Vesicovaginal	
- Urethrovaginal	- Anovaginal
- Vesicouterine	

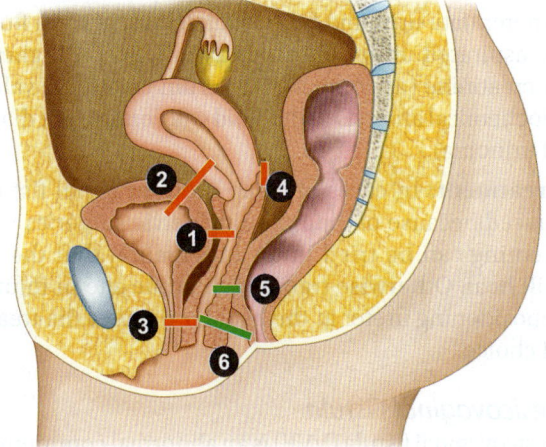

Fig. 19.5: Various types of genital fistulae: 1. Vesicovaginal fistula, 2. Vesicouterine fistula, 3. Urethrovaginal fistula, 4. Ureterovaginal fistula, 5. Rectovaginal fistula, 6. Anovaginal fistula.

Urinary Fistulae

Ureterovaginal fistula

It is an abnormal communication between the ureter and the vagina. Urine in this case flows directly from the ureter into the vagina without passing into the bladder.

This results from either direct injury (clamping, ligation, transection) or devascularization of pelvic ureters during pelvic surgeries.

Clinical presentation: Most of the patients present with continuous urine leakage from vagina. Abdominal pain, flank pain, fever and paralytic ileus may also develop as a result of seepage of urine into the peritoneal cavity. History of recent pelvic/gynecological surgery should be asked for.

Diagnostic tests:

- Speculum examination: This will reveal urine leak in the vagina. Fistulous opening might or might not (in cases of small fistulae) be evident.
- Three-tampon test of Moir: In this clinical test 3 small cotton tampons are kept in high, mid and lower vagina respectively. Bladder is then filled with diluted methylene blue. Patient is asked to walk around for about 15 minutes. After this tampons are carefully removed and examined. Topmost tampon being wet with urine but no swab with methylene blue stain confirms ureterovaginal fistula (Table 19.3).

- Excretory urography: Extravasation of radiopaque dye from the ureter will confirm the diagnosis.
- Cystoscopy: Visualization of drainage of urine from the ureteric orifices helps to ascertain integrity of ureters. Thus in case of ureteric fistula, efflux of urine would not be demonstrable from ureteric orifice on cystoscopic examination.

Ultrasound: To rule out hydroureteronephrosis or urinoma (localized collection of urine in the peritoneal cavity. To differentiate urinoma from loculated ascites, the fluid can be aspirated under ultrasound guidance. A higher level of creatinine (as compared to serum creatinine value) on biochemical analysis of this fluid will confirm the diagnosis of urinoma.

Treatment: In cases of clean ureterovaginal fistulae as caused because of injury during pelvic surgeries ureteric stenting can be tried in an anticipation that the fistula will heal. Otherwise transaction at the site of injury and repositioning ureter at the bladder dome is the treatment of choice.

Vesicovaginal Fistula

Vesicovaginal fistula (VVF) is an abnormal communication between the bladder and the vagina. This is the commonest type of genital fistula seen in gynecological practice.

Types: Based on the anatomical location VVF are of three types:

1. Supratrigonal or high fistula
2. Trigonal or Low/midvaginal fistula
3. Massive (a+b)

Clinical presentation: Continuous urinary leakage.

Diagnosis:
- Speculum examination: This will reveal urine leak in the vagina. Fistulous opening usually is seen. In cases of small fistulae retrograde filling of bladder with diluted methylene blue dye will help to establish the diagnosis.
- Three-tampon test of Moir: In this clinical test 3 small cotton tampons are kept in high, mid and lower vagina respectively. Bladder is then filled with diluted methylene blue. Patient is asked to walk around for around 15 minutes. After this tampons are carefully removed and examined. Middle swab being blue with methylene blue stain confirms VVF (Table 19.3).
- Cystoscopy: Cystoscopy will locate the defect in the bladder, which will help to plan the management.

Management:

Prolonged bladder catheterization: In selected cases this may help by giving rest to the bladder thus facilitating healing.

- Surgical repair: It can be done either vaginally or abdominally. The success rate is better when the repair is delayed for the time till the surrounding tissues are no longer indurated and infected (usually 3 months), especially in cases of obstetric fistulae.
- Vaginal repair: This is usually the preferred method of VVF repair, as the peritoneal cavity is not entered. In this a circular incision is made around the fistulous opening in the vaginal wall, to excise the fistulous track. Then vagina and bladder wall are widely separated all around, by flap-splitting method. After adequate mobilization of vagina and bladder wall the edges are approximated in two layers without tension. Water tight closure is ensured by instilling diluted methylene blue in the bladder, which should not leak to vagina once the closure is perfect.
- Abdominal repair: This is required in cases massive VVF, previous surgical failures or radiation fistula. Interposition of omental flap between the bladder and vagina facilitates healing (Fig. 19.6).

Table 19.3: Three swab test: How to interpret?

	Observation	Interpretation
1.	Topmost swab: Wet (but not blue)	Ureterovaginal fistula
2.	Middle swab: Blue	Vesicovaginal fistula
3.	Lower swab: Blue (upper two are dry)	Transurethral incontinence (No fistula)

Note: Ureterovaginal fistula will have leakage only during micturition, not otherwise

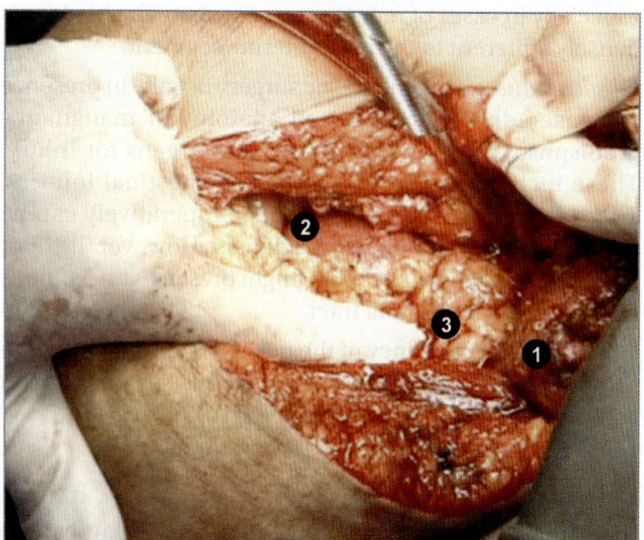

Fig. 19.6: Abdominal method of VVF repair by interpositioning of omental flap to facilitate healing. 1. Bladder, 2. Uterus, 3. Omental flap.

Urethrovaginal Fistula

It is a rare entity causing urinary leakage from the vagina only at the time of micturition. This fistula might be caused by obstructed labor, or instrumental deliveries.

Vesicouterine Fistula

Vesicouterine fistula is an abnormal communication between bladder and the lower uterine segment. It is caused usually because of bladder injury during cesarean section.[12] Patient typically presents with Youssef classical triad: cyclical hematuria (menouria), amenorrhea and urinary continence.

Transabdominal surgical repair is standard treatment. Meticulous practice of obstetric and surgical principles during cesarean section can prevent the formation of these fistulae.[13]

Fecal Fistulae

- Fecal fistula either rectovaginal or anovaginal are rare. The most common causes are obstetric trauma, local infection, and rectal surgery. It can also be caused by gynecological or anorectal malignancies and as a complication of radiation therapy.
- Diagnosis is clinical based on history and examination.
- Imaging and scopy might help to discover the primary cause.
- Treatment is surgical excision of fistulous tract and closure. Approach can be endoanal, transvaginal, transperineal or abdominal.

REFERENCES

1. Mostwin J BA, Haab F, et al. Pathophysiology of urinary incontinence, fecal incontinence, and pelvic organ prolapse. In: Abrams P, Cardozo L, Khoury S, Wein A (Eds). Incontinence, Plymouth (UK): Health Publications, Ltd. 2005:61.
2. Resnick NM, Yalla SV. Management of urinary incontinence in the elderly. The New England Journal of Medicine. 1985;313(13): 800-5.
3. Pandey D, Anna G, Hana O, Christian F. Correlation between clinical presentation and urodynamic findings in women attending urogynecology clinic. Journal of Mid-life Health. 2013;4(3):153-9.
4. Scarpero H. Urodynamics in the evaluation of female LUTS: when are they helpful and how do we use them? The Urologic Clinics of North America. 2014;41(3):429-38.
5. Dumoulin C H-SE, Mac Habée-Séguin G. Pelvic floor muscle training versus no treatment, or inactive control treatments, for urinary incontinence in women. Cochrane Database of Systematic Reviews. 2014 (5).
6. Hersh L, Salzman B. Clinical management of urinary incontinence in women. American Family Physician. 2013;87(9):634-40. PubMed PMID: 23668526. Epub 2013/05/15. eng.
7. Burgio KL, Locher JL, Goode PS, Hardin JM, McDowell BJ, Dombrowski M, et al. Behavioral vs drug treatment for urge urinary incontinence in older women: a randomized controlled trial. JAMA. 1998;280(23):1995-2000.
8. Cody JD JM, Richardson K, Moehrer B, Hextall A. Oestrogen therapy for urinary incontinence in post-menopausal women. Cochrane Database of Systematic Reviews. 2012 (10).
9. Rao SS. Diagnosis and management of fecal incontinence. American College of Gastroenterology Practice Parameters Committee. The American Journal of Gastroenterology. 2004;99(8):1585-604.
10. Andrews V, Shelmeridine S, Sultan AH, Thakar R. Anal and urinary incontinence 4 years after a vaginal delivery. International Urogynecology Journal. 2013;24(1):55-60.
11. Rezvan A, Jakus-Waldman S, Abbas MA, Yazdany T, Nguyen J. Review of the diagnosis, management and treatment of fecal incontinence. Female pelvic medicine & reconstructive surgery. 2014.
12. Rajamaheswari N, Chhikara AB. Vesicouterine fistulae: our experience of 17 cases and literature review. International Urogynecology Journal. 2013;24(2):275-9.
13. Rao MP, Dwivedi US, Datta B, Vyas N, Nandy PR, Trivedi S, et al. Post caesarean vesicouterine fistulae-- Youssef syndrome: our experience and review of published work. ANZ Journal of Surgery. 2006;76(4):243-5.

CHAPTER 20

A Simplified Approach to Breast Diseases for Obstetricians and Gynecologists

SS Prasad

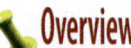
Overview

- Breast symptoms are quite common and often the affected presents to their gynecologists.
- Majority of the breast symptoms are due to underlying benign etiology.
- Increasing incidence of breast cancer in young females and increasing age at childbirth have contributed to overall increase in pregnancy associated breast cancer.
- Acute mastitis and lactational breast abscess are common problems. Early diagnosis of mastitis and prompt initiation of appropriate antibiotics reduce the risk of evolution of lactational breast abscess thereby significantly reducing the morbidity.

INTRODUCTION

Most women seek consultation for breast-related symptoms at some point during their lifetime. More often the anxious lady concerned about the possibility of breast cancer consults her family physician or gynecologist for her breast-related symptoms. On most occasions the symptoms will have a benign cause. However, it is of paramount importance to thoroughly evaluate and rule out breast cancer. This Chapter aims to give an overview of significance and approach to breast-related symptoms and discusses briefly about common breast diseases.

RELEVANT ANATOMY AND PHYSIOLOGY

The breast spans from 2nd or 3rd rib to 6th or 7th rib. It transversely extends from the lateral border of sternum to anterior axillary line. A small part of breast called axillary tail of Spence extends beyond the anterior axillary line. The breast is composed of 15–20 lobes. Each lobe is drained by a major lactiferous duct. These ducts open into the ampulla of nipple. Histologically, breast is composed of glandular elements and stromal elements. The lymphatics of the breast drain into axillary, internal mammary and supraclavicular group of lymph nodes.

The development, differentiation and functioning of the breast is under the influence of various hormones. While estrogen is responsible for the development of ductal system, progesterone accounts for lobular development and differentiation of epithelium. The hormone prolactin promotes lactogenesis which can be physiological in late pregnancy and lactation and pathological in prolactinomas. During pregnancy, under the influence of increased circulating levels of estrogens and progestins, the breast enlarges. This is due to proliferation of ductal and lobular elements. Other changes that occur in breast during pregnancy include, darkening of skin of nipple areolar complex with prominent accessory areolar glands called tubercles of Montgomery. With the onset of menopause, the proportion of connective tissue including adipose tissue increases, while the glandular components like ducts and alveoli involute. Such a change in breast structure during pregnancy renders breast for effective screening by mammography in perimenopausal age group.

COMMON BREAST-RELATED SYMPTOMS

Mastalgia

The term Mastalgia means "breast pain". Breast pain is a very common symptom. A vast majority of women suffer

from this symptom at some point in their lifetime. While few patients may have an underlying cause (e.g. Mastitis), in most others the etiology is poorly understood. Mastalgia can be:
- Cyclical mastalgia which has characteristic association with the woman's menstrual cycle
- Non-cyclical mastalgia—where no such association can be found.

When a patient presents with mastalgia, a thorough clinical evaluation and investigations are required to rule out an underlying malignancy. In patients with no demonstrable underlying causes, treatment options include:
- Reassurance
- Wearing properly fitting brassiere
- Reducing caffeine intake
- Evening primrose oil, Vitamin E and Vitamin B6 can be tried with varying degrees of success
- When these interventions prove futile, pharmacotherapy with nonsteroidal anti-inflammatory drugs, danazol, bromocriptine and tamoxifen can be tried
- In extreme cases, surgical excision of tender spots can be employed as the last resort.

Breast Lump

Breast lump is the most common concern that brings the patient to the physician. When a patient presents with a lump in her breast, the entire exercise of evaluating the lump is mostly centered on confirming or refuting a possible breast cancer. A painless lump, short history with rapid growth in a postmenopausal woman should be considered malignant unless proved otherwise. Such lumps are evaluated with mammogram, ultrasonogram and appropriate biopsy.

Nipple Discharge

Nipple discharge can be:
- Physiological or pathological
- Unilateral or bilateral
- From single duct or multiple ducts
- Bloody or non-bloody
- Spontaneous or self-induced.

Physiological nipple discharge can occur during pregnancy and lactation due to normal hormonal changes related to pregnancy and lactation. Hormone mediated pathological nipple discharge can occur in pituitary tumor (prolactinoma), hypothyroidism and drugs (antidepressants, antihypertensives, antidopaminergics). Bloody nipple discharge can be encountered in duct papilloma and breast cancer. Green or brownish discharge is common with duct ectasia. Depending upon the type of presentation, for a patient with nipple discharge, following option should be considered.

- Mammogram to look for malignancy
- TSH levels and prolactin levels in bilateral spontaneous milky discharge
- MRI of brain when prolactin levels are elevated
- Ductography, ductoscopy and excision of lactiferous ducts in instances of bloody discharge from single duct.

INVESTIGATIONS FOR BREAST DISEASES

Mammography

Mammogram is a very effective tool to evaluate breast lesions. Mammography can be screening mammography or diagnostic mammography. Screening mammography employs two views namely craniocaudal and mediolateral oblique. Diagnostic mammogram can make use of additional views like 90°–lateral view or spot compression view to obtain more information about the lesions. A mammogram takes into account asymmetry, shape of the lesion, margins, architectural distorsions and calcification patterns to evaluate the nature of then breast lesions.

The mammographic findings in breast lesions have been standardized in system termed "Breast Imaging Reporting and Database System", commonly abbreviated as BIRADS. Depending upon mammographic findings breast lesions have been categorized (Table 20.1). Although originally described for mammography, the scope of BIRADS has been widened to encompass ultrasonography and MRI findings as well.

Ultrasound Scan

Ultrasonography of breast or sonomammography complements conventional mammogram. It is of particular

Table 20.1: Mammographic findings in breast lesions.

Category	Findings	Recommendations
0	Need additional imaging evaluation	Additional imaging needed
1	Negative	Continue annual screening mammograms
2	Benign finding	Continue annual screening mammograms
3	Probably benign	Initial short-term follow-up (usually six month) mammogram (<2% chance of malignancy)
4	Suspicious abnormality	Biopsy should be considered (2%–95% chance of malignancy)
5	Highly suggestive of malignancy	Requires biopsy (>95% chance of malignancy)
6	Known cancer	Biopsy-proven malignancy

use in characterizing cystic lesions and various echogenic qualities of solid lesions. Ultrasonography can further aid in targeted fine needle aspiration cytology (FNAC) or aspiration of a breast cyst.

Magnetic Resonance Imaging

Magnetic resonance imaging (MRI) is off late a commonly used imaging modality for breast pathologies. MRI of the breast can be particularly helpful in the following situations.

- To evaluate patients who have undergone breast conservation surgery for breast cancer wherein MRI can be of immense value to discriminate scar from recurrence
- To assess the multifocality and multicentricity in a patient diagnosed with lobular breast cancer
- MRI can be helpful in assessing the extent of ductal carcinoma in situ
- MRI is the best investigation to image the breasts of women with implants
- MRI is a good screening tool for women belonging to high-risk category for breast cancer.

Fine Needle Aspiration Cytology

A 21 G or 23 G needle may be used to obtain cytological sample from a breast lesion or a suspicious area. Such a procedure is a minimally invasive modality and can be very accurate if the operator and the cytologist are well-experienced. The main limitations of FNAC in breast lesions are:

- A risk of false negative report
- Failure to differentiate in situ from invasive carcinoma.

Core Needle Biopsy

Here a reasonable amount of tissue can be sampled and a histological evaluation including hormone receptor assay is possible.

The combination of a meticulous clinical examination, appropriate breast imaging and cytological/histological assessment can establish the diagnosis of the breast disease in most cases. Such an assessment employing three pronged approach is termed "Triple assessment" for breast lesions.

COMMON BENIGN BREAST DISEASES

Aberrations of Normal Development and Involution

Breast is a dynamic organ. During various phases in the life of a woman, her breasts show different degrees of differentiation and involution. Thus, a spectrum of changes occur in breasts during a woman's lifetime. Mild exaggeration of such changes is termed "disorder". Severe exaggerations of these changes constitute "disease". Aberrations of normal development and involution (ANDI) can be more clearly explained in the following instances:

- During early reproductive phase of an woman, normally the breast shows lobular and stromal development. Mild exaggeration of such developments results in "disorders" like fibroadenoma and adolescent hypertrophy. Severe exaggeration of breast development results in diseases like giant fibroadenoma and gigantomastia.
- Similarly during reproductive phase and involution phase one can come across benign breast conditions like macrocysts, duct ectasia and incapacitating mastalgia which are nothing but exaggeration of normal phenomenon.

Fibrocystic Disorder

This entity has also been described as fibrocystic disease. It is more frequent in 30–50 years age group. These patients present with a "lumpy breast". One of the lumps may be "dominant". Every effort should be made in such cases to rule out an associated malignancy. After thorough evaluation, patient may be reassured of the benign nature of her ailment. Also most treatment options recommended for mastalgia can also be tried for fibrocystic disorder; none of them give consistent results.

Fibroadenoma

Fibroadenomas are benign lesions comprising of both epithelial and stromal components derived from terminal duct lobular unit (TDLU). They have been considered as a type of ANDI. Although, they can occur in any age group, they are somewhat common in the age group of 20–40 years. Clinically they are discrete, small (usually less than 3 cms), mobile, firm to hard lumps. On ultrasound scan they are seen as lobulated wider than tall masses. The diagnosis can be established by core needle biopsy. They can be left alone if small. Larger fibroadenomas and those showing rapid growth can be enucleated. Fibroadenomas larger than 6 cms are termed "giant fibroadenomas" which need to be distinguished from phyllodes tumor.

Phyllodes Tumor

Phyllodes tumor have clinical features similar to larger fibroadenomas. They are differentiated from fibroadenomas by their rapid growth and larger size. These tumors may be benign, borderline or malignant. Malignant phyllodes tumor behaves like sarcomas and have propensity for hematogenous spread, commonly to lungs. Even benign phyllodes tumors can be troublesome because of their high tendency for recurrences. Hence, they are excised with a margin of at least 1 cm. If obtaining 1 cm margin is difficult because of a large tumor, simple mastectomy is acceptable option.

Duct Ectasia

It is benign condition characterized by shortening and dilatation of the lactiferous ducts. The affected patients present with nipple discharge, "slit-like" nipple retraction or occasionally a lump. The condition is mostly otherwise asymptomatic, usually self-limiting and does not require surgery.

Periductal Mastitis

It is a type of non-lactational mastitis. It is more common among young women who smoke. This condition is thought to be due to alteration in bacterial flora and accumulation of toxic metabolites in lactiferous ducts among smokers. This condition needs antibiotic therapy with aspiration or surgical drainage of pus if present.

BREAST CANCER

The Chapter on breast disease is grossly incomplete without a note on breast cancer. However, a detailed account of breast cancer is beyond the scope of this chapter. Enthusiastic readers are requested to refer appropriate literature to learn more about the same, some of which have been quoted in list of references. The entire clinical discussion of a patient with breast symptoms can be summarized to either confirming or refuting the possibility of breast cancer. As a primary physician who is the first medical professional evaluating the patient, the gynecologist should be aware of the following aspects of breast cancer.

Risk Factors for Breast Cancer

Risk factors for breast cancer may be categorized as, hormonal risk factors and non-hormonal risk factors. Any factor which increases the exposure of breast to estrogen increases the risk of breast cancer. Conversely those factors which are associated with reduction in exposure of breast to estrogen reduce the risk of breast cancer. Thus, early menarche, late menopause and older age at first live birth increase the risk for breast cancer. Late menarche, early menopause and multiparity reduce the risk of breast cancer. Exercise and longer lactation period offer protection against breast cancer. Exposure to radiation, obesity and alcohol consumption increases the risk for breast cancer.

BRCA Mutations

BRCA 1 gene is located on chromosome arm 17q. *BRCA 2* is located on chromosome 13q. BRCA mutations are associated with hereditary breast and ovarian cancers. It is important to remember that eliciting history of breast or ovarian cancer in first, second or third degree relative from both paternal and maternal sides is essential to suspect possible BRCA mutations. Such information is particularly relevant in early onset breast and ovarian cancer. Consulting genetic counselor for further testing goes a long way in taking appropriate measures for early detection or prevention of breast cancer.

Screening for Breast Cancer

Table 20.2 shows screening recommendations for breast cancer by various organizations.

Breast Cancer in Pregnancy

Pregnancy-associated breast cancer (PABC) is defines as breast cancer occurring durig pregnancy or within 1 year following child birth. Breast cancer is one of the commonest cancers occurring during pregnancy. With the trend of increasing age at child birth the incidence of breast cancer in pregnancy is also on the rise. Diagnosis of breast cancer is particularly difficult in pregnancy. This is because the physiological changes in breast during pregnancy like hypertrophy, engorgement, nodularity and nipple discharge may camouflage the cancer rendering clinical diagnosis a serious challenge. The obstetrician being the primary physician evaluating such a patient should have a very high degree of suspicion and low threshold to consider the patient for imaging and cytopathological studies. With adequate abdominal shielding the risk of radiation exposure to fetus can be significantly reduced. Ultrasound scan can complement mammography and can provide valuable information on primary tumor as well as regional lymph nodes.

Table 20.2: Screening recommendations for breast cancer by various organization.

Organization	Breast self-examination (BSE)	Clinical breast examination (CBE)	Mammography
American College of Obstetricians and Gynecologists	Consider for high-risk patients	For 20–39 years—every 1–3 years For 40 years and older—annually	Aged 40 year and older annually
American Cancer Society	Optional for those aged 20 years and older	For 20–39 years—every 1–3 years For 40 years and older annually	Aged 40 year and older annually
National Comprehensive Cancer Network (NCCN)	Recommended	For 20–39 years—every 1–3 years For 40 years and older—annually	Aged 40 year and older annually

Treatment of breast cancer during pregnancy should be individualized and should concur as far as possible with the guidelines recommended for non-pregnant patients. If diagnosed in first trimester the patient may be offered the option of termination of pregnancy. However, the decision to terminate the pregnancy is a personal one and should be considered keeping in mind the risks for the fetus arising from treatment of cancer and the ability to care for the baby in the background of stress of breast cancer treatment. While surgical and chemotherapeutic options can be considered with reasonable safety from second trimester onwards, radiotherapy is deferred till the completion of pregnancy. Although, all the usually practiced surgical procedures for breast cancer can be considered in pregnancy, mastectomy has slight advantage of not requiring immediate adjuvant radiotherapy. Anthracycline and taxane-based chemotherapy can be reasonably safe from second trimester onwards. Hormonal manipulation with tamoxifen and selective estrogen receptor modulators are deferred till completion of pregnancy. Use of trastuzumab in HER-2-neu positive patients is contraindicated during pregnancy.

When compared stage to stage the outcome of breast cancer in pregnancy is not significantly different from non-pregnant patients. Rather than pregnancy per se the delay in diagnosis and initiation of treatment might adversely affect the outcome of the disease.

BREAST PROBLEMS IN PREGNANCY AND LACTATION

Acute Mastitis and Lactational Breast Abscess

Edematous epithelium or casein milk precipitate blocks the nipple pore. Such a block may be seen as a "white spot". This can result in pain due to cramping of duct or contraction of myoepithelial units. A worse eventuality is milk stasis progressing on to mastitis or breast abscess. Sore nipple, cracked nipple and superficial skin infection in the region of nipple areola complex results in staphylococcal colonization. This could progress on to cellulitis, mastitis and breast abscess. Continued milk synthesis combined with inadequate drainage will lead to stasis. Secondary bacterial infection of the pent up milk will result in mastitis and subsequent breast abscess.

An ultrasound scan of the affected breast complemented with needle aspiration under local anesthesia is the most useful investigation. Analysis of the aspirate can differentiate mastitis, breast abscess, galactocele and the very rare possibility of inflammatory breast cancer.

Acute mastitis may be treated with appropriate antibiotics. Antibiotics like ampicillin, amoxicillin which are effective against *Staphylococcus* and *Streptococcus* are commonly used. Erythema, tenderness and fluctuant lump are features of breast abscess. While most breast abscesses can be managed by ultrasound image-guided aspiration, surgical drainage is often required in a multiloculated breast abscess. Occasionally, the causative organism may be highly virulent methicillin resistant *Staphylococcus* which requires treatment with reserve antibiotics like linezolid. An important aspect of management of management of infectious conditions in a lactating breast is regular emptying of breast using a suction pump.

Galactocele

A galactocele is collection of milk in an obstructed lactiferous duct which gets dilated. It may be found in lactating women or women with recent history of lactation. It may mimic malignancy, particularly in the older child bearing women. Therefore, every effort should be made to rule out malignancy. Simple aspiration can be both diagnostic and therapeutic.

BIBLIOGRAPHY

1. A companion to specialist surgical practice. In: Dixon JM (ed). 5th edn. Elsvier; 2014.
2. ACS Surgery 7/editorial chair, Stanley W. Wshley; associate editors, William G. Cance, et. al. 2014. Decker Intellectual Properties, Inc.
3. Schwartz's Principles of Surgery/editor-in-chief, F. Charles Brunicardi; associate editors, Dana K. Anderson….et al. 9th edition. The McGraw-Hill Companies, Inc.

CHAPTER 21

Instruments Used in Obstetrics and Gynecology

Rajesh Bhakta

Overview

☐ Route instruments used in Obstetrics and Gynecology is explained with the indications, complications.

SIM'S VAGINAL SPECULUM

This instrument is a bivalve speculum with groove. One end is smaller than the other. A trough runs along the entire length of the instrument so that secretions or blood collecting in the concave blade drain off along the trough (Fig. 21.1).

Uses
- For exposing and inspecting the vaginal wall and cervix
- For collecting discharge from vagina and cervix for microscopy
- Used in dilatation and curettage, fractional curettage, intrauterine contraceptive device (IUCD) insertions, etc.
- To detect vesicovaginal fistula, vaginal wall prolapse like cystocele, enterocele, etc.

CUSCO'S VAGINAL SPECULUM

This instrument has two blades hinged so that they can open and close around a transverse axis, which can be opened out and adjusted to the size of the vagina by means of the screw hence, it is self-retaining (Fig. 21.2).

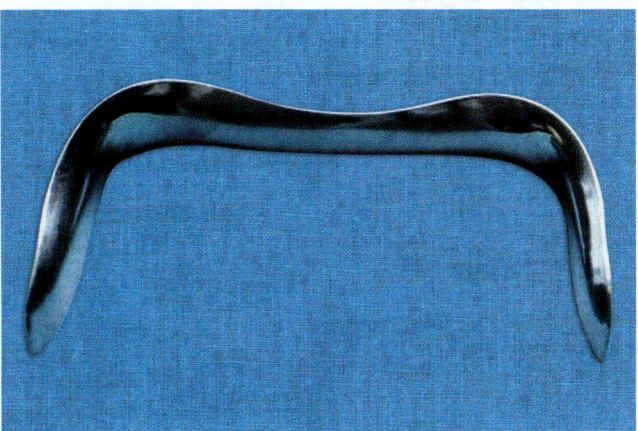

Fig. 21.1: Sim's vaginal speculum.

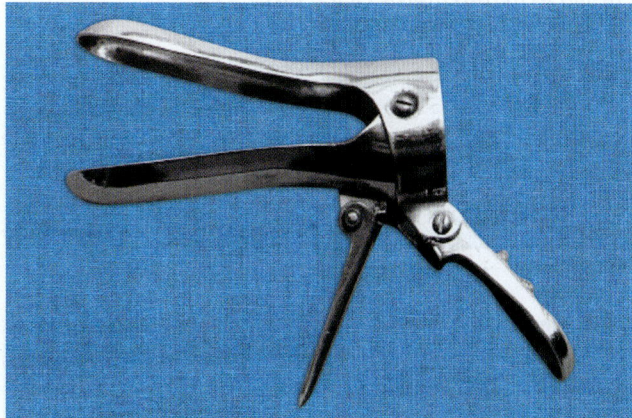

Fig. 21.2: Cusco's vaginal speculum.

Uses

- Inspection of vagina and cervix
- Useful in Pap smear, cervical biopsy, high vaginal swab, etc.

Advantages

- It is self-retaining.
- Gives good exposure as it can be adjusted to the size of the vagina.

Disadvantage

Though, the exposure of the vagina and cervix is good, the space available to carry out the procedure is limited by the rim of the instrument at the introitus.

SIM'S ANTERIOR VAGINAL WALL RETRACTOR

This instrument has loop shaped ends with transverse serrations on either surface. The loops make an angle of 15° with the shaft and are angled in opposite directions (Fig. 21.3).

Uses

- To retract the lax vaginal wall to expose the cervix along with Sim's speculum
- To visualize cervix, cystocele, any growth on vagina
- To visualize site of fistula like vesicovaginal fistula, etc.

UTERINE SOUND

This instrument is long about 30 cm with rounded tip. There may be markings on the back side which may be in centimeter or inches. The uterine end is angulated and curved to fit into uterus (Fig. 21.4).

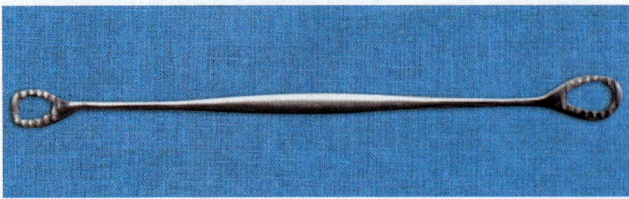

Fig. 21.3: Anterior vaginal retractor.

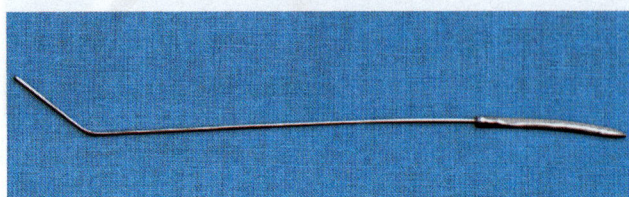

Fig. 21.4: Uterine sound.

Uses

Diagnostic

- To determine the uterocervical length, position of the uterus
- In diagnosis of cervical elongation
- To determine the location of the displaced intrauterine contraceptive device (IUCD) by doing an X-ray with sound in situ in the lateral plane
- To diagnose cervical stenosis.

Therapeutic

- To drain pyometra in case of carcinoma cervix/endometrium
- Asherman's syndrome to remove adhesions.

Complications

Perforation of uterus causing bleeding and infection of the peritoneal cavity.

VULSELLUM FORCEPS

This instrument has multiple sharp teeth at the end which when locked gives a firm grip on the cervix. Usually 20 cm in length, may be curved or straight (Fig. 21.5).

Uses

- To grasp or hold the anterior or posterior lip of the cervix in operations.
- To steady the cervix to get firm grip on cervix as to any instrument inside the uterus during procedure like dilatation and curettage.

Disadvantages

- Discomfort or pain
- Trauma to cervix especially in pregnancy.

TENACULUM

Long handle with one sharp point on each blade of the forceps. It causes least injury to cervix. It is applied by catching the anterior lip of the cervix transversely (Fig. 21.6).

Use

- To hold cervix in nulliparous women

Complications

- Discomfort or pain
- Bleeding rarely.

CHAPTER 21 Instruments Used in Obstetrics and Gynecology

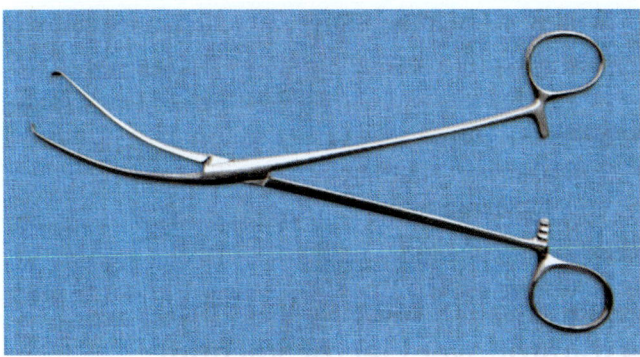

Fig. 21.5: Vulsellum forceps.

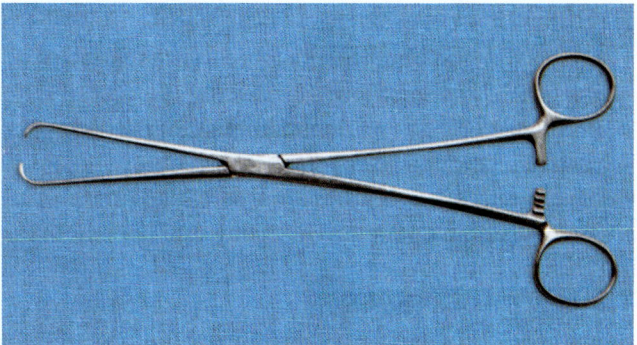

Fig. 21.6: Tenaculum.

CERVICAL DILATORS

Hegar's Dilator

They are double ended or single ended metal dilators with a suitable curve for the uterocervical canal in pregnant uterus. They are supplied with a set available in gradually increasing numbers (Fig. 21.7).

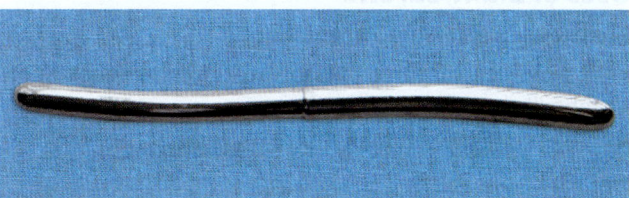

Fig. 21.7: Hegar's dilator.

Uses

Used mainly for the obstetrical indications:
- To dilate the internal os of cervix in cases of abortion or in medical termination of the pregnancy for suction and evacuation
- To dilate the cervix during the elective cesarean section for the draining of lochia
- To diagnose the incompetent cervical os by passing the number 8 dilator in a non gravid uterus.

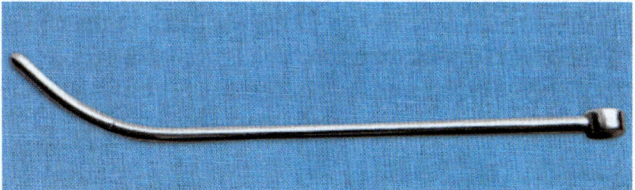

Fig. 21.8: Mathew-Duncan dilator.

Mathew-Duncan Dilator

They are single ended metal dilators used for dilatation in cases of gynecological condition. They are angled at a point 2.5 inches from the tip indicating the normal length of the uterocervical canal (Fig. 21.8).

Uses

Used mainly in the gynecological condition:
- As a preliminary to any intrauterine operations like endometrial curettage, removal of polyp, hysteroscopy, etc.
- To establish drainage in pyometra.

Complications

- Perforation—commonest site of perforation is in lateral wall of internal os on the posterior part. Next common site is fundus of the uterus
- Cervical incompetence.

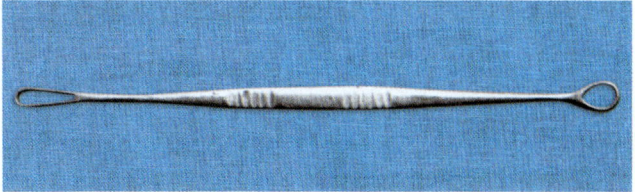

Fig. 21.9: Sim's double ended uterine curette.

UTERINE CURETTE

Sim's Double Ended Uterine Curette

The ends of the curette may be blunt and sharp or both ends sharp or both blunt. The loops are of various sizes: small, medium, large (Fig. 21.9).

Uses of Sharp Curette

Used for gynecological conditions for both diagnostic and therapeutic purposes.

SECTION 1 — General Gynecology

Diagnostic Conditions
- In dysfunctional uterine bleeding (DUB) for histopathology of endometrium
- In suspected cases of tuberculous endometritis
- In patients with postmenopausal bleeding
- Suspected cases of endometrial carcinoma
- Before certain operations like Fothergill's operation.

Therapeutic Conditions
In patients with DUB where bleeding is profuse and not responding to hormones.

Uses of Blunt Curette
Mainly used in obstetrical conditions:
- To curette retained bits of products in incomplete abortion
- To curette the retained bits of placenta.

SUCTION CANNULA
The cannula is made up of metal or plastic. Usually 25 cm long, has a round tip with two subterminal openings. Its proximal end is grooved for fitting the rubber tube which connects it to the vacuum source. It is available in different sizes ranging from 4 mm to 12 mm and the size indicates the external diameter of the cannula in millimeters (Fig. 21.10).

Uses
- For suction evacuation after cervical dilatation in case of first trimester medical termination pregnancy
- Completion of incomplete abortions during the first trimester termination of pregnancy
- Used for suction evacuation of vesicular mole.

Complications
- Uterine perforation and its complications
- Hemorrhage from incomplete evacuation
- Infection.

MANUAL VACUUM ASPIRATOR
Manual vacuum aspiration is a method of uterine evacuation that involves use of hand-held plastic aspirator providing a vacuum source attached to a cannula (Fig. 21.11).

Uses
- First trimester abortion
- Incomplete abortion
- Endometrial biopsy.

Advantage of Manual Vacuum Aspirator over Electric Vacuum Aspirator and D and C
- Low cost and does not require electricity
- Less cervical dilatation and less pain
- Fewer incidences of complications like perforation.

AYER'S SPATULA
Spatula made up of wood or plastic is so shaped that one end rounded and the other end used for scraping squamocolumnar junction. The blunt round end is used to take a high lateral vaginal wall scrape and the other portion of the one end will fit into the external os. The endocervical brush is also used along for collection of cells for cytology screening (Fig. 21.12).

Uses
- To take smear directly from the cervix or Pap smear (surface biopsy)
- For screening of carcinoma cervix.

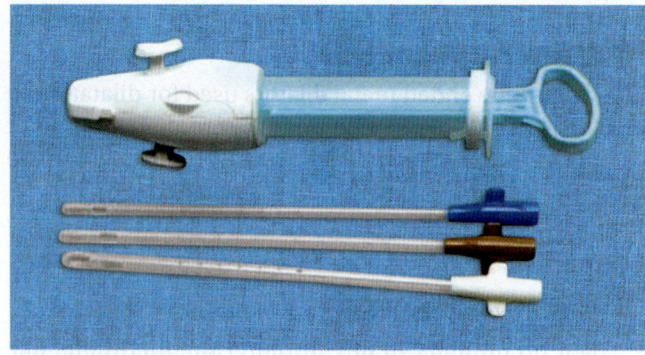

Fig. 21.11: Manual vacuum aspirator.

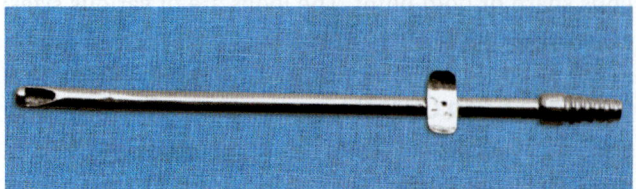

Fig. 21.10: Suction cannula.

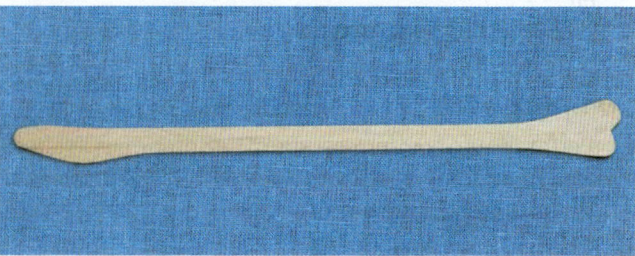

Fig. 21.12: Ayer's spatula.

PUNCH BIOPSY FORCEPS

This instrument is curved and 27.5 cm long with the end so shaped that a small bit of tissue can be removed or punched out (Fig. 21.13).

Uses
- Used to take the biopsy from the cervix, vulva, vagina, etc.
- The site of the biopsy is either suspected are or after applying iodine or colposcopic guided or if there is growth then from the edge of the growth.

ENDOMETRIAL BIOPSY CURETTE

This instrument is 23 cm long, with external diameter of 2 mm, tubular and curved near the tip to facilitate entry into the endometrial cavity. It has subterminal opening with a sharp edge (with four notches in succession) in its distal part such that during withdrawal of the instrument pressing against the uterine wall a strip of endometrium will be removed (Fig. 21.14).

Indication of Use
Endometrial biopsy in detecting the hormonal pattern of endometrium in DUB, diagnosis of anovulation, corpus luteal deficiency.

Disadvantage
Endometrial biopsy is not adequate for the diagnosis of endometrial tuberculosis or carcinoma because the strip of the endometrium removed may not be representative of the entire endometrium.

Advantage
Procedure can be carried out as an OP basis and does not require anesthesia or dilatation of the cervix.

RED RUBBER CATHETER

It is made up of India rubber. It is a soft rubber tubing with a solid distal end beyond the eye for easy introduction (Fig. 21.15).

Indications
- Urinary retention during pregnancy, labor, puerperium
- Prior to application of the forceps or vacuum
- Used as a tourniquet during myomectomy
- Nasopharyngeal or oropharyngeal suctioning in eclampsia.

FOLEY'S CATHETER

This is a self-retaining urinary catheter made up of latex rubber. The catheter has two channels, a channel for drainage of urine and one for inflating the subterminal bulb which makes the catheter self-retaining (Fig. 21.16).

Indications
Obstetrics
- Retroverted gravid uterus with retention of urine
- Whenever monitoring the urine output in cases like eclampsia, abruptio, cesarean section, etc.
- Cord prolapse where the bladder is inflated so that the presenting part is displaced up to relieve the compression of the cord.
- In method of induction of labor as a cervical ripening agent

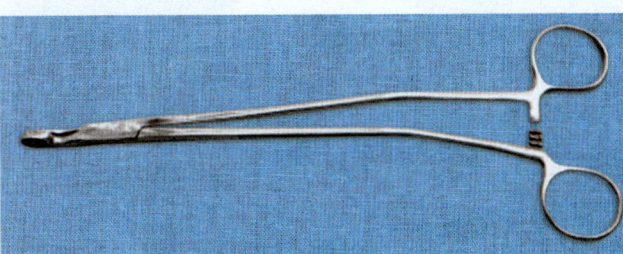

Fig. 21.13: Punch biopsy forceps.

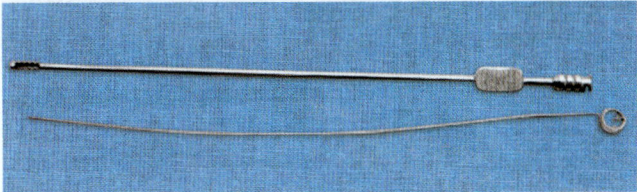

Fig. 21.14: Endometrial biopsy curette.

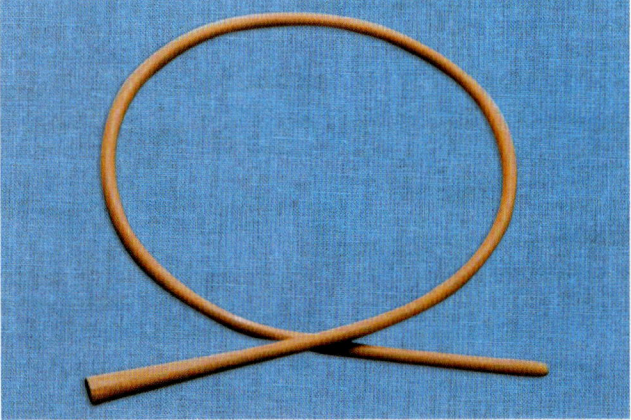

Fig. 21.15: Red rubber catheter.

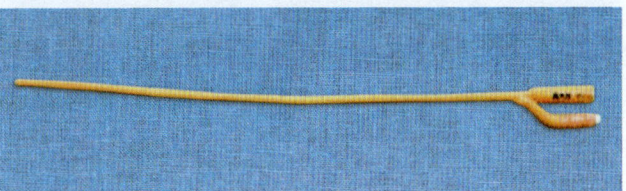

Fig. 21.16: Foley's catheter.

SECTION 1 General Gynecology

- Induction of 2nd trimester abortion
- In atonic postpartum hemorrhage to enhance uterine contraction and retraction.

Gynecology

Following gynecological operations:
- Surgery on uterovaginal prolapse—3 days.
- Abdominal hysterectomy—24 hours.
- Vesicovaginal fistula repair—7 days.
- Wertheim's operation—14 days.
- Repair of bladder injury—7 days.
- Tubal patency test like laparoscopic chromopertubation or hysterosalpingography pediatric Foley's catheter (No. 8 F) is used to push the dye.

Complications

Urinary tract infection.

LEECH WILKINSON'S CANNULA

This instrument is 28 cm long with a fixed spiral cone at one end and a luer-lock mount at the other. The cannula is put at the external os after exposing the cervix using the Sim's speculum. It is rotated clockwise so that its tip advances in the cervical canal and cannula gets fixed in the cervix. The spiral cone achieves airtight fit and prevents leak of any dye back into the vagina (Fig. 21.17).

Indications for Use

- Hysterosalpingography (HSG)
- Chromopertubation during laparoscopy.

SHIRODKAR'S HOOK

This instrument is shaped somewhat like a uterine sound but has a hook at its end (Fig. 21.18).

Uses

It is used for removing intrauterine contraceptive device in which the thread is missing or removing the intratubal prosthesis inserted at the time of cornual implantation of the fallopian tube.

PESSARY (HODGE, SMITH OR RING PESSARY)

Smith-Hodge Pessary

It has a double curve with its lower end is either flattened or square. Its upper end is much broader than the lower end.

Ring Pessary

It is made up of plastic or rubber, may be solid or hollow (Fig. 21.19).

Indications

Temporary correction of uterine prolapse in following situations:
- To allow decubitus ulcer on the cervix to heal before the corrective surgery
- Uterine prolapse during pregnancy
- As a part of pessary test.

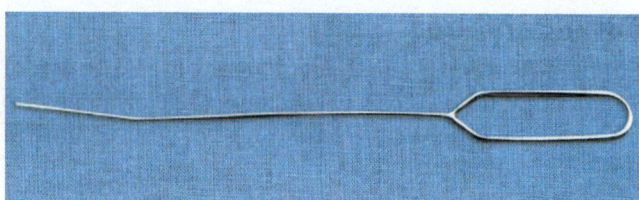

Fig. 21.18: Shirodkar's hook.

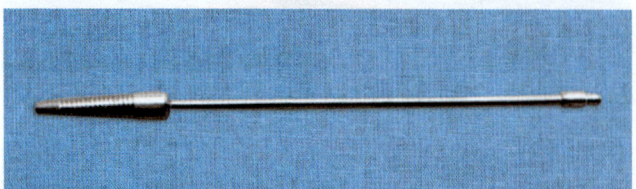

Fig. 21.17: Leech Wilkinson's cannula.

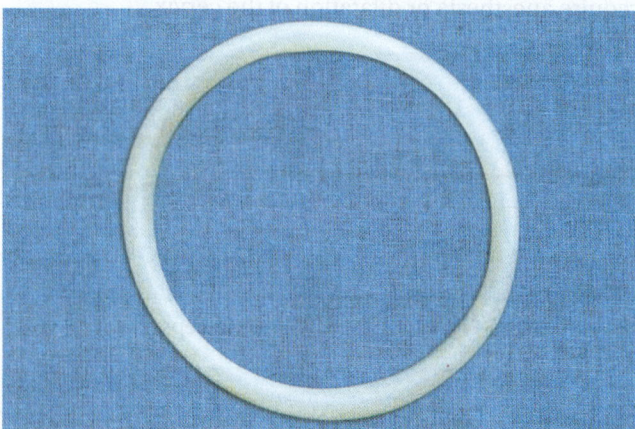

Fig. 21.19: Ring pessary.

Complications of Pessary

- Vagintis
- Vaginal ulceration
- Hemorrhage from the ulcerated vagina
- Granulations in the vagina causing leukorrhea
- Vesicovaginal or rectovaginal fistula with prolonged use.

DOYEN'S RETRACTOR

This instrument is made up of steel with a curved blade with depth and a uniform curvature with a handle. The broad retracting surface achieves good retraction. The solid blade compresses the cut edges of the abdominal wall and achieves a reduction in the blood loss from the injured vessel (Fig. 21.20).

Indications

- Used for retraction of the abdominal wall suprapubically during the abdominal operations like cesarean section, hysterectomy, etc.
- Also used to retract the bladder during the lower segment cesarean section.

RICHARDSON'S TETRACTOR

This retractor has an L-shaped blade. Its bent portion has a shallow curve, concave outwards. The blade is long which makes it suitable for retraction at the depth.

Uses

It is best suited for the retraction of the bladder away from the cervix and vagina during abdominal hysterectomy.

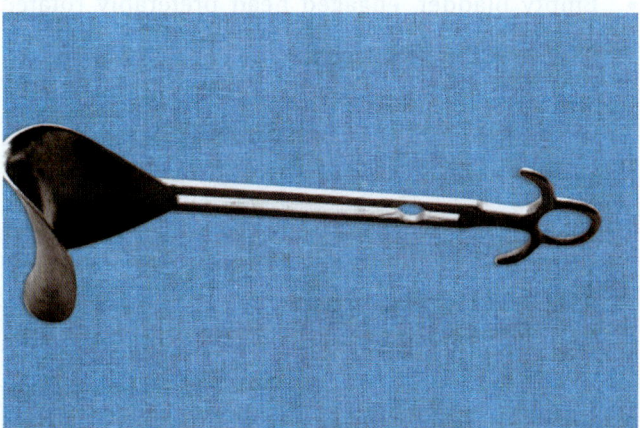

Fig. 21.20: Doyen's retractor.

EPISIOTOMY SCISSORS

These scissors have angled blades. Its angle makes it convenient to use to prevent handle to put against the patient's buttock. Episiotomy is given when the head is crowning. Episiotomy widens and shortens the birth canal (Fig. 21.21).

UMBILICAL CORD CUTTING SCISSOR

This instrument is 10.5 cm long. The blades are broad and curved and on closing they meet at their tips leaving gap in between. This ensures a firm grip on the umbilical cord when the cord is being cut (Fig. 21.22).

KOCHER'S ARTERY FORCEPS

This instrument may be straight or curved, has a single tooth at the tip hence ensures firm grip. It is used for grasping and crushing the pedicle containing vessels during the abdominal and vaginal operations (Fig. 21.23).

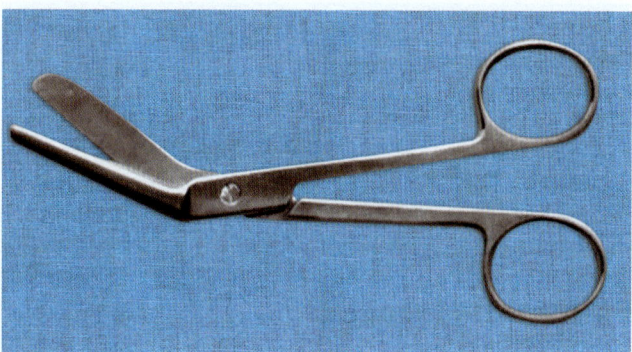

Fig. 21.21: Episiotomy scissor.

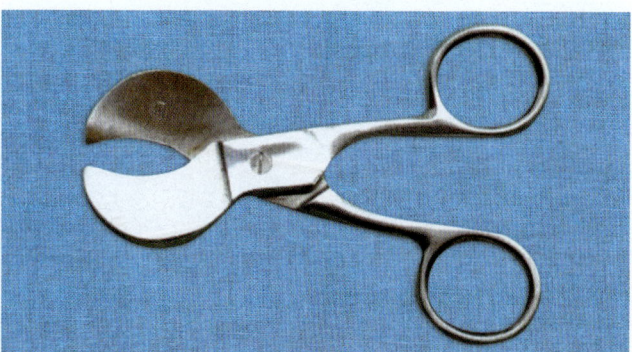

Fig. 21.22: Umbilical cord cutting scissor.

SECTION 1 General Gynecology

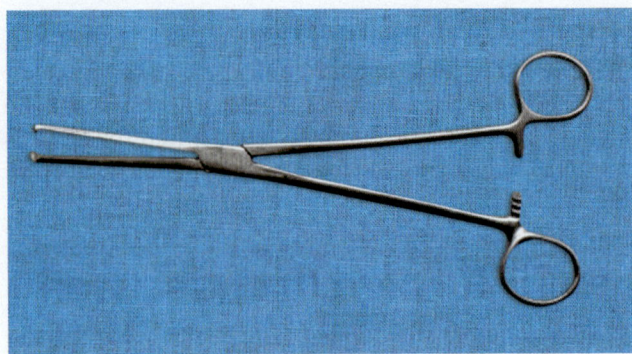

Fig. 21.23: Kocher's artery forceps.

Uses
For clamping the pedicles during the hysterectomy.

GREEN-ARMYTAGE'S FORCEPS
This instrument has triangular tips used for grasping the edges of the uterine incision. A ratchet lock makes the grip firmer (Fig. 21.24).

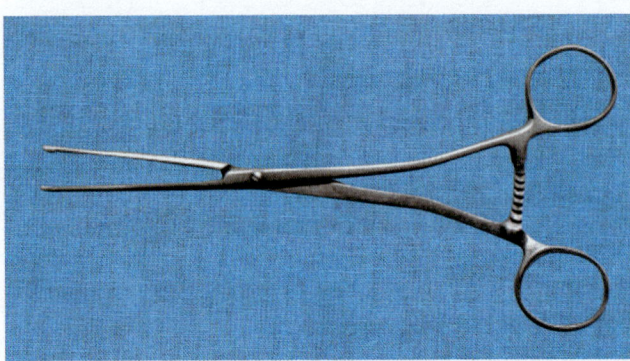

Fig. 21.24: Green-Armytage's forceps.

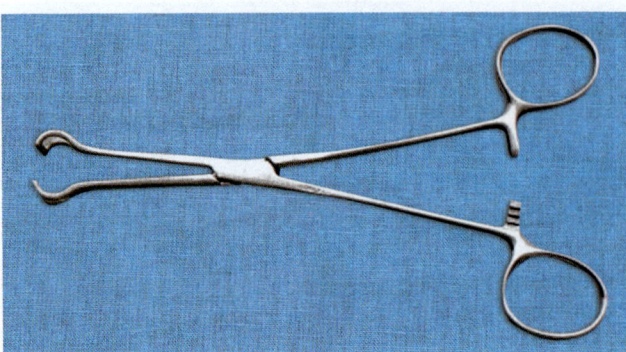

Fig. 21.25: Babcock's forceps.

Uses
It is used as a hemostatic for controlling multiple bleeding points during the cesarean section from the cut edges of uterine incision without damaging the uterine wall.

It may be used instead of sponge holding forceps to trace the cervix for cervical tear.

BABCOCK'S FORCEPS
This forceps is 15–25 cm long, with fenestrated triangular-shaped blades and grooved jaws. They ensure firm grip on the tube without crushing or damaging its blood supply and mucosa (Fig. 21.25).

Uses
- To hold or fix the hold fallopian tube, in operations like tubectomy, tuboplasty.
- For handling the appendix, intestine, ureters, etc.

FORCEPS
Is an instrument designed to assist and expedite delivery of the fetal head. Consist of two metallic halves that articulate with each other at lock. Each halve consists of blade, shank, lock, handle (Fig. 21.26).

Prerequisites for Outlet Forceps Application
- **F**ully dilated and effaced cervix
- **O**ccipitoanterior position
- **R**upture of membranes
- **C**ephalopelvic disproportion should be ruled out
- **E**mpty bladder, engaged head preferably rotated completely

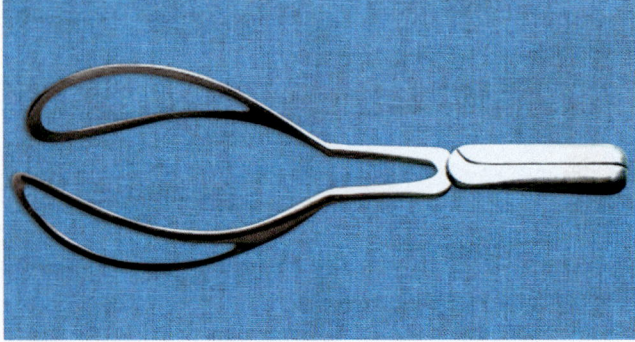

Fig. 21.26: Forceps.

- **P**osition is ideally occipitoanterior
- **S**tation of the head at + 3.

Indications of the Forceps
Fetal Indications
- Fetal distress in second stage if no contraindication for vaginal delivery
- After coming head of breech
- Low-birth weight baby/preterm babies.

Maternal Indications
- Heart disease complicating pregnancy
- Previous cesarean pregnancy
- Severe preeclampsia.

Labor
- Delay in the second stage due to uterine inertia.

Complications
Maternal
- Extension of the episiotomy to involve rectum or towards vault
- Vaginal lacerations
- Postpartum hemorrhage
- Pelvic hematoma.

Fetal
- Intracranial hemorrhage due to over compression of the fetal head
- Cephal hematoma
- Fracture skull
- Facial palsy
- Abrasion of the soft tissue of the face or scalp by the blade of the forceps.

VACUUM DELIVERY (VENTOUSE)
The vacuum extractor has been designed to assist the delivery by applying traction to a suction cup attached to the fetal scalp. The original metal cups have undergone many modifications and softer, less traumatic and safer, Silastic cups have been made available. This has made vacuum very useful especially when the station of the head is high and not well-rotated and deflexed.

MALMSTROM CUP
Cup is made up of stainless steel. Cup has flattened hemisphere whose margins are incurved so that the diameter at the rim is materially smaller than the greatest diameter of the cup. The cup is available in four sizes 30, 40, 50, 60 in diameter (Fig. 21.27).

VACUUM EXTRACTOR
Equipment consists of vacuum pump, vacuum bottle with a pressure gauge, rubber tube to connect vacuum bottle to the pump, traction handle.

Indications for the Ventouse
Refer indications for forceps above.

Contraindications for Ventouse
- Premature babies
- Cephalopelvic disproportion
- Breech and face presentation
- Station of the head above zero
- Intrauterine fetal death
- Lack of expertise in the procedure.

Prerequisites
Refer prerequisites of forceps above.

SPONGE HOLDING FORCEPS
This forceps is 22.5 cm long, straight and has ring shaped tip which is serrated, with a lock (Fig. 21.28).

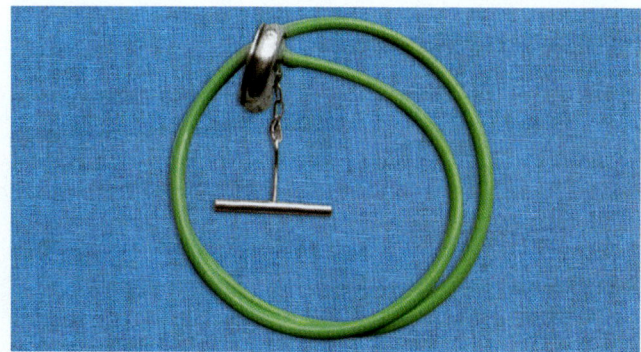

Fig. 21.27: Malmstrom cup.

SECTION 1 *General Gynecology*

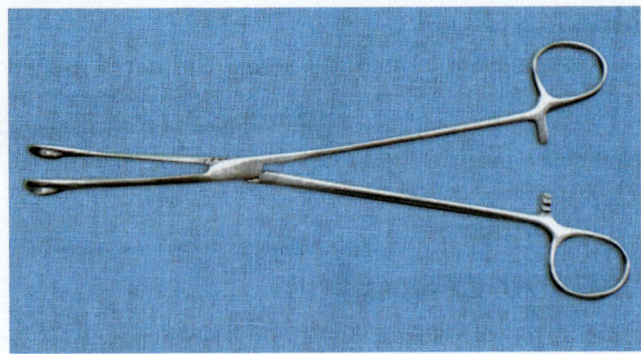

Fig. 21.28: Sponge holding forceps.

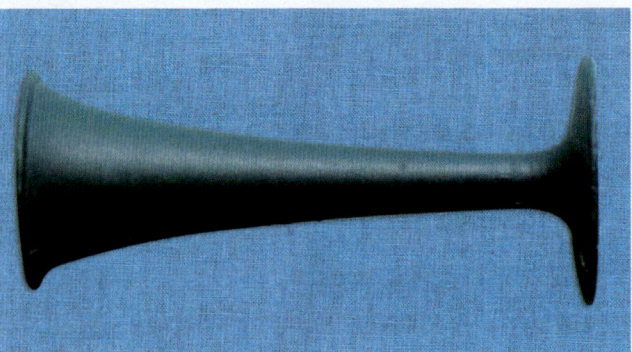

Fig. 21.29: Pinard's fetal stethoscope.

Uses
- For holding sponge to swab-out cavities like vagina
- For painting antiseptic over abdomen, vagina and clean the parts for asepsis
- For grasping cervix in cases of obstetrical conditions.

Used as a sponge stick to push/mobilize the bladder down during the abdominal hysterectomy.

PINARD'S FETAL STETHOSCOPE

It is funnel shaped and has a broad flat disc with a central perforation attached at the narrow end of the funnel at the right angles to the long axis of the funnel (Fig. 21.29).

Indications

Used to hear fetal heart sounds in the antenatal and intranatal period.

LAMINERIA TENT

It is stem of a sea weed which is dried and compressed measuring about 5.5–6 cm long. It is used as a slow dilator of the cervix as it swells up due to hygroscopic action (absorbs water). Usually more than one tent is introduced to prevent dumbling of the end. Commonly three sizes are available—small (3–5 mm), medium (5–7mm), large (>7 mm).

CHAPTER 22

Ultrasound and Color Doppler in Gynecology

Neharika Malhotra Bora, Rishabh Bora, Narendra Malhotra, Jaideep Malhotra, Sonal Panchal

Overview

- The 3D ultrasound offers a clear additional benefit for accuracy of gynecological anatomical scanning. 3D TVS probes give sculpture like pictures of the uterus, endometrial cavity and ovaries.
- Volume estimation of a lesion is important and tumor volume is most prognostic, this is possible by VOCAL software in 3D machines.
- Today advancement in 3-D technology and in 3D PD vascular studies is occurring at a very rapid pace and it is estimated the modality of choice for gynecological imaging for the future is and will be three-dimensional ultrasound.
- Transvaginal ultrasound is a very good, reliable, reproducible, easy, safe method to evaluate the female pelvis and very accurate for gynecological diagnosis.

ULTRASONOGRAPHY IN GYNECOLOGY

High-resolution transvaginal sonography (TVS) has been widely available since mid 1980 and has gained acceptance as an integral part of gynecologic and easily obstetric sonographic examinations. In many ultrasound laboratories, the standard examination of female pelvis consists of transvesical-transabdominal (TAS) combined with TVS and in some cases, transvaginal color flow Doppler (TVCFD) (Figs. 22.1 and 22.2).

Patient need not be fasting unless an upper abdomen scan is also asked for. TAS is performed first which provides a wider field for view and overview of pelvic organs. For a TVS, patient is asked to void immediately before examination. The transvaginal approach by passes attenuating tissue

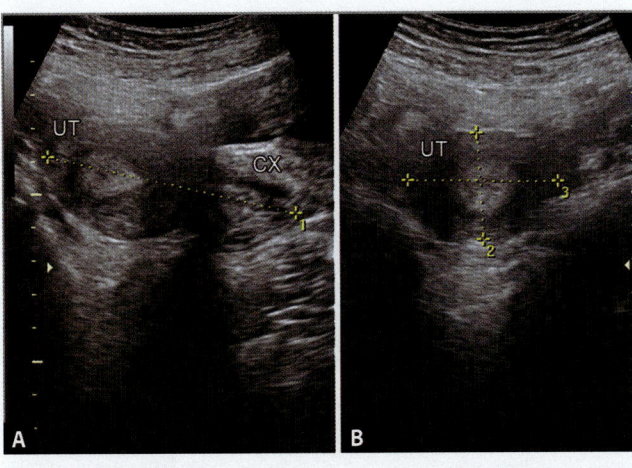

Figs. 22.1A and B: Transabdominal scan shows the uterus as a pear-shaped structure on (A) longitudinal scan and (B) transverse scan.

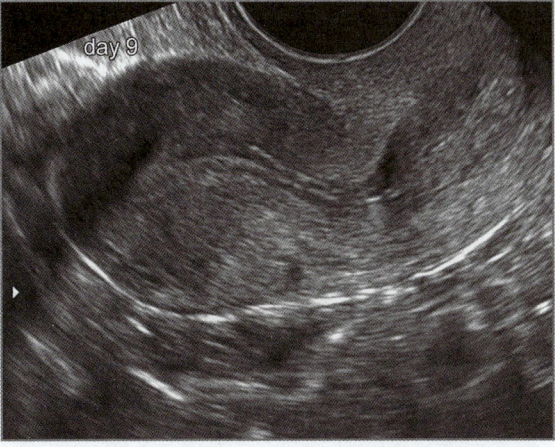

Fig. 22.2: Transvaginal scan shows the anteverted uterus. Triple layered endometrium is well seen.

and allows a high frequency probe to be placed close to 'target organs'. Scanning is performed with patient supine, thighs abducted and knees flexed. Probe is covered with a condom or sheath containing small amount of gel. Probe is inserted gently with slight push towards rectum. Four types of probe movements are required: (i) Pushing and pulling, (ii) Rotation, (iii) Rocking or upwards and downwards, (iv) Side-to-side or 'Panning'. Today fingertip and finger-cap probes are also available. TVS probe may be disinfected by Cidex.

NORMAL FEMALE PELVIS

Female pelvis consists of true and false pelvis. Female genital organs lie within true pelvis (Fig. 22.3).

UTERUS

It is a pear-like organ between urinary bladder anteriorly and rectosigmoid posteriorly. It consists of two major parts: the body or corpus and the cervix. Isthmus separates the body and cervix.[1] Fundus of the uterus is the superior portion of the uterus between the insertion of the tubes (Fig. 22.4).

The ratio of the length of body and cervix varies with age. Before menarche, the corpus is approximately one-half the length of cervix; in nulliparous women, the corpus and cervix are of approximately equal length, and in multiparous women, the corpus is about twice the length of the cervix.

Uterus measures about 8 × 4 × 4 cm in childbearing age, which increases by about 1 cm in multiparous women. After menopause uterus atrophies.[2]

Uterus consists of: (i) Myometrium: It is homogenous in echotexture with smooth margins. (ii) Endometrium: It is seen as a hyperechoic band in the center of the uterus. The total thickness of it represents the anterior and posterior opposed layers. Normal endometrial thickness and appearance varies with phase of menstrual cycle. Endometrial fluid when present should not be included in the measurement (Fig. 22.5).

OVARIES

Ovaries are ellipsoidal; position is variable especially in multiparous women. In nulliparous female, ovaries are situated in the ovaries fossa (also known as fossa of Waldeyer).[3] The ovarian fossa is situated on the lateral pelvic wall and is bounded anteriorly by the obliterated umbilical artery, ureter and internal iliac artery posteriorly and the external iliac vein superiorly (Fig. 22.6).

Ovaries in girls younger than 2 years of age are typically less than 1 mL in volume. After menarche, ovaries generally measure 30 × 20 × 20 mm (Fig. 22.7).

FOLLICULOGENESIS

In proliferative phase of menstrual cycle, multiple small follicles 10 mm in diameter are seen. A dominant follicle

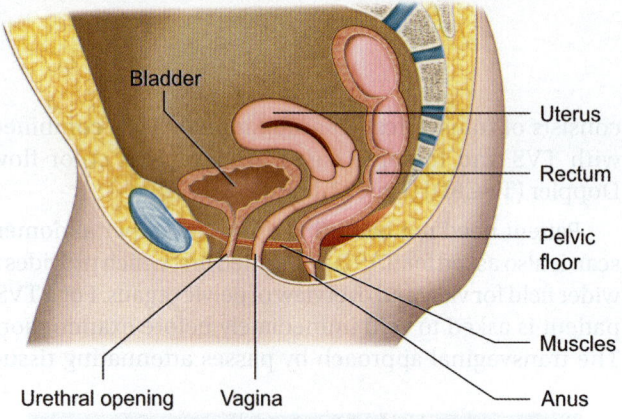

Fig. 22.3: Normal female pelvic floor.

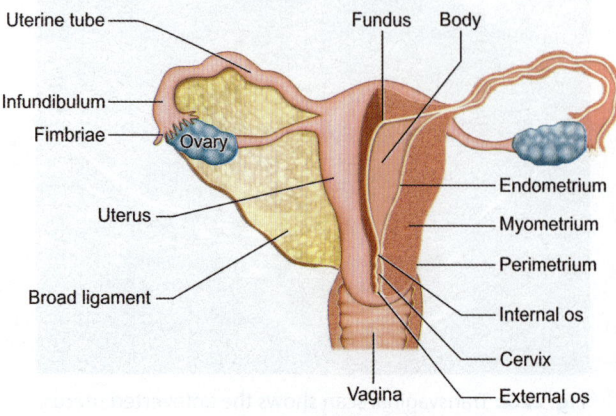

Fig. 22.4: Uterus.

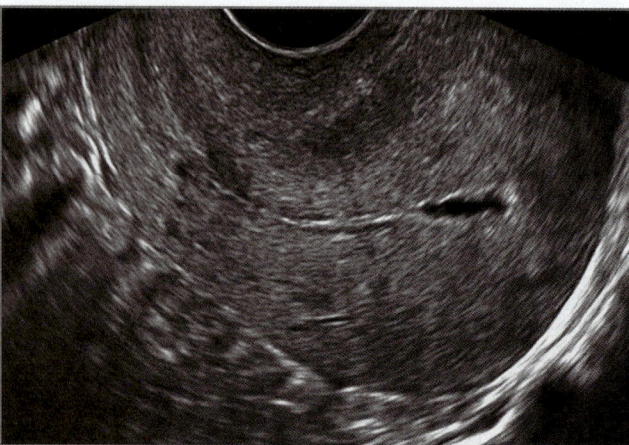

Fig. 22.5: Transvaginal scan. Retroverted uterus, thin layer of fluid is seen in endometrial cavity.

CHAPTER 22 Ultrasound and Color Doppler in Gynecology

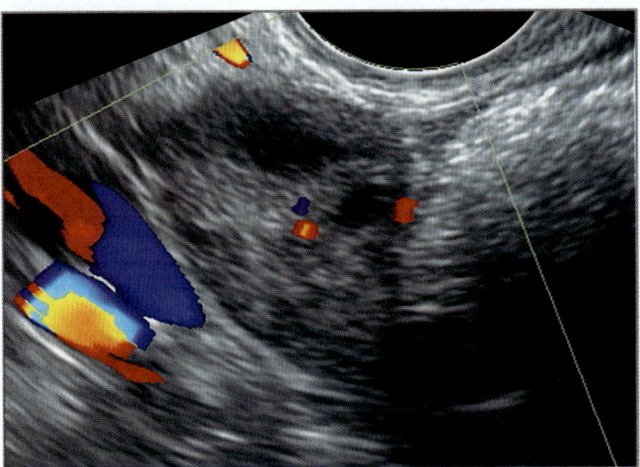

Fig. 22.6: Normal ovary bounded laterally by the iliac vessels, floor is formed by the obturator internus muscle.

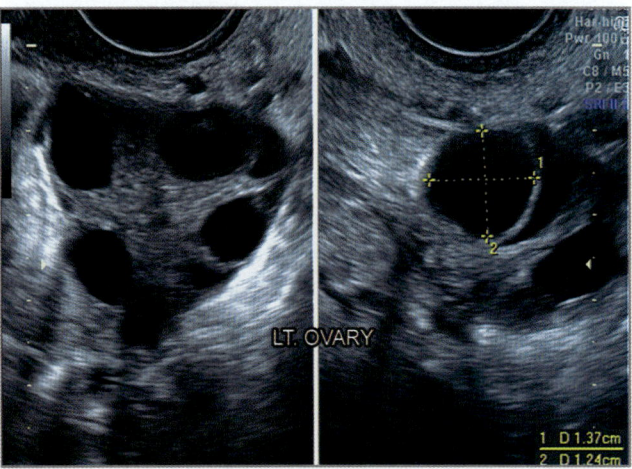

Fig. 22.7: Transvaginal scan shows the dominant follicle in left ovary.

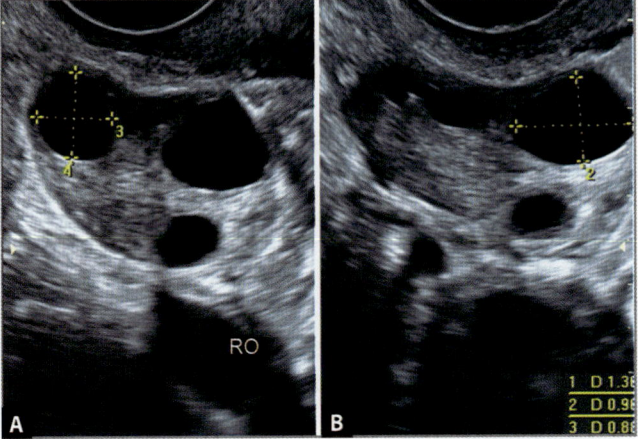

Figs. 22.8A and B: Folliculogenesis.

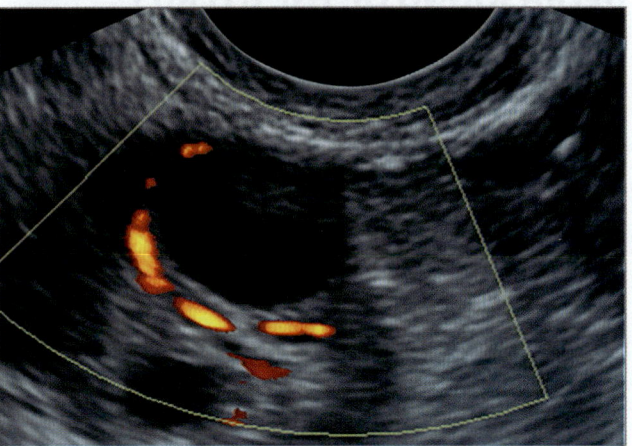

Fig. 22.9: Dominant follicle showing perifollicular flow.

develops in midcycle which measures up to 20 mm in diameter. After ovulation corpus luteum develops (Figs. 22.8 to 22.10).

FALLOPIAN TUBES

These originate from the lateral uterine angles towards their respective ovaries. These measure approximately 7–12 cm in length and are a few mm wide.[1] Normal fallopian tubes are normally not visualized by ultrasound unless abnormal or surrounded by fluid.

POUCH OF DOUGLAS

Also known as cul-de-sac or rectouterine pouch. Small amount of fluid may be physiological within the sac (Fig. 22.11).

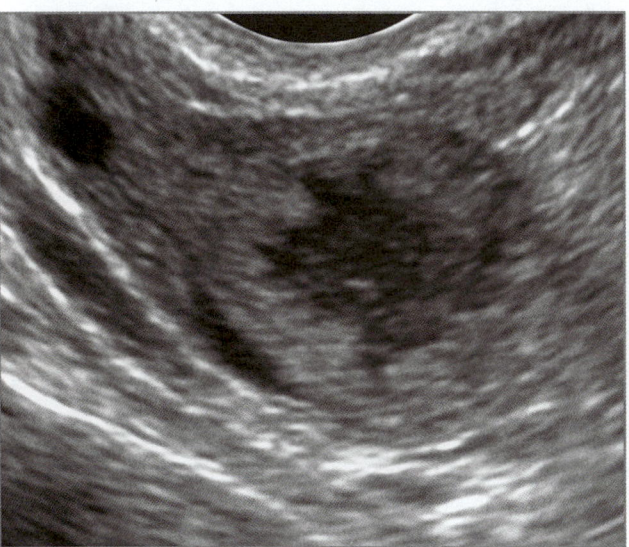

Fig. 22.10: Corpus luteum.

SECTION 1 General Gynecology

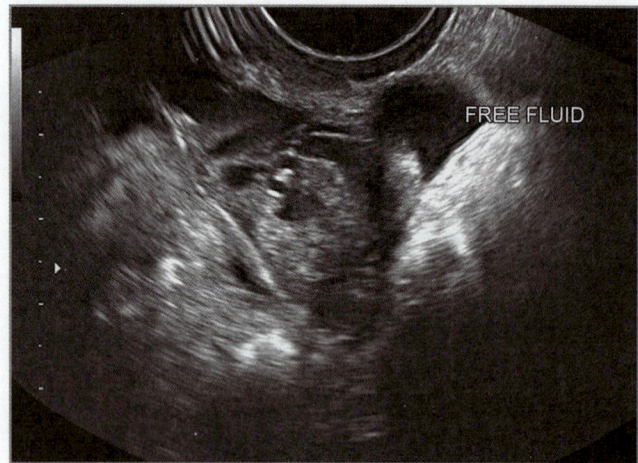

Fig. 22.11: Small amount of ovulatory free fluid in cul-de-sac.

ULTRASOUND OF THE UTERUS

Sonographic evaluation of uterus comprises checking for (Fig. 22.12):

- Size
- Shape
- Position
- Surface
- Mobility
- Tenderness on probe pressure.

Parts of uterus evaluated include:

- Myometrium
- Endometrium
- Uterine cavity
- Uterine size:
  - Small (hypoplastic)/absent uterus may be seen associated with congenital syndromes.
  - Uterine atrophy is seen in older females (postmenopausal).
- Uterine shape (Fig. 22.13): Abnormal uterine shape may be seen with congenital malformations which result from defects in lateral fusion of müllerian ducts or subsequent incomplete septal resorption.[4] These include:
  - Uterus didelphys: Two uteri, two cervix and may be a septated vagina
  - Bicornis bicollis: Two uteri and two cervix
  - Bicornuate (Unicollis) uterus: Two uteri with partially fused lower segment (Fig. 22.14)
  - Septate uterus: Thick or thin fibrous septa divides the myometrial component
  - Arcuate uterus: Fundal dimpling is seen (Fig. 22.15).
  - Unicornis uterus with rudimentary horn
  - T-shaped uterus.

DISEASES OF THE MYOMETRIUM

Benign Conditions

- Adenomyosis (Figs. 22.16 to 22.19)
- Myometritis
- Myometrial calcification (Fig. 22.20).

Benign Tumors

- Leiomyoma (Figs. 22.21 to 22.25)
- Arteriovenous malformation (Figs. 22.26 and 22.27).

Malignant Tumor

- Sarcomatous change in leiomyoma

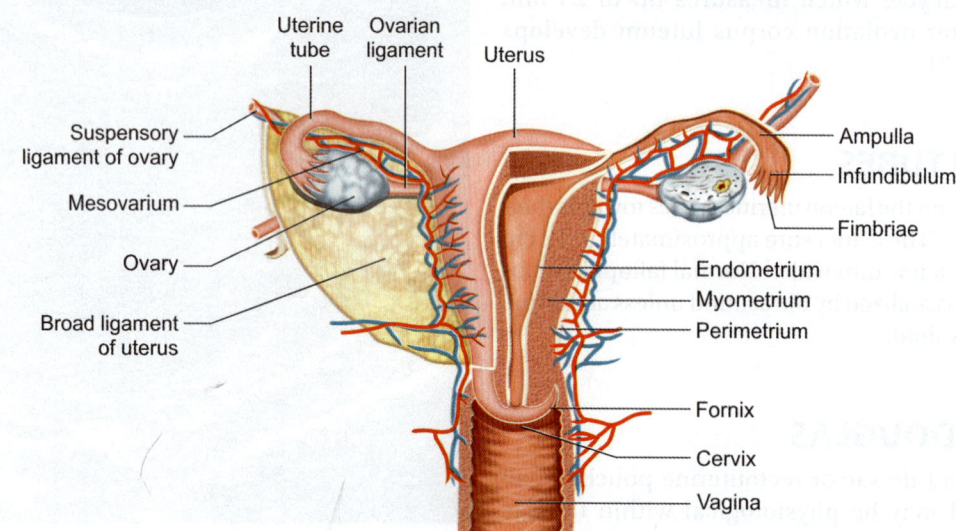

Fig. 22.12: Uterus and adnexa.

CHAPTER 22 Ultrasound and Color Doppler in Gynecology

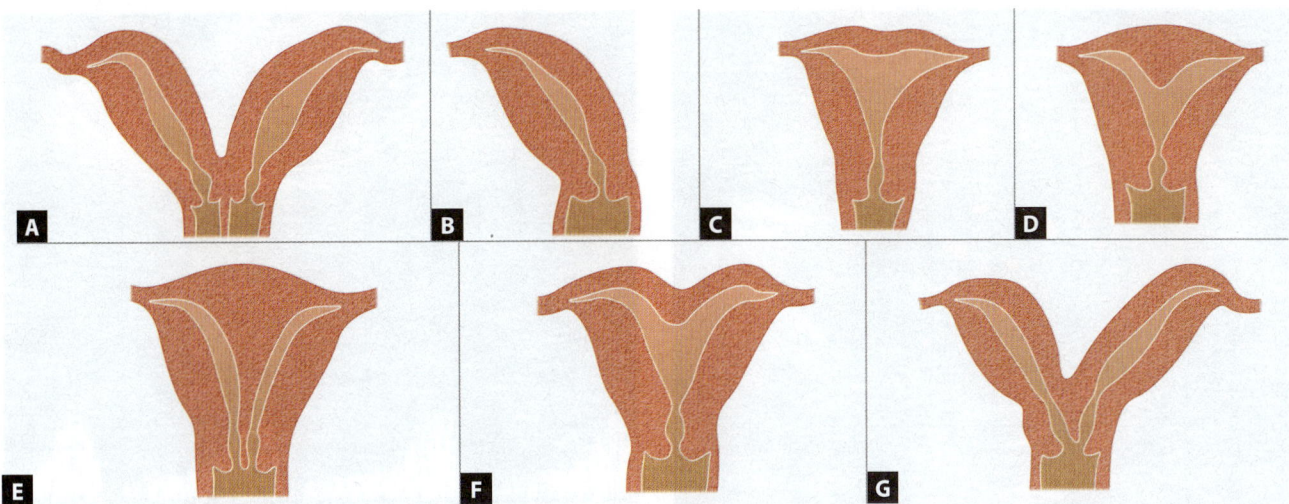

Figs. 22.13A to G: Abnormal uterine shapes. (A) Didelphic; (B) Unicornuate; (C) Arcuate; (D) Septate (partial); (E) Septate (complete); (F) Bicornuate (partial); (G) Bicornuate (complete).

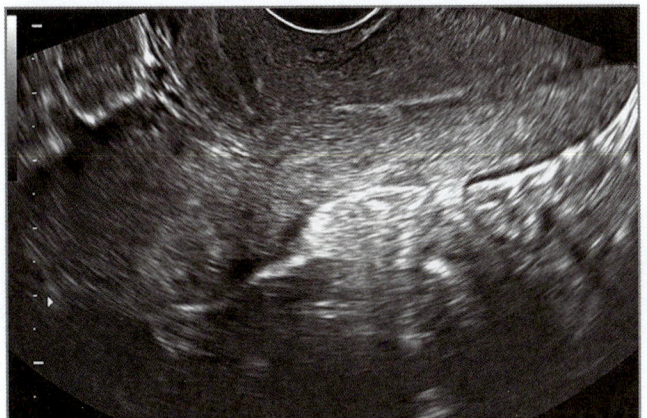

Fig. 22.14: Bicornuate (unicollis) uterus.

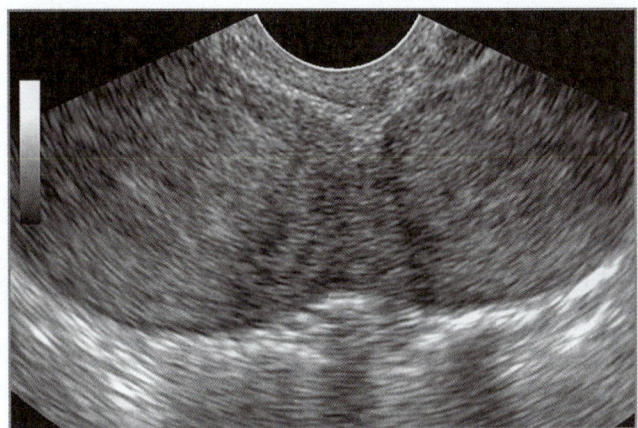

Fig. 22.15: Arcuate uterus showing fundal dimpling.

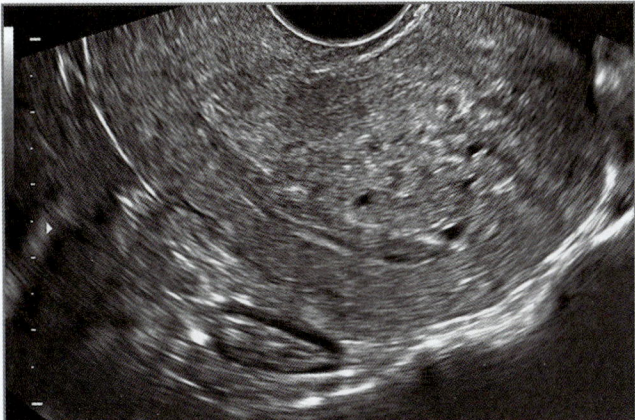

Fig. 22.16: Adenomyosis: Retroverted uterus showing thickened posterior endometrium with ill-defined endometrial myometrial interface and tiny subendometrial myometrial cysts.

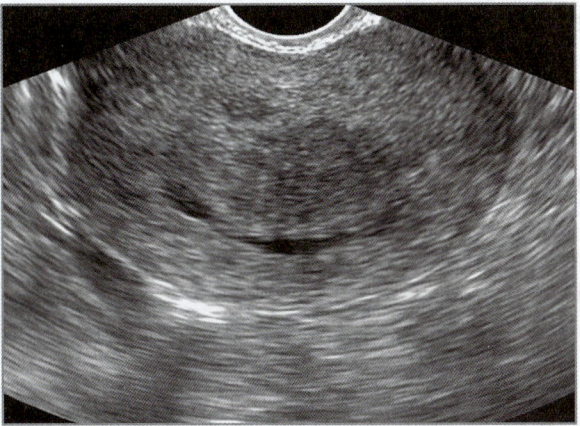

Fig. 22.17: Transvaginal scan. Adenomyoma: Ill-defined hypoechoic mass in the anterior myometrium. Small amount of fluid is seen within the endometrial cavity.

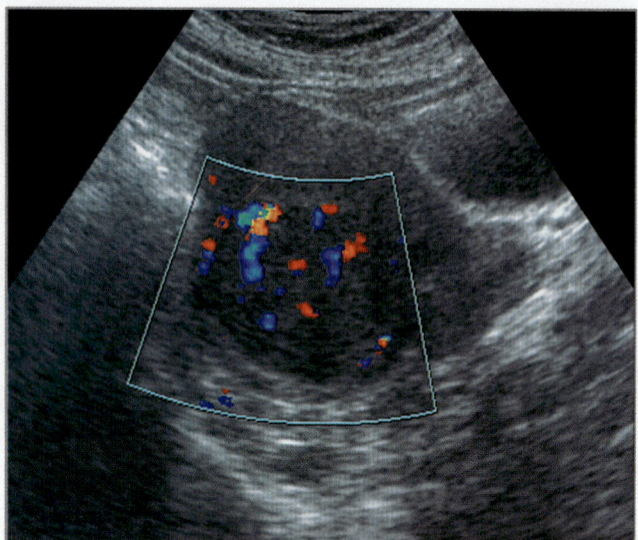

Fig. 22.18: Scattered vascularity in the ill-defined, hypoechoic mass in suggestive of adenomyoma.

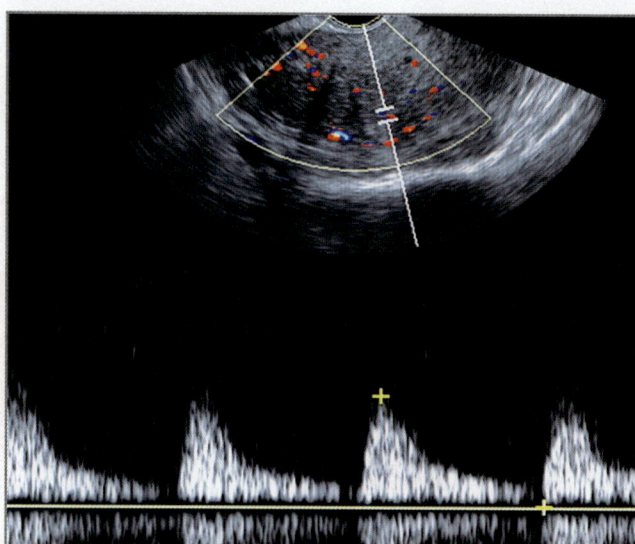

Fig. 22.19: Spectral analysis shows low velocity, high resistance flow velocity waveform pattern.

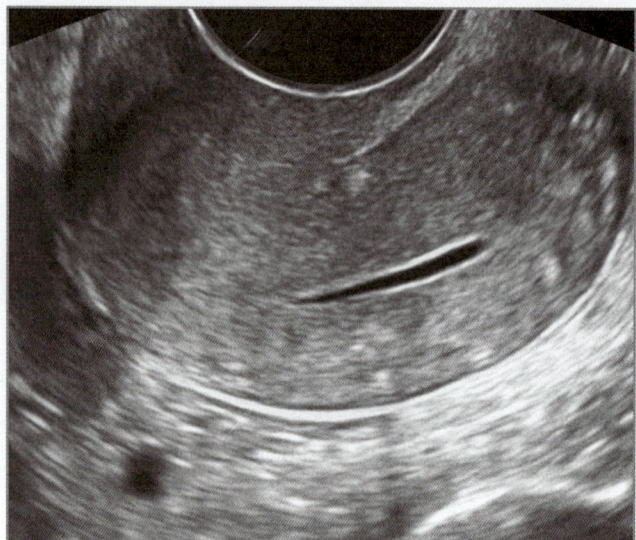

Fig. 22.20: Myometrial calcification. Small amount of fluid is seen in the endometrial cavity.

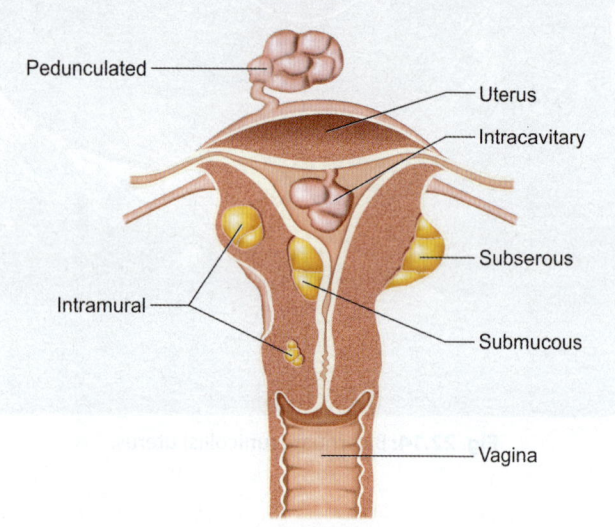

Fig. 22.21: Uterine fibroids.

DISEASES OF THE ENDOMETRIUM

Benign Condition
- Endometritis (Fig. 22.28).

Benign Tumors
- Endometrial hyperplasia (Fig. 22.29)
- Endometrial polyps (Figs. 22.30 and 22.31).

Malignant Tumor
- Endometrial tumors (Fig. 22.32)

DISEASES OF THE UTERINE CAVITY
- Endometrial fluid (Fig. 22.19)
- Intrauterine contraceptive devices (Fig. 22.33)
- Synechiae (Asherman's syndrome).

Benign Condition

Adenomyosis (Figs. 22.16 to 22.19)

Ultrasonographic Appearance
- Diffuse uterine enlargement with no alteration in echotexture or uterine contour

CHAPTER 22   *Ultrasound and Color Doppler in Gynecology*

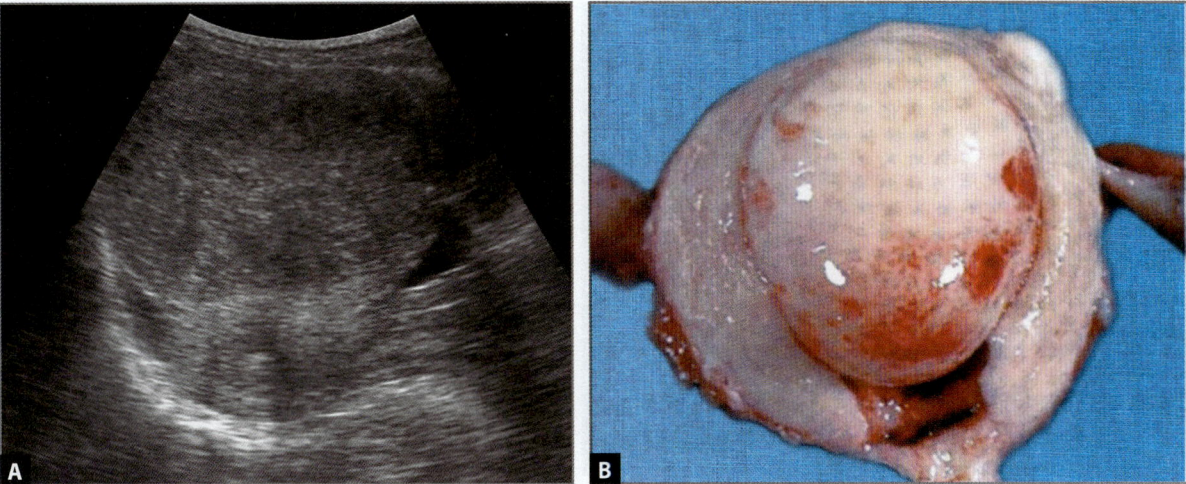

Figs. 22.22A and B: Transabdominal scan. Leiomyoma: (A) Well-circumscribed mass with hypoechoic periphery; (B) Gross specimen of the same.

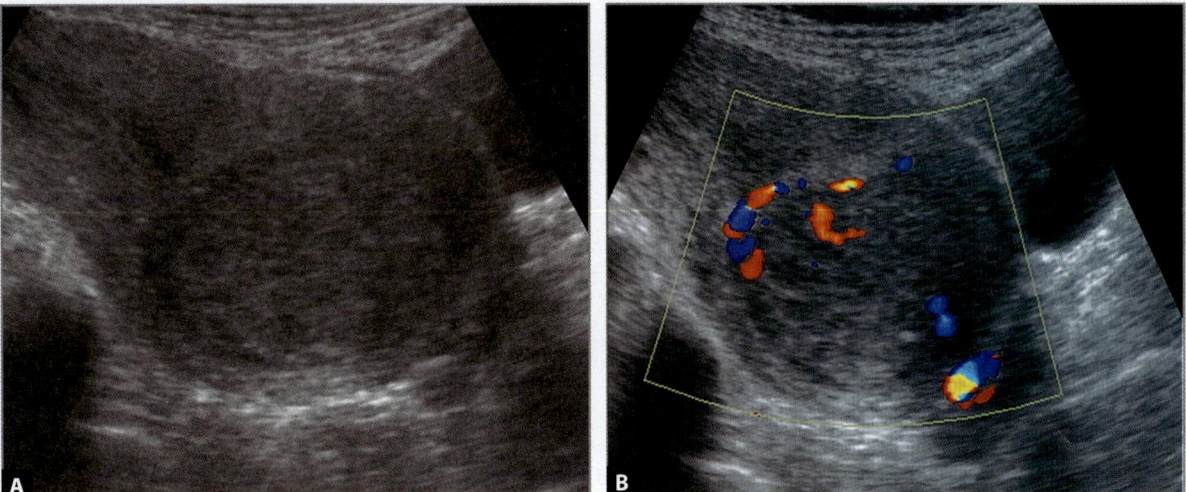

Figs. 22.23A and B: Transabdominal scan: (A) Cervical leiomyoma; (B) Color flow mapping shows peripheral vascularity.

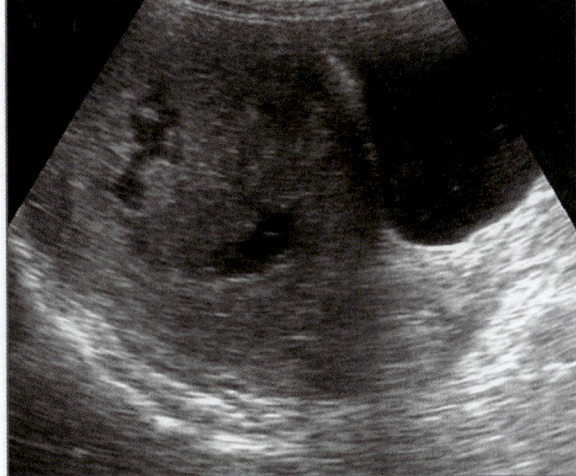

Fig. 22.24: Transabdominal scan. Leiomyoma with cystic degeneration.

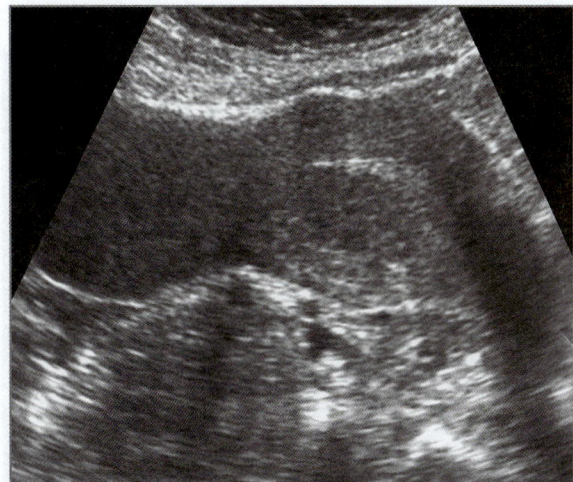

Fig. 22.25: Transabdominal scan showing a subserosal myoma arising from the fundus of the uterus.

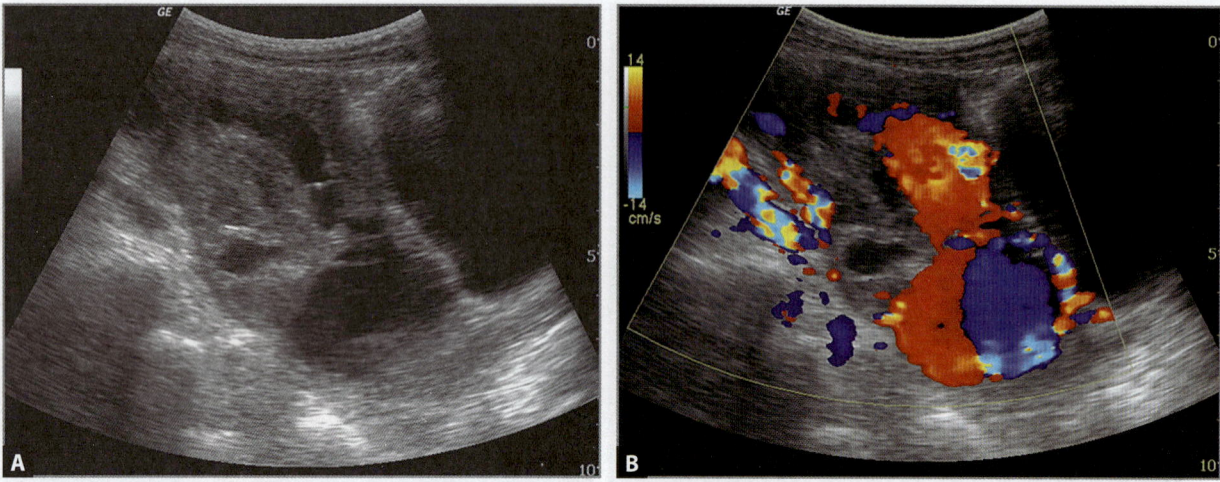

Figs. 22.26A and B: Sagittal sonogram showing enlarged vessels within the myometrium. After a dilatation and curettage, an arteriovenous malformation developed.

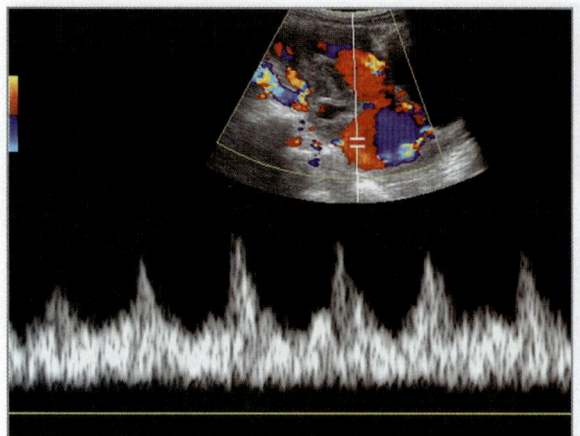

Fig. 22.27: Same patient. Doppler ultrasound confirms expected low resistance flow with high peak systolic velocities.

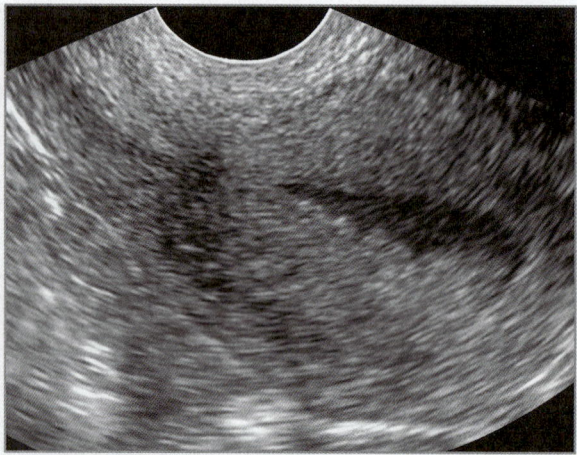

Fig. 22.28: Transvaginal scan showing irregular endometrial outline and fluid within the endometrial cavity. Findings are suggestive of endometritis. The most common cause of chronic endometrial infection is *Mycobacterium tuberculosis*.

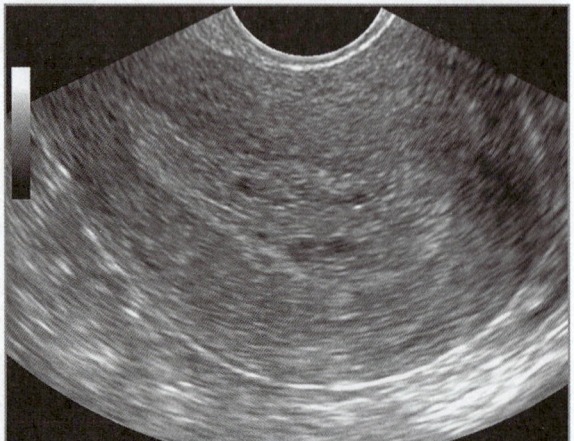

Fig. 22.29: Transvaginal scan showing a thickened endometrium with tiny cystic areas suggestive of endometrial hyperplasia.

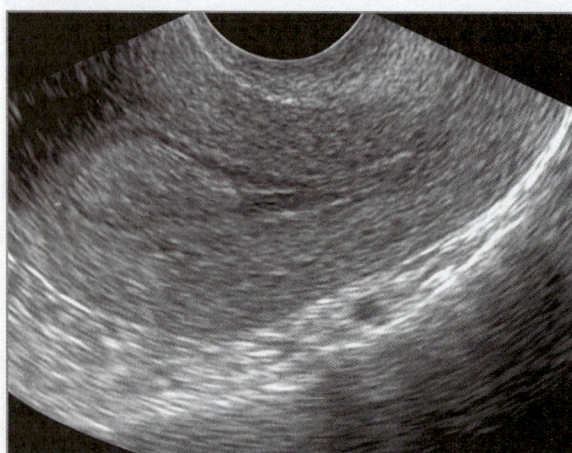

Fig. 22.30: B-mode trasvaginal scan showing a nodular echogenic lesion within the endometrium suspected to be an endometrial polyp. Histopathology confirmed a polyp.

CHAPTER 22 Ultrasound and Color Doppler in Gynecology

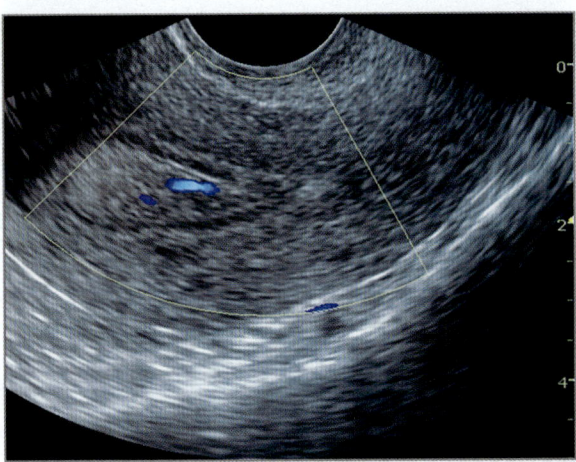

Fig. 22.31: Transvaginal color Doppler sonogram showing a single vessel penetrating to the endometrial polyp. This vessel corresponds to the polyps' pedicle.

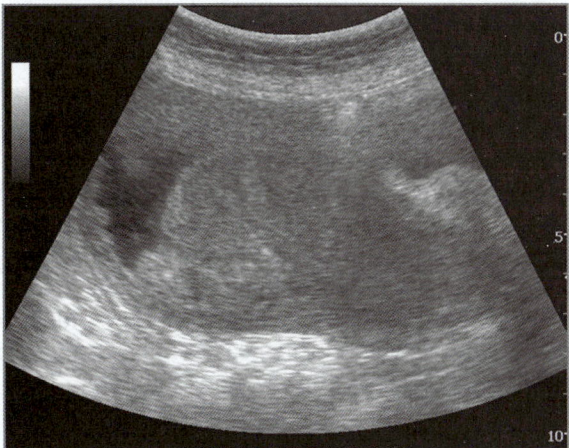

Fig. 22.32: Transabdominal scan of a postmenopausal patient with enlarged and heterogenous uterus. It was difficult to delineate an endometrial echo. Note the presence of intracavitary fluid. Endometrial malignancy.

- Focal adenomyosis: Poorly defined area of abnormal echotexture within myometrium[5]
- Focal or diffuse speckled appearance of the myometrium (salt and papper appearance)
- Cystic areas at endom-myom interface
- Increased thickness of posterior myometrium as compared to anterior myometrious
- Ill-defined, focal abnormal texture lesion defined as adenomyoma
- Scattered vascularity on color flow imaging
- Additional ovarian lesions (endometriotic cysts) may be seen.

Myometritis

Ultrasonographic findings include:
- Multiple bright spots within myometrium
- Fluid in endometrial cavity
- Fluid within pouch of Douglas
- Probe tenderness
- Blood flow pooling.

Myometrial Calcification

- Most common cause—calcified myoma
- Less common cause—arcuate artery calcification (see Fig. 22.20).

Benign Tumor

Leiomyoma

These may be submucosal (5–10%) which displace/distort the endometrium. Most common type is intramural (within the wall of uterus), subserosal myomas distort the uterine cavity. Panmural myomas extend through and from the outer surface to the endometrial cavity (Figs. 22.21 to 22.25). Few myomas may have a pedicle.

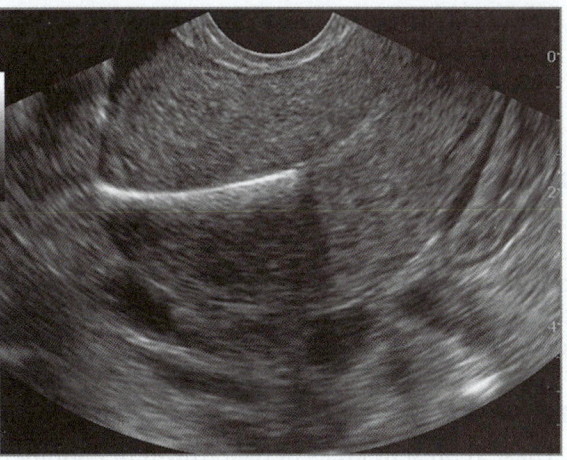

Fig. 22.33: Transvaginal scan showing an IUCD perforating the myometrium.

- Ultrasonography appearance depends on age, site, size and composition of the tumor.[6]
- When muscular component predominates, lesion is a well-defined, concentric mass with poor sound through transmission (Isoechoic fibroids difficult to see by USG)
- Increasing echogenicity marks the start of fibrous degeneration. With further ageing, myomas undergo cystic degeneration (e.g. hemorrhagic, proteolytic) seen as an anechoic mass with posterior enhancement
- Highly echogenic portions with acoustic shadowing is seen from areas of calcification or from myxomatous and lipomatous change.

Arteriovenous Malformation (see Figs. 22.25 and 22.26)

These may appear on gray scale imaging as subtle myometrial inhomogeneity, tubular spaces within the myometrium, intramural uterine mass, endometrial or cervical mass or sometimes as prominent parametrial vessels. Their appearance is nonspecific. These anechoic, tubular spaces fill with color on color flow imaging and show low resistance flow with high peak systolic velocities on spectral analysis. Venous flow also shows high flow velocities and systolic velocity peaks similar to an arterial pattern, which suggests arteriovenous shunting.[7]

Rare Condition
- Sarcomatous change within leiomyoma
- Ultrasound appearance is identical to that of benign tumors.

Endometritis
- Occurs with pelvic inflammatory disease and in postpartum patients
- Sonographically endometrium is echogenic or irregular with small amount of endometrial fluid (see Fig. 22.28).

Endometrial Hyperplasia

It is the most common cause of vaginal bleeding in both pre- and postmenopausal women, results from unopposed estrogen stimulation. Sonographically the endometrium is diffusely or focally thickened. Diagnosis is confirmed by endometrial biopsy (see Fig. 22.29).

Endometrial Polyp (see Figs. 22.29 and 22.30)
- These represent areas of overgrowth of endometrial glands and stroma covered by endometrial epithelium
- They usually arise from the fundus and are multiple in 20% cases
- Presents with vaginal bleeding or mucus discharge
- Appear sonographically as areas of increased endometrial thickening. TVS shows focal irregularity of the endometrial stripe, endometrial myometrial interface however is preserved
- Sonohysterography confirms the diagnosis.

Endometrial Tumor
- Seen in postmenopausal women with postmenopausal bleeding
- The telltale sign or endometrial carcinoma on ultrasound is not simply thickening of the endometrium but rather focal irregularity and myometrial distortion (see Fig. 22.32).
- Most of endometrial carcinoma are either diffusely or partially echogenic, 10–15% may be isoechoic

- Sonography is helpful in assessing superficial or deep invasion and in follow-up management.[8]

Endometrial Fluid
- Physiological (menstrual phase, normal early pregnancy)
- Pathological (abnormal pregnancy—missed abortion, ectopic pregnancy, molar pregnancy)
  - Infection
  - Obstruction
    - Malignant
    - Cervical stenosis.

Intrauterine Contraceptive Devices (see Fig. 22.33)

Ultrasound helps to locate the position of IUCD when string is not felt. It is seen as bright reflector within the uterus.

Synechiae (Asherman Syndrome)
- Intrauterine fibrous adhesions cross the endometrial cavity
- Synechiae form a mesh or Spider's web within the uterine lumen, may cause infertility, hypo- or amenorrhea, better seen with sonohysterography
- Fibrous strands may calcify, with a characteristic sonographic appearance.

SONOHYSTEROGRAPHY (FIGS. 22.34 TO 22.37)

This is done by using saline contrast, which is pushed through the cervix by a pediatric Foley's or feeding tube under transvaginal scan visualization. This is an excellent, easy, noninvasive, quick and reliable method to evaluate uterine cavity for Asherman's disease, polyps, submucus fibroids, focal lesions or even malignancy.

ULTRASOUND AND PUERPERIUM
- Postpartum uterus should return to near normal size within 6–8 weeks after delivery
- Postpartum ultrasound is visually requested if there is clinical concern about retained product or endometritis.
  - **Ultrasonography:** The cavity may look normal
  - Echogenic mass within cavity suggestive of retained products
  - Heterogenous mass may be due retained bits, blood clot, necrotic or injected material in the absence of placental tissue (Fig. 22.38)[9]

CHAPTER 22 Ultrasound and Color Doppler in Gynecology

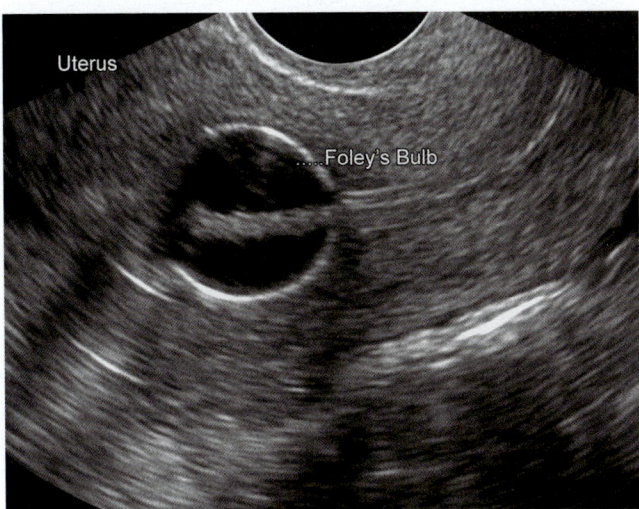

Fig. 22.34: Sonosalpingography. Foley's bulb *in situ*.

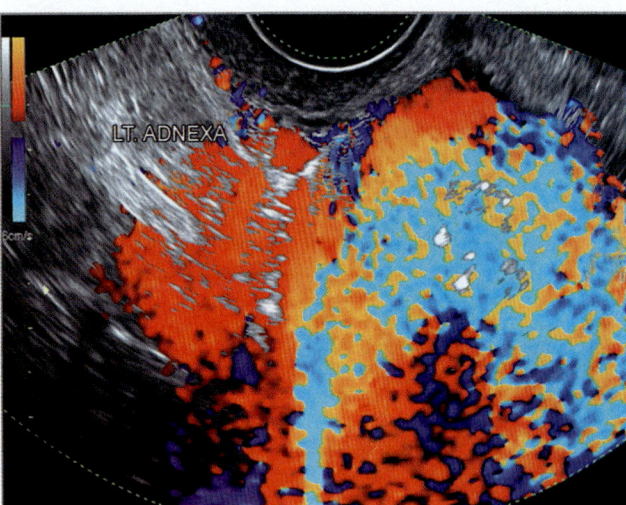

Fig. 22.35: Sonosalpingography. Free flow in pelvis seen as color bruit on color flow mapping (Waterfall sign).

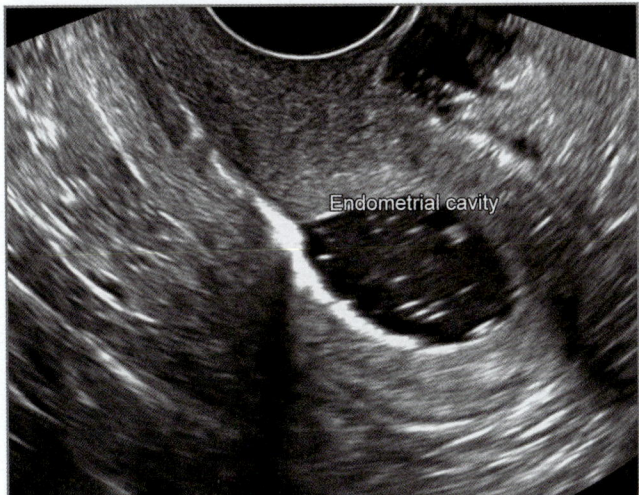

Fig. 22.36: Sonosalpingography. Fluid outlining a normal endometrial cavity.

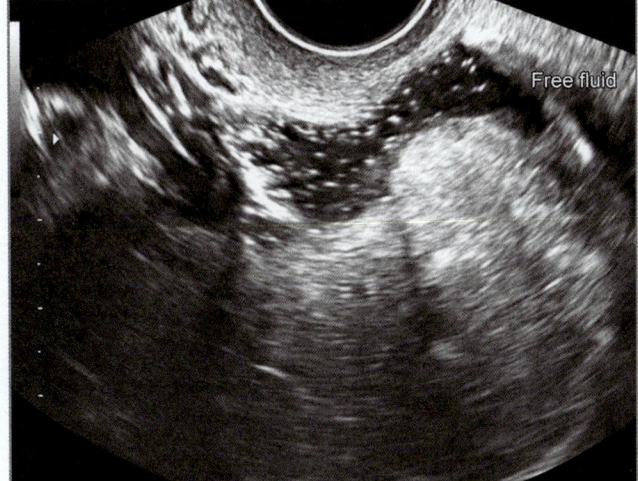

Fig. 22.37: Sonosalpingography. Free fluid seen in cul-de-sac after the procedure.

- Fluid within endometrial cavity blood or infection.
- Gas within cavity:[10] It may be a normal finding in puerperium, atleast until the end of 3rd postpartum week. May indicate infection.

DISEASES OF CERVIX
- *Nabothian cysts:* These are obstructed and hence dilated inclusion cysts, of no clinical relevance. May be seen at the interval os level and in the stroma, could indicate cervicitis
- *Cervical fibroids:* Are well-defined, hypoechoic masses (Fig. 22.39).
- *Cervical cancer:* Ultrasound is not especially useful in the diagnosis of cervical malignancy. USG serves to document the complications of advanced cervical disease and its treatment. For example, ultrasound

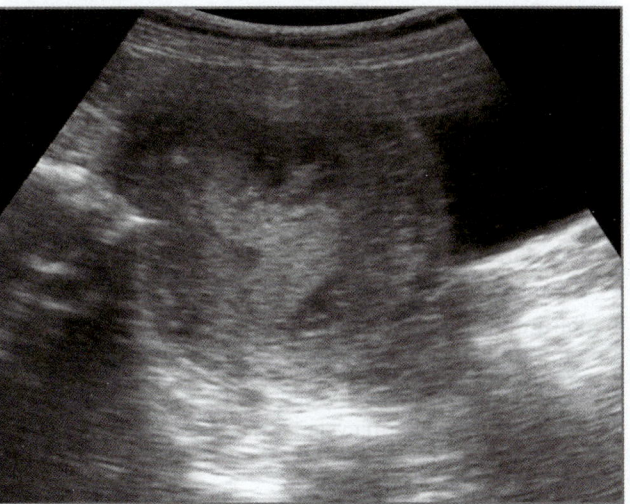

Fig. 22.38: Transabdominal scan showing the retained bits.

SECTION 1 General Gynecology

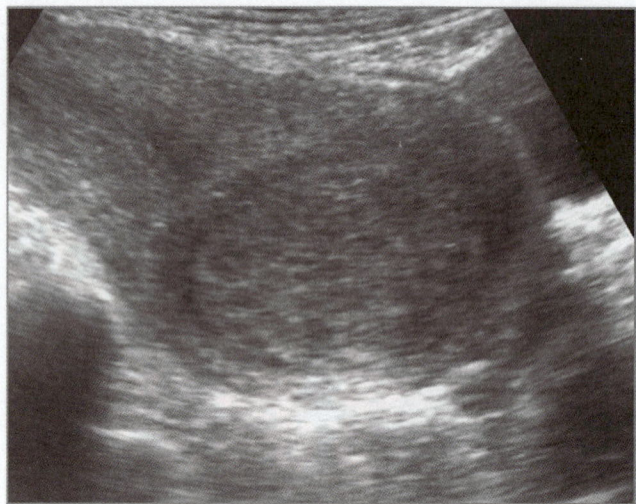

Fig. 22.39: Transabdominal scan. A cervical leiomyoma.

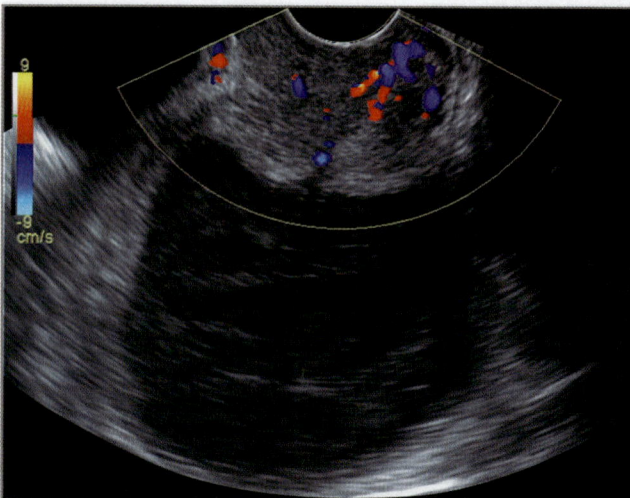

Fig. 22.40: Transvaginal scan showing bulky inhomogenous cervix with increased vascularity. Carcinoma cervix with pyometra.

can document cervical stenosis and intrauterine fluid retention or hydronephrosis (Fig. 22.40).
- Ultrasound also can calculate volume of mass and staging and 5-year survival.

VAGINA

The most common lesion visualized with sonography are Gartner's duct cysts. Transverse vaginal septums may present as amenorrhea with hematocolpos (Fig. 22.41).

OVARIAN SONOGRAPHY

Benign cystic lesion of ovarian and paraovarian structures.
- Functional cysts
  - Follicular cysts
  - Corpus luteum cysts
  - Corpus luteum of pregnancy
  - Theca lutein cysts
- Surface epithelial inclusion cysts
- Rete cysts
- Hyperreactio luteinalis
- Ovarian hyperstimulation syndrome (OHSS)
- Polycystic ovarian syndrome
- Ovarian remnant syndrome
- Neonatal ovarian cysts
- Paratubal and paraovarian cysts
- Endometriosis and endometriomas
- Pelvic inflammatory disease
- Peritoneal inclusion cysts.

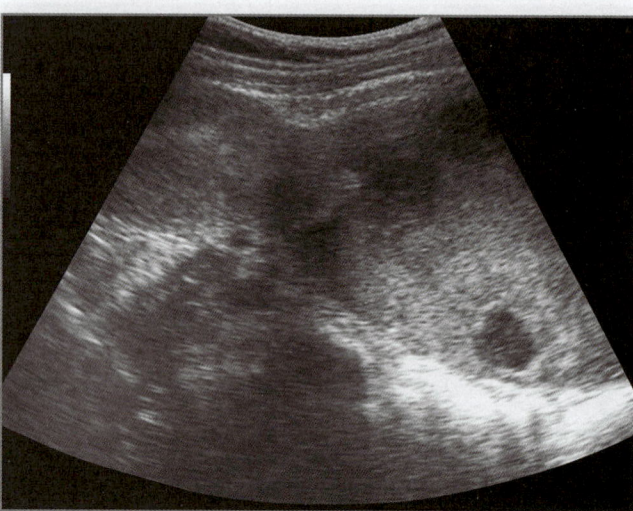

Fig. 22.41: Transabdominal scan showing distended vagina with fluid containing low level echoes within suggestive of hematocolpos. Small uterus is seen on the right.

Ovarian vascular lesions
- Ovarian torsion
- Massive ovarian edema
- Ovarian venous thrombosis.

Ovarian neoplasms (Fig. 22.42)
- Surface epithelial stromal tumors
  - Serous tumors
  - Mucinous tumors
  - Epidermoid
  - Clear cell tumors
  - Transitional cell (Brenner) tumors.

CHAPTER 22: Ultrasound and Color Doppler in Gynecology

- Germ cell tumors
  - Mature cystic teratomas (ovarian dermoid cysts)
  - Mature solid teratoma
  - Immature teratoma
  - Dysgerminoma
  - Yolk sac tumors
- Sex cord—stromal tumors
  - Fibroma
  - Thecoma
  - Granulosa cell tumors
  - Sertoli-Leydig cell tumors.
- Metastatic tumors.

Benign Cystic Lesion of Ovarian and Paraovarian Structure (Fig. 22.43)

Functional Cysts

- **Follicular cysts:** Thin walled, unilocular 3–8 cm in size. Usually regress spontaneously[11] (Fig. 22.44)
- **Corpus luteum cysts:** Commonly complicated by hemorrhage. Thick walled with echogenic contents (Fig. 22.45)
- **Corpus luteum of pregnancy:** Corpus luteum of pregnancy may become enlarged and cystic. Needs follow-up ultrasound and monitoring
- **Theca lutein cysts:** Usually multilocular results from overstimulation by high levels of circulating human chorionic gonadotropin (hCG) in trophoblastic disease.

Surface Epithelial Inclusion Cysts

These result from cortical invaginations of ovarian surface epithelium. Mostly seen in postmenopausal women, usually multiple cysts.

Rete Cysts

Rare origin, located within ovarian hilus. Indistinguishable from other simple cysts.[11]

Hyperreacto Luteinalis

Ovarian enlargement resulting from the presence of multiple luteinized follicle cysts, secondary to hCG stimulation.[12]

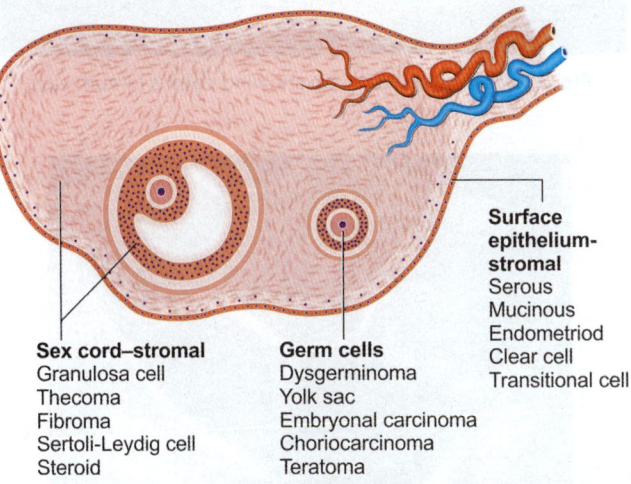

Fig. 22.42: Ovarian neoplasm.

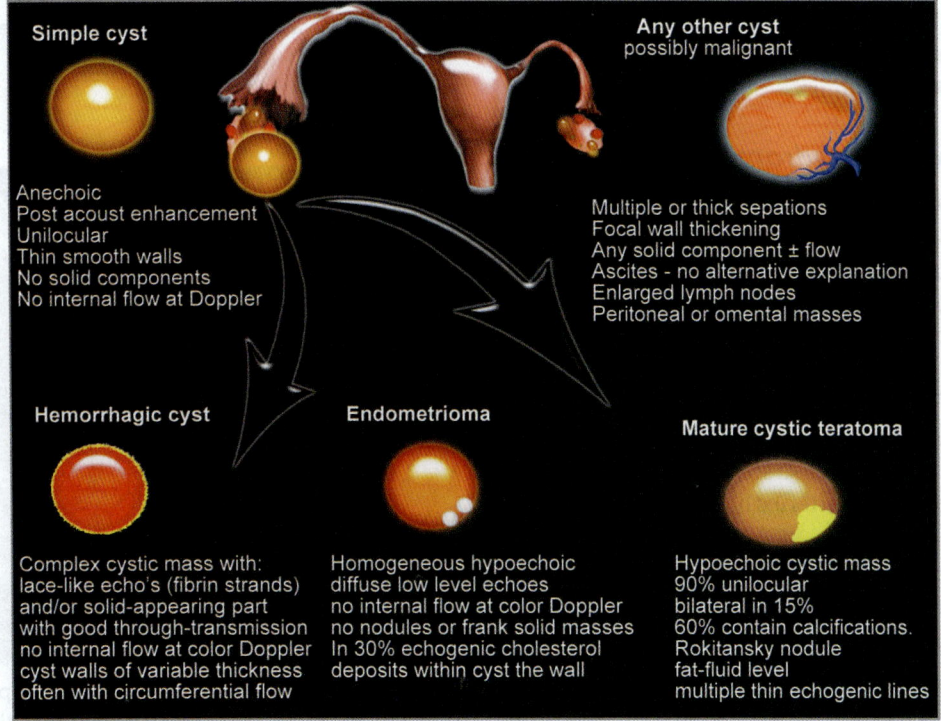

Fig. 22.43: Lesions of ovary.

SECTION 1 General Gynecology

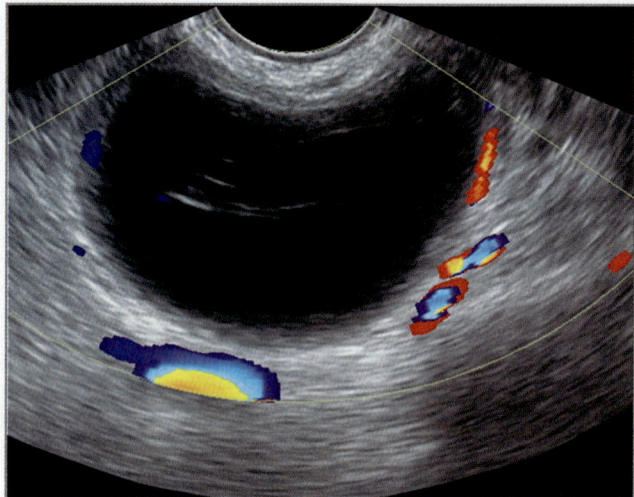

Fig. 22.44: Transvaginal scan showing a follicular cyst.

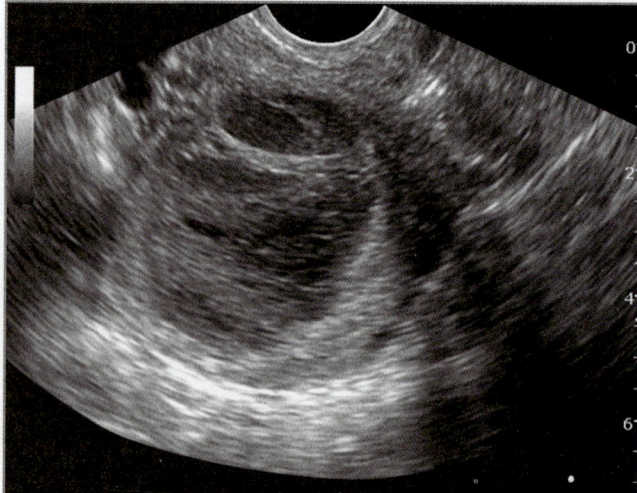

Fig. 22.45: Transvaginal scan showing corpus luteum cyst.

Self-limiting condition USG shows bilaterally enlarged ovaries containing multiple cysts. Cysts may be simple or have hemorrhagic contents.

Ovarian Hyperstimulation Syndrome

Seen in women undergoing ovulation induction, after administration of gonadotropins followed by hCG or rarely clomiphene alone (Fig. 22.46).

Ultrasonography: Mild to moderate OHSH is characterized by cystic ovarian enlargement (>5 cm in diameter) and a small amount of pelvic fluid. Severe OHSS is characterized by cystic ovarian enlargement with abdominal distension and discomfort or pain with or without nausea and vomiting or diarrhea. Ascites and pleural effusion are seen.[13]

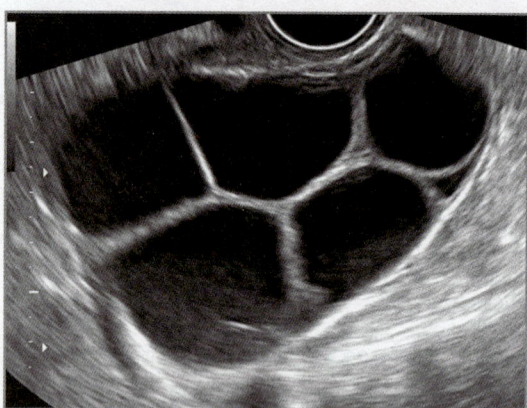

Fig. 22.46: Ovarian hyperstimulation. Enlarged ovary showing multiple enlarged follicles.

Polycystic Ovarian Syndrome

Seen in 16–22% of women in their reproductive years and in up to 50% of women presenting to infertility clinics.

Ultrasonography: Typical polycystic pattern is defined by the presence of 10 or more cysts measuring 2–18 mm in diameter in a single plane arranged peripherally around an increased amount of central stroma (Garland sign) (Necklace sign)[14] (Fig. 22.47).

Greater ovarian stromal blood flow velocity and lower impedance have been demonstrated in women with PCO. The impedance of uterine arteries has been demonstrated to be increased.

Ovarian Remnant Syndrome

It is a complication of oophorectomy in patients with distorted anatomy resulting from adhesions and endometriosis, making surgical dissection difficult, residual ovarian tissue may form a cystic or complex mass.

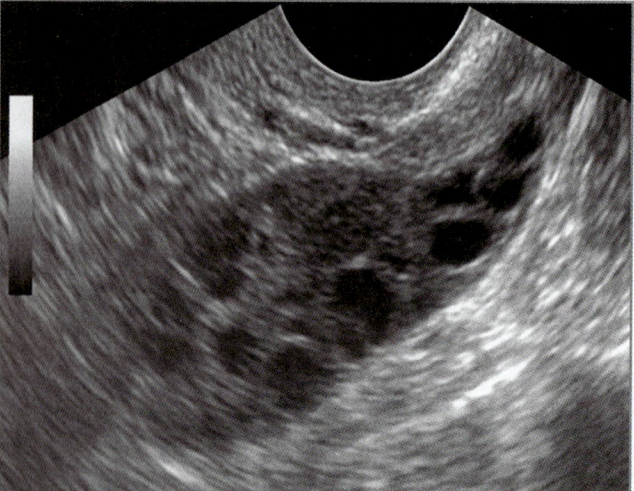

Fig. 22.47: Transvaginal sonogram of the polycystic ovaries showing small cysts scattered throughout the entire ovarian parenchyma (Garland sign).

Paratubal and Paraovarian Cysts

These arise from the mesonephric and paramesonephric structures. Most common in IIIrd and IVth decade may be multiple. Morphologically, these cysts are indistinguishable from simple functional cysts. They may be complicated by hemorrhage, torsion or rupture.

Endometriosis

It is the presence of endometrial tissue outside the endometrium and myometrium. Ovaries, uterine ligaments, rectovaginal septum, cul-de-sac and pelvic peritoneum are the most common sites.

USG: Endometriomas have a variety of appearances ranging from an anechoic cyst to a cyst containing diffuse low level echoes with or without solid components to a solid appearing mass.[15] Presence of a fluid-fluid level, punctate or linear bright echogenic foci in the wall of the cyst favors the diagnosis of endometrioma. TVS does not detect endometriotic implants[15] (Fig. 22.48).

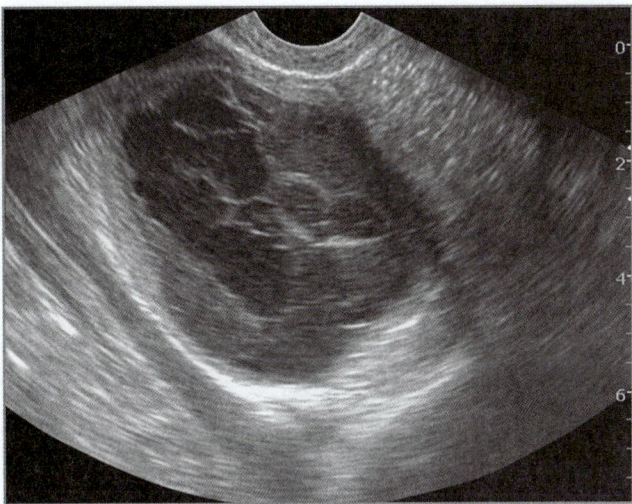

Fig. 22.48: Transvaginal scan demonstrating a multilocular endometriotic cyst.

Pelvic Inflammatory Disease

Ovarian involvement in pelvic inflammatory disease (PID) is almost always secondary to salpingitis.

Sonographic findings may be normal early in the disease course. Timor Tritsch et al. described the sonographic findings as[16] (Figs. 22.49 to 22.51):

- Thickening of tube wall ≥ 5 mm
- **Cogwheel sign:** Cogwheel-shaped structure seen in cross-section of tube in acute salpingitis
- Incomplete septa correlating with folds or kinds in dilated tube
- **Beads-on-a-string sign:** Hyperechoic mural nodules within fluid tube representing flattened and fibrotic endosalpingeal folds
- **Tubo-ovarian complex:** Ovary cannot be separated from the tube by pushing with the vaginal probe
- **Tubo-ovarian abscess:** Conglomerate mass or fluid collection
- Cul-de-sac fluid.[16]

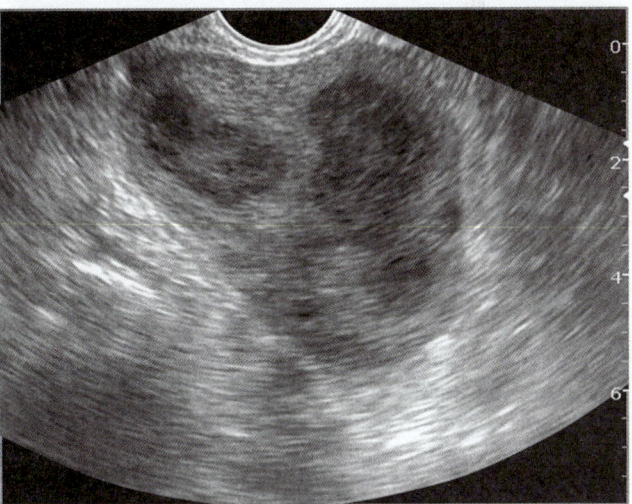

Fig. 22.49: Transvaginal scan of a complex adnexal mass that could be interpreted as a tubo-ovarian abscess.

Peritoneal Inclusion Cysts

These are formed by trapping of fluid (which is normally produced by active ovaries) within peritoneal adhesions. A history of trauma, abdominal surgery, PID or endometriosis is common. USG shows the ovary surrounded by septations and fluid and lies inside or in the wall of a large ovoid or irregular anechoic cyst.

Ovarian Vascular Lesions

- **Ovarian torsion:** Usually caused by ovarian (particularly dermoid) and paraovarian cysts. Sonographic

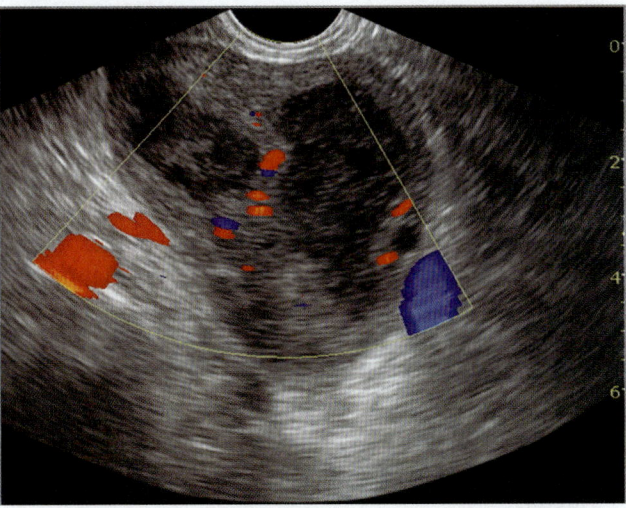

Fig. 22.50: Transvaginal color Doppler scan. Same patient shows vessels within the ovarian parenchyma.

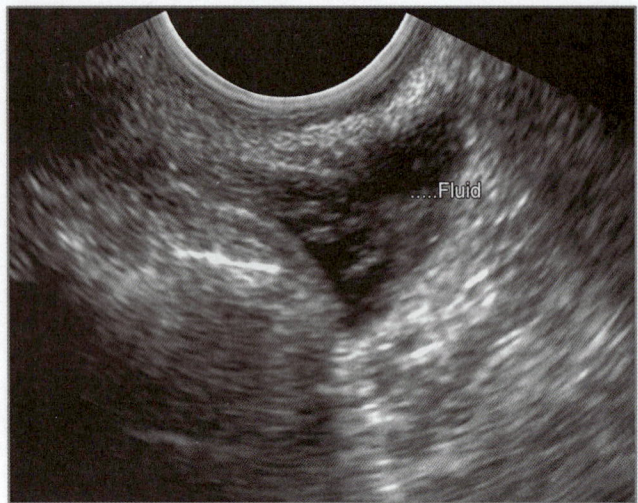

Fig. 22.51: Transvaginal sonogram. Same patient shows septated fluid in the pouch of Douglas suggestive of infective etiology.

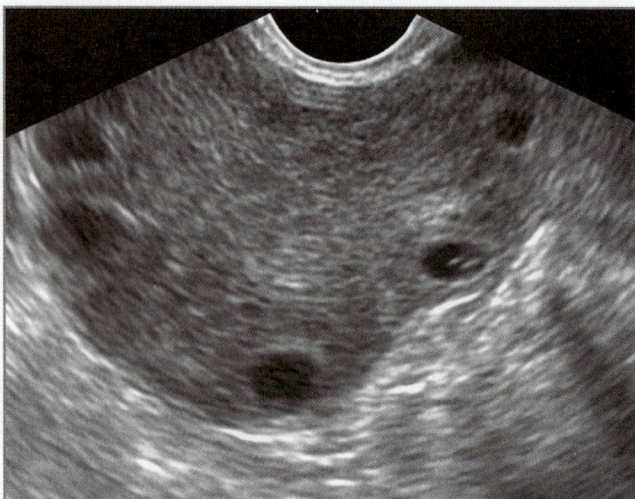

Fig. 22.52: Transvaginal scan showing an enlarged ovary with echogenic stroma, peripheral tiny follicles with echogenic walls.

appearance depends on the duration, degree of torsion and any associated intraovarian mass.[17] USG shows a cystic, solid or complex mass with or without pelvic fluid, thickening of wall. These findings however are nonspecific. Enlargement of ovary with absent or markedly diminished ovarian flow is a specific finding (Fig. 22.52).

- **Massive ovarian edema:** Accumulation of edema fluid within ovarian stroma, most likely due to torsion of the ovary. A definitive diagnosis of massive ovarian edema cannot be made on preoperative imaging but should be considered in the differential diagnosis of a solid extrauterine mass in the appropriate clinical setting.[18]
- **Ovarian venous thrombosis:** Occurs most often postpartum, may also follow pelvic operations, pelvic trauma—sonographically thrombosed vein appears as an anechoic to hypoechoic tubular mass extending superiorly from the adnexa with absence flow on Doppler.[19] A perivenous phlegmon with increased vascularity may be seen.

Ovarian Neoplasms

Surface Epithelial Stromal Tumors

- **Serous tumors:** Benign serous cystadenomas appear as sharply marginated, anechoic masses that may be large and are usually unilocular. Internal thin-walled septations and papillary projections may be seen (in borderline tumors)[11] (Fig. 22.53).
  Serous cystadenocarcinomas are usually multilocular, containing multiple papillary projection and septations, echogenic material is occasionally seen within the loculi.

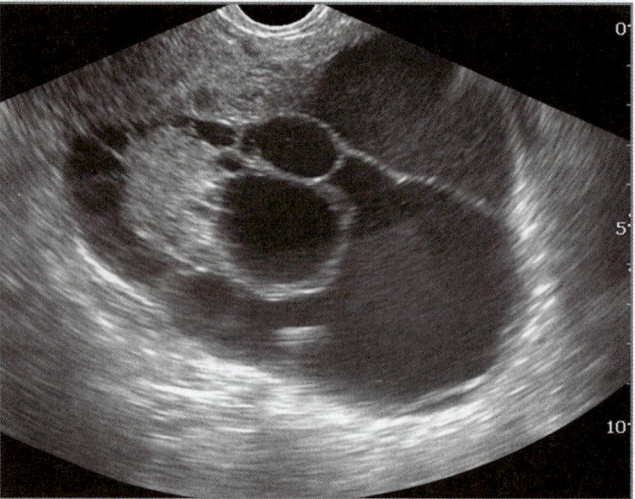

Fig. 22.53: Transvaginal scan showing a multilocular ovarian tumor presenting thick septa and echogenic content. Serous cystadenoma.

- **Mucinous tumors:** Sonographically, mucinous cystadenomas have thicker and more numerous septations and frequently contain fine, gravity-dependent echoes produced by thick contents (Fig. 22.54).[20]
  Mucinous cystadenocarcinomas usually appear as large, multiloculated cystic lesions containing echogenic material and papillary excrescences (Figs. 22.55A and B).
  Pseudomyxoma peritonei is by far the most common manifestation of atypically proliferating mucinous tumors.
- **Endometrioid tumors:** USG—These tumors are seen as cystic masses containing papillary projection.

CHAPTER 22 Ultrasound and Color Doppler in Gynecology

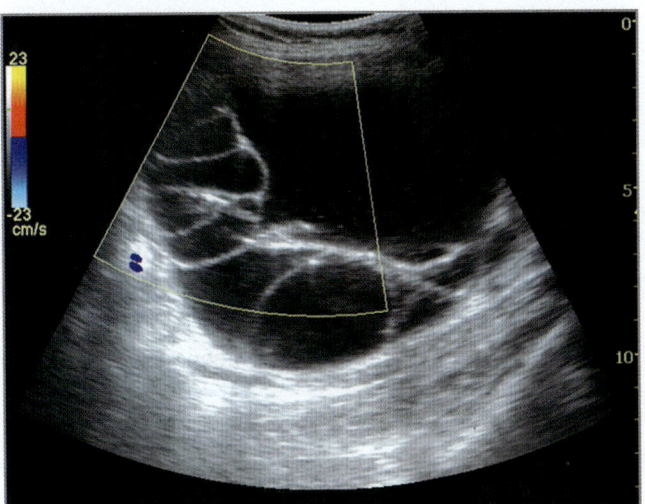

Fig. 22.54: Benign mucinous tumor. A multiloculated cyst is demonstrated with multiple thick septa. No definite flow could be demonstrated on color flow mapping.

- **Clear cell tumors:** Sonographic features of clear cell tumors are nonspecific, usually seen as complex, predominantly cystic masses
- **Transitional cell tumors (Brenner's tumor):** These are usually small (1–2 cm), hypoechoic and solid. Extensive calcification may be seen, cystic areas are unusual.

Germ Cell Tumors

- **Mature cystic teratomas (Ovarian dermoid):** USG features include the presence of regional diffuse bright echoes with or without posterior acoustic shadowing, hyperechoic lines or dots, shadowing echodensity and a fluid-fluid level[21] (Figs. 22.56 and 22.57)
- **Immature teratomas:** These are rare malignant tumors, usually large and predominantly solid
- **Struma ovarii:** This term is used for tumors (mature cystic teratomas) containing thyroid tissue
- **Dysgerminoma:** Sonographically, the presence of a solid ovarian mass with a multilobulated appearance separated by fibrovascular septa, is highly suggestive
- **Yolk sac tumors:** Similar in appearance to that of dysgerminomas.

Sex Cord—Stromal Tumors

- **Fibromas:** Meig's syndrome complicates about 1% of ovarian fibromas and is defined as ascites and pleural effusion accompanying a fibrous ovarian tumor usually a fibroma. Two typical appearances have been described sonographically.[21] The first has features similar to that of uterine fibroid. Second appearance is that of a hypoechoic mass with substantial attenuation
- **Thecoma:** Sonographically, these tumors are similar in appearance to fibromas

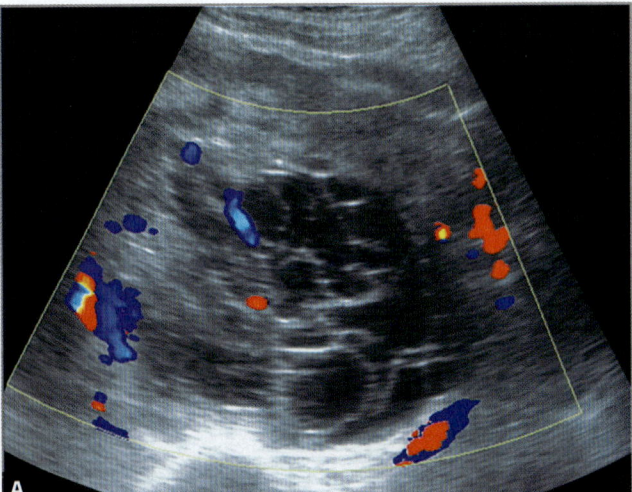

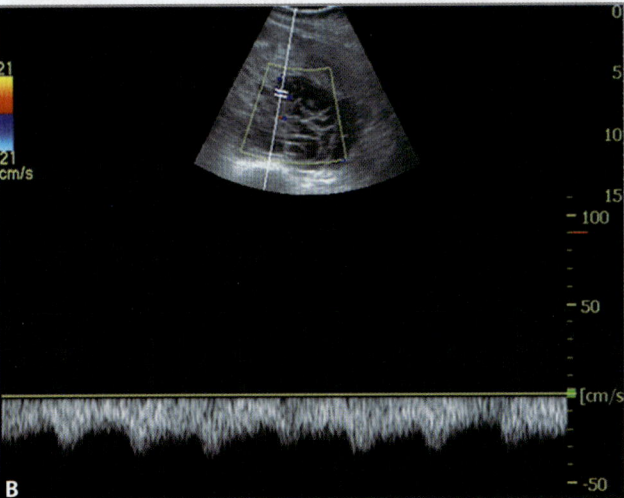

Figs. 22.55A and B: (A) Transabdominal scan showing a complex adnexal mass with thick septae. Vascularity is seen within the septa; (B) Transvaginal color Doppler scan. Spectral shows low resistance, high diastolic flow. Histology confirmed a malignant tumor.

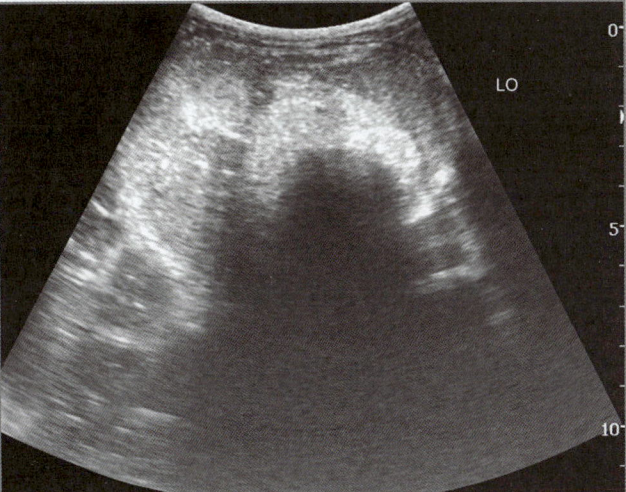

Fig. 22.56: Transvaginal scan of an adnexal mass showing dense echopattern with an echogenic tubercle and posterior shadowing, a dermoid tumor.

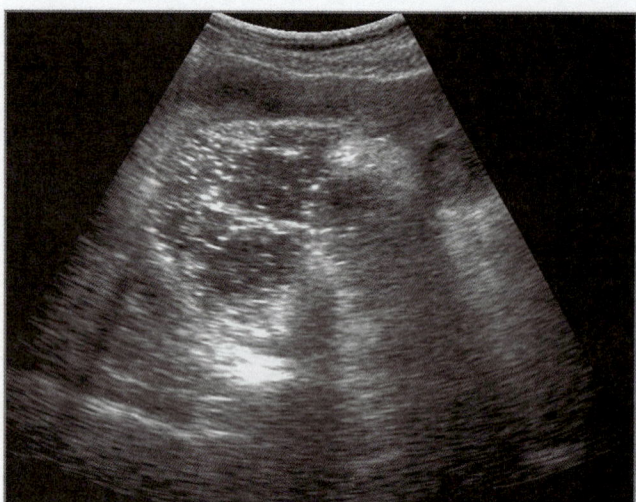

Fig. 22.57: Transabdominal sonogram showing a cystic solid ovarian lesion. Multiple hyperechoic lines and dots characteristic of a dermoid cyst. Note the regional diffuse bright echoes with posterior shadowing.

- **Granulosa cell tumors:** Sonographically small tumors are predominantly solid, having an echogenicity similar to that of fibroids. Large ones resemble cystadenomas and are multiloculated and cystic
- **Sertoli-Leydig cell tumors:** Similar in appearance to granulosa cell tumors.

Metastatic Tumors

Tumor spread to ovaries is by several routes:

- **Direct spread:** Carcinomas of fallopian tube and uterus colonic carcinomas and retroperitoneal sarcomas
- Through the lumen of fallopian tube onto the surface of ovary. Uterine corpus carcinoma.
- Distant site metatatic deposits via blood and lymphatics
- Transcoelomic dissemination with surface implantation.[11]

Ultrasonography: Bilateral ovarian enlargement by solid masses is highly suggestive. These masses may contain hypoechoic areas that represent cystic degeneration or necrosis.

Ovarian lymphoma: Solid hypoechoic masses.

EVALUATION OF AN OVARIAN MASS

- **Morphologic parameters:** Benign tumors are usually unilocular, well-defined borders, thin walls or septa. Malignant tumors are multilocular, have thick or irregular walls or septa, poorly defined borders, mural nodules, solid components and echogenic elements.[22]
- **Doppler parameters:** Neovascularity is a feature of malignant tumors and is characterized by 1000 impedance, high velocity flow. Most authors used a cut-off for malignancy of less than 0.4 for RI and 1.0 for PI.
- **Color flow mapping:** Peripheral vascularization appears to be more common in benign tumors, whereas malignant tumors tend to have more centrally located vessels.

Arrangement of vessels is also a helpful discriminator because benign masses tend to have regularly spaced vessels, whereas malignant tumors demonstrate random distribution of vessels.[23]

Absence of diastolic notch has been associated with malignant tumors.

GESTATIONAL TROPHOBLASTIC DISORDERS

- **Complete hydatidiform mole (CHM):** Snowstorm appearance on sonography without associated embryonic or fetal structure, large sonolucent areas result from stasis of maternal blood between the molar villi. Theca lutein cysts are seen. High serum β-hCG levels combined with sonographic appearance is highly indicative of the disease. Doppler shows high velocities and low resistance flow in uterine arteries (Figs. 22.58A and B).[24]

  A complete mole may coexist with a normal fetus and placenta in cases of molar transformation of one ovum in a dizygotic twin pregnancy.[25]

- **Partial hydatidiform mole (PHM):**[26] Refers to the combination of a fetus with localized placental molar degeneration. In 90% of cases, partial moles are triploid, having inherited 2 sets of chromosomes from the father and one from the mother. Partial mole presents on ultrasound as an enlarged placenta containing multicystic, avascular sonolucent spaces (Swiss cheese appearance). Fetus shows symmetric IUGR and myoformations.
- **Invasive hydatidiform mole:** It is defined as the penetration of molar villi from a CHM or PHM into the myometrium or the uterine vasculature. Sonographically, it appears as focal areas of increased echogenicity within the myometrium.[27] The lesion is heterogenous, often containing fluid-filled cavities.
- **Placental site trophoblastic tumor:** It is the rarest form of GTD. Sonographically, it is similar in appearance to invasive mole.
- **Choriocarcinoma:** It is a highly malignant tumor that metastasizes to lungs, liver and brain. Sonographically, it appears as a solid, echogenic mass with cystic areas suggestive of hemorrhage and summary.

Pelvic sonographic imaging is the technique of choice for evaluation of pelvic organs and is a very commonly performed examination. For vaginal bleeding and pelvic

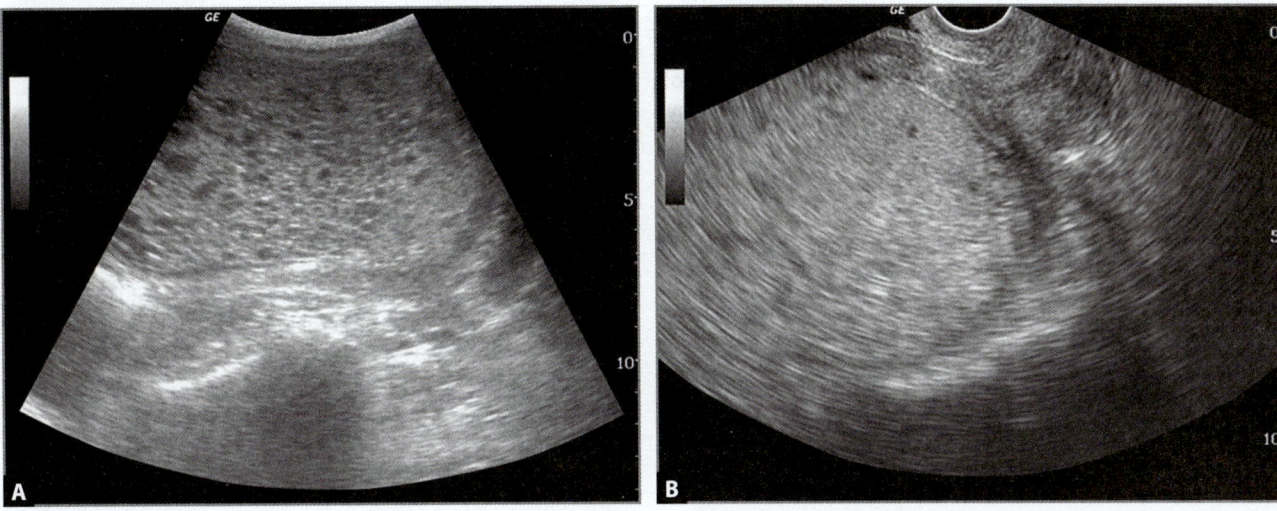

Figs. 22.58A and B: A patient in her 15th week of pregnancy came to the clinician with uterine size larger than dates. Transvaginal sonogram: (A) Longitudinal; (B) Transverse showed an enlarged uterus completely filled with grape-like clusters. No fetal pole was seen suggestive of a complete hydatidiform mole.

pain, the main roles are to determine the presence of lesion, its origin and whether surgery is required. Where there is difficulty, a tailored MRI examination can be helpful.

PELVIC KIDNEY

Rarely, ectopic kidney is visualized in the pelvis and may mimic abnormal T-O masses.

REFERENCES

1. Burnett LS. Anatomy. In: Jones HWIII, Wentz AC (Eds). Novak's textbook of gynecology, 11th edition Baltimore: Williams and Wilkins; 1988;40.
2. Platt JF, Bree RL, DavidsonD. Ultrasound of the normal nongravid uterus: correlation with gross and histopathology. J Clinical Ultrasound. 1990;18:15.
3. Splanchnology: Reproductive organs of the female. In: Williams PM, Warwick R (Eds). Gray's Anatomy, 36th edition Edinburgh: Churchill Livingstone; 1980;1423.
4. Wagner BJ, Woodward PJ. Magnetic resonance evaluation of congenital uterine anomalies. Semin Ultrasound CT MR. 1994;15(1):4.
5. Reinhold C, Atri M, Mehio A, et al. Diffuse uterine adenomyosis: morphologic criteria and diagnostic accuracy of endovaginal sonography. Radiology. 1995;197(3):609.
6. Cramer SF, Patel A. The nonrandom regional distribution of uterine leiomyomas: A clue to histogenesis? Hum Pathol. 1992;23(6):635.
7. Mungen E, Yergok YZ, Ertekin AA, et al. Color Doppler sonographic features of uterine arteriovenous malformations: Report of two cases. Ultrasound Obstet Gynecol. 1997;10(3):215.
8. DelMaschio A, Vanzulli A, Sironi S, et al. Estimating the depth of myometrial involvement by endometrial carcinoma: Efficacy of transvaginal sonography vs MR imaging. AJR J Roentgenol. 1993;160:533.
9. Carlan SJ, Scott WT, Pollock R, et al. Appearance of the uterus by ultrasound immediately after placental delivery with pathologic correlation. J Clin Ultrasound. 1997;25(6):301.
10. Wachsberg RH, Kurtz AB. Gas within the endometrial cavity at postpartum US: A normal finding after spontaneous vaginal delivery. Radiology. 1992;183(2):431.
11. Kurman RJ. Blaustein's pathology of female genital tract. 4th edition New York: Springer- Verlag; 1994.
12. Wajda KJ, Lucas JG, Marsh WL. Hyperreactio luteinalis. Benign disorder masquerading as an ovarian neoplasm. Arch Pathol. Lab Med. 1989;113:921.
13. Brinsden PR, Wada I, Tan SL, et al. Diagnosis, prevention and management of ovarian hyperstimulation syndrome. Br J Obstet Gynecol. 1995;102:767.
14. Matsunga I, Hata T, Kitao M. Ultrasonographic identification of polycystic ovary. Asia Oceania J Obstet Gynecol. 1985;11:227.
15. Kupfer MC, Schwimer SR, Lebovic J. Transvaginal sonographic appearance of endometriomata: Spectrum of findings. J Ultrasound Medicine. 1992;11:129.
16. Timor-Tritsch IE, Lerner JP, MonteagudoA, et al. Transvaginal sonographic markers of tubal inflammatory disease. Ultrasound Obstet Gynecol. 1998;12:56.
17. Rosado WM Jr, Trambert MA, Gosink BB, et al. Adnexal Tortion: Diagnosis by using Doppler sonography. AJR Am J Roentgenology. 1992;159:1251.

18. Roberts CL, Weston MJ. Bilateral massive ovarian edema: a case report. Ultrasound Obstet Gynecol. 1998;11:65.
19. Baran GW, Frisch KM. Duplex Doppler evaluation of puerperal ovarian vein thrombosis. AJR Am J Roentgenology. 1987;149:321.
20. Fried AM, Kenney CM, Stigers KB, et al. Benign pelvic masses: sonographic spectrum. Radiographics. 1996;16:321.
21. Atri M, Nazarnia S, Bret P, et al. Endovaginal sonographic appearance of benign ovarian masses. Radiographics. 1994;14:747.
22. Rottem S, Levit n, Thaler I, et al. Classification of ovarian lesions by high frequency transvaginal sonography. J Clin Ultrasound. 1990;18:359.
23. Fleischer AC, Rodgers WH, Kepple DM, et al. Color Doppler sonography of ovarian masses: A multiparameter analysis. J Ultrasound Medicine. 1993;12:41.
24. Elston CW. Trophoblastic tumors of the placenta. In: Fox H (Ed). Pathology of the placenta. Philadelphia: WB Saunders; 1978;369.
25. Stellar MA, Genesst DR, Bernstein MR, et al. Natural history of twin pregnancy with complete hydatidiform mole and coexisting fetus. Obstet Gynecol. 1994;83:35.
26. Jeffers MD, O'Dwyer P, Curran B, et al. Partial Hydatidiform mole: a common but underdiagnosed condition. Int J Gynecol Pathol. 1993;12:315.
27. Fleischer AC, James AE, Krause DA, et al. Sonographic patterns in trophoblastic disease. Radiology. 1978;126:215.

CHAPTER 22: Ultrasound and Color Doppler in Gynecology

3D ULTRASOUND IN GYNECOLOGY

INTRODUCTION

Ultrasound has revolutionized obstetrics and gynecology practice. It is now impossible to even conceive an obstetric unit without ultrasound. The impact of ultrasound was seen a little less in gynecological diagnosis till the advent of transvaginal probe (Fig. 22.59).

2D ultrasound of female pelvis has been established from several decades limited by only certain views of pelvis. In order to have a clear view of anatomy, previously we were dependent on our mental ability to create a 3D image. Now 3D has change and enhanced the capability of ultrasonography.

With Professor Katrochwil inventing the TVS probe, the practise and diagnosis of gynecological pelvic problems became the main indication of ultrasound.

Today 3D scanning has added another dimension to imaging. Now all three planes of the scanned organ can be depicted on the screen with 3D reconstruction and with computer software of the machine, various modes like virtual organ computer-aided analysis (VOCAL) (for volume estimation), niche mode for sectional anatomy, extended view for a wide scanning, color 3D-PD for vessel orientation and angiographic images of lesion's vascularity.

In the last three decades, diagnostic ultrasound has come a long way from static "dinosaurs" type of ultrasound scanners to amazing real-time three-dimensional sonographic machines (Fig. 22.60).[1]

Transabdominal scanning gives an overview of the pelvis, transvaginal scanning depicts details, TVS color Doppler gives information about physiological blood supply to the scanned organs and 3D gives sculpture like images while 3D-4D-PD gives an angiographic picture of the vascular connections of the pelvic mass (Table 22.1).[2]

To assess a pelvic lesion by ultrasound the following features have to be evaluated:
- Organ of origin: Uterus, ovary, tubes, and bowel
- Internal contents: Cystic, solid, mixed
- Associated findings like ascites, hydronephrosis
- Color Doppler for flow studies

Table 22.1: Pelvic masses (Sonographic differential diagnosis).

Cystic	Complex	Solid
Completely cystic • Physiological ovarian cysts • Cystadenomas • Hydrosalpinx • Endometrioma • Paraovarian cyst • Hydatid cyst of Morgagni	**Predominantly cystic** • Cystadenomas • Tubo-ovarian abscess • Ectopic pregnancy • Cystic teratoma	**Uterine** • Leiomyoma • Sarcoma • Endometrial carcinoma
Multiple cysts • Endometrioma • Multiple follicular	**Predominantly solid** • Cystadenoma (Solid) • Germ cell tumor	**Extrauterine** • Solid ovarian tumor
Septated • Cystadenoma (carcinoma) • Mucinous • Serous • Papillary		

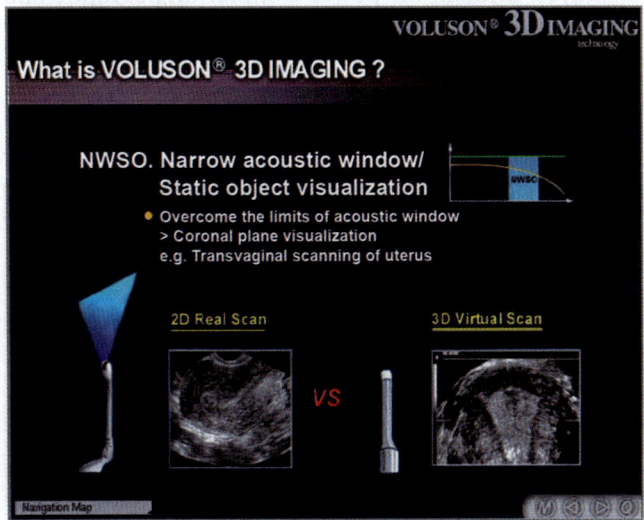

Fig. 22.59: 3D ultrasound in imaging pelvic masses.

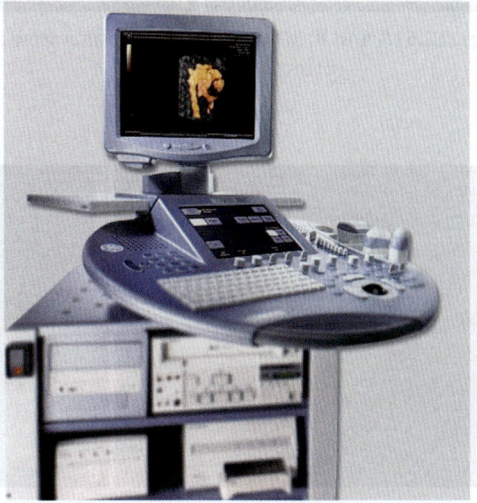

Fig. 22.60: 3D machine with real-time 4D.

- 3D reconstruction of the lesion
- 3D power Doppler for vascularity of the lesion.

Common Practical Difficulties

It is important to remember that any information using color Doppler or 3D is of little value if vessel/organ sampled is incorrectly identified.

All major vessels have characteristic waveforms. All organs have their own unique appearance.

UTERINE LESIONS

Three-dimensional ultrasound provides simultaneous display of coronal, saggital and transverse planes. Volume data can be viewed using a standard anatomic orientation demonstrating entire volume and continuity of curved structure in a single image[3] (Fig. 22.61).

When three perpendicular planes are simultaneously displayed on screen, sagittal plane is chosen for volume measurements, while the other two planes are used to ensure that the entire pathology is included in the measurement (Fig. 22.62).

3D surface rendering mode allows exploration of the outer or inner contour of the lesion while the "niche aspect" presents detection and analysis of the selected sections of the uterine lesion (Fig. 22.63).

Three-dimensional ultrasound offers improved visualisation of the lesions, more accurate volume estimation, retrospective review of stored data, assessment of tumor invasion, and using rendered images, it can identify more accurate location of abnormalities needing surgical intervention (Fig. 22.64).

Three-dimensional sonohysterography is very useful in the evaluation of the uterine cavity and is more informative than normal 2D sonohysterography for submucous myoma and polyps[4,5] (Fig. 22.65).

3D power Doppler gives information about normal blood supply and also abnormal tumor vascularity. 3D power Doppler helps in accurate examination of small vessels (Fig. 22.66).

3D OF ENDOMETRIUM

3D ultrasound can simultaneously assess the endometrial volume and low vessel flow endometrial perfusion for use as a predictive marker for implantation endometrial scoring (Fig. 22.67).

ENDOMETRIAL VOLUME

Assessment done by 3D ultrasound is a reliable and reproducible method.[6] By using VOCAL the endometrial volume and perfusion can be assessed.

ENDOMETRIAL PERFUSION

First the endometrial volume and endometrial vessels are displayed through 3D power Doppler angiography and vascularization index (VI), flow index are calculated by VOCAL.

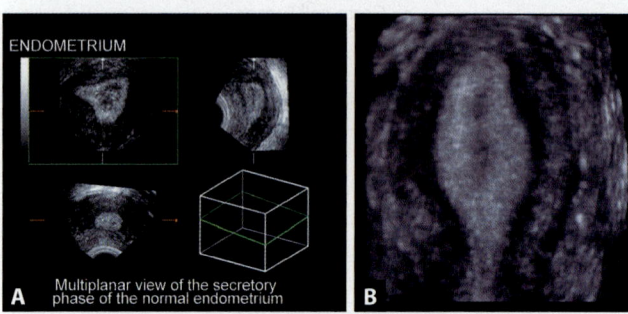

Figs. 22.61A and B: 3D uterus (A) multiplanar view and; (B) reconstructed view.

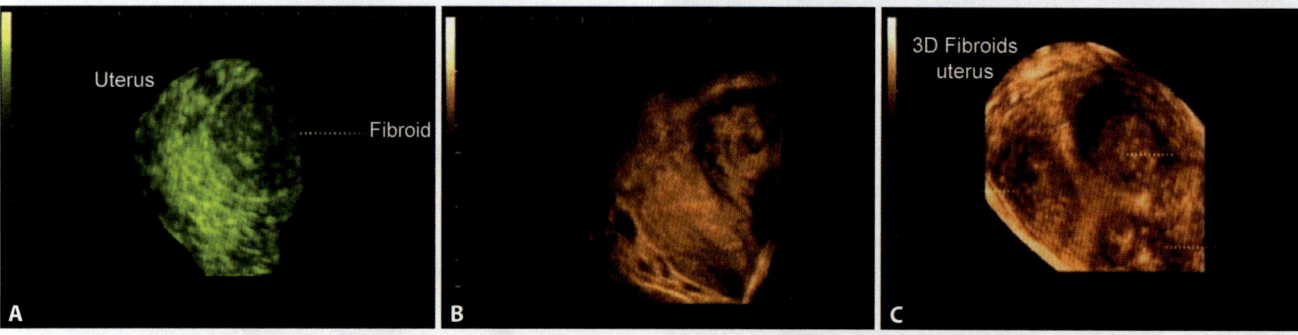

Figs. 22.62A to C: 3D fibroids.

CHAPTER 22 Ultrasound and Color Doppler in Gynecology

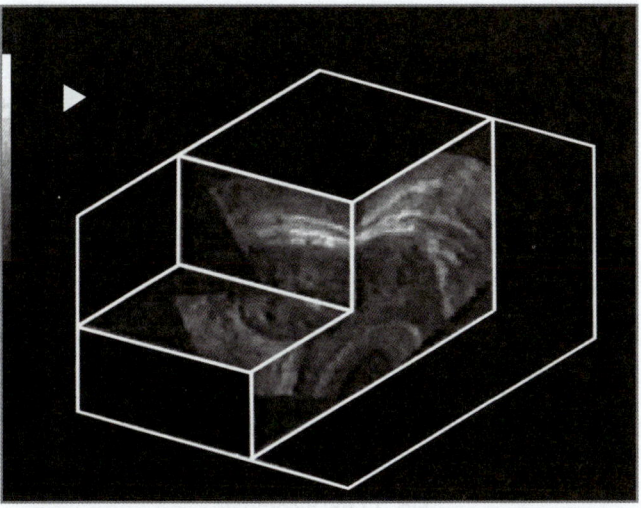

Fig. 22.63: Niche mode uterus area showing a fibroid.

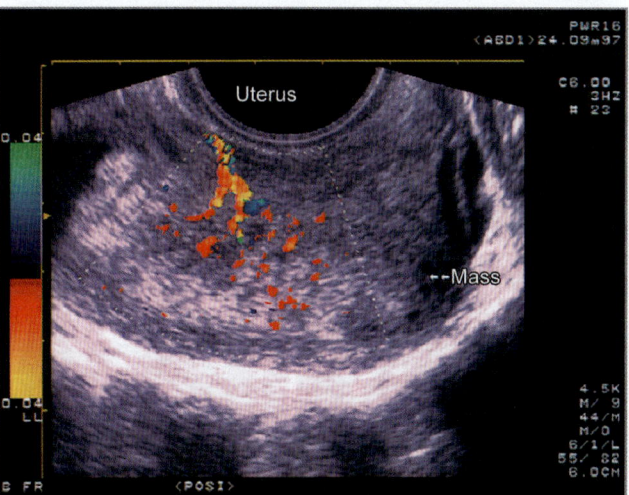

Fig. 22.64: Color fibroid.

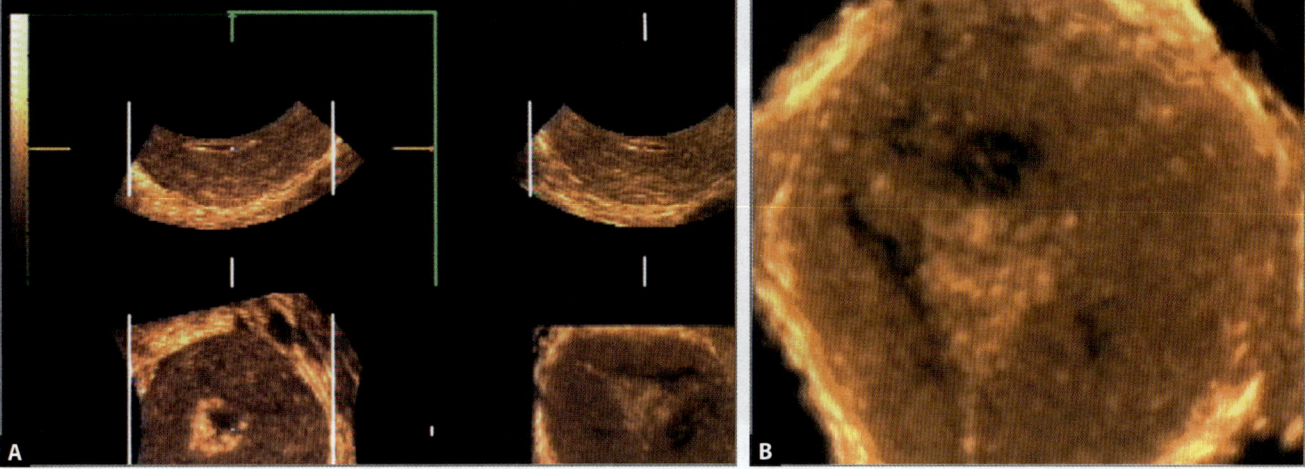

Figs. 22.65A and B: 3D cavity.

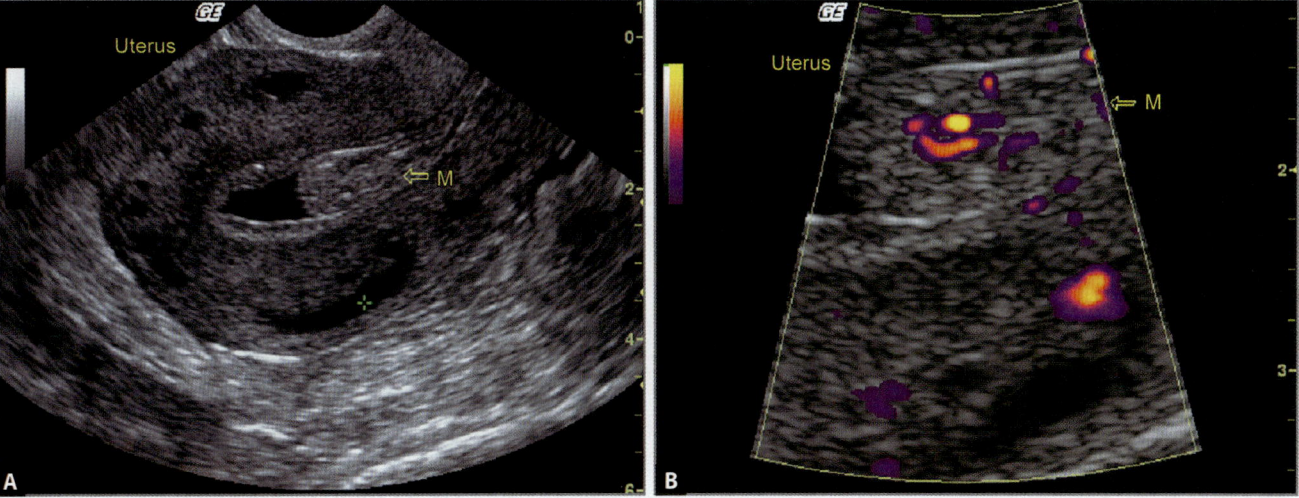

Figs. 22.66A and B: Uterine polyp.

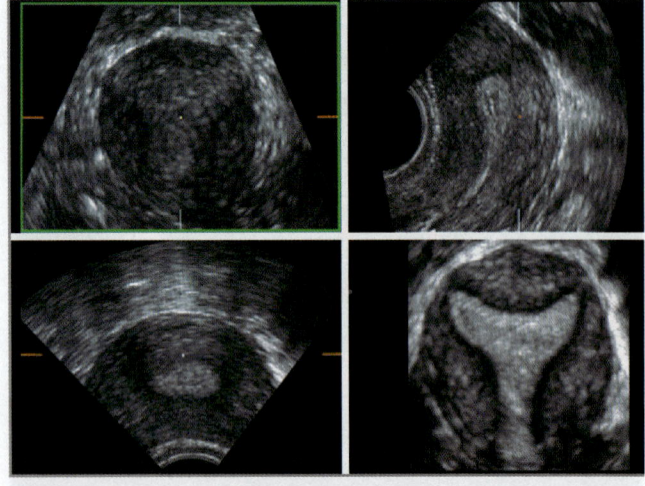

Fig. 22.67: Arcuate uterus.

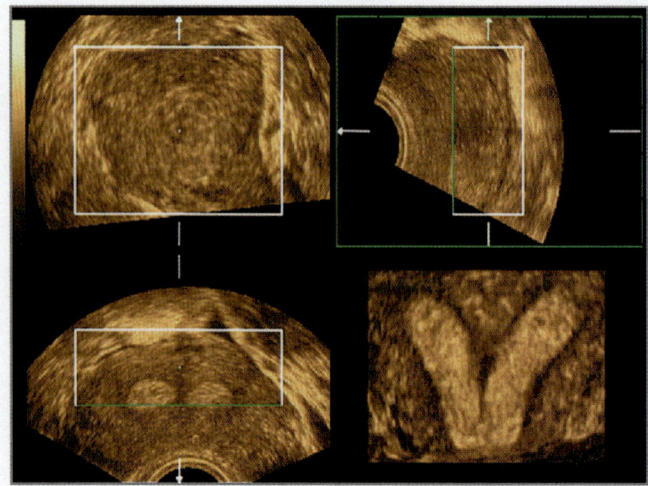

Fig. 22.68: Bicornuate.

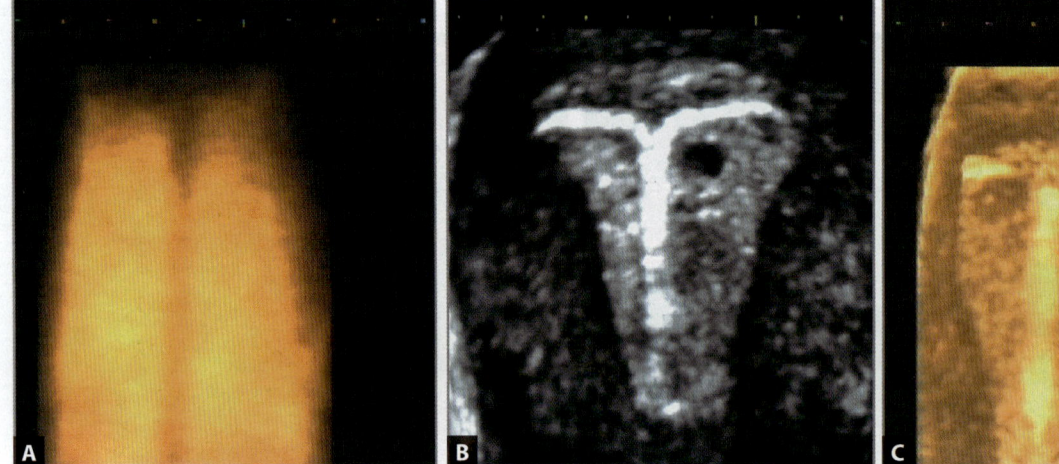

Figs. 22.69A to C: 3D reconstruction and multiplanar scanning of the uterus.

OVARIAN LESIONS

Transvaginal sonography can provide a good, detailed delineation of normal and abnormal ovaries. The 3D provides display of all three planes on the screen and volume measurements can be performed by using computer program VOCAL.

Surface rendering mode will give clear picture of ovarian surface lesions, and niche aspects helps in analysis of selected ovarian sections.

With 3D small intraovarian lesions can be assessed more accurately and 3D power Doppler helps in accurate analysis of intraovarian helical vessels[7,8] (Figs. 22.68 to 22.73).

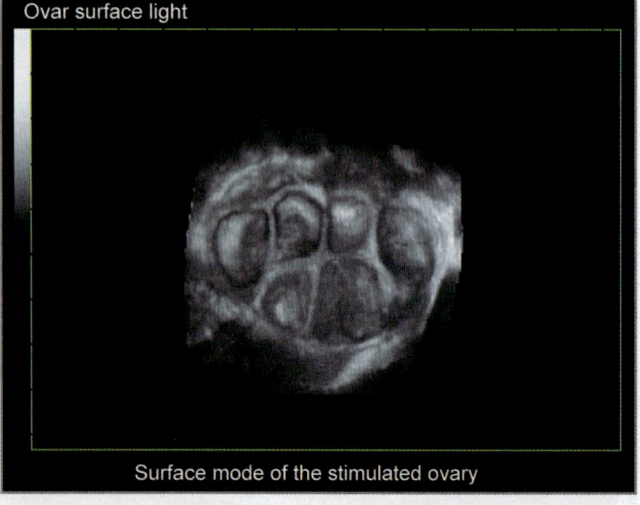

Fig. 22.70: 3D ovarian surface.

CHAPTER 22 *Ultrasound and Color Doppler in Gynecology*

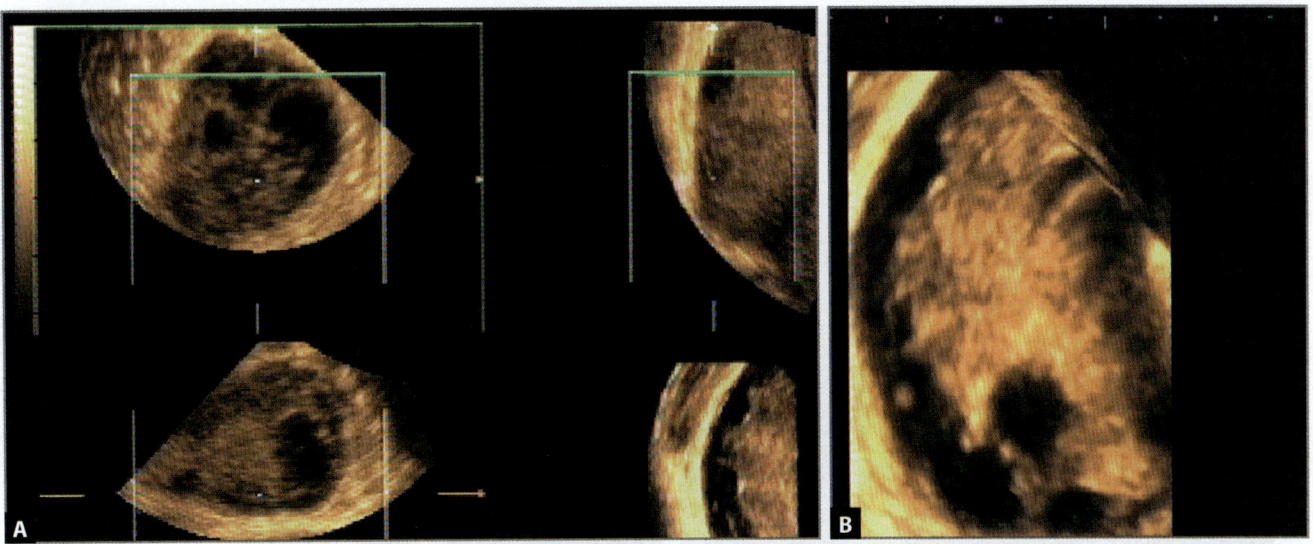

Figs. 22.71A and B: 3D polycystic ovarian disease (PCOD).

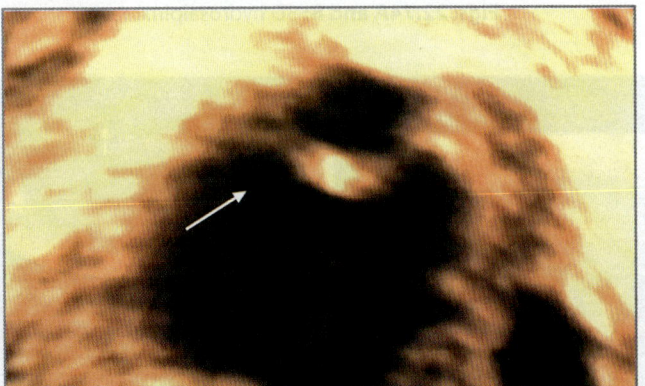

Fig. 22.72: 3D follicle.

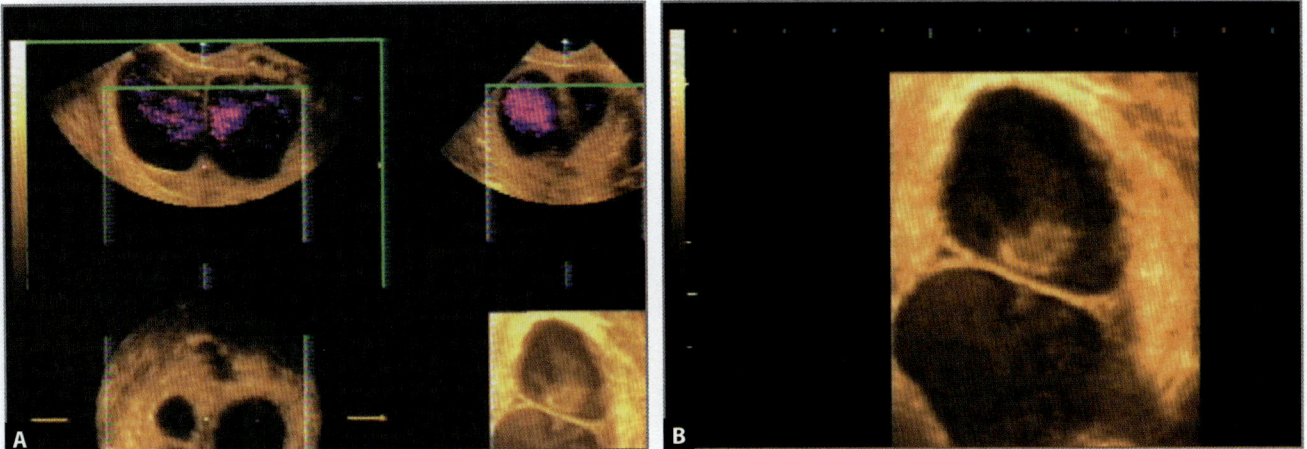

Figs. 22.73A and B: Ovarian cyst.

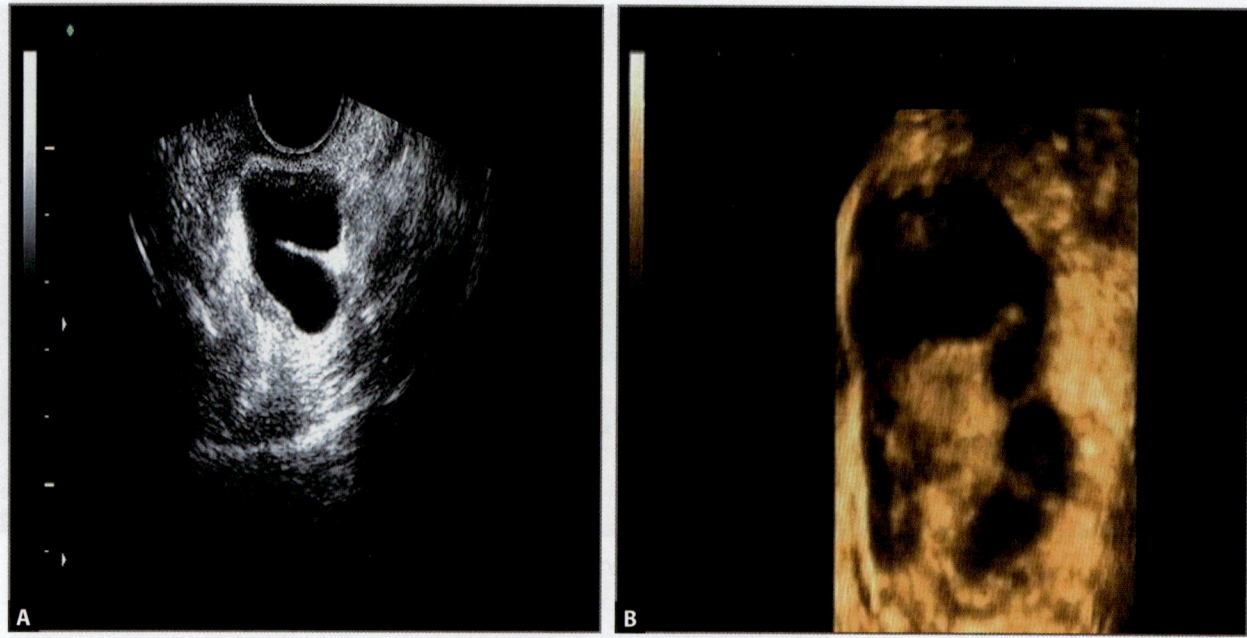

Figs. 22.74A and B: 3D hydrosalpinx.

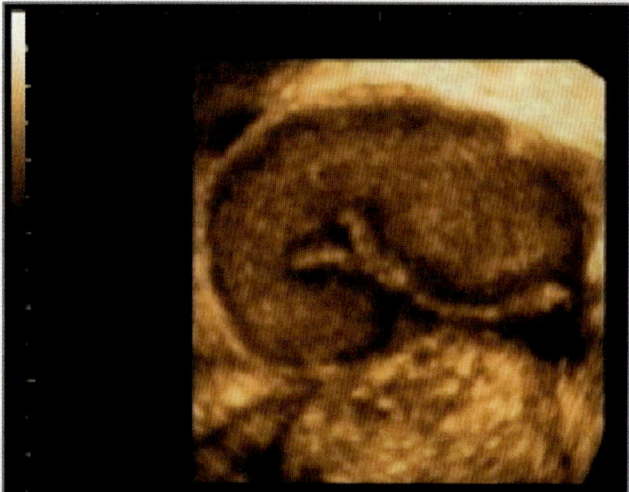

Fig. 22.75: Pyosalpinx.

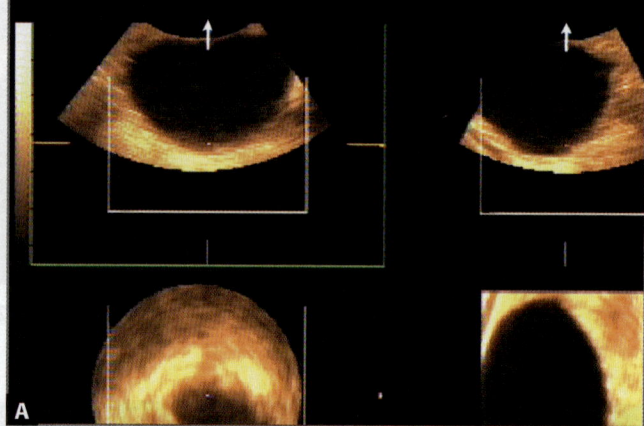

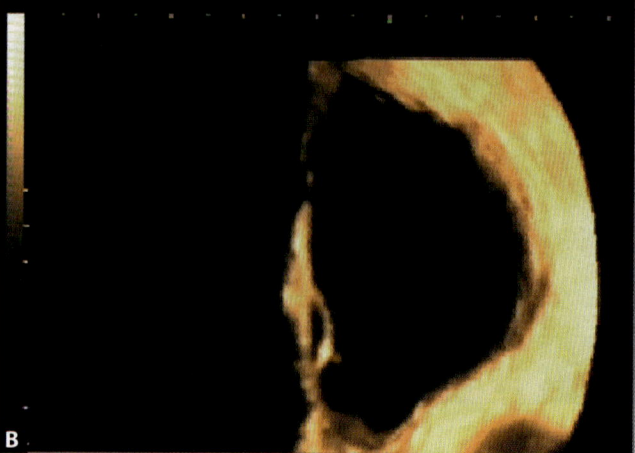

Figs. 22.76A and B: Endometrioma.

OTHER ADNEXAL LESIONS

3D also helps to accurately analyze lesions of the fallopian tubes and complex tubo-ovarian masses and abscess (Figs. 22.74 to 22.76).

Typical characteristic of tubal inflammatory disease has been described as Timor-Tritsch criteria.[9]

- Tubal wall thickening >5 mm (100% of acute and 3% chronic cases)
- Cogwheel sign (86% acute and 3% chronic cases)
- Incomplete septa
- Beads on a string sign

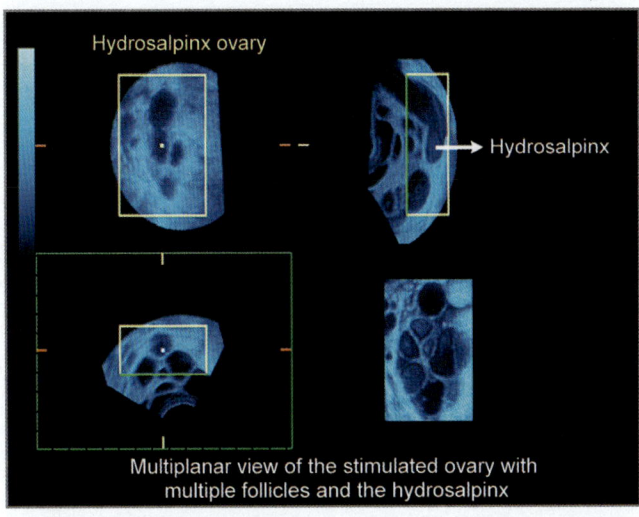

Fig. 22.77: Multiplanar display of adnexa.

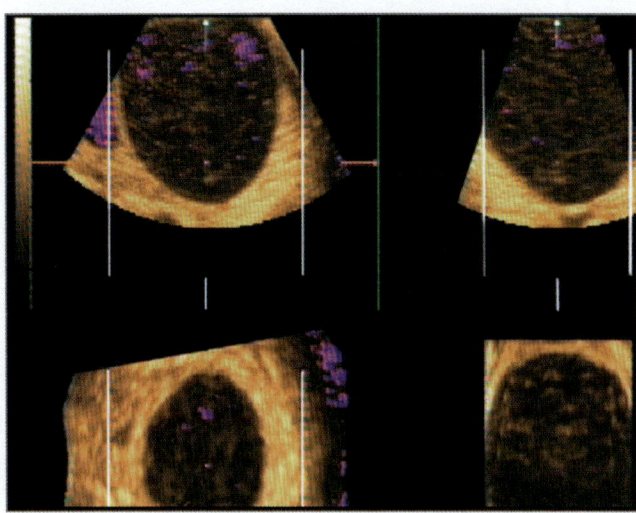

Fig. 22.78: Hemorrhagic cyst.

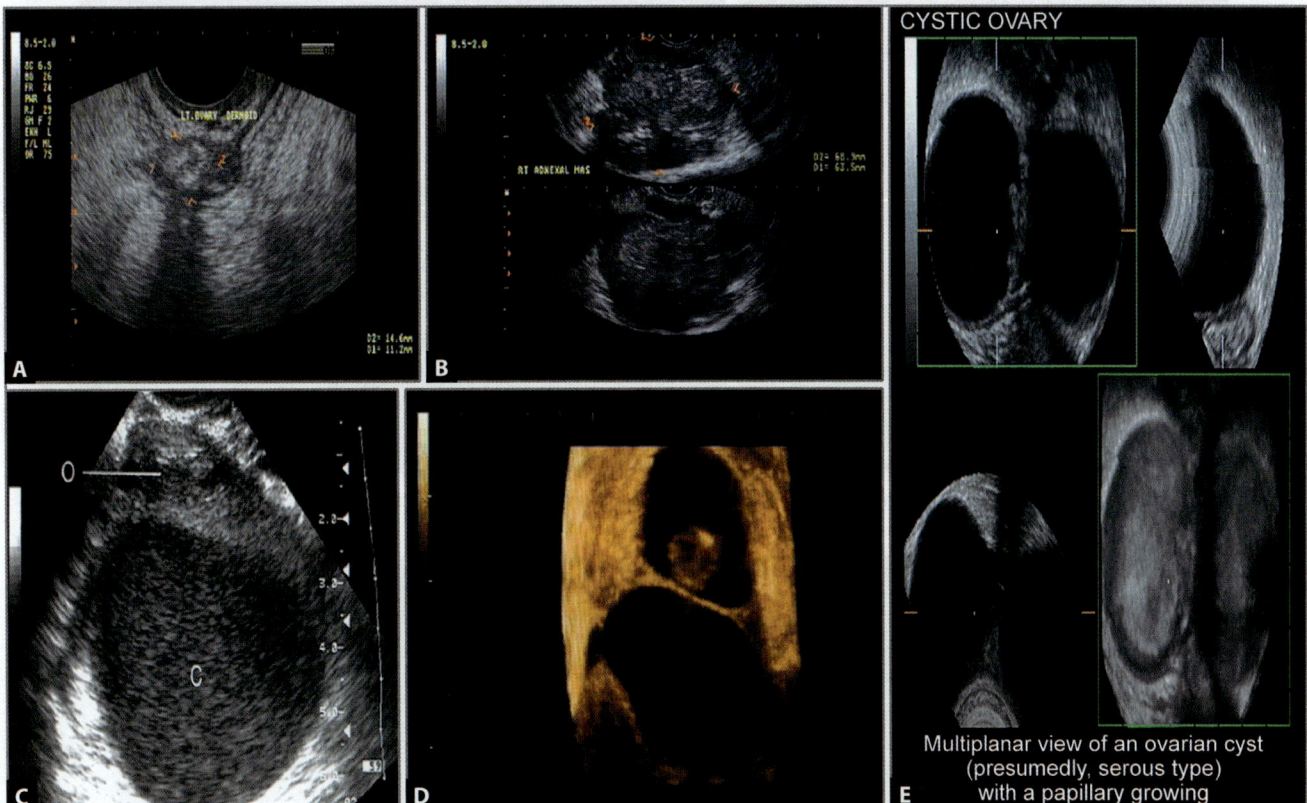

Figs. 22.79A to E: Abnormal ovaries.

- Tubo-ovarian complex (push pull sign) (sliding sign)
- Tubo-ovarian abscess
- Cul-de-sac fluid (50% acute and 10% chronic cases).

All of these signs are more accurately depicted by 3D reconstruction and multiplanar scanning (Figs. 22.77 to 22.79).

ENDOMETRIOSIS

Although, the ultrasound findings of endometriosis are nonspecific but the differentiation of an endometriotic cyst from a functional hemorrhagic cyst is possible by showing multiple thick walls, homogeneity of echogenic content and multiplicity of lesion.[10] Also on observation for several cycles, hemorrhagic cysts tend to disappear. Use of color Doppler imaging, CA 125 and 3D characterization of the cyst does not improve the diagnostic accuracy of a 2D, B mode, high-resolution transvaginal scan (Figs. 22.80 and 22.81).

PARAOVARIAN CYSTS

3D scanning will accurately depict cysts not arising from the ovaries like paraovarian cyst, peritoneal cyst or cyst of Morgagans[11] (Figs. 22.82A and B).

OVARIAN DERMOID CYSTS

Kurjack's morphologic scoring system for dermoids by transvaginal color and 3D of the lesion gives almost a sensitivity of 93% and specificity 99%.[12]

OTHER OVARIAN MASSES (FIGS. 22.83 AND 22.84)

Borilla-Musoles et al.[13] have found 3D US superior in:

- Evaluating papillary projections
- Characterizing cystic walls
- Identifying the extent of capsular infilteration
- Calculating tumor volume.

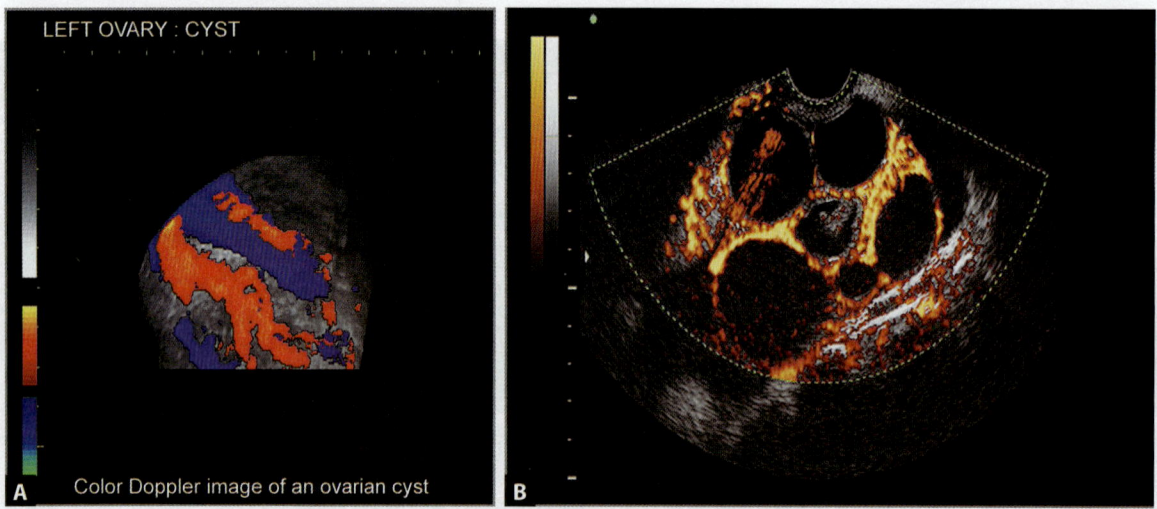

Figs. 22.80A and B: Color 3D picture of ovarian cyst and surface blood vessels.

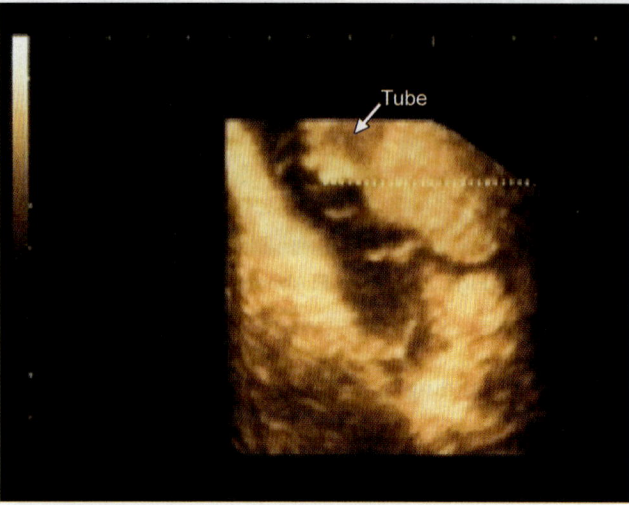

Fig. 22.81: Normal fallopian tube 3D.

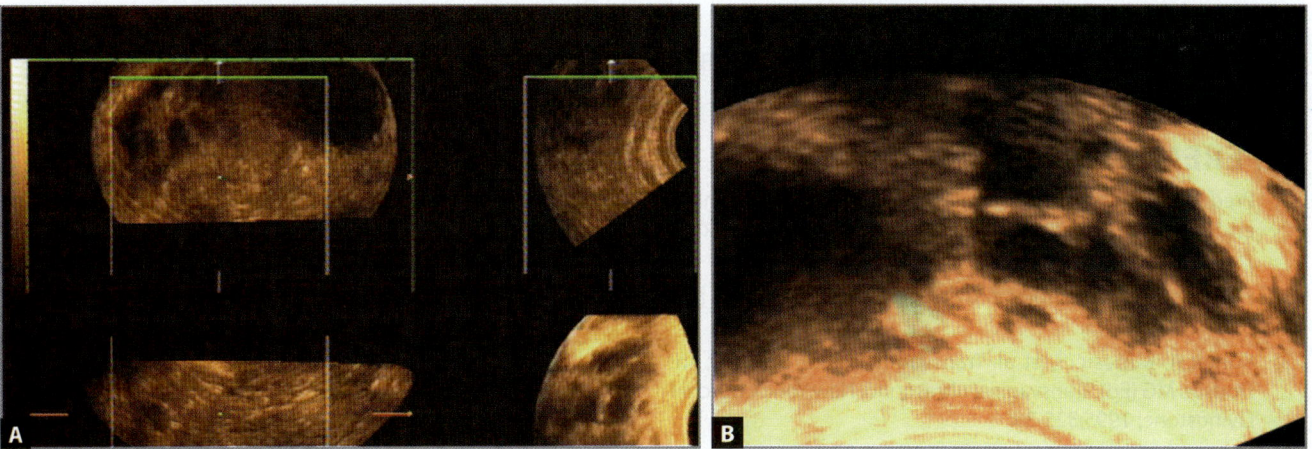

Figs. 22.82A and B: Paraovarian cyst.

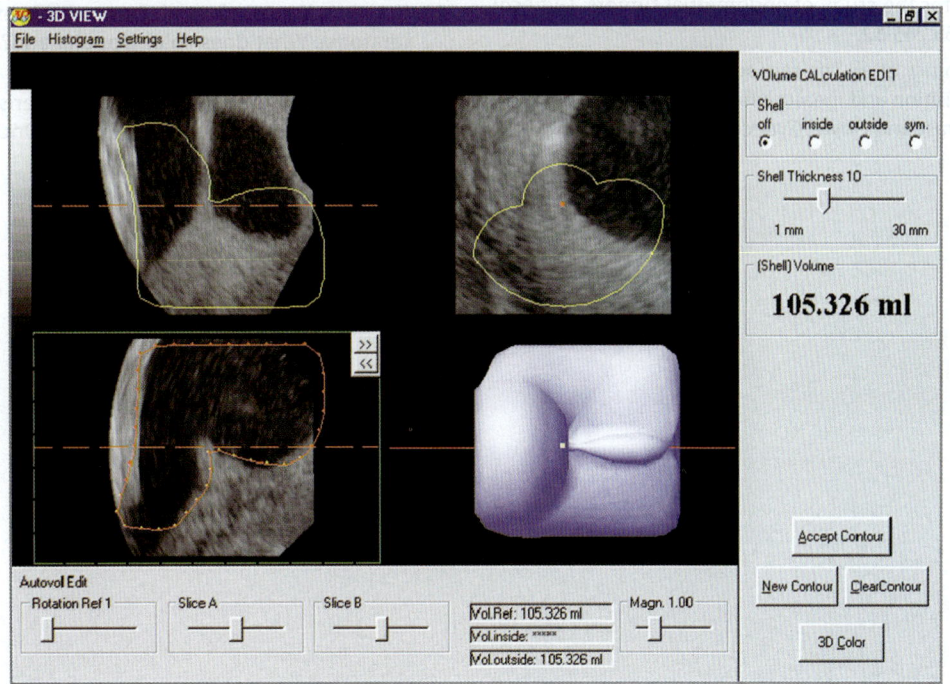

Fig. 22.83: Volume measurement.

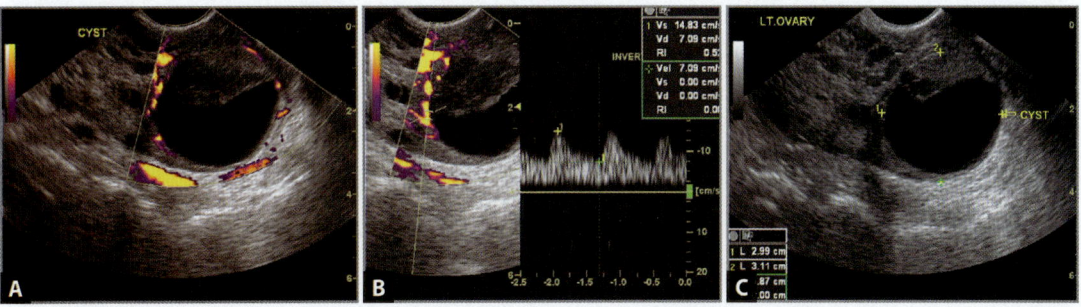

Figs. 22.84A to C: Benign ovarian cyst.

ACKNOWLEDGMENTS

I am thankful to Dr BI Patel, Dr Kuldeep Singh and Dr Bhupendra Ahuja for providing some of the photographs.

REFERENCES

1. Predanic M. Advanced sonographic assessment of benign endometrial disease. Chapter 40, Donald Textbook of Transvaginal Sonography, 2005.
2. Flascher AC. Sonography in gynecology and obstetrics: just the facts, 2004;95.
3. Kurjak A, Kupesic S, et al. Transvaginal color Doppler. In: Dodson MG (Ed). Transvaginal ultrasound. New York: Churchill Livingstone; 1995;325-39.
4. Momtag M, El E Brashi A. 3D sonohysterography in the evaluation of the uterine cavity. Syllabus Las Vegas, Oct. 1999.
5. Borilla–Musoles F, Raga F, et al. Three-dimensional hysterosonography for the study of endometrial tumors. Gynecol Oncol. 1997;65:245-52.
6. Raine – Fenning, et al. The reproducibility of endometrial volume acquisition and measurements with VOCAL imaging program. Ultrasound Obstel Gynecol. 2002;19:69-75.
7. Fleisher AC, et al. Color Doppler sonography of benign and malignant ovarian masses. Radiographics. 1992;12:879-85.
8. Kurjak A, et al. Transvaginal color Doppler sonography in assessment of pelvic tumor vascularity. Ultrasound Obstet Gynecol. 1993.
9. Timor-Tritsch, et al. Transvaginal sonographic markers of tubal inflammatory disease. Ultrasound Obstet Gynecol. 1998; 12:56-66.
10. Atri M, et al. Endovaginal sonographic appearance of benign ovarian masses. Radiographics. 1994;14:747-60.
11. Karbin CD, et al. Paraovarian cystadenomas and cystadenofibromas: sonographic characteristic in 14 cases. Radiology. 1998;208:459-62.
12. Kurjak A, Kupesic S, et al. Preoperative evaluation of cystic teratoma. What does color Doppler add? J Clin ultrasound. 1997;25:309-16.
13. Borilla-Musoles F, et al. Three-dimensional ultrasound evaluation of ovarian masses. Gynecol Oncol. 1995;59:129-35.

CHAPTER 23

Gynecological Operations

AP Manjunath, Jayaraman Nambiar

Overview

- Abdominal hysterectomy carries an increased morbidity compared with vaginal hysterectomy but has an advantage of adequate exposure especially in patients with malignancy and other intra-abdominal diseases.
- Ovaries are generally left behind if they are grossly normal and if the patient is below 40 years. After the age of 40, ovaries are removed with the consent of the woman to prevent the occurrence of ovarian carcinoma at a later date.
- There are various operative interventions available for vaginal prolapse. These operations are aimed at the restoration of normal anatomy.
- Laparoscopy has several clear advantages over laparotomy. In recent years, the spectrum of gynecological indications for operative laparoscopy has expanded dramatically.

ABDOMINAL HYSTERECTOMY

Abdominal hysterectomy is a common operation performed in gynecology. Abdominal hysterectomy is performed three times more commonly than vaginal hysterectomy.[1] Abdominal hysterectomy carries an increased morbidity compared with vaginal hysterectomy but has an advantage of adequate exposure especially in patients with malignancy and other intra-abdominal disease.

Types of Abdominal Hysterectomy

Subtotal Hysterectomy

Here the body of uterus is removed and the cervix is left behind. This is generally done in cases of emergency like postpartum hemorrhage and in cases where approach to lower part of uterus is difficult as in cases of adhesions.[2]

Total Abdominal Hysterectomy

In total abdominal hysterectomy, the uterus and cervix is removed. This is usually done in cases of benign uterine pathology when the patient's age is less than 40 years.

Total Abdominal Hysterectomy with Bilateral Salpingo-oophorectomy

Here the uterus and cervix is removed along with the adnexa. It is also known as pan abdominal hysterectomy. It is generally done for patients above the age of 50 years and in some centers above the age of 40 years.

Radical Hysterectomy (Wertheim's Hysterectomy)

This is a special surgery done in cases of cervical malignancy. Here the uterus, cervix, parametrium, adnexa and upper third of vagina are removed. The removal of ovaries is optional depending on the age of women. Grossly, normal ovaries are generally preserved if the woman is less than 40 years of age.

The draining pelvic lymph nodes are also removed in addition to the removal of above structures for complete treatment of cervical cancer.

Indications for Abdominal Hysterectomy

Common indications for hysterectomy include fibroid uterus, dysfunctional uterine bleeding (DUB) and endometriosis. Other indications include pelvic inflammatory disease and malignancies of genital tract. Hysterectomy may also be performed for cases of severe intraepithelial neoplasia (CIN III) of the cervix if the patient is not willing for ablative therapies. Hysterectomy may be performed as an emergency procedure to control atonic postpartum bleeding.

Preoperative Preparations for Hysterectomy

Prior to surgery, a detailed history and physical examination should be undertaken. Apart from detailed gynecological history, careful urological and gastrointestinal history should be taken. These organs lie close to the uterus and previous surgery in these systems may make gynecological operations difficult. Details regarding previous gynecological operations should be carefully asked as these procedures may make the surgery difficult. Thorough gynecological examination should be done. Apart from this assessment of cardiovascular system and other systems should be undertaken which may make anesthesia difficult. Investigations preoperatively include a full blood count, platelet count, fasting blood sugar, renal function tests, liver function tests, chest X-ray and ECG. Patients should be subjected to routine HIV and HBsAg screening. Adequate amount of blood should be arranged before surgery depending on the blood loss expected during the procedure. In situations where adhesions or other intrabdominal disease is suspected a preoperative consultation with urologist or general surgeon need to be taken.

Choice of Incision

Incisions for abdominal hysterectomy may be a subumbilical midline incision or a suprapubic transverse incision. A midline incision is used when there is a large uterus to be removed or there is malignancy. Transverse incisions do not provide adequate exposure and are generally reserved for benign uterine pathology and when the uterine size is not big. A transverse incision produces a more cosmetic and stronger scar (Figs. 23.1 to 23.3).[3]

When operating for huge fiborids, a Maylards muscle cutting incision can be used. Huge fibroids can be removed through a Maylards incision instead of a midline incision.

Prophylactic Oophorectomy at the Time of Hysterectomy

Ovaries are generally left behind if they are grossly normal and if the patient is below 40 years. After the age of 40, ovaries are removed with the consent of the woman to prevent the occurrence of ovarian carcinoma at a later date.[4]

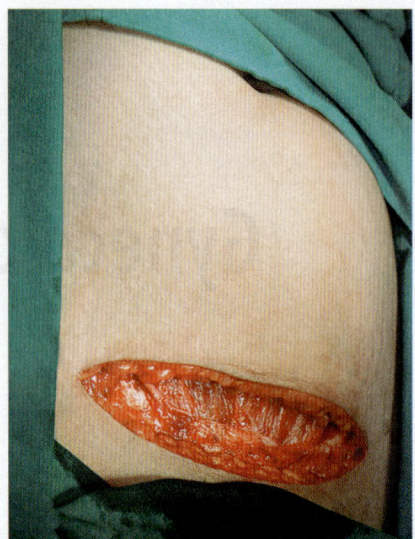

Fig. 23.1: Pfannenstiel transverse abdominal incision.

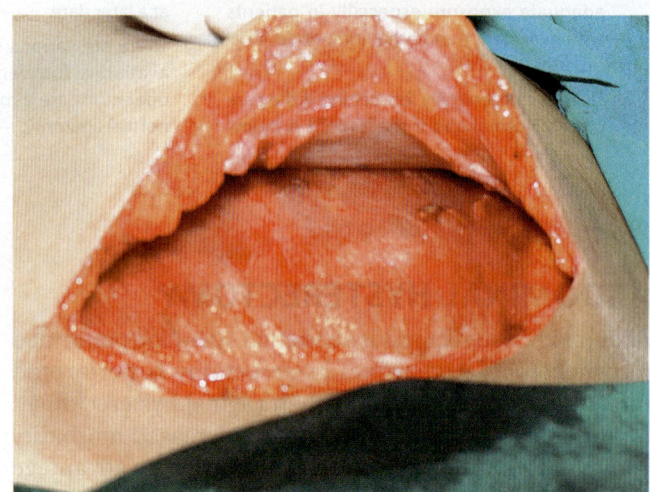

Fig. 23.2: Rectus sheath opened.

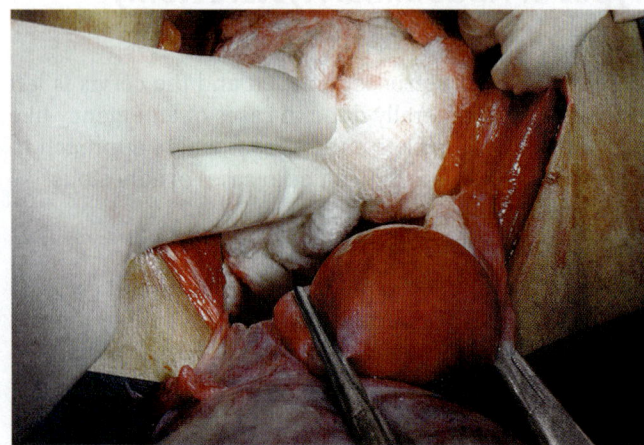

Fig. 23.3: Intestines pushed back by packing the abdomen.

CHAPTER 23 Gynecological Operations

Steps of Abdominal Hysterectomy

The operation begins with placement of clamps by the side of the uterus. Alternatively, uterus may be held with a bulldog clamp at the fundus and lifted up from the pelvis.

This clamp apart from lifting the uterus, tubes and ovaries out of the pelvis also helps in dissection and hemostasis (Fig. 23.4). The round ligaments are clamped, cut and ligated (Figs. 23.5A to D). The incision on the anterior leaf of broad ligament is now extended anteriorly to the midline of uterus. Next, the bladder is separated from the lower uterine segment by sharp dissection and pushed down (Figs. 23.6A and B). If tubes and ovaries have to be conserved, tubes and ovarian ligament are clamped, cut and ligated close to uterus after making a window in the posterior leaf of broad ligament (Fig. 23.7). If ovaries have to be removed, the infundibulopelvic ligament is clamped cut and ligated (Figs. 23.8A and B). Next structure that is clamped is uterine vessels (Figs. 23.9A to D). One should remember three cardinal rules in clamping uterine vessels:

- The clamp is placed at the level of internal cervical os
- It is placed at right angle to the lower uterine segment
- The lowest clamp is placed initially.

If these principles are followed, the injury to the ureter is avoided. Ureters lie close to the cervix as they travel

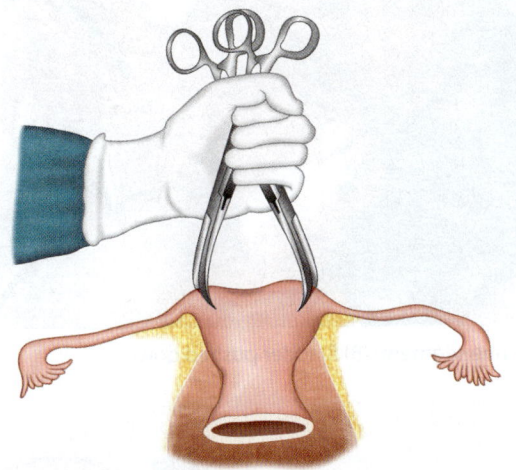

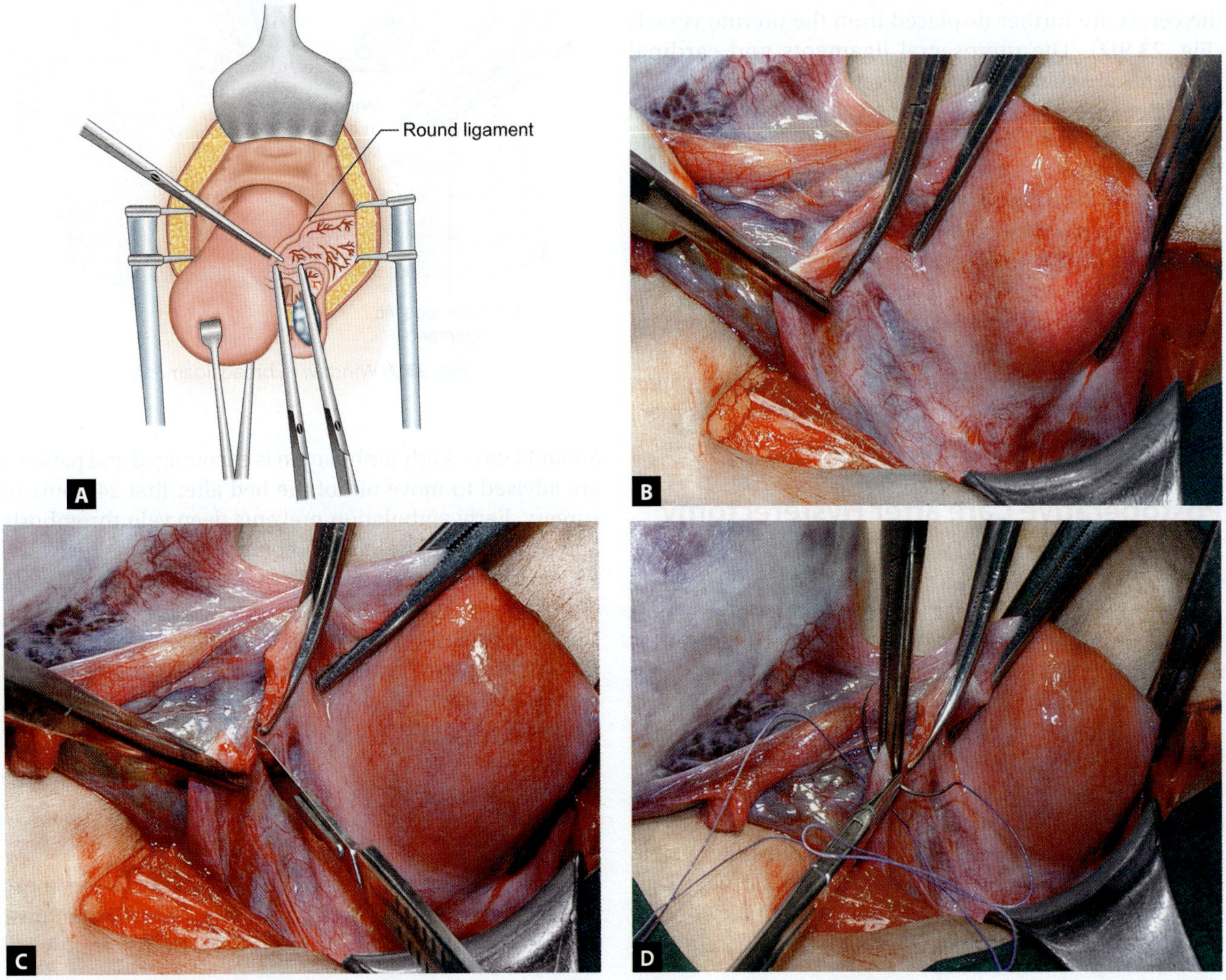

Fig. 23.4: Clamps applied at the cornual structure.

Figs. 23.5A to D: (A) Round ligament clamping; (B) Round ligament clamped; (C) Round ligament cut; (D) Round ligament sutured.

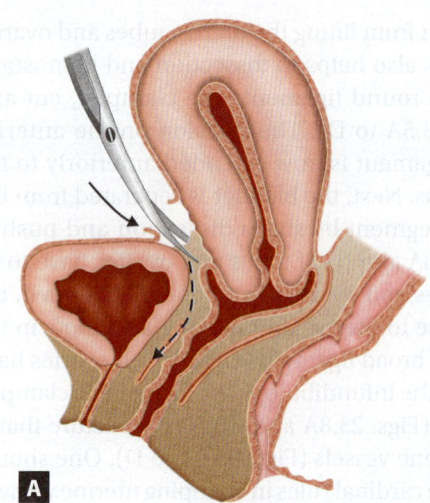
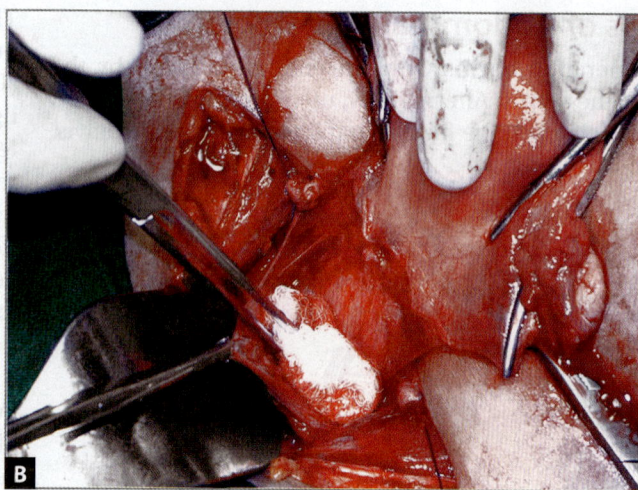

Figs. 23.6A and B: (A) Bladder separated from lower uterine segment; (B) Bladder pushed down.

through the pelvis. One should carefully palpate and identify the ureter during its course through pelvis. By gentle upward uterine traction and downward mobilization of bladder, the ureters that usually lie 2 cm and lateral to the cervix are further displaced from the uterine vessels (Fig. 23.9D). The uterosacral ligaments and cardinal ligaments are clamped cut and ligated (Figs. 23.10A to C). After the surgeon has determined that the bladder and rectum have been completely dissected away from the vagina (Figs. 23.11A and B), the anterior vaginal fornix is opened and the incision is extended circumferentially close to the cervix to maintain the length of the vagina. Straight clamps are placed on lateral vaginal angles and the uterus and cervix are removed and angles sutured (Figs. 23.12A to C). Vaginal angles are supported with uterosacral and cardinal ligaments to prevent vault prolapse in later life. Vaginal vault is closed with interrupted 0 chromic catgut sutures (Figs. 23.13A and B). Prior to closing the abdomen, all the stumps should be inspected for hemostasis.

Postoperative Care after Hysterectomy

Patient is kept in the postoperative ward to closely monitor vital signs and urine output in the postoperative period. Patient is kept nil by mouth for the first 24 hours after surgery. Intravenous fluids are administered in this period to maintain fluid and electrolyte balance. In case the operation has involved handling of the bowel, patient may be kept nil by mouth for a longer time till peristalsis returns. Postoperative pain relief is achieved with pethedine intramuscularly every 8 hours. When the surgery has been done under epidural anesthesia, the same may be continued for postoperative pain relief. Urinary retention is common after pelvic surgeries and continuous bladder drainage is usually kept for first 24 hours. If there has been bladder injury during the surgery, a catheter should be kept for a longer time for

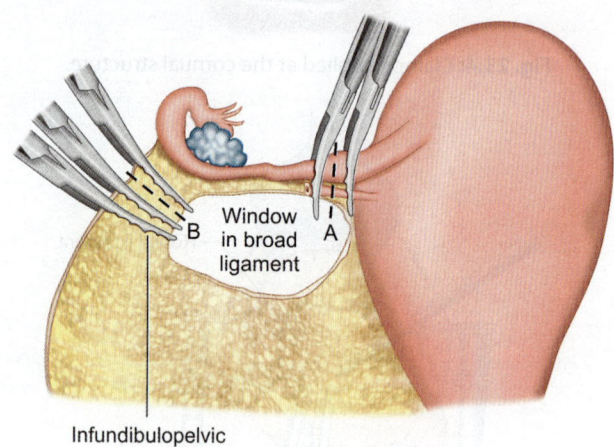

Fig. 23.7: Window in broad ligament.

about 14 days. Early ambulation is encouraged and patients are advised to move out of the bed after first 24 hours of surgery. Early ambulation prevents deep vein thrombosis and induces a sense of well-being and hastens recovery. Patient after hysterectomy can resume their household work in 3–4 weeks. However, heavy activities like lifting weight should be delayed for 6 weeks after hysterectomy. Coitus should be delayed for 6 weeks after hysterectomy. Patient is called for postoperative check-up 6 weeks after hysterectomy to assess the healing and complete recovery.

Postoperative Complications

Hemorrhage

One of the most dangerous complications of hysterectomy is the bleeding that occurs in the immediate postoperative period usually within the first 24 hours following

CHAPTER 23 Gynecological Operations

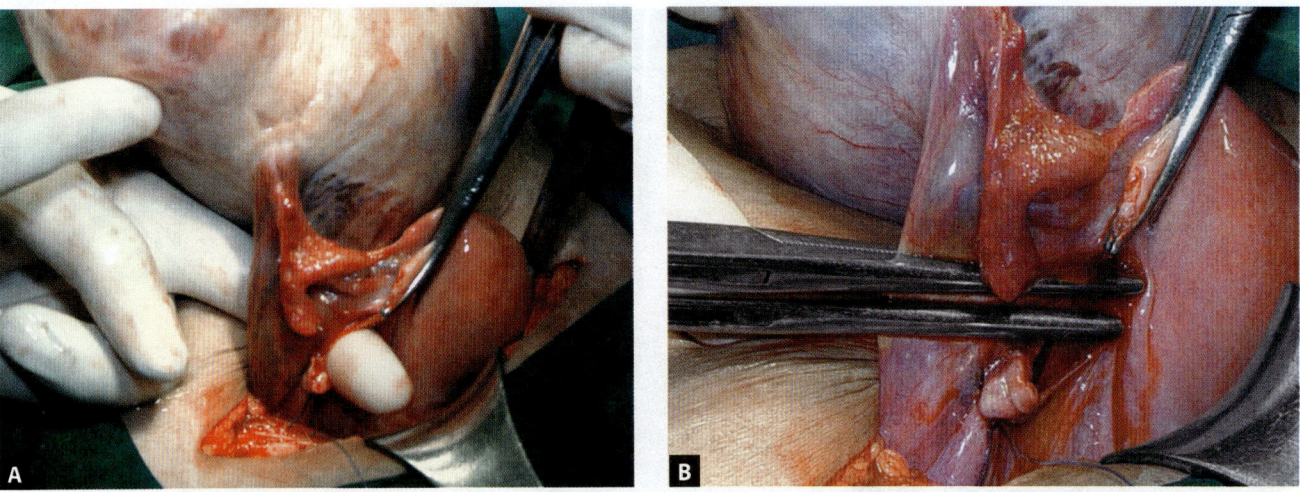

Figs. 23.8A and B: (A) Infundibulopelvic liagment; (B) Infundibulopelvic ligament clamped and later cut and ligated.

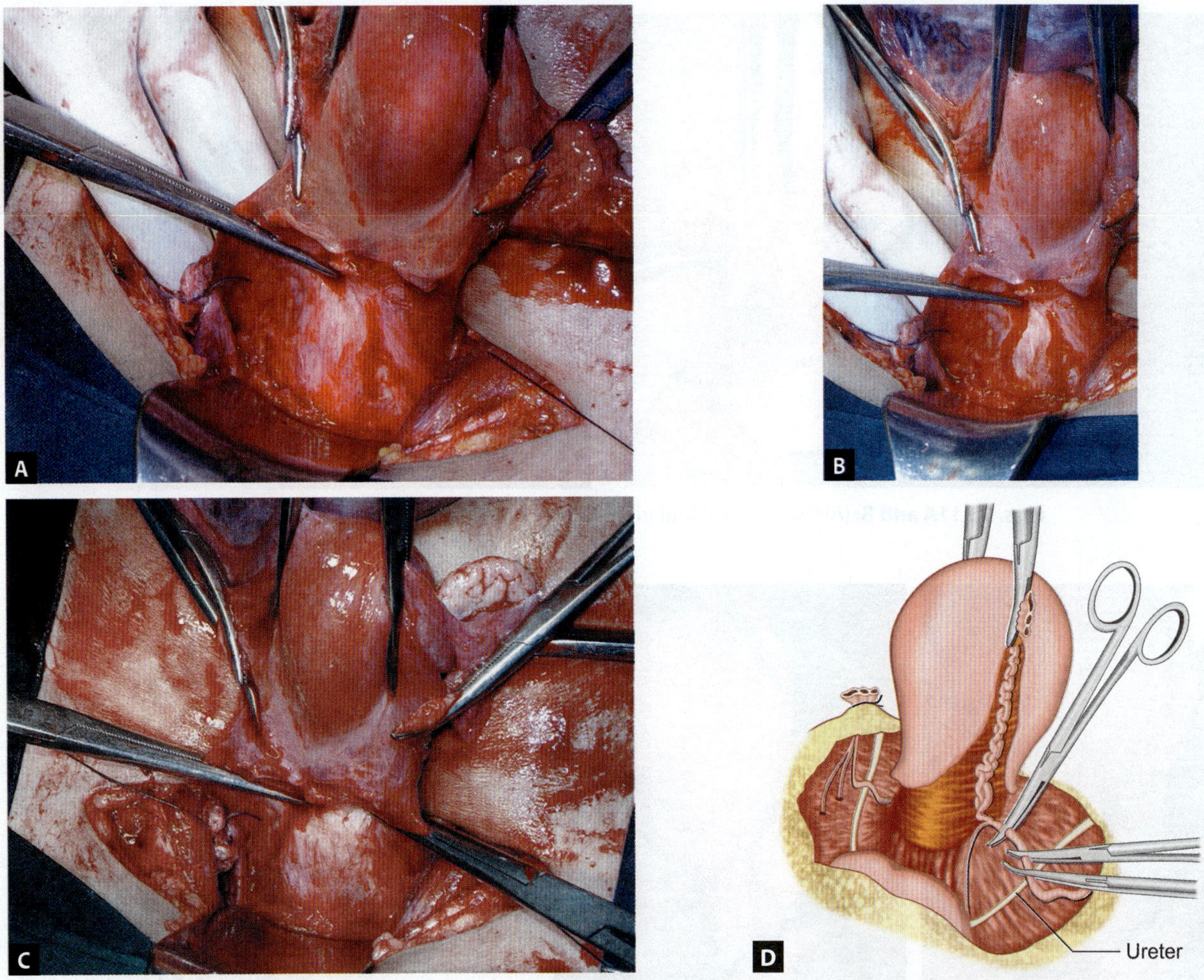

Figs. 23.9A to D: (A) Uterine artery ligation; (B) Uterine arteries ligation; (C) Both sides uterines clamped; (D) Clamping of uterine vessels.

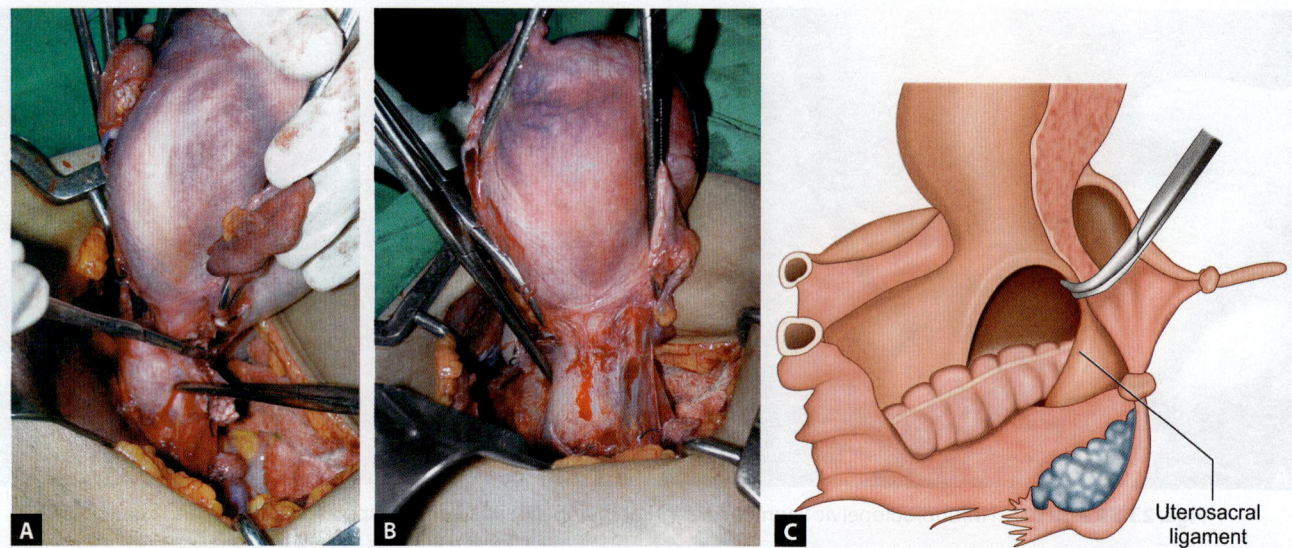

Figs. 23.10A to C: (A) Mackenrodt's ligament clamped; (B) Mackenrodt's ligament; (C) Clamping uterosacral and cardinal ligament complex.

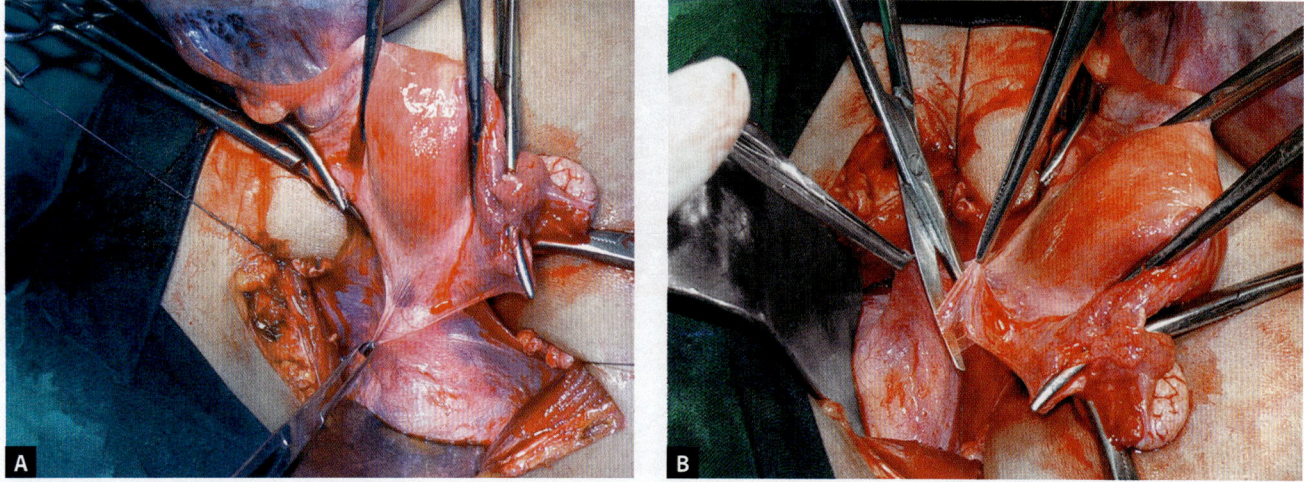

Figs. 23.11A and B: (A) Uterovesical fold identified by the loose fold and cut; (B) UV fold cut.

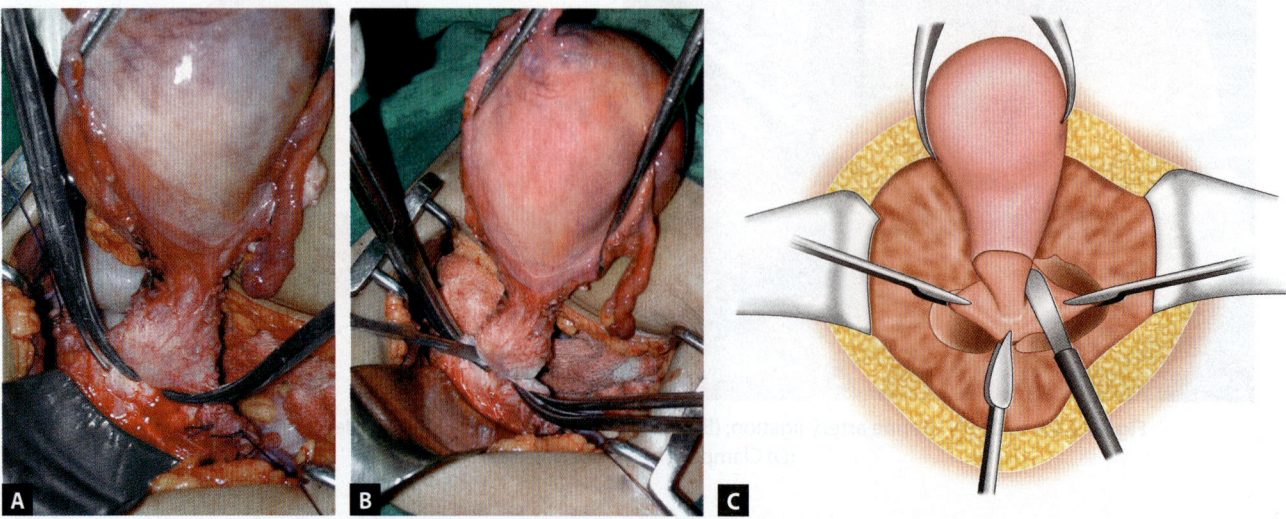

Figs. 23.12A to C: (A) Vaginal angles clamped; (B) Vaginal angles cut; (C) Uterus and cervix removed.

CHAPTER 23 Gynecological Operations

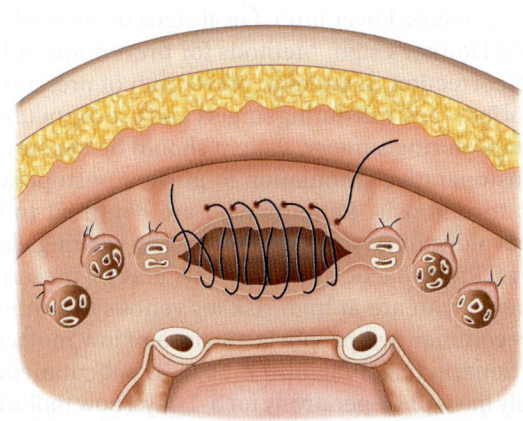
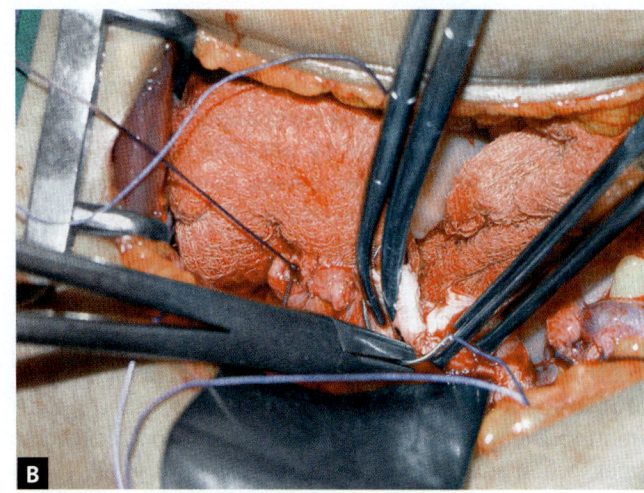

Figs. 23.13A and B: (A) Closure of vaginal vault; (B) Vault closure.

hysterectomy. This is manifested in the postoperative period by hypotension, tachycardia and altered sensorium. This needs exploration and suturing of the bleeding points in the vault under anesthesia. If bleeding is intraperitoneal, it may need relaparotomy and suturing of bleeding points. Bleeding which occurs late after hysterectomy is called secondary hemorrhage. It usually occurs between 8 and 14 days following hysterectomy and is usually due to infection and separation of the slough at the vault. Bleeding is usually small in amount and it needs to be treated with systemic antibiotics. Suturing is generally not recommended for secondary bleeding as bleeding is generalized and not limited to a particular point. If bleeding is of concern, vaginal packing under anesthesia is recommended.[5]

Postoperative Fever

Slight rise of temperature is very common following a hysterectomy within the first 48 hours after hysterectomy. This is usually due to absorption of products of tissue damage and absorption of blood in the pelvis. This usually subsides as blood and other tissue damage is absorbed. If the surgery was done under general anesthetic, pulmonary atelectasis can be the cause of the rise in temperature in the first 48 hours. More serious rise in temperature accompanied by systemic and localizing signs need investigation. Most common causes of temperature elevations include urinary tract infection (UTI), infection of abdominal wound or pelvic peritonitis, which needs to be treated.

Urinary Tract Injuries

Injuries to urinary tract occur in about 0.5–1% cases of abdominal hysterectomy. Injuries to bladder occur when entering the abdominal cavity and when bladder is dissected from the lower uterine segment especially when there are adhesions between the bladder and lower

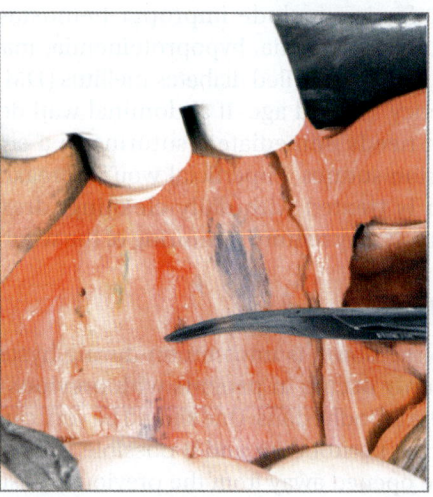

Fig. 23.14: Identifying the ureter on the medial leaf of broad ligament. The artery forceps points towards the ureter.

uterine segment due to previous lower segment cesarean section. Injuries to bladder should be repaired with 2-0 or 3-0 interrupted or continuous sutures. The first layer should include the bladder mucosa and the second layer, the muscularis. The course of ureter is such that it is liable to get damaged during hysterectomy. Ureters are liable to get injured during situations where there is a large uterus, large pelvic mass and in cases of extensive adhesions as seen in pelvic inflammatory disease or endometriosis. In such cases where ureteric injury is expected, a preoperative intravenous pyelogram (IVP) may be undertaken. One should be careful in applying hemostatic clamps blindly in the presence of bleeding. Ureteric injuries should be repaired with the help of an urologist. When difficulty is anticipated, the ureter may be dissected during the surgery to prevent injury. Ureter is exposed by opening the broad ligament and identifying ureter on the medial leaf of broad ligament (Fig. 23.14).[6]

If ureteric injury is suspected intraoperatively, a Urologist must be called in. Injuries in upper and middle part of ureter are repaired by end-to-end anastomoses. Injuries in the lower part may need implantation of ureter into bladder as it may not be possible to mobilize the ureter for end-to-end anastomoses. Sometimes ureteric injury may not be evident on table and may be recognized first time in the postoperative period as lion pain, fever or fistula. Retroperitoneal fluid collection may be seen in ureteric injury. Contrast CT scan is one of the investigations to identify the ureteric injury. The management of uretic injury recognized in the postoperative period involves relief of obstruction by percutaneous nephrostomy or retrograde stenting. Delayed repair should be undertaken after several weeks when edema around the ureter has subsided.

Wound Dehiscence and Infection

Factors that can predispose to wound dehiscence and wound infection include improper hemostasis at the time of surgery, anemia, hypoproteinemia, malignancy, obesity, poorly controlled diabetes mellitus (DM), vitamin C deficiency and old age. If abdominal wall dehiscence occurs, it needs immediate resuturing in a single layer with tension sutures. Superficial wound breakdown and infection is treated with daily cleaning, dressing and antibiotics. It may require resuturing of the wound.

Bowel Injuries

Injury to the bowel is uncommon during hysterectomy. It commonly occurs in patients with previous surgeries when there are adhesions. One should be very careful when opening the peritoneum and if possible the peritoneum should be opened away from the previous incision taking care to avoid the bowel. Intra-abdominal bowel adhesions if present should be carefully dissected with sharp dissection with the help of a general surgeon. If bowel injuries are recognized during surgery, it should be closed with 3-0 absorbable sutures in 2 layers. Larger lacerations on bowel need to be closed transversely to prevent narrowing of the bowel lumen.

Deep Venous Thrombosis

Postoperative venous thrombosis is more common in western races than in the Afro-Asian races. General incidence of postoperative venous thrombosis is said to be around 3–5%. Factors that can predispose to venous thrombosis include age more than 45 years, obesity, immobilization after surgery, dehydration, anemia, malignancy, injury to vein walls by pressure or hypoxia. There is a familial predisposition to deep vein thrombosis. Deep vein thrombosis (DVT) generally occurs 7–14 days after the operation and symptoms include calf pain and stiffness in the legs, which is often dismissed by the patient as a muscle ache. Within 2–3 days after the pain, the limb edema develops which begins in the foot and ankle and may involve the whole lower limb. Local signs include edema, pain and Homan's sign. Methods for prevention of DVT include correction of anemia, prevention of pressure on popliteal fossa and calf during surgery and use of pneumatic calf pumps during surgery. Patient should be encouraged early postoperative ambulation to prevent postoperative venous thrombosis. Patients who are confined to bed should avoid venous stasis in their legs by wearing elastic stockings. Prophylactic anticoagulants may be prescribed for patients who are at high risk for venous thrombosis. Usual recommended prophylactic dose of low molecular weight heparin (e.g. Fragmin) is 5000 IU subcutaneously on a daily basis postoperatively for 5–7 days. Low molecular weight heparin, which can be used as a once daily dose with little need for monitoring, is becoming popular.

Remote Complications

Remote complications that can follow a hysterectomy include vault prolapse, incisional hernia and menopausal symptoms if ovaries have been removed at the time of hysterectomy. Vault prolapse can be prevented by giving proper attention to vault suspension at the time of hysterectomy and obliterating an enterocele with culdoplasty sutures. The symptoms of surgical menopause are more severe than a natural menopause.

Vaginal Operations

There are various operative interventions available for vaginal prolapse. These operations are aimed at the restoration of normal anatomy. Preoperative evaluation includes fitness for major surgery, any problem to control micturation or defecation, and the surgeon should be fully aware of the sexual activity of the patient and desire to preserve fertility. These evaluations will enable the surgeon to choose the particular operation and modify the techniques to suit the individual patient. Various operations are listed below:

- Anterior colporrhaphy
- Colpoperineorrhaphy
- Manchester operation (Fothergill's operation)
- Extended Manchester operation (Shirodkar's vaginal repair)
- Vaginal hysterectomy with pelvic floor repair
- Le Fort's operation
- Shirodkar's sling operation
- Abdominal cervicopexy (Purandare).

Anterior Colporrhaphy or Operations for Cystocele

It is done in almost all cases of prolapse. It may be combined with other operative treatments of prolapse.

Objectives
- To mobilize bladder
- To return bladder to normal anatomical position
- To prevent the recurrence of bladder descent.

Surgical technique has been explained under vaginal hysterectomy with pelvic floor repair.

Posterior Colpoperineorrhaphy

Objectives
- Reduction of gaping of introitus
- Reconstruction of the perineal body
- Reinforcement of pelvic diaphragm by approximation of levator ani muscle
- Correction of rectocele.

Surgical technique has been explained under vaginal hysterectomy with pelvic floor repair.

Manchester Operation (Fothergill's Operation)

Objectives
- Amputation of vaginal portion of cervix
- Approximation of cardinal ligament in front of the cervical stump. This shortens the ligaments and elevates and displaces the cervix posteriorly. This backward displacement encourages anteversion and helps prevent prolapse of the uterus
- This operation is always combined with anterior repair. Posterior repair is common but not obligatory.

Extended Manchester Operation (Shirodkar's Vaginal Repair)

Shirodkar modified the Manchester operation, where the cervix is not amputated. The uterosacral ligaments were dissected from posterolateral aspect of the uterus and brought forward and stitched in front of the uterus. Here pouch of Douglas is routinely opened to get the greater length of uterosacral ligaments and also to correct the enterocele if present. Because the cervix is not amputated, the pregnancy complications are minimized.[7]

Vaginal Hysterectomy with Pelvic Floor Repair

This procedure is done on women who have completed their family, who also suffer from other pathologies like DUB, fibroids, cervical dysplasia or who have complete procedentia and in postmenopausal women. It must be emphasized that removal of uterus in itself does not cure prolapse. Uterus is not at fault. The main objective is to repair and reinforce the weakened tissues of pelvic floor. Hysterectomy is incidental as it is technically easier to do pelvic floor repair if uterus is removed and the ligaments are available to reinforce the repair.

Principles
There are three pedicles, which are clamped, cut and ligated from below upwards:
- The cardinal and uterosacral ligament complex
- Uterine vessels
- Tubo-ovarian and round ligament bundle.

The two peritoneal pouches, the anterior uterovesical pouch and posterior cul-de-sac pouch need to be opened to facilitate the procedure.

Surgical Technique

Vaginal Hysterectomy

With the patient in dorsolithotomy position, appropriate preparation and draping of the surgical field is accomplished. Circular incision is made around cervix. Blunt and sharp dissection is carried out between anterior cervix and posterior bladder wall (vesicocervical plane) to separate bladder from the cervix (Fig. 23.15). Dissection is continued till anterior peritoneum (uterovesical) is reached and opened. Then posterior cervical fascia is dissected. Similar dissection is carried out separating posterior vaginal wall from cervix till pouch of Douglas is reached and opened (Fig. 23.16). Next step is to clamp cut and ligate the uterosacral cardinal ligament complex close to the cervix on both sides (Fig. 23.17). This stump of uterosacral cardinal ligament complex is held long with the stitches to carry out prophylactic cooptation to prevent future enterocele and vault prolapse.

Then uterine vessels are doubly clamped and doubly ligated (Fig. 23.18). Now the uterus is attached only with round ligament, ovarian ligament and infundibulopelvic ligament. The fundus of the uterus is eventrated and brought outside the introitus. Now clamps are applied close to the body of uterus to ligate cornual structures, i.e. round ligament, ovarian ligament, and fallopian tube (Fig. 23.19).

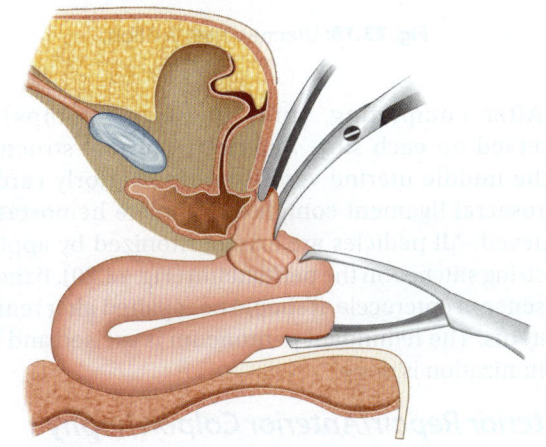

Fig. 23.15: Bladder separation in vesicocervical plane.

SECTION 1 General Gynecology

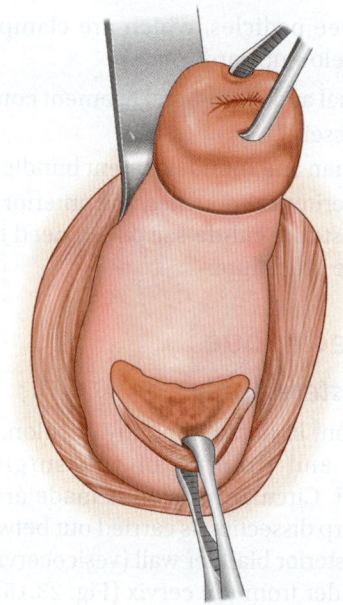

Fig. 23.16: Pouch of Douglas is opened.

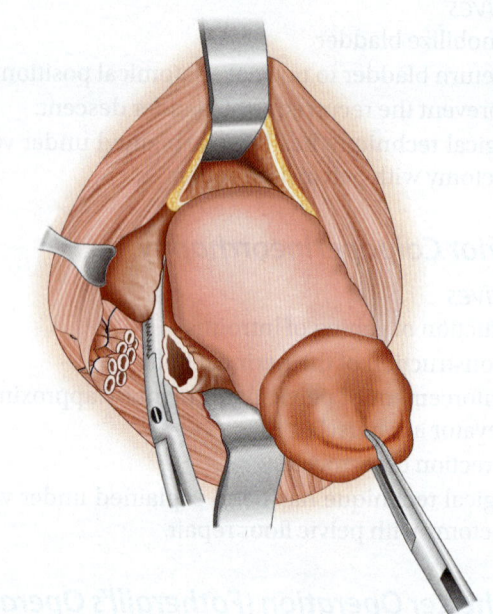

Fig. 23.17: Clamping uterosacral cardinal ligament complex.

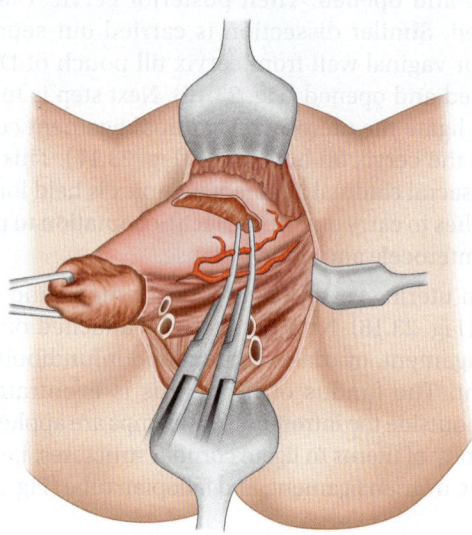

Fig. 23.18: Uterine vessel ligation.

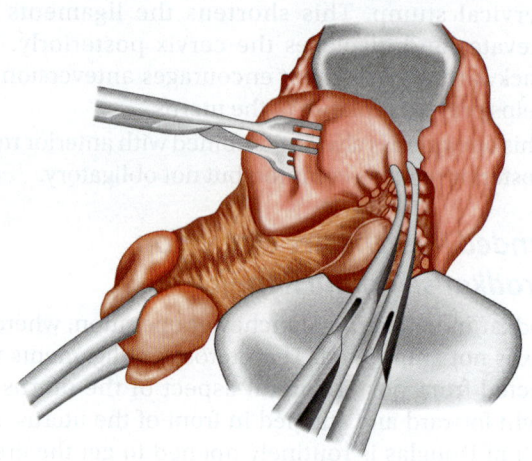

Fig. 23.19: Clamping cornual structures.

After completing, three pedicles (stumps) are observed on each side. Anteriorly cornual structures, in the middle uterine vessels and posteriorly cardinal uterosacral ligament complex. Complete hemostasis is achieved. All pedicles are extraperitonized by applying perstring stitches on the peritoneum (Fig. 23.20). If there is presence of enterocele, it should be repaired after removal of uterus. The redundant peritoneum is excised and high peritonization is done.

Anterior Repair/Anterior Colporrhaphy

Cystocele repair immediately follows vaginal hysterectomy. Two Allis forceps are applied to the lower edge of cystocele (free cut edge of vagina where ultimately the vaginal cuff will be closed) and one at the suburethral sulcus (Fig. 23.21). Now bladder is separated from the vagina in the midline with blunt as well as sharp dissection, till the point corresponding to the urethrovesical junction is reached. Bladder is pushed gently upwards and medially with a gauze in the vesicovaginal plane bilaterally. Interrupted bladder buttressing stitches are applied with 2-0, absorbable material (Fig. 23.22). The bladder-buttressing stitches are tied so that the cystocele is reduced. Redundant vaginal skin is trimmed and then incision is closed with continuous 3-0 sutures. Plication of cardinal uterosacral ligament complex pedicle into the vaginal wall is accomplished to

CHAPTER 23 Gynecological Operations

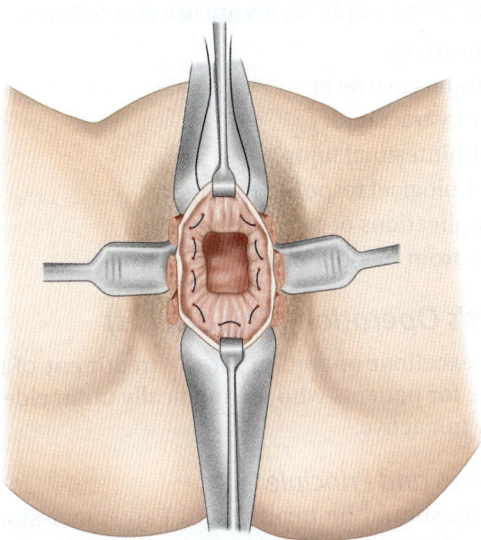

Fig. 23.20: Three pedicles seen at vaginal vault.

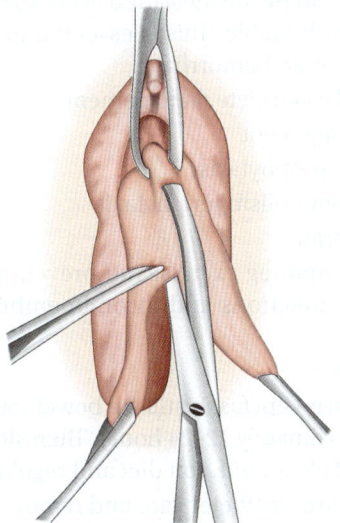

Fig. 23.21: Cystocele repair.

prevent subsequent development of vault prolapse. The vaginal cuff is closed.

Posterior Repair/Posterior Colpoperineorrhaphy

Two Allis tissue forceps are placed at the lateral aspect of mucocutaneous junction and one at the point above the rectocele. An incision along the mucocutaneous junction is made. Rectovaginal space is opened by sharp as well as blunt dissection. Full thickness of posterior vaginal wall is transected along the midline. The rectovaginal space is opened bilaterally by sharp and blunt dissection to expose the perirectal facial tissue. Care is taken to avoid inadvertent damage of the rectum. Lateral margin of the lower vaginal cut edge is separated sharply from the underlying levator ani (pubococcygeus) muscle bilaterally. The perirectal fascia is plicated in the midline over the rectum throughout its entire length. Excessive posterior vaginal skin is excised. Levator ani is plicated in the midline with one or two interrupted stitches (Fig. 23.23). Posterior vaginal skin is closed with running suture. Perineal skin incision is closed.

Vaginal packing is done with roller gauze soaked with glycerin acriflavine. Foley's catheter is inserted for continuous bladder drainage for 24–48 hours.

Postoperative Care
The principles of postoperative care are:
- Monitoring of vital signs:
  - Temperature, pulse, blood pressure and urine output

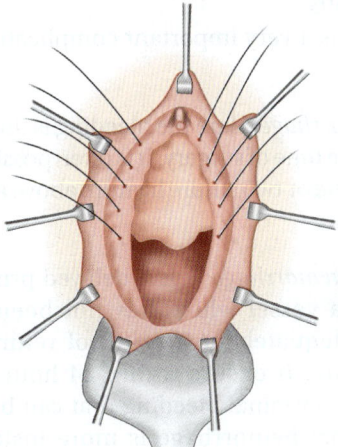

Fig. 23.22: Bladder buttressing stitches.

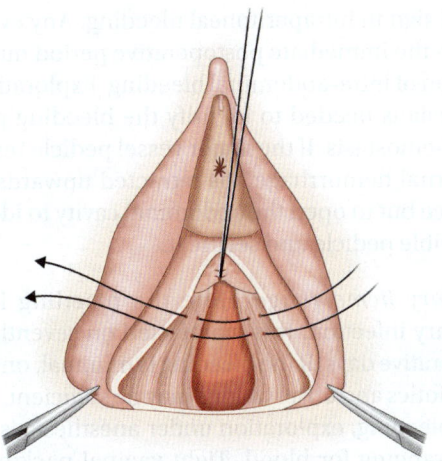

Fig. 23.23: Levator ani plication.

- Pulse and BP are measured every 15 minutes till the patient is stable. This is essential to recognize the reactionary hemorrhage.
- Fluid and electrolyte management
- Pain management
- Antibiotic prophylaxis
- Thromboembolism prophylaxis
- Physiotherapy:
  - Chest and leg exercises to prevent postoperative chest infections and thromboembolism, respectively.
- Nutrition:
  - Patient is kept fasting till the bowel sounds are heard (approximately 12–24 hour). Then slowly start with sips of clear fluid, soft diet and regular diet.
- Bladder care—catheter care and remove catheter after 24–48 hour later.

Vaginal packing removed after 12–24 hours of surgery.

Complications

Hemorrhage is a very important complication of vaginal hysterectomy.

Primary hemorrhage: Here the bleeding is due to technical difficulty at the time of surgery. It is often possible to control bleeding by one or two suture ligature above and below the bleeding point.

Reactionary hemorrhage: It is a delayed primary hemorrhage from a vessel which has not been secured or secured inadequately as a result of return of normal blood pressure. It occurs within 24 hours of surgery. Most often it is vaginal bleeding that can be recognized easily. Internal hemorrhage is more insidious and is a dangerous condition because the patient would have suffered considerable blood loss before the diagnosis and active intervention. Abdomianl distension is a very delayed sign in intraperitoneal bleeding. Any evidence of shock in the immediate postoperative period must raise a suspicion of intra-abdominal bleeding. Exploration under anesthesia is needed to identify the bleeding point and secure hemostasis. If the major vessel pedicle responsible for internal hemorrhage has retracted upwards, there is no choice but to open the abdominal cavity to identify the responsible pedicle and secure it.

Secondary hemorrhage: Here the bleeding is due to secondary infection. It is manifested on seventh to tenth postoperative days. If the bleeding is minimal, only change of antibiotics and observations may be sufficient. If there is severe bleeding, exploration under anesthesia is required after arranging for blood. Tight vaginal packing will be sufficient in most of the cases. Rarely, internal iliac artery ligation is required to control the hemorrhage.

Postoperative complications are listed as follows:
- Hemorrhage
- Postoperative fever
- Urinary tract injury
- Gastrointestinal injury
- Psychological response to surgery
- Complications of general anesthesia
- Risks from blood transfusions.

Le Fort's Operation (Colpocleisis)

It is an excellent operation for the treatment of uterine prolapse for patients who are medically unfit, elderly and sexually not active.

Objectives and Principle
- Cervix should be healthy and Pap smear should be normal
- It is performed using local, epidural or spinal anesthesia
- There is no need for general anesthesia
- Approximates the anterior and posterior vaginal wall
- Small tunnel on either side for drainage of discharge
- Minimal pain or complications
- About 90 to 95% cure rate
- It is not a suitable operation for a woman who is sexually active.

Shirodkar's Abdominal Sling Operation

This operation is for nulliparous prolapse or congenital prolapse where supporting ligaments of pelvis are congenitally very weak. This is technically a difficult operation. One should have a sound anatomical knowledge to perform this surgery.

Objective
An 18-inch mersilene tape is attached to the posterior surface of supravaginal portion of the cervix and the free ends of the tape are brought extraperitoneally on either side of pelvis towards the sacral promontory. On the right side, the tape is carried extraperitoneally along the brim of the true pelvis. On left side, the sigmoid colon prevents the direct extraperitoneal passage of tape. It may interfere with blood supply by kinking the sigmoid colon. It can be overcome by creating a psoas loop. By traction on free ends of the tape, the uterus can be pulled up to its correct location in the pelvis. The free ends of tapes are stitched to the anterior sacral ligaments and periosteum of sacral promontory.

Purandare Cervicopexy (Abdominal Cervicopexy)

Objective
Abdomen is opened by low transverse incision and two strips of anterior rectus sheet are prepared and brought

CHAPTER 23 Gynecological Operations

down into the pelvis extraperitoneally and stitched to the front of the uterus. Whenever intra-abdominal pressure raises, the strips pull the cervix anteriorly towards symphysis pubis and prevents its prolapse.

LAPAROSCOPY

Definition

The word laparoscopy simply means visual examination of the abdomen by means of a laparoscope (a small telescope). It is also called as "belly button surgery", endoscopy, or keyhole surgery. It is a surgical technique involving small incisions in the abdomen that allows direct visualization and remote handling of pelvic organs.

Laparoscopy was described several decades ago. It was used as a diagnostic and simple operative procedure. Recent advances in optics, electronics and physics have allowed the development of excellent visualization system, which provide brilliant views of entire pelvis and abdominal cavity. These new systems provide close-up and magnified views far superior to those obtained at conventional open surgery. Video laparoscopy offers superb visualization technique and with the accessories like laser, bipolar cautery and harmonic scalpel, it is possible to perform almost every type of surgery laparoscopically, which were traditionally performed by laparotomy.

Laparoscopy has several clear advantages over laparotomy, which are highlighted in Box 23.1.

Currently, laparoscopy accounts for large proportion of all gynecological procedures.

This keyhole surgery will be an added advantage in women's health care if the principles are followed regarding the selection of cases keeping in mind the contraindications and prerequisites.

Box 23.1: Advantages of laparoscopy over laparotomy

- Avoidance of large painful skin incision
- Less intraoperative blood loss
- More precise surgery because of superior view
- Less tissue handling and trauma
- Shorter hospital stay
- Less infective morbidity
- Avoid use of retractors and packs
- Less postoperative pain and less analgesic requirement
- Quicker mobilization
- More rapid return to full activities.
- More rapid convalescence
- Reduced postoperative adhesion formation
- Cosmetic
- Reduced cost

General Guidelines

Basic prerequisites for laparoscopic surgery:
- Adequate surgical skills
- Appropriate equipments
- Proper indications based on the risk and benefits.

Laparoscopy is generally performed under general anesthesia. However, laparoscopic tubal ligation and other minor diagnostic tests can be performed under sedation and local anesthesia.

Indications for Laparoscopy

Diagnostic Laparoscopy

- Evaluation of acute abdomen: Laparoscopy is a valuable tool for diagnosis of acute abdomen or acute pelvic pain, in which the differential diagnosis includes ectopic pregnancy, pelvic inflammatory disease, adnexal torsion, and appendicitis
- Elective diagnostic laparoscopy: The most common indications for this category are pelvic pain and infertility. In infertile patients, it permits evaluation of tubal and peritoneal factors. A thorough evaluation of severity of pelvic adhesions and extent of endometriosis which allows selection of appropriate treatment. Table 23.1 gives the overview of various indications.

Operative Laparoscopy

In recent years the spectrum of gynecological indications for operative laparoscopy has expanded dramatically. The definite indications are ectopic pregnancy, pelvic adhesions, endometriosis, benign ovarian masses, and tubal sterilization. Most surgeries done through laparotomy can now be done with opertaive laparoscopy. These include ectopic pregnancies, ovarian cystectomy, ovariotomy, hystercetomy and myomectomy.

Laparoscopic hysterectomy is gaining acceptance as a mode of surgery for benign disease. Laparoscopic radical hysterectomy for malignant disease also being done. In laparoscopic hysterectomy pedicles either coagulated with bipolar cautery, Harmonic scalpel or ligated with intraperitoneal knots. American Association of Gynecologic Laparoscopists (AAGL) has classified laproscopic hysterectomy depending on the structures removed during laparoscopy. The classification is described in Box 23.2.

Laparoscopy is increasingly being used for management of ectopic preganacies. Both conservative procedures like Salphongostomy, Salphingotomy and Salphnigenctomy can be done through laparoscope. Ovarian cysts can be removed through laparoscopy. Myomectomy can be done through laparoscope. For huge fibroids, size may be reduced with preoperative GnRH before laparoscopic myomectomy. Endometriosis can be effectively treated

Table 23.1: Indications for laparoscopy.

Diagnostic laparoscopy	Operative laparoscopy
Infertility	• Tubal sterilization
• Chromotubation for tubal patency	• General adhesiolysis
Pelvic pain	•Ovariolysis and salpingolysis
• Endometriosis	• Fimbrioplasty and salpingostomy
• Pelvis inflammatory disease	• Salpingostomy or linear salpingotomy
• Ectopic pregnancy	• Ovarian cystectomy and oophorectomy
• Unexplained pain	• Ovarian drilling for PCOD
Assessment of pelvic masses	• Adnexectomy
• Ovarian cysts	• Ovarian biopsy
• Fibroids	
• Pelvic adhesions	Advanced operative laparoscopy
Fertility problems	• Laparoscopic assisted vaginal hysterectomy (LAVH)
• Location of misplaced IUCD	• Myomectomy
• Prior to reversal of sterilization	• Burch procedure
• Primary amenorrhea	• Pelvic and para-aortic lymphadenectomy
• Congenital anomalies of genital tract	• Laparoscopic radical hysterectomy
Second look procedures	
• After cancer treatment	
• After infertility surgery	

(IUCD: Intrauterine contraceptive device; PCOD: Polycystic ovarian disease)

by Laparoscope. Endometriotic deposits can be vaporized. Endometroitic cystectomy can also be done through laparoscope.

Contraindications

Contraindications to laparoscopy include bowel obstruction, ileus, peritonitis, intraperitoneal hemorrhage, diaphragmatic hernias and severe cardiorespiratory disease.

Other relative contraindications are massive obesity, inflammatory bowel disease, large intra-abdominal masses and advanced intrauterine pregnancy (Table 23.2).

Techniques of Laparoscopy

- "Closed" laparoscopy—employing a Veress needle to create pneumoperitoneum followed by blind insertion of the first trocar
- "Open" technique where the fascia and the peritoneum are surgically opened and the trocar inserted under direct visualization.

Box 23.2: Laparoscopic hysterectomy as per AAGL classification.

Laparoscopic Hysterectomy is classified as follows by AAGL (American Association of Gynecologic Laparoscopists)
Type 0: Laparoscopic-directed preparation for vaginal hysterectomy
Type 1: Dissection up to but not including uterine arteries
Type 2: Type I + uterine artery occlusion and division, unilateral or bilateral
Type 3: Type II + portion of cardinal-uterosacral ligament complex only, unilateral or bilateral
Type 4: Type II + total cardinal-uterosacral ligament complex, unilateral or bilateral

Note: In Type 0 to 3, the operation is completed vaginally. In Type 0, the operation is done vaginally only a preliminary laparoscopic evaluation of pelvis is done. In Type 1, the upper pedicles are divided laparosocpically above the uterine A. In Type 2, dissection up to uterine A is done through laparoscope. In Type 3 upper pedicles, uterine A and part of cardinal ligament complex is divided laparoscopically. In Type 4, the operation is completed laparoscopically. In laparoscopic hysterectomies, uterus is lifted out of the pelvis with the help of a uterine manipulator. Pedicles are usually coagulated with bipolar forceps and cut. Ultraound energy source or vessel sealers can also be used to divide the pedicles. The operation is completed vaginally.[8]

In Type 4, laparoscopic hysterectomies after division of cardinal uterosacral ligament complex both anterior and posterior colpotomy is performed and uterus delivered. The vaginal vault is closed with laparoscopic assistance. Laproscopic hysterectomy has a slightly higher complications and longer operating time when compared with abdominal hysterectomy.

Table 23.2: Contraindications for laparoscopy.

Absolute	Relative
• Generalized peritonitis	• Large pelvic or abdominal masses of >26 weeks size
• Class IV cardiac disease	• Intrauterine pregnancy of >16 weeks
	• Hypovolemic shock
	• Intestinal obstruction
	• Chronic pulmonary disease
	• Previous laparotomy

The various instruments required for laparoscopy are shown in Table 23.3.

Veress Needle and Primary Trocar Insertion (Close Laparoscopy)

The patient is placed in dorsolithotomy position. The patient must be in the complete horizontal position (not Trendelenburg). The site of abdominal entry is intraumbilical or subumbilical, since it is a natural location for scar concealment and also this point offers the advantage of attenuation of the layers of abdominal wall and least vascularity (Fig. 23.24). When laprsocopy is done for large pelvic masses, a supraumbilical entry is preferred.

CHAPTER 23 Gynecological Operations

Table 23.3: Equipment for laparoscopy.

Basic equipment	Ancillary instruments	Hemostatic instruments
Laparoscope	Probes	Electrocoagulation
Veress needle	Forceps	Laser
Trocars	Scissors and scalpels	Suture
Gas insufflators	Aspirators and irrigators	Clips and staples
Light source	Morcellators	Chemical substances
Cameras	Harmonic scalpel	

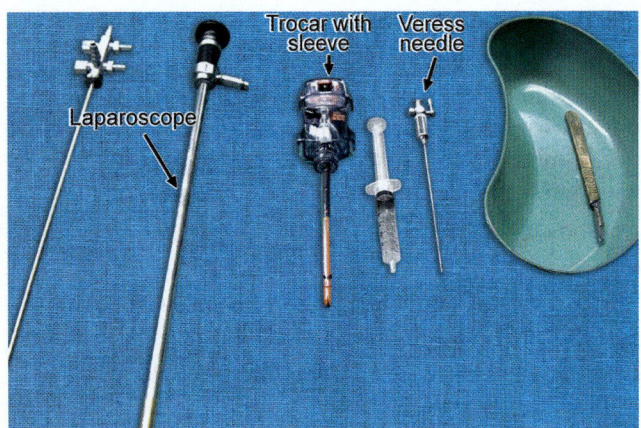

Fig. 23.25: Basic instruments for laparoscopy.

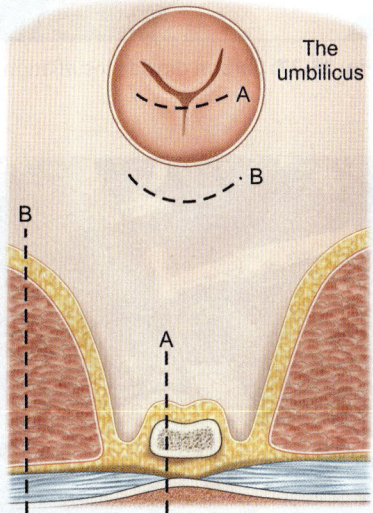

Fig. 23.24: Site of abdominal entry. Cross-section view of the umbilical area. A—At the umbilicus the rectus sheath and peritoneum is underneath. B—Just below the umbilicus there is subcutaneous fat, anterior rectus sheath, rectus muscle, posterior rectus sheath and peritoneum.

First step of laparoscopy is to achieve pneumoperitoneum with carbon dioxide gas using Veress needle. Veress needle is a relatively small gauge instrument with a spring-loaded tip and is used for initiation of pneumoperitoneum (Fig. 23.25).

This device consists of sharp needle containing within its lumen a spring-loaded gas-carrying channel. When the needle is inserted through the skin, the blunt-ended gas channel is forced against its spring and into the central channel of the needle exposing the cutting edge of the needle. This sharp edge easily penetrates all the layers of abdominal wall. When the tip enters the abdominal cavity, the gas channel with its perforations is released and protrudes beyond the sharp bevelled needle tip to permit the free flow of gas. A small subumbilical incision is made. The Veress needle is placed by the controlled entry. The lower anterior abdominal wall is elevated by manually grasping the skin and subcutaneous tissue to maximize the distance between the umbilicus and the retroperitoneal vessels. The Veress needle is inserted towards the hollow of the sacrum at a correct angle of 45° aimed towards the uterine fundus (Fig. 23.26). When the Veress needle is placed through the umbilicus into the peritoneal cavity, avoidance of both the retroperitoneal vessels and the intestinal tract is of paramount importance.

Correct placement of the Veress needle may be confirmed by a number of methods, such as the hanging drop test, injection and aspiration of fluid through the Veress needle, or measurement of intra-abdominal pressure with carbon dioxide insufflation and the hissing sound caused by air rushing through the Veress needle. Once the Veress needle is in place, carbon dioxide gas is insufflated (Fig. 23.27). Tympani percussed over the liver is a clinical sign of proper intraabdominal insufflation.[9]

Umbilical Trocar Insertion

After a pneumoperitoneum has been achieved with a Veress needle, the primary trocar with sleeve is placed at a similar angle to the Veress needle (Fig. 23.28). Intra-abdominal trocar placement is accomplished by hearing a rush of gas through the trocar sheet. Then laparoscope is

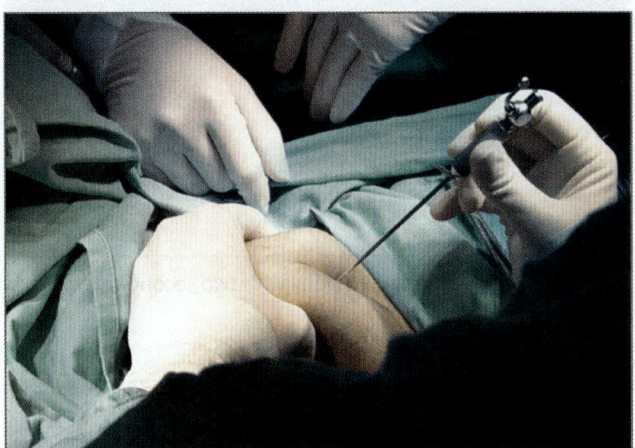

Fig. 23.26: Insertion of Veress needle.

SECTION 1 General Gynecology

inserted through the trocar sheet to visualize and confirm intraperitoneal access (Fig. 23.29).

Secondary trocar sites are chosen for manipulatory and operative instruments. Care should be taken to avoid injury to the inferior epigastric vessels. Operative laparoscopy with two secondary trocars is shown in Figure 23.30.

The complications of laparoscopy are summarized in Box 23.3.

The evolving role of laparoscopy in the field of operative gynecology has a dramatic effect on clinical practice. Laparoscopic surgery is an important technique in the armamentarium of gynecologic surgeon. It is safe, cost-effective, and patient-friendly.

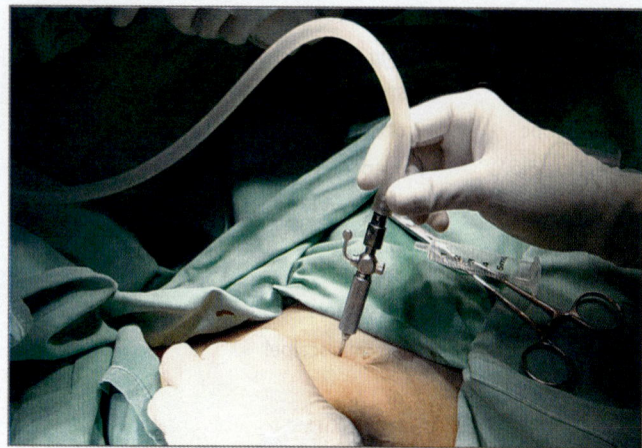

Fig. 23.27: Carbon dioxide insufflation.

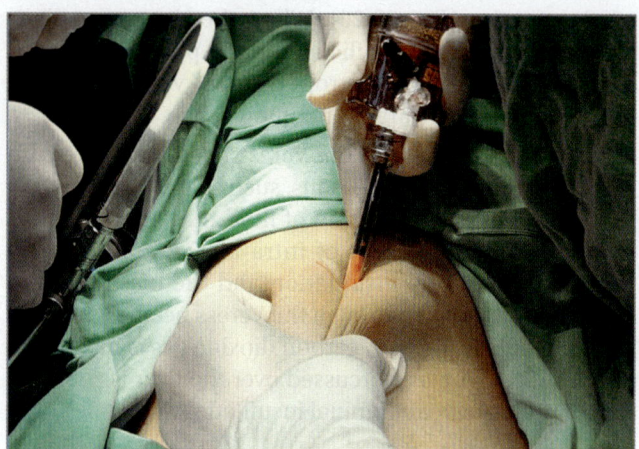

Fig. 23.28: Umbilical trocar insertion.

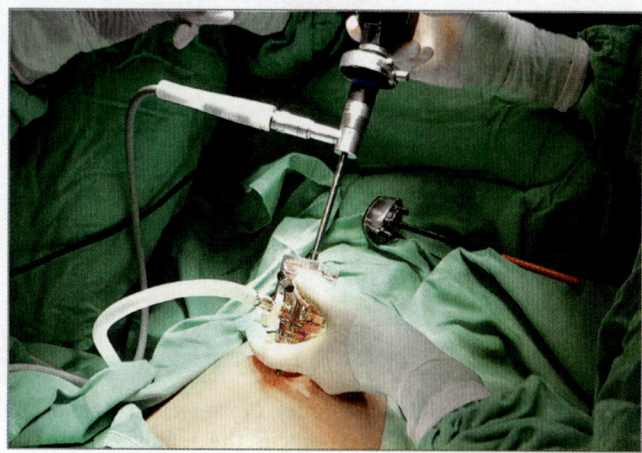

Fig. 23.29: Insertion of laparoscope through trocar.

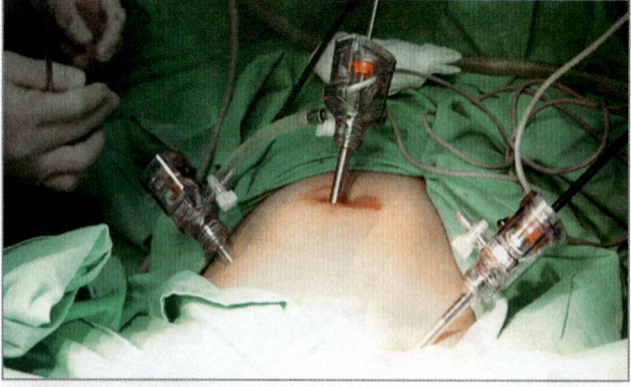

Fig. 23.30: Operative laparoscopy with two secondary trocars.

Box 23.3: Complications of laparoscopy.

- Major vessel trauma
- Ileum and/or colon perforation
- Bladder perforation
- Inferior epigastric vessel damage
- Incisional hernia
- Hematomas
- Surgical emphysema
- Venous gas embolism
- Ureteric damage
- Pulmonary embolism
- Anesthetic problem

HYSTEROSCOPY

Hysteroscopy involves passage of a rigid or flexible instrument into the uterine cavity and visualization of uterine cavity. Various diagnostic and therapeutic procedures can be performed through the hysteroscope (Fig. 23.31).

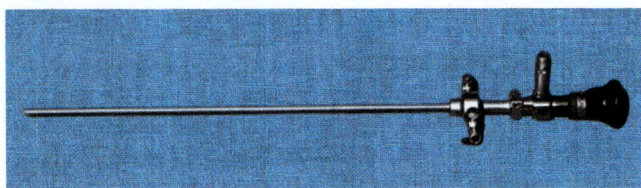

Fig. 23.31: Hysteroscope.

Box 23.4: Indications for hysteroscopy.

- Abnormal uterine bleeding
- Endometrial polyp
- Submucus myoma
- Uterine septum
- Asherman's Syndrome
- Retained IUCD

Procedure for Hysteroscopy

The basic procedure of hysteroscopy involves insertion of hysteroscope via the cervix, if needed after cervical dilatation, distension of the uterine cavity and visualization of uterine cavity. Diagnostic hysteroscopy can be done under paracervical block. Operative hysteroscopy is generally performed under regional or general anesthesia. Most hysteroscopic procedures need cervical dilatation and this may be achieved with insertion of a laminaria tent 3–8 hours prior to the procedure and/or by using Hagar's dilators at the time of surgery. Mispostol 400 micrograms vaginally 4 hours before the procedure can also be used to dilate the cervix. Media that are used to distend the uterine cavity include carbon dioxide, normal saline, Dextran 70 and low viscosity fluids, such as 1.5% glycine and 3% sorbitol. Carbon dioxide cannot be used in the presence of bleeding and can cause gas embolism if intrauterine pressure exceeds 100 mm Hg. Dextran 70 is a hyperosmolar solution and if it gets into the circulation it may draw water into the systemic circulation and cause fluid overload and circulatory failure. It can also induce an allergic response and coagulopathy. Not more than 500 mL of Dextran 70 should be infused at a time during hysteroscopy.[10] Dextran 70 does not mix with blood and is a good media during operative hysteroscopy. Dextran 70 can cause pulmonary edema, anaphylactic reaction and may also effect Platelet function. Normal saline is a safe medium and can be used safely even in large volumes if needed as it does not generally cause electrolyte imbalances. But normal saline cannot be used in cases that require electrosurgical procedures. Low viscosity fluids like glycine and sorbitol can sometimes cause electrolyte imbalances, but they are compatible with electrosurgical procedures. There should be meticulous monitoring of inflow and outflow of fluids during hysteroscopic procedures. If there is a fluid deficit of more than 750 mL during the procedure, the procedure must be abandoned.[11]

Indications for Hysteroscopy

Hysteroscopy has diagnostic and therapeutic uses. Common diagnostic indications include evaluation of abnormal uterine bleeding, infertility evaluation and recurrent pregnancy losses. Hysteroscopy is indicated in abnormal uterine bleeding especially if a diagnosis cannot be established by curettage. Hysteroscopy allows directed biopsy in cases of endometrial hyperplasia. In patients with infertility when hysterosalpingography suggests intrauterine abnormalities, this can be confirmed with hysteroscopy as this allows better visualization of endometrial cavity. Intrauterine pathology like Asherman's syndrome and septum can be resected hysteroscopically at the same time. Many therapeutic procedures can be performed with hysteroscopy. Intrauterine contraceptive device if embedded in the uterine cavity may be removed with hysteroscope. Sepatte uterus can be cause of preterm labor and second trimester abortion. Septum can be resected with hysteroscopy. Small submucus fibroids may be resected with a loop electrode. Intrauterine synechiae as seen in Asherman's syndrome may be divided under hysteroscopic vision. Functional polyp within the endometrial cavity can be removed with hysteroscopy. Endometrial ablation in patients with abnormal uterine bleeding can be achieved with electrosurgical resection or with laser. But the relief of menorrhagia with endometrial ablation is not as promising as it was originally thought to be. Hysterectomy rates after endometrial ablation is around 24%. Cornual tubal block can be corrected by tubal canalization through Hysteroscope. Indications for Hysteroscopy is summarized in Box 23.4.

Complications of Hysteroscopy

Complications during Hysteroscopy are rare with an incidence of 1-2/1000 cases.[12] Complications of hysteroscopy include perforation, bleeding, thermal trauma and complications related to distension media. Vasovagal shock can occur during hysteroscopy. Uterine perforation is suspected if the operative view suddenly disappears, the fluid deficit suddenly increases, or the hysteroscope suddenly inserts farther than the fundus. Perforation during hysteroscopy warrants termination of the procedure and laparotomy in case there is damage to other intra-abdominal structures like bowel or urinary tract. It is better to do hysteroscopy under laparoscopic guidance when doing hysteroscopic myomectomy and septal resection to prevent perforation of uterus. Bleeding during hysteroscopy is generally due to damage to the myometrial vessels during resection. This needs either electrocoagulation of the bleeding vessel or balloon tamponade of uterine cavity with Foley catheter. Injection of dilute vasopressin has also been tried locally to control bleeding from the myometrial vessels. Thermal injuries can occur during electrosurgical procedures of endometrium. If there is thermal injury to surrounding structures this may need laparotomy and repair of the defect. Complications related to distension media have been already described above.

REFERENCES

1. Howard W. J III. Abdominal hysterectomy.In:Rock JA, Howard WJ III, (Eds). Ti Lindes Operative Gynaecology. 10th edition Philadelphia: Lippincott Williams & Wilkins;2008.p.729.
2. Howard WJ III. Abdominal hysterectomy.In: Rock JA, Howard WJ III, (Eds). Ti Lindes Operative Gynaecology. 10th edition Philadelphia: Lippincott Williams & Wilkins;2008.p.730.
3. Hoffman B, Schorge J, Schaffer J, Halvorson L, Bradshaw K, Cunningham F. Willimas Gynaecology. 2nd edition. New York. McGraw-Hill Education LLC;2012.pp.1020-23.
4. Fong YF, Lim FK, Arulkumaran S. Prophylactic oophorectomy: a continuing controversy. Obstet Gynecol Surv. 1998; 53:493.
5. Harris WJ. Early complications of abdominal and vaginal hysterectomy. Obstet Gynecol Surv. 1995;50(11):795-805.
6. Harkki-Siren P, Sjoberg J, Titinen A. Urinary tract injuries after hysterectomy. Obstet Gynecol. 1998;92:113.
7. Shaikh R, Sardesai S. Shirodkar's extended manchester repair: a conservative vaginal surgery for genital prolapse in young women and reinforcement of weak uterosacral ligaments with merselene tape: retrospective and prospective study. International Journal of Recent Trends in Science and Technology. 2014;10(2):263-6.
8. Olive DL, Parker WH, Cooper JM, Levine RL. The AAGL Classification System for Laparoscopic Hysterectomy. The Journal of the American Association of Gynecologic Laparoscopists. 2000;7(1):9-15.
9. Howard WJ III. Abdominal hysterectomy.In:Rock JA, Howard WJ III, (Eds). Ti Lindes Operative Gynaecology. 10th edition. Philadelphia: Lippincott Williams & Wilkins;2008.pp.325-6.
10. Worldwide AAMIG, Munro MG, Storz K, Abbott JA, et al. AAGL Practice Report: Practice Guidelines for the Management of Hysteroscopic Distending Media: (Replaces Hysteroscopic Fluid Monitoring Guidelines. J Am Assoc Gynecol Laparosc. 2000;7:167-168.). J Minim Invasive Gynecol. 2013;20:137-148.
11. Munro MG, Storz K, Abbott JA, et al. AAGLPractice Report: Practice Guidelines for the Management of Hysteroscopic Distending Media: (Replaces Hysteroscopic Fluid Monitoring Guidelines. J Am Assoc Gynecol Laparosc. 2000;7:167-168.). J Minim Invasive Gynecol.2013;20:137-148.
12. Jansen FW, Vredevoogd CB, van Ulzen K, et al. Complications of hysteroscopy: a prospective, multicenter study. Obstet Gynecol. 2000;96:266–70.

FURTHER READING

1. Rock JA, Howard WJ III. Ti Lindes Operative Gynaecology. 10th Edition. Lippincott Williams and Wilkins; 2008.
2. Lopes T, Nick MS, Naik R, John M. Monaghan Bonney's Gynaecological Surgery, 11th Edition. Wiley-Blackwell; 2011.

CHAPTER 24

General Surgical Problems in Gynecology

Krishnendu Mukherjee

Overview

- Acute abdominal pain in pregnancy, symptomatic diseases of the breast and urinary or fecal incontinence often present first to the gynecologist.
- General surgical disorders may coexist with gynecological diseases or may masquerade as one.
- Lower abdominal pain in females often poses diagnostic dilemma. The gynecological clinicians would most often consider the following differential diagnoses. Acute or recurrent appendicitis, ureteric colic, urinary tract infections, irritable bowel syndrome, inflammatory bowel disease (IBD), i.e. Crohn's disease, ulcerative colitis, indeterminate colitis, infective enteritis/colitis; tuberculosis, hernias, etc.
- The pelvic surgeon must have accurate knowledge of the course of the ureters and be proficient in locating the ureter at different sites and steps of pelvic dissection. Identification of ureteral injury is of paramount importance, because primary repair has the best chance of success.
- Intestinal injuries are particularly prone to occur in the presence of adhesions, usually from previous surgical procedures. Endometriosis, multiple surgeries, previous intraperitoneal sepsis and previous irradiation for malignancy increase the density of adhesions.

INTRODUCTION

The overlap of general surgery in the practice of obstetrics and gynecology is appreciated by all clinicians. Acute abdominal pain in pregnancy, symptomatic diseases of the breast and urinary or fecal incontinence often present first to the gynecologist. These topics have been dealt with elsewhere in this textbook. The present Chapter shall focus on other areas where knowledge and understanding of general surgical principles is essential to the good practice of obstetrics and gynecology.

CATEGORIES OF GENERAL SURGICAL PROBLEMS IN GYNECOLOGY

General surgical disorders may coexist with gynecological diseases or may masquerade as one. During the course of pregnancy or treatment for a gynecological condition, surgical problems may be precipitated.

Three broad categories can be identified, which encompass these areas:

- Diagnostic dilemmas in females presenting with lower abdominal pain
- Extra-abdominal general surgical problems in pregnancy
- Operative surgical considerations with relevance to iatrogenic injuries of nonreproductive organs or structures during the course of pelvic surgery in females.

Diagnostic Considerations in Lower Abdominal Pain

Lower abdominal pain in females often poses diagnostic dilemma. The gynecological clinicians would most often consider the following differential diagnoses.

- Acute or recurrent appendicitis
- Ureteric colic, urinary tract infections (UTI)
- Irritable bowel syndrome (IBS)
- Inflammatory bowel disease (IBD), i.e. Crohn's disease, ulcerative colitis, indeterminate colitis
- Infective enteritis/colitis; tuberculosis, hernias, etc.

While a typical presentation of acute appendicitis is a straightforward diagnosis, not all cases will present with the usual features. History of "shifting pain" should be carefully sought in all cases as it is highly suggestive of acute appendicitis. In the absence of signs of peritoneal inflammation, the diagnosis becomes more difficult. It is rational to perform full blood count and urinalysis. However, one should bear in mind that polymorphonuclear leukocytosis is neither specific for, nor invariable in appendicitis. Microscopic hematuria or pyuria also does not negate or refute a diagnosis of appendicitis. High resolution ultrasonography performed by an experienced sonologist may be able to demonstrate an inflamed appendix directly (luminal gas shadow) and it should be used in the evaluation of lower abdominal or right iliac fossa (RIF) pain. Though an invasive procedure, laparoscopy is useful in distinguishing acute appendicitis from other pathologies.

Low grade, persistent (chronic) RIF pain is not a feature of recurrent appendicitis. The pain in this condition is typically recurrent in fashion and localized in the RIF and adjoining areas. Only if, repeated clinical assessment and other investigations fail to resolve the problem and provided acute abdominal signs are absent, a barium study may be performed. Barium enema is preferable to barium follow through. Though nonfilling of the appendix is suggestive, but not diagnostic of appendicits, a completely filled appendicular lumen rule out the diagnosis. Reproduction of the crampy abdominal pain during performance of a double contrast barium enema is highly suggestive of irritable bowel syndrome (IBS). Laparoscopy may not help in diagnosing recurrent appendicitis but visualization of the pelvis and distal small bowel may be helpful in the final assessment.

Irritable bowel syndrome is a common condition. These patients often complain of pellet-like stools, tenesmus and a myriad of nonspecific abdominal symptoms in addition to pain. Though a psychosomatic component is common, these patients do not usually have any recognizable psychiatric morbidity. Presence of systemic symptoms (e.g. low-grade fever), extra-abdominal manifestations (e.g. oral aphthous ulcers), mucous diarrhea with rectal bleeding should raise the possibility of inflammatory bowel disease. Even in the absence of these features, IBS should not be diagnosed without full evaluation and it is customary to perform colonoscopy and small bowel barium enema (which is preferable to barium follow through) or double balloon enteroscopy, in these patients.

In the presence of pregnancy, evaluation of abdominal pain of nonacute nature poses special difficulties because conventional radiology and laparoscopy are both relatively contraindicated. Hence, for example, gallstones detected by ultrasonography need to be treated by the conventional cholecystectomy as opposed to the laparoscopic procedure. Symptoms of biliary tract disease can be reduced by adherence to a low-fat diet and operation should be advised in the second trimester of pregnancy. Management of asymptomatic gallstones detected in pregnancy evokes controversy. Since, pregnancy itself increases the lithogenicity of gallbladder bile, operation is the preferred option in the second trimester or soon after delivery.

Unlike intestinal colic, ureteric colic is not a colicky pain. The pain is usually constant with exacerbations and classically, radiates from loin to groin though the later is by no means invariable. The pain is produced by increasing luminal pressure in the upstream collecting system and is mediated by prostaglandins. Hence, the pain responds well to nonsteroidal anti-inflammatory agents. Urinalysis demonstrates hematuria in 85% of cases and a straight X-ray of the kidney, ureter, bladder (KUB) demonstrates calculi in over 80% of patients. Ultrasonography may not demonstrate the stone but usually shows the dilatation of the pelvicalyceal system and the ureter. Combining the three investigations in the said order, a diagnostic accuracy of nearly 100% can be achieved.

Dysuria and hypogastric pains are common manifestations of urinary tract infections (UTI), and rarely, may be the first manifestation of a gynecological or bladder malignancy. In postmenopausal women, the frequent coexistence of bladder neck obstruction and vaginal dryness predispose to UTI. However, in recurrent UTI, especially if abacterial pyuria is repeatedly demonstrated, one must consider the possibilities of tuberculous cystitis, interstitial cystitis and carcinoma-in situ of bladder. Appropriate workup should include culture for acid fast bacilli (AFB) and cystoscopy.

Extra-abdominal General Surgical Problems in Pregnancy

Anorectal Diseases

The actual frequency of proctological diseases in pregnancy is poorly documented; it is estimated, however, that 85% primi or multiparae with anorectal disorders develop them during or after their first pregnancy.[1]

Proctological diseases provoked or aggravated by pregnancy are:
- Congestion of anal canal and anal varices
- Changes in stool movements
- Hemorrhoids and their complications
- Acute perianal hematoma (thrombotic "piles")
- Anal neuralgias
- Pruritus ani.

Increased tendency to constipation is almost universal in pregnancy. Dietary adjustments are crucial and specific dietary advice is more rewarding than general statements like "increasing fiber intake". Bran and wheat cereals, apricot, dessicated coconut, peas, spinach and lentils are high in fiber. Osmotic laxatives (e.g. lactulose) can be prescribed in pregnancy.

CHAPTER 24 General Surgical Problems in Gynecology

Table 24.1: Different degrees of hemorrhoids, signs and treatment.

	Signs	Treatment options
First degree	Internal hemorrhoids	• Injection sclerotherapy (e.g. oily phenol)
Second degree	Larger, may prolapse, but reduces spontaneously	• Laser photocoagulation, injection sclerotherapy
Third degree	Prolapse, requiring digital repositioning	• Hemorrhoidectomy (stapled or conventional)
Fourth degree	Permanently prolapsed	• Hemorrhoidectomy (stapled or conventional)

Topical preparations containing astringents, anti-inflammatory (e.g. corticosteroids) and local anesthetic agents are popularly used to treat anorectal problems. Though there is little evidence of their efficacy, temporary symptomatic relief may be achieved. They may, however, aggravate pruritus ani by causing maceration of perianal skin. Most anorectal disorders in pregnancy will respond to adequate bed rest (decrease of perineal congestion), suitable diet and judicious use of laxatives. Hygiene is important. The hypersecretory state of the vagina with modified pH of secretions and extension of vaginal mycosis predisposes to pruritus ani. Secondary bacterial infections are common. Treatment of vaginal mycoses, endoanal application of antifungals, maintaining dry perianal skin, dusting with antiseptic powder will help to alleviate pruritus ani. Local nystatin is useful in thrush; its systemic absorption from the gastrointestinal tract is negligible. All patients should be advised on regular nail clipping.

Hemorrhoids present with rectal bleeding which is fresh, painless and usually not mixed with motions. Internal hemorrhoids are not palpable by digital rectal examination and need to be visualized with a protoscope. Since hemorrhoidal bleeding exacerbates the anemia of pregnancy and since early cases can be dealt with by nonoperative means, hemorrhoids should be treated energetically in pregnancy. Topical creams have little to offer in hemorrhoids except short-term relief. The advent of stapled hemorrhoidectomy has challenged conventional wisdom on pathology of hemorrhoids. The procedure which is less painful and helps earlier return to normal activities can be performed under low regional anesthesia, like the conventional operation. It may be performed even for some 2nd degree hemorrhoids but may not be appropriate in the presence of large external components (Table 24.1).

Acute Perianal Pain

The common causes of acute perianal pain are listed in Box 24.1.

Box 24.1: Cause of acute perianal pain.

- Acute perianal hematoma
- Anal fissure
- Prolapsed thrombosed internal hemorrhoids
- Anal neuralgias
- Anorectal suppuration (abscess)

Pregnancy carries a higher than usual incidence of the first four causes of acute perianal pain.

- Acute perianal hematoma is a common condition often referred to by the misnomer, "external thrombotic pile" because it is not a true hemorrhoid. It presents with a typical globular and exquisitely tender swelling on the perianal margin. The condition is very painful. The 'clot' can be evacuated by a simple incision drainage under a local anesthetic with dramatic symptomatic relief. The natural history of this condition is benign. The pain usually settles and swelling shrinks to a skin tag over 1–2 weeks. Hence, for patients presenting late, intervention may not be required
- Fissures are usually posterior splits in the anoderm but anterior fissures are relatively more common in women. Spasm of the external sphincter precludes examination and heightens the pain. Acute anal fissures can be treated by local application of glyceryl trinitrate cream. However, in pregnancy the consequent hypotension may be detrimental. Hence, it must be used with caution only in hospitalized states with adequate supervision and bedrest. Fissures are best treated by a subcutaneous lateral sphincterotomy of the internal sphincter. Conventional manual anal stretching (Lord's procedure) should be avoided whenever possible; however, a gentle anal stretch may ameliorate the pain of prolapsed thrombosed hemorrhoids which must be distinguished from acute perianal hematoma[2]
- *Hemorrhoids* have been discussed above
- *Anal neuralgias,* attributed to the stretching of pelvic neural plexuses, usually presents with constant burning pain which, often radiates to the thighs, vagina and sacral region. A psychogenic component may be prominent. Exacerbations occur during impaction of solid feces; such acute periods should be treated with enemas followed by long-term administration of laxatives
- *Condyloma accuminatum* may be aggravated during pregnancy. Severe cases need electrocoagulation as podophyllin is contraindicated in pregnancy.

Venous Disorders

Pregnancy is a hypercoagulable state and deep vein thrombosis (DVT) is not uncommon. Recent studies have identified genetic susceptibility to protein C resistance in pregnancy and these women have a higher incidence of

DVT.[3] The risk of potentially fatal pulmonary embolism dictates that DVT should be diagnosed and treated urgently. Heparin is safe in pregnancy as it does not cross the placental barrier but Warfarin is best avoided in pregnancy.

Varicose veins are also common in pregnancy. Though distressing symptoms are rare, there may be a slight predisposition to DVT. Venous disorders are best investigated by Duplex Doppler imaging and patency of deep venous flow can be accurately judged in most patients. Varicose veins are best managed conservatively with elastic compression stockings and adequate bed rest with elevation of feet.

Operative Surgical Considerations

In the course of difficult pelvic surgery, inadvertent injuries are prone to occur to the ureter, intestine and major blood vessels.

Ureteric Injuries

The pelvic surgeon must have accurate knowledge of the course of the ureters and be proficient in locating the ureter at different sites and steps of pelvic dissection. The ureter is posterior to the ovarian vessels at the origin of the infundibulopelvic ligament. During ligation of the ovarian vessels, it can be inadvertently incorporated in the pedicle and it is at this site the ureter is most commonly injured during pelvic surgery.[4] The ureter continues in the base of the broad ligament and courses under the uterine artery and is 0.7–1.5 cm lateral to the uterine isthmus. While ligating the uterine vessels at this situation, the ureter is again vulnerable to injury. The ureter traverses the parametrium lateral to the cervix, ultimately entering the bladder trigone at the level of anterior vaginal fornix. This is the third common site of ureteric injury, left side being commoner than the right side (Fig. 24.1).

The common causes of iatrogenic ureteral injury are outlined in Box 24.2.

Identification of ureteral injury is of paramount importance, because primary repair has the best chance of success. Unrecognized traumas lead to delayed diagnosis usually with the formation of fistulae, infected urinomas or obstructive uropathy, which presents with fever, flank pain and ileus in the postoperative period. Presence of mild hematuria should arouse suspicion of urinary tract injuries. In the postoperative period, these injuries are best investigated by intravenous urography. Partial injuries may be dealt with by stenting the ureter by a double J stent passed over a guidewire, either from below by cystoscopy or from above through a percutaneous nephrostomy (Table 24.2). Ureteric repairs or reimplantations should be performed with interrupted sutures of absorbable variety, e.g. polyglycolic acid or polydioxanone. The repair should

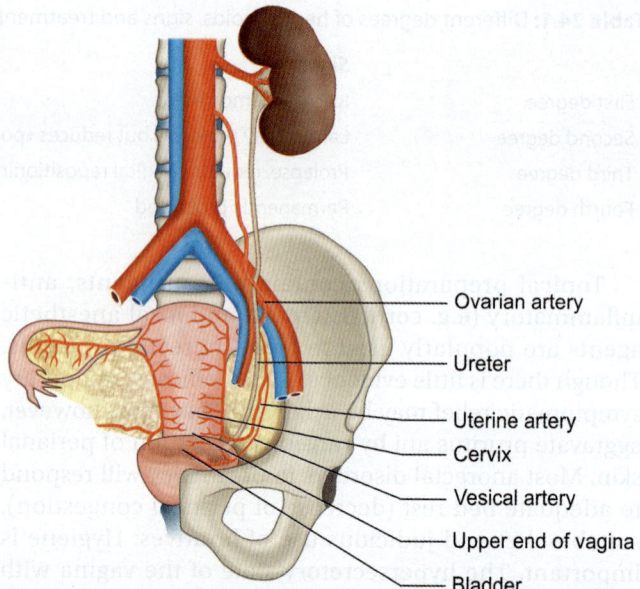

Fig. 24.1: Common sites of ureteral injury during pelvic operations Posterior to ovary (ovarian fossa), coursing under the broad ligament anterior to uterine vessels. Anterolateral to fornix of vagina and lateral to cervix.

Box 24.2: Common causes of ureteric injury.

- Abdominal hysterectomy
- Vaginal hysterectomy
- Salpingo-oophorectomy
- Laparoscopy (rarely)
- Cystocele repair

Table 24.2: Surgical techniques for ureteral reconstruction.

Procedure	Ureteral defect
Ureteroureterostomy	1–3 cm
Ureteroneocystostomy alone	3–5 cm
Uretoneocystostomy with psoas hitch	5–10 cm
Ureteroneocystostomy with Boari flap	10–15 cm

be drained extraperitoneally. A double J stent may be used to splint the anastomosis, and it is customary to keep the bladder decompressed with an indwelling catheter for 6–7 days. Ureteroneocystostomy (ureteric reimplantation) is generally performed by a tunnelled antireflux procedure. Additional length of the bladder may be obtained by mobilization of the dome and suturing the ipsilateral extension to psoas major muscle ('the psoas hitch') as per diagram (Figs. 24.2A to C). Avoidance of tension is crucial as tension at the site of ureteric anastomoses predisposes to stenosis.[5] Bladder injuries are best-repaired in two layers and decompression is maintained with a catheter for 10–12 days.

CHAPTER 24 General Surgical Problems in Gynecology

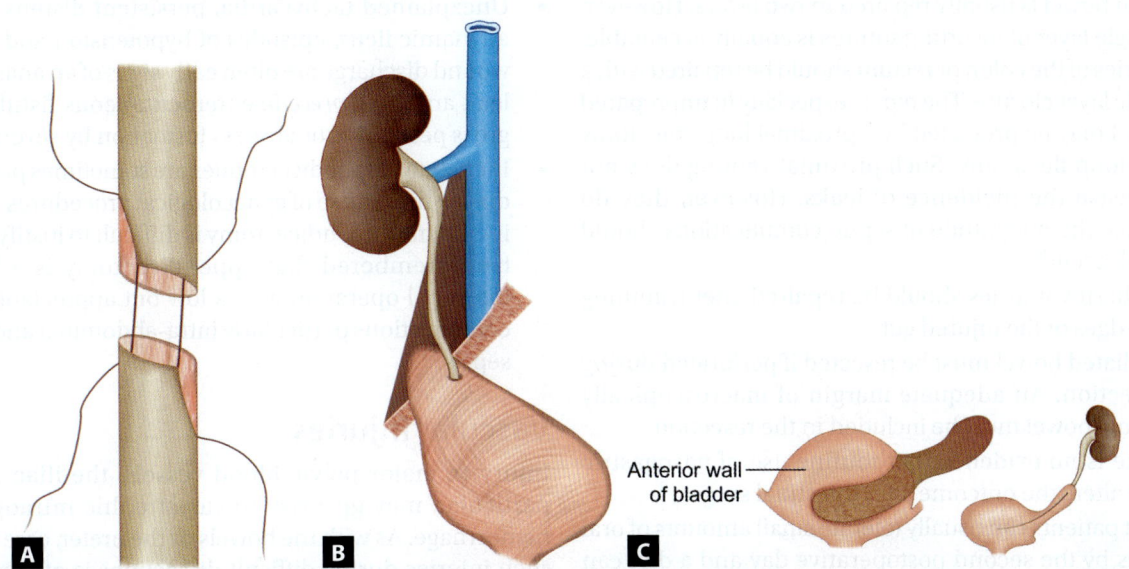

Figs. 24.2A to C: (A) End-to-end ureteroureterostomy (note the obliquity and spatulated ends); (B) Ureteroneocystostomy with psoas hitch (the dome of bladder is fully mobilized), contralateral superior vesical pedicle may be divided; (C) Ureteroneocystostomy with Boari flap (the flap is based posterolaterally on the ipsilateral superior vesical artery. Base of flap: 4 cm in width, tip of flap: 3 cm, in width).

Bowel Injuries

Intestinal injuries are particularly prone to occur in the presence of adhesions, usually from previous surgical procedures. Endometriosis, multiple surgeries, previous intraperitoneal sepsis and previous irradiation for malignancy increase the density of adhesions. In surgery involving resection for pelvic cancers, particularly ovarian carcinoma, en-bloc resection of loops of small intestine may be necessary if they are involved with tumor.

It is salutary to consider the possibility of adhesions and bowel injuries before the operation. A knowledge of the pathology of the individual patient should alert the discerning clinician of technical difficulties. Resection of a large chocolate cyst in the presence of pelvic endometriosis or resection of a bulky tubo-ovarian mass may lead to inadvertent injury of the rectosigmoid, necessitating a proximal colostomy. It is difficult to site a colostomy with perfection in an anesthetized, supine patient. Such a patient may therefore, benefit from a preoperative physical evaluation to select the site of a stoma should the eventuality arise. A stoma should avoid the creases produced by abdominal fat rolls, which can only be assessed by sitting the patient up. Stoma should also be at least 4 cm away from bony prominences (e.g. anterior superior iliac spine), the umbilicus and surgical scars.

Key Points

- It is important to anticipate difficult pelvic dissections, adhesions and possible bowel injury
- Repair of intestinal injuries or resections of bowel are contaminated procedures. Appropriate antisepsis protocols should be employed, e.g. change of gloves and wound drapes and use of fresh instruments for wound closure
- Perioperative antibiotics are best administered by the intravenous route at or before induction of anesthesia. A second-generation cephalosporin is usually adequate. Anti-anaerobic cover must be added as soon as possible if bowel injuries have occurred. Continuing prophylactic antibiotics beyond the first postoperative day confers no additional benefit[6]
- Bowel preparation may be considered preoperatively, if left colonic or rectal injury is anticipated. It has no role in small bowel resections or right colonic repairs
- Adhesions are best separated under direct vision with blunt tipped fine dissection scissors. Interloop adhesions of small bowel need not be separated. All adhesions distal to the site of an intestinal repair, however, must be carefully lysed; presence of distal obstruction is the single most important factor contributing to anastomotic leaks. All bands must be divided. Bands originating from the mesentery and crossing the ileum and attached inside the pelvic cavity should be ligated before division as rarely, they harbor blood vessels[7]
- Whenever possible synthetic absorbable sutures [(e.g. polyglactin 910 (Vicryl) or polyglycolic acid or polydioxanone (PDS)] should be chosen over chromic catgut

- Small bowel is usually repaired in two layers. However, a single layer of inverting sutures is equally acceptable. Injuries of the colon or rectum should be repaired with a single layer closure. The repair, especially in unprepared bowel may be protected by a proximal loop colostomy or a loop ileostomy. Such proximal venting does not decrease the incidence of leaks. However, they do reduce the magnitude of septic complications should a leak occur[8]
- Diathermy injuries should be repaired after trimming the edges of the injured gut
- Irradiated bowel must be resected if perforated during dissection. An adequate margin of macroscopically normal bowel must be included in the resection
- There is no evidence that routine use of nasogastric tube alters the outcome after intestinal surgery[9]
- Most patients can usually tolerate small amounts of oral fluids by the second postoperative day and a diet can usually be introduced by the fourth day. There is no evidence that withholding oral feeds in the postoperative period lessens the incidence of anastomotic leak[10]
- Intraperitoneal drains may be used in left colonic or rectal repairs. Closed system of drainage employing soft tube drains avoiding direct contact with the suture line is preferable. Following small bowel resections the abdomen need not be drained
- All mesenteric gaps should be closed
- Peritoneal wash (lavage) is not necessary unless gross macroscopic contamination has occurred. Sterile normal saline is adequate for lavage; strong antiseptic solutions, e.g. povidone iodine should be avoided
- It is rational to avoid over infusion of sodium in the early postoperative period, though clear evidence to justify this is unavailable
- Unexplained tachycardia, persistent distension with adynamic ileus, episodes of hypotension and copious wound discharge are often early signs of an anastomotic leak and may *precede* enterocutaneous fistulation or gross peritonitis or abscess formation by several days
- Incidental appendicectomies are sometimes performed during the course of gynecological procedures. Routine incidental appendicectomy is difficult to justify. It must be remembered that appendicectomy is a "major" intestinal operation with a low but appreciable risk of complications particularly intra-abdominal and wound sepsis.[11]

Vascular Injuries

Injury to major pelvic blood vessels, the iliac veins in particular, may give rise to catastrophic intraoperative hemorrhage. As with the bowels or the ureter, care to avoid such injuries during difficult dissections is of paramount importance. Proximal and distal control of the vessel makes repair of injuries easier and safer. A selection of vascular clamps and appropriate suture materials (5-0 or 6-0 Prolene) should be available in the operating room. Panic laden attempts to apply hemostatic forceps to injured vessels causes greater injury and laceration. Bleeding can be usually controlled with localized pressure with a finger or small swab while proximodistal dissection is continued to mobilize the vessel to perform an anastomosis or repair without tension on the vessel.

CONCLUSION

Understanding the principles, which underlie general surgical problems and operative surgery, will significantly help obstetricians and gynecologists in their own field of work.

REFERENCES

1. Marti MC. Pregnancy and proctological disease, Surgery for anorectal diseases. Springer-Verlag; 1989;305-09.
2. Hancock BD. Hemorrhoids and Anal fissures, ABC of colorectal disease. BMJ publishing group; 1998. pp. 24-26.
3. Barbieri RL, Repke JT. Medical disorders during pregnancy, Harrison's Principles of Internal Medicine, 15th edn. McGraw Hill; 2001. pp. 25-30.
4. Montz FJ, Berek JS. Gynecologic Pelvic Procedures. Maingot's Abdominal Operations, 10th edn. Appleton and Lange; 1997. pp. 2133-49.
5. Franke JJ, Smith JA. Surgery of the ureter. Campbell's Urology, 7th edn. WB Saunders company; 1998. pp. 3069-72.
6. Bellinger EP. Surgical infections. Sabiston Textbook of Surgery, 15th edn. WB Saunders Company; 1997. p. 43.
7. Mukherjee K, Fryer L, Stephenson BM. Mesodiverticular bands. British Jour Surg. 1997;84(1):43.
8. Fielding LP. Lessons from the Large Bowel Cancer Project 1976. pp88. Recent Advances in Surgery. Vol 3 Churchill Livingstone; 1998. pp. 143-57.
9. Savassi-Rocha PR, Conceicao SA, Ferreira JT, et al. Evaluation of routine use of nasogastric tube in digestive operations by a prospective controlled study. Surg Gynecol Obstet. 1992;174: 317-20.
10. Bickel A, Shtamler B, Mizrahi S. Early oral feeding following removal of narogastric tube and gastrointestinal operations. Arch Surg. 1992;127:287-9.
11. Hayes RJ. Incidental appendectomis; current teaching. JAMA. 1977;238:31.

CHAPTER 25

Genital Tuberculosis

Prashanth K Adiga, Pratap Kumar

Overview

- About 75% of patients belong to the age group between 24 and 45 years.
- Fallopian tubes the most common structures involved in female genital tuberculosis.
- Infertility is the presenting symptom in 43–74% of patients.
- Patients with endometrial tuberculosis usually present with menstrual symptoms.
- High index of suspicion is the first step in the diagnostic process of genital tuberculosis.
- Endometrial aspirate, biopsy or curettage in the premenstrual phase—required for making a diagnosis of endometrial tuberculosis.
- Mantoux test has sensitivity of 55% and specificity 80% in patients with genital tuberculosis.
- Hysterosalpingogram is contraindicated in women where genital tuberculosis is suspected.
- Surgery is indicated where medical therapy has failed to resolve symptoms and in the presence of a persistent pelvic mass.

INTRODUCTION

Genitourinary tuberculosis is still a major health problem in many developing countries including India, and had been declared by World Health Organization (WHO) as 'public health emergency' in 1993.[1] Tuberculosis (TB) has a devastating impact in developing countries with 13 countries accounting for 75% of the cases. The most common type of extrapulmonary tuberculosis is genitourinary tuberculosis, accounting for 27% (range 14–41%) worldwide.[2] In India, the incidence of genital tuberculosis is nearly 18%.[3]

INCIDENCE

It is estimated that 1% of infertile women, aged between 20 to 40 years in United States and 18% in India suffer from genital tuberculosis.[4] Genital tuberculosis in females is found in 0.75 to 1% of gynecological admissions in India.[5] Cases occur more frequently (62%) in postmenopausal women in developed countries than in developing countries, where only 28% of cases were in the postmenopausal category.[6]

PATHOLOGY

The causative organism of genital TB is *Mycobacterium tuberculosis* in 90–95% of cases. In 5–10% of cases, *Mycobacterium bovis* is the responsible organism. Genital TB occurs mostly secondary to pulmonary tuberculosis. The bacilli reach the genital tract by three principle routes, i.e. (1) hematogenous spread in 90% of cases, with the primary focus being the lung, lymph nodes or skeletal system, (2) descending direct spread and (3) lymphatic spread. Direct inoculation during sexual intercourse with patients with genitourinary tuberculosis, rarely can result in the spread of the disease. In females, the genital organs commonly affected are as follows:

- Fallopian tube (95–100%)
- Endometrium (50–60%)
- Ovaries (20–30%)
- Cervix (5–15%)
- Myometrium (2.5%)
- Vulva/vagina (1%).[7]

Female genital tuberculosis begins in the endosalpinx and can spread to the peritoneum, endometrium, ovaries, cervix, and vagina.[8] The appearance of the tube may vary. In some cases, the tubes may appear normal. When the infection is active, the tubes appear red and edematous. In chronic infection, they appear fibrosed. Adhesions may occur between the tubes and the ovaries and the other pelvic organs with loss of fimbrial structure. Patent ostia along with grossly diseased fallopian tubes are suggestive of tuberculous salpingitis.

Endometrial involvement may result in an endometrial ulcer or accumulation of caseous material to form pyometra. Complete or partial adhesions may form depending upon the degree of endometrial involvement.

The ovaries may be involved by direct infection from a neighboring structure, such as the bowel. However, in most instances, infection spreads from the tubes and the process extends to the surface of the ovaries. Adhesions with the fimbria or formation of unilateral or bilateral adnexal masses may be seen.

The cervix is involved by spreading from the endometrium or as part of the hematogenous infection. Ulceration and necrosis is present that can easily be confused with a cervical carcinoma.

Vulval and vaginal tuberculosis is usually associated with ulceration and has an appearance very similar to that of a chancre. The lesion may appear brown or red and may have a surrounding area of induration. They have raised edge around the central ulcer.

CLINICAL FEATURES

Genital tuberculosis can occur in any age group. The majority of patients are in the reproductive age group. Seventy-five percent of patients belong to the age group between 24 and 45 years.[9] Postmenopausal women account for 7 and 11% of cases of genital TB. The clinical manifestation of genital TB is listed in the Table 25.1.[7]

Table 25.1: Clinical manifestation of genital tuberculosis.

Symptoms	Percentage of total
• Infertility	43–74
– Primary	55–78
– Secondary	11–72
• Normal menstrual function	50–88
• Oligomenorrhea	54
• Amenorrhea	14
• Menorrhagia	19
• Abdominal pain	42.5
• Dyspareunia	5–12
• Dysmenorrhea	12–30

Majority of women are diagnosed during the work up for infertility. The patient may have constitutional symptoms like:
- Fever
- Night sweat
- Weight loss.

In acute phase, the clinical picture might be similar to that of acute pelvic inflammatory disease with pelvic pain, fever and vaginal discharge.

The abdominal and vaginal examinations may be normal. Occasionally, a pelvic mass may be felt and adnexal tenderness might be elicited.

Tuberculosis of the endometrium: The most common presenting symptoms are:
- Menstrual disturbance
- Oligoamenorrhea
- Pelvic pain.[10]

Postmenopausal women may present with postmenopausal bleeding, pyometra or leukorrhea.[11,12]

Tuberculosis of the cervix: Patient present with postmenopausal bleeding and/or chronic discharge. On inspection of the cervix, there is often ulceration and necrosis that can easily be confused with a cervical carcinoma.

Tuberculosis of the vulva: Patient presents usually with ulceration and has an appearance very similar to that of a chancre (tuberculous chancre).

Diagnosis

Genital tuberculosis is an elusive diagnosis and a high index of suspicion is the first step in the diagnostic process. Genital TB should be considered in a women presenting with unexplained infertility, amenorrhea not explained by other causes, pelvic infection that does not respond to ordinary treatment and, in postmenopausal women with bleeding, persistent leukorrhea and pyometra where endometrial neoplasia has been ruled.

The following investigations may help in establishing the diagnosis of genital TB.

Blood Picture

Complete blood count with ESR may show (a) anemia, (b) leukocytosis with lymphocytosis, and (c) raised ESR.

Chest X-ray

X-ray chest may help to exclude or confirm coexisting respiratory tract TB.

Mantoux or Tuberculin Test

A positive Mantoux or tuberculin test (>10 mm of induration) indicates that the person is, or has been infected with

M. tuberculosis. This has a sensitivity of 55% and specificity 80% in patients with genital TB.[13]

In populations with a high incidence of tuberculosis and where BCG is given routinely, the Mantoux test is often falsely positive. The Mantoux test may be negative in patients with active tuberculosis if the patient has overwhelming clinical disease, is severely immune compromised, has coincidental viral infection or is malnourished.

Endometrial Aspirate, Biopsy or Curettage

This is the easiest and most commonly performed test for the diagnosis of genital TB. This is performed in the premenstrual phase of the menstrual cycle. One part of the aspirate/biopsy is sent for histopathology examination in formalin. The other part of the specimen is sent for acid-fast bacilli (AFB) smear, culture, guinea pig inoculation. Microscopic examination of acid-fast bacilli (AFB) requires the presence of at least 10,000 organisms per milliliter in the sample. Culture is more sensitive, requiring only 100 organisms per milliliter, but it takes about 8 weeks to grow on Lowenstein-Jensen medium. Liquid culture with radiometric growth detection, such as BACTEC-460 or nonradiometric (CO_2) growth detection, such as BacTAlert 3D provides more:

- Rapid growth (average 10–14 days)
- Specific identification of *Mycobacterium tuberculosis*
- Rapid drug susceptibility testing the therapy.[14]

Polymerase Chain Reaction

Polymerase chain reaction (PCR) is a rapid and sensitive molecular biological method for detecting tuberculosis DNA. This method can detect fewer than 10 organisms in the clinical specimen compared with 10,000 necessary for smear positivity.

Disadvantages of PCR:
- Cannot differentiate between live and dead bacilli
- Can give false-negative results due to contamination with heparin or to a high salt concentration of the specimen which may interfere with PCR results.

Imaging Modalities

Abdominal and pelvic ultrasound, computed tomography (CT) and magnetic resonance imaging (MRI) are used where there is a pelvic or an abdominal mass and the presence of ascites. These modalities are useful where malignancy is suspected.

Ultrasound features of wet tuberculosis (with ascites) include:[7]

- Septate ascites (Fig. 25.1)
- Particulate ascites
- Loculated fluid
- Thickened peritoneum
- Thickened omentum
- Endometrial involvement and adnexal masses.

Ultrasound features of dry tuberculosis (no ascites) are:

- Adnexal mass (Fig. 25.2)
- Adhesions and loculated fluid (Fig. 25.1)

CT Scan

This is a useful modality for pelvic and abdominal masses especially when the lesion may resemble malignant ovarian tumor. CT scan features include:

- Ascites
- Omental and mesenteric infiltration
- Smooth thickening of the parietal peritoneum.[15]

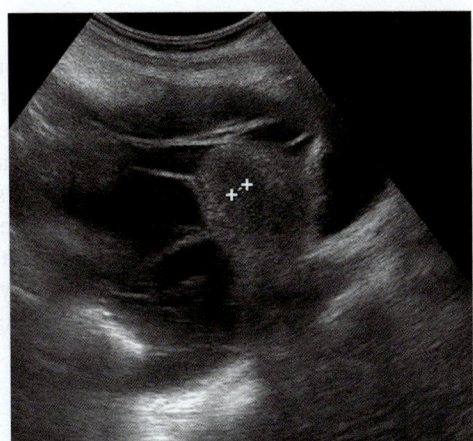

Fig. 25.1: Adhesions between the uterus and the peritoneum with ascites.

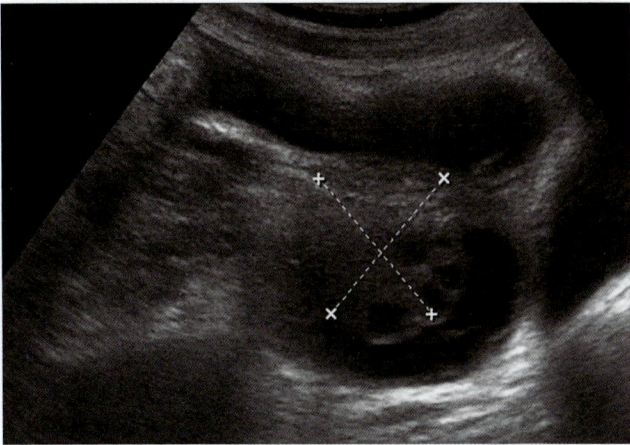

Fig. 25.2: Adnexal mass. The ovary is well-demarcated with adhesions and fluid around it.

MRI

MRI scan has better resolution than a CT scan and may avoid necessity of laparotomy as the differential diagnosis is usually from an ovarian tumor.

Hysterosalpingogram

Hysterosalpingogram (HSG) is one of the frequently performed tests for evaluation of infertility. HSG should not be performed where tuberculosis is diagnosed by other means, as this can disseminate the disease.[16]

Hysterosalpingogram features suggestive of tuberculosis of the fallopian tubes are listed below:
- Calcification showing as linear streaks
- Tufted tubal outline or tubal diverticula
- Tubal occlusion, especially at the transit between the isthmus and the ampulla, multiple occlusions causing beaded appearance or a rigid pipe stem appearance
- Hydrosalpinx showing as tubal dilatation with thick mucosal folds
- Peritubal adhesions giving the tube a "corkscrew" appearance, a per tubal halo or loculated spillage of contrast medium
- The rare finding of enterotubal fistulae—most common between the sigmoid colon and fallopian tube.

HSG findings for endometrial tuberculosis are nonspecific and are characterized by:
- Synechiae formation
- Distorted uterine contour
- Venous and lymphatic intravasation.

Laparoscopy

Laparoscopy is a more invasive procedure, and allows for visualization of the fallopian tubes, ovaries and peritoneal cavity, but also gives the opportunity to biopsy tuberculous lesions.[10] Laparoscopy should be done carefully to avoid injury to an adherent bowel loop. The following features may be found on laparoscopy.[10]
- Tubercles on the peritoneal surface (Fig. 25.3)
- Inflamed or blue-colored uterus
- Salpingitis or oophoritis or tubo-ovarian mass
- Tubal occlusion with hydrosalpinx. Dye dripping (instead of free flowing) from the fimbreal opening on chromopertubation
- Free peritoneal fluid looking like blood
- Ceseation in the pouch of Douglas
- Frozen pelvis
- Omental adhesions.

Hysteroscopy

Hysteroscopy should be combined with laparoscopy to exclude/confirm endometrial involvement. The endometrium may be pale looking. The cavity may be partially or completely obliterated by adhesions of varying grade. The cavity may be shrunken.

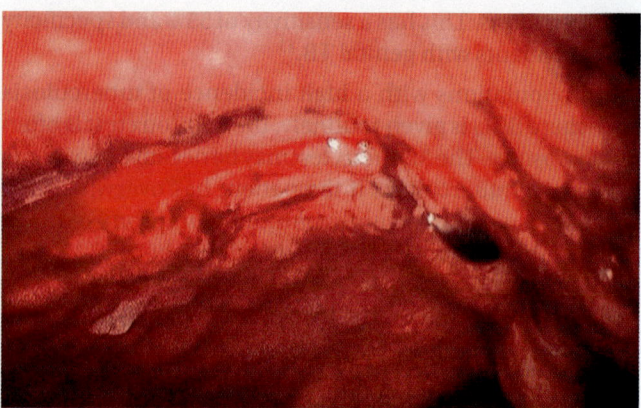

Fig. 25.3: Laparoscopic picture with the presence of tubercles on the peritoneal surface.

Analysis of the Ascitic Fluid

Tapping of the ascitic fluid should be done and send for analysis for biochemistry and cytology, microscopy for AFBs, TB culture and serology. This is helpful to differentiate between a malignant ovarian tumor and TB when there is ascites with adenexal mass.

The laboratory findings consistent with tuberculous ascites are:
- Lymphocytic exudates
- Absence of malignant cells
- High total protein content (>25 g/L)
- Small serum-ascites albumin gradient (<11 g/L)
- Lactate dehydrogenase (LDH) above 90 U/L
- Adenosine deaminase (ADA) above 30 IU/mL.[17-19]

Treatment

Medical

The current treatment regime is quadruple chemotherapy with isoniazid, rifampicin, pyrazinamide and ethambutol. Genitourinary tuberculosis responds to short courses of treatment as it carries lower mycobacterial load than pulmonary infection. A four-drug regimen consisting of isoniazid, ethambutol, rifampicin and pyrazinamide is used for the first 2 months, followed by triple or dual therapy. The total duration of treatment should be six months to a year.[20-22] Excellent cure rates are reported for all of the standard treatment regimens.

Surgery

Surgery may be indicated where medical therapy has failed to resolve symptoms and in the presence of a persistent pelvic mass. In these patients, total abdominal hysterectomy is the operation of choice, while bilateral salpingo-oopherectomy is done if the ovaries are damaged as well.[23-25]

REFERENCES

1. World Health Organization. Global tuberculosis control report, 2007. Available from: http://www.who.int/tb/publications/global_report/2007/en/index.html
2. Das P, Ahuja A, Datta Gupta S. Incidence, etiopathogenesis and pathological aspects of genitourinary tuberculosis in India: A journey revisited. Indian J Urol. 2008;24:356-61.
3. Marjorie P, Holenarsipur RV. Extrapulmonary tuberculosis. An overview. Am Fam Physician. 2005;72:1761-8.
4. Vithalani N, Udani PM, Vithalani N. A study of 292 autopsies proved cases of tuberculosis. Indian J Tuber. 1982;29:93-7.
5. Arora R, Rajaram P, Oumachigui A, Arora VK. Prospective analysis of short course chemotherapy in female genital tuberculosis. Int J Gynecol Obstel. 1992;38:311.
6. Marcus SF, Rizk B, Fountain S, Brinsden P. Tuberculous infertility and in vitro fertilization. Am J Obstet Gynecol. 1994;171(6):1593-96.
7. Gatoni DK, Gitau G, Kay V, Ngwenya S, Lafong C, Hasan A. Female genital tuberculosis. Obstet Gynecol. 2005;7:75-9.
8. Simon HB, Weinstein AJ, Pasternak MS, Swartz MN, Kunz LJ. Genitourinary tuberculosis. Clinical features in a general hospital. Am J Med. 1977;63:410-20.
9. Qureshi RN, Sammad S, Hamd R, Lakha SF. Female genital tuberculosis revisited. J Pak Med Assoc. 2001;51:16-8.
10. Botha MH, Van der merwe FH. Female genital tuberculosis. SA Fam Pract. 2008;50(5):12-6.
11. Gatongi DK, Kay KV. Endometrial tuberculosis presenting with postmenopausal pyometra. J Obstet Gynaecol. 2005;25(5):518-20.
12. Maestre MA, Manzano CD, Lopez RM. Postmenopausal endometrial tuberculosis. Int J gynaecol obstet. 2004;86(3): 405-06.
13. Raut VS, Mahashur AA, Sheth SS. The Mantoux test in the diagnosis of genital tuberculosis in women. International Journal of Gynecology & Obstetrics. 2001;72:165-69.
14. Haas DW. Mycobacterial disease. In: Mandell GL, Benetton JE, Dolin R (Eds). Principles of practice of infectious diseases. Philadelphia, PA: Churchill Livingstone; 2000. pp. 2576-607.
15. Zissin R, Gayer G, Chowers M, Sapiro-Feinberg M, et al. Computerized tomography finding in abdominal tuberculosis. Reports of 19 cases. Isr Med Assoc J. 2001;3:414-8.
16. Tripathy SN, Tripathy SN. Infertility and pregnancy outcome in female genital tuberculosis. Int J Gynaecol Obstet. 2002;76:159-63.
17. Piura B, Rabinovich A, Leron E, Yanai-Inbar I, Mazor M. Peritoneal tuberculosis-an uncommon disease that may deceive the gynecologist. Eur J Obstet Gynecol Reprod Biol. 2003;110(2):230-5.
18. Gurbuz A, Karateke A, Kabaca C, Kir G, Cetingoz E. Peritoneal tuberculosis simulating advanced ovarian carcinoma: Is clinical impression sufficient to administer neoadjuvant chemotherapy for advanced ovarian cancer? Int J Gynecol Cancer. 2006;16 (Suppl 1):307-12.
19. Protopapas A, Milingos S, Diakomanolis E, et al. Miliary tuberculous peritonitis mimicking advanced ovarian cancer. Gynecol Obstet Invest. 2003;56(2):89-92.
20. Chong VH, Rajendran N. Tuberculosis peritonitis in Negara Brunei Darussalam. Ann Acad Med Singapore. 2005;34(9):548-52.
21. Bilgin T, Karabay A, Dolar E, Develioglu OH. Peritoneal tuberculosis with pelvic abdominal mass, ascites and elevated CA 125 mimicking advanced ovarian carcinoma: A series of 10 cases. Int J Gynecol Cancer 2001;11(4):290-4.
22. Mahdavi A, Malviya VK, Herschman BR. Peritoneal tuberculosis disguised as ovarian cancer: an emerging clinical challenge. Gynecol Oncol. 2002;84(1):167-70.
23. Chowdary NN. Overview of tuberculosis of the genital tract of the female genital tract. J Indian Med Assoc. 1996;94:345-6.
24. Figueroa-Damian, Martinez-Velazco I, Villagranazesati R, Arredondo-Garcia JL. Tuberculosis of the female reproductive tract. Effect on function. Int J fertile Menopausal Stud. 1996;41:430-6.
25. Sutherland AM. Surgical treatment of tuberculosis of the female genital tract. Br J Obstet Gynaecol. 1980;87(7):610-2.

CHAPTER 26

Uterine Displacements including Retroversion and Uterine Inversion

Akhila Vasudeva, Pratap Kumar

Overview

- Uterus is normally in an anteverted and anteflexed position.
- About 20% of women have retroverted uterus which is mobile and neither causes any symptom, nor warrants any treatment.
- Fixed retroversion may be caused by pelvic pathologies, including endometriosis and pelvic inflammatory disease.
- Acute uterine inversion mostly results from mismanagement of third stage of labor.
- Acute uterine inversion requires prompt recognition, resuscitation, and repositioning, to prevent maternal mortality and morbidity.
- Chronic uterine inversion may represent late puerperal cases.
- Chronic uterine inversion needs to be differentiated from submucus fibroid polyp protruding into the vagina.
- Chronic inversion often requires surgical correction, either abdominally or vaginally.

INTRODUCTION

Uterus is situated between bladder anteriorly and rectum posteriorly in the female pelvis. Uterus is not a fixed organ in the pelvis. Its position is altered by several physiological changes like filling and emptying of the bladder, changes in posture, increased intra-abdominal pressure and filling of the rectum. Usually, cervix and uterus do not lie in line with the vaginal axis. Common position of the uterus is that of anteversion and anteflexion. Anteversion means that cervix (along with the uterus) is bent forwards at its junction with vagina (Fig. 26.1). Anteflexion means that uterine body is bent forwards in relation to the axis of the cervical canal. Similarly, retroversion and retroflexion indicate backward inclination of cervix and uterus. Usually when there is retroversion, retroflexion is also present (Figs. 26.2 and 26.3). Supravaginal portion of the cervix is relatively fixed and any displacement is usually rotation of the organ around this axis, in other words, bending of the corpus on the cervix.[1]

UPWARD DISPLACEMENT OF THE UTERUS

Rarely, uterus can be displaced upwards such that external os cannot be reached by the examining fingers since it

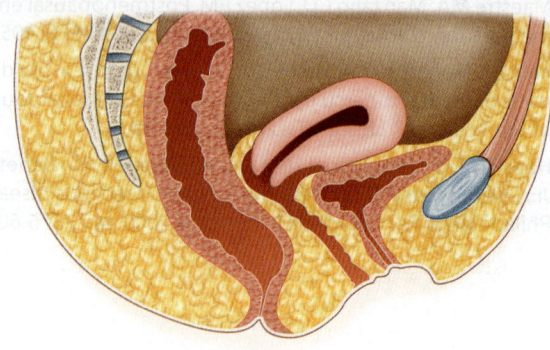

Fig. 26.1: Anteverted uterus.

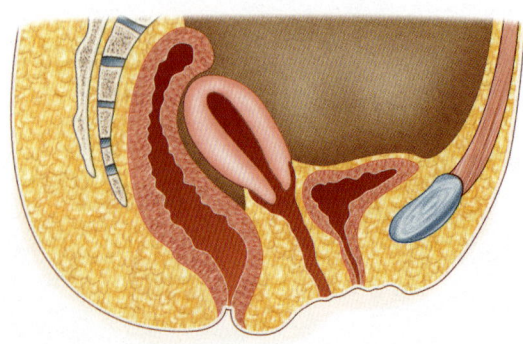

Fig. 26.2: Retroverted uterus.

CHAPTER 26 Uterine Displacements including Retroversion and Uterine Inversion

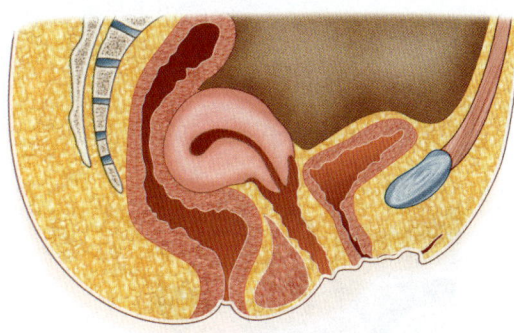

Fig. 26.3: Retroverted and retroflexed uterus.

lies above the level of upper border of pubic symphysis. Following can cause such a displacement of the uterus:[1]
- Vaginal/paravaginal tumor.
- Hematocolpos.
- A collection of blood/pus in the pelvis.
- A broad ligament myoma or a low cervical myoma.
- Any tumor impacted in the pouch of Douglas.

Treatment of the cause corrects this displacement of the uterus.

LATERAL DISPLACEMENT OF THE UTERUS[1]

At times, uterus is laterally deviated as a whole or tilted to one side, so that corpus points to one direction and cervix points to the other direction. Following can cause lateral displacement of the uterus:
- A broad ligament tumor or a hematoma/pus collection
- Adhesions pulling the uterus to one side, may be following severe pelvic inflammatory disease or tuberculosis
- Operative removal of one adnexa
- Unicornuate/bicornuate deformity
- Idiopathic.

Other displacements also have been described in the literature, example, forward displacement of the uterus as a whole due to tumor or fluid collection in the pouch of Douglas, acute anteflexion occurring commonly in early pregnancy when the fundus is heavy and supravaginal cervix is soft and atonic.

RETROVERSION

Uterus is found retroverted in about 15–20% of the women. Usually it is asymptomatic, and uterus would be mobile without any pathology. Uterine retroversion is common in certain physiological conditions like in puerperium, and this corrects itself spontaneously once pelvic muscle tone improves. Retrodisplacement is quite common in fetuses and young children.

Degrees of Retroversion[2]

First Degree
Fundus is vertical and points towards sacral promontory (also called uterus in midposition).

Second Degree
Fundus lies in the sacral hollow but not below the level of internal os.

Third Degree
Fundus lies below the level of internal os, flexed deeply into the cul-de-sac, pressing against the rectum.

Pathological conditions where uterus is found retroverted:
- Uterine prolapse: It is not clear whether retroversion is the cause of prolapse or whether prolapse causes retroversion.
- Tumors in the anterior pelvis: Myomas or ovarian cysts situated anteriorly can push the uterus backwards. Fibroid, even if in the posterior wall, can cause retroversion due to the heaviness.
- Fixed retroversion: Here adhesions or adherent tumors fix the uterus in a retroverted position, thus causing retroverted and fixed uterus. Common causes are pelvic inflammatory disease, endometriosis.

SYMPTOMS OF RETROVERSION

Symptoms earlier attributed to retroversion like dysmenorrhea, dyspareunia, infertility, etc. are no longer thought to be due to retroversion *per se*. It is now understood that the symptoms are mostly due to the disease causing retroversion like endometriosis or pelvic inflammatory disease.

Dyspareunia

Of all the symptoms earlier attributed to retroversion, deep dyspareunia is the one which could be the result of retroversion *per se*, it could also be the result of the disease which caused it, like endometriosis. It is said that uterine body or the prolapsed ovaries in the pouch of Douglas, may cause deep dyspareunia or dull aching pain lasting several hours after the coitus.[3] However, dyspareunia is present in minority of the women having retroverted uterus, depending possibly on the length of vagina. This symptom is position dependent and change of coital position may reduce or prevent this problem.[1]

Infertility

Infertility is usually the result of disease that caused fixed retroversion. However, there is a possibility that in cases of acute retroversion, cervix is anteriorly situated and away from the pool of motile sperms which are usually in the posterior fornix. Also, external os can be closed by the anterior vaginal wall at the end of coitus. However, a postcoital test is needed to confirm that motile sperms are not reaching the cervical canal and that is the reason for infertility.[3] Dyspareunia, chronic backache and infrequent coitus may also contribute to infertility.

DIAGNOSIS

Mostly when the uterus is anteverted, Cusko's speculum inserted with an angle of about 30° posteriorly (downwards), would reach the cervix because cervix is situated either midway or posteriorly in the vagina. Face of the cervix points towards posterior vaginal wall. In cases of acute retroversion, speculum examination reveals that cervix is anteriorly situated and comes into view unusually easily. Cervix is directed upwards and forwards. Some more signs noticeable in retroverted uterus are that anterior vaginal wall and cervix appear to be almost continuous to each other, and there is a shallow anterior fornix. Vagina too sometimes appears shorter than usual.

Bimanual examination is required to confirm the position of the uterus, and commonly, uterine body is felt easily between the examining hands in anteverted uterus (Fig. 26.4). In cases of retroverted uterus, uterine body is felt in the pouch of Douglas, and this moves along with movements of the cervix (Fig. 26.5). It is difficult to assess the size of the uterus in cases of acute retroverted uterus. Third degree retroverted uterus which cannot be brought forward by vaginal examination, is best examined by rectovaginal examination.

Differential Diagnosis

- A tubal or an ovarian mass prolapsed into pouch of Douglas or adherent to the back of the uterus
- Feces or other mass impacted in the rectum
- A tumor in the pouch of Douglas like chocolate cyst/pelvic hematocele/abcess
- Fibroid in the posterior wall of the uterus.

It is important to perform pelvic examination after patient empties her bladder. Identifying position of the uterus is important during pelvic examination, especially prior to performing certain procedures like IUCD insertion and insertion of uterine sound, etc. If retroversion is not identified, intrauterine manipulations like sounding during or outside pregnancy, or attempts at IUCD insertion, can lead onto perforation of the uterus through the anterior wall.

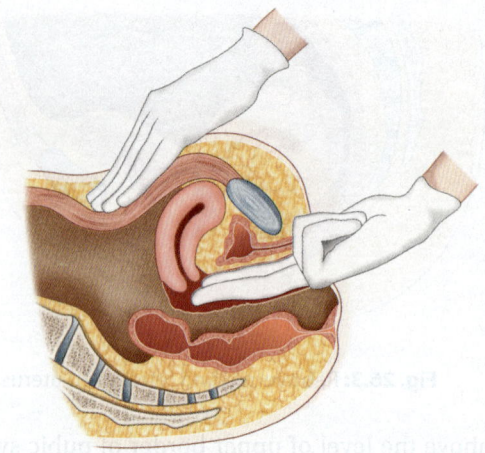

Fig. 26.4: Bimanual examination in an anteverted uterus.

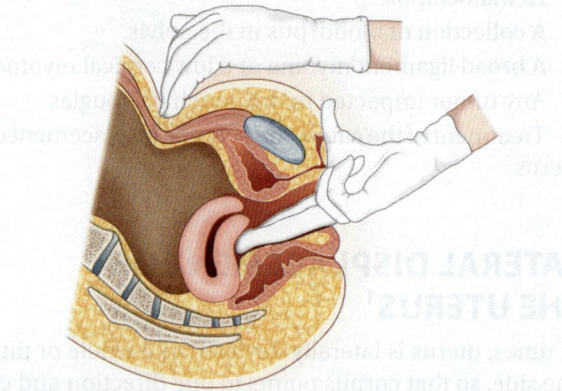

Fig. 26.5: Bimanual examination in a retroverted uterus.

MANAGEMENT

Asymptomatic mobile retroversion does not require any treatment, and treatment of symptomatic fixed retroversion is directed towards the disease that caused such a retroversion.

Rarely, if retroversion is the reason for dyspareunia and chronic pelvic pain, following treatment modalities can be tried:

- *Pessary treatment:* Uterus is bimanually replaced into anteverted position (done by pushing the cervix backwards and pushing the fundus forwards), and a Smith-Hodge pessary is inserted in the vagina to keep the uterus in anteverted position. Pessary acts by stretching the uterosacral ligaments so as to pull the cervix backwards. Pessary is usually retained in place for 3 months and then removed. If the pessary relieves the symptoms, and the symptoms recur after removing the pessary, operative treatment for retroversion may be justified or the patient may continue to use the pessary if she is comfortable with it. A properly fitted pessary does not interfere with coitus. This is known as the 'pessary test'. If the patient is symptomatic despite the pessary, operative correction of retroversion is not justified.

- *Surgery:* Fixed retroversion needs surgical management of the underlying condition which has caused such a retroversion, e.g. endometriosis or pelvic inflammatory disease. At the end of such a surgery, additional procedures for ventrosuspension of the uterus is done. Following certain surgeries, prophylactic ventrosuspension is done to prevent formation of severe pelvic adhesions, e.g. myomectomy and tuboplasty. Rarely, these procedures are done in patients who have symptoms due to retroversion alone and pessary test is positive.
- *Gilliam's ventrosuspension:* Round ligaments normally do not play a role in maintaining anteversion and anteflexion, but they are sometimes used in correcting retroversion during surgery. Round ligaments are first held by nonabsorbable sutures close to the cornu. They are brought out through the internal inguinal ring, suspended and anchored to the anterior rectus sheath close to the anterior superior iliac spine. Thus, round ligaments are drawn up against the anterior abdominal wall, maintaining uterus in the anteverted position. However, round ligaments have considerable capacity to stretch and a permanent correction can never be guaranteed.
- Plication and shortening of the round ligaments using nonabsorbable sutures.
- *Baldy Webster operation:* Round ligaments are taken posteriorly through anterior and posterior leaves of broad ligament, and sutured together to the posterior surface of the uterus, thus shortening the round ligament and anteverting the uterus.
- At laparotomy, shortening of the uterosacral ligaments can be done along with modified Gilliam's operation but care must be taken to avoid kinking/ligating the ureter.

These procedures can be done laparoscopically also. While laparoscopically evaluating chronic pelvic pain/dysmenorrhea and dyspareunia, round ligament plication and uterosacral ligament plications have been attempted as corrective measures for uterine retroversion, with reported improvement in symptoms.[4-6] However, these procedures are not widely performed and there are not many randomized trials to prove their efficacy.

RETROVERTED GRAVID UTERUS

Uterus is retroverted in early pregnancy in upto 15% of the pregnancies. Spontaneous correction of the retroverted uterus usually takes place by 10th week of pregnancy. This spontaneous correction succeeds even in presence of adhesions, since adhesions undergo softening and stretching in pregnancy. Very rarely, retroverted gravid uterus gets impacted in the pouch of Douglas after 12-14th week of pregnancy. This condition is seen in 1:3000 pregnancies and is associated with adverse pregnancy outcome, if diagnosis is missed or delayed.[7] These women present with acute urinary retention, which requires immediate catheterization, followed by bimanual vaginal examination along with ultrasound, to confirm the diagnosis. This kind of impaction is likely to occur when the pelvis is very small with overhanging sacral promontory, or in presence of a posterior wall leiomyoma. Rarely incarcerated uterus can cause sacculation of uterus.[7] Indwelling catheter and knee chest positioning can correct the problem in many cases. If not, next step would be to attempt manual repositioning.[8] Smith-Hodge pessary has been advocated by some to correct this condition. However if discovered later on, expectant management is preferred.[7] MRI is helpful in delineation of anatomy. Cesarean section is the method of delivery.

UTERINE INVERSION

Here, uterus is turned inside out. It is a rare condition, occurs in 1 in 30,000 cases, but it requires prompt recognition and management to avoid mortality and morbidity.

This condition can be classified in several ways. In terms of duration, uterine inversion can be described as: (a) acute, which occurs within 24 hours of delivery; (b) subacute, which occurs beyond 24 hours of delivery yet within 4 weeks; and (c) chronic, which occurs beyond 4 weeks of delivery. Inversion can be puerperal or obstetrical, or non-puerperal/gynecological.

Inversion may vary in degree from mere dimpling of the fundus to a degree in which whole uterus and cervix turns inside out (Figs. 26.6A to D).

First degree: Uterine fundus inverts into uterine cavity but fundus does not descend beyond the internal os.

Second degree: Uterine fundus protrudes beyond the internal os and lies in the vagina.

Third degree: Complete inversion of the uterus, and fundus protrudes out of introitus, with or without vaginal inversion.

ACUTE INVERSION

Most acute inversions are puerperal. Incidence is said to be 1 in 2000 to 1 in 20,000.[9] Most acute inversions are due to mismanagement of third stage of labor, however, spontaneous inversions also occur. Certain factors predispose the woman to develop inversion, like primiparity, uterine inertia and atony, fundal attachment of placenta, erect posture during confinement, precipitate labor, macrosomic infant, sudden emptying of the

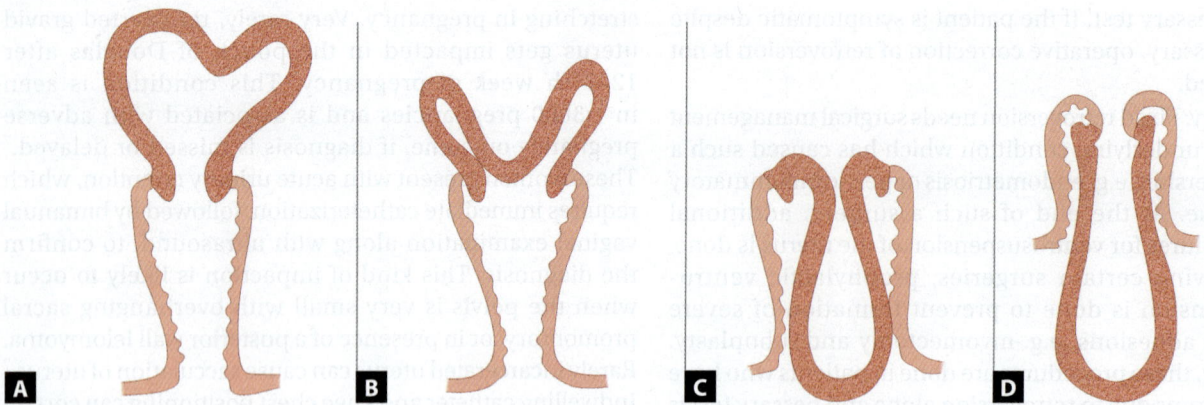

Figs. 26.6A to D: Degrees of uterine inversion.

overdistended uterus, magnesium sulphate, uterine anomalies, morbidly adherent placenta, and short cord.[9]

However, certain factors like squeezing the relaxed uterus immediately following delivery of the baby, Crede's method of expulsion of placenta, increased intra-abdominal pressure with relaxed uterus, e.g. coughing/sneezing/straining or traction on the cord before signs of placental separation or cord traction in cases of morbidly adherent placenta can all cause puerperal inversion of the uterus.

Presentation

This condition is associated with severe pain and postpartum hemorrhage. Most common presentation is that of a PPH (94% of the cases have PPH).[10] About 40% of the women would be in hypovolemic shock. However, amount of shock is out of proportion to the amount of bleeding because there is severe neurogenic shock associated with pulling of the ligaments, though this disproportionate shock is not proven by the recent studies.[9,10] Condition can be quickly fatal.

Diagnosis

Patient would be pale, restless, and in shock. Abdominal and vaginal examination findings would vary depending on the degree of inversion. Uterine fundus is not palpable or there is a dimple at the fundus. At times, uterine fundus may have a reasonably normal contour also. Placenta and the cord are still attached in this situation. A fleshy mass is palpable in the vagina, associated with shallow fornices, which usually represents the fundus of the uterus. Cervical rim may or may not be palpable.

PREVENTION OF PUERPERAL INVERSION

Proper management of third stage of labor is important to prevent acute inversion. Cord should not be pulled on when the placenta is still attached specially when the uterus is not yet contracted. Crede's method of expressing the placenta when the uterus is still relaxed should not be done. Fundal pressure should not be applied without seeing signs of placental separation, cord traction should not be given without manual support by left hand and while not have administered uterotonics.

MANAGEMENT

Management depends on the circumstances in which inversion is diagnosed. Resuscitative measures should be taken immediately and large bore IV cannula inserted, fluids/blood products should be arranged and transfused, analgesics given, urinary catheterization done. Measures to replace inverted uterus should be taken simultaneously because antishock measures do not work until uterus is repositioned. If the inversion happens in presence of a doctor or a trained nurse, or if patient arrives half an hour to one hour after the episode, uterus should be immediately reposited back by applying firm constant pressure, starting from the part which has inverted last (one closest to the cervical rim), progressing slowly upwards, replacing fundus back into its position at the end with or without the attached placenta. Applying pressure on the fundus with a vaginal hand directed towards the umbilicus is called as Johnson's maneuver. Uterine relaxants used simultaneously help in repositioning the uterus. Some have advocated applying counter traction on the cervix using a ring forceps.

No attempt should be made to pull on the placenta before positioning the uterus back, except for two exceptional circumstances:

- When the cervical ring is too narrow to reduce the inverted mass along with the placenta
- When the part of placenta is already separated.
  Earlier removal of placenta may lead onto the following complications:
- Opening up of maternal sinuses which aggravates bleeding and predisposes to infections

- Tearing and perforation of the uterine wall
- Difficulty in removal due to morbid adherence of the placenta.

Once uterus is reposited, oxytocics are started, manual removal of placenta is done and operator's hand is withdrawn along with placenta as the uterus contracts in response to oxytocics.

However, when a patient is referred with inversion, there would be congestion, edema, increasing cervical contraction, and reposition is possible only with general anesthesia with halothane and uterine relaxation. Also, vaginal manipulations under these circumstances may exacerbate vasovagal shock. However, if the uterus is projecting outwards, it should be replaced back in the vagina with moist packing with or without vaginal plugging devices. This will reduce traction on infundibulopelvic ligaments and may improve the neurogenic shock.

R Vijayaraghavan, et al. have reported a case wherein manual reposition of inverted uterus was facilitated with the help of laparoscopic assistance.[11]

Other method which has been tried with success is O Sullivan's hydrostatic pressure, in which sterile irrigating fluid is taken in a can situated at a height 3 to 4 feet above the level of vagina, it is infused into the vagina using a suitable cannula, closing the vaginal introitus either using hand as a cup or a vacuum cup, thus slowly building up hydrostatic pressure in the vagina. As much as 3 liters of fluid may be needed to reposition the uterus back into position. Hydrostatic pressure built in the vagina lifts up the uterus towards umbilicus, causing traction on the round ligaments, which slowly brings about repositioning of the uterus.

As a last resort, laparotomy may have to be done. In the Huntington procedure, the cup of the uterine inversion is identified at laparotomy; Allis forceps are placed within the dimple of the inverted fundus and gentle upward traction is exerted on the clamps, with a further placement of forceps on the advancing fundus. The process is repeated until the procedure is complete.[12] If this technique fails, Haultain's technique is employed. This involves incising the cervical ring posteriorly with a longitudinal incision and facilitates uterine replacement by the Huntington method. After replacement is complete, the uterus is repaired in two or three layers.

Very occasionally, hysterectomies have been done in older women, when all the measures failed and uterus could not be repaired.

Rarely, acute recurrent puerperal uterine inversions are seen. Several techniques have been proposed to tackle the problem, including balloon tamponade, brace sutures, and "holding the cervix" method.[13,14]

Simultaneous to repositioning the uterus, prompt management of shock, replacement of blood products, and appropriate coverage with antibiotics are essential to prevent maternal mortality/morbidity.

The current consensus is that early diagnosis of uterine inversion and prompt corrective action can completely prevent maternal mortality. The major morbidity is transfusion related. Laparotomy for uterine inversion is rarely necessary provided attempts at repositioning are initiated promptly.[10]

When acute inversion has been encountered and tackled in one delivery, there is a high-risk of recurrence in the third stage of next delivery, for which woman has to be watched for carefully. Active management of third stage of labor would facilitate effective uterine contraction, bring about placental delivery, and prevent recurrence of the problem.

CHRONIC INVERSION

Chronic inversion is rare, often results from late puerperal cases where initial stages of inversion has been overlooked and shock and hemorrhage produced by incomplete inversion was minimum. This kind of inversion can also occur in the puerperium, and presents several weeks or months later, when gynecological symptoms develop.

Inversion can be due to a fundal submucosal myomatous polyp, or rarely a fibroma or a fibrosarcoma which soften the uterine wall leading onto chronic inversion. When a malignant tumor is associated with chronic inversion, it is usually a sarcoma (often a sessile tumor) rather than a carcinoma, because sarcoma causes the softening of uterine wall, and also forms a mass protruding into the cavity bringing about uterine contractions, leading on to inversion.[15]

Spontaneous inversion is sometimes seen in old age, especially if the cervix has been amputated at a high level.

Overall, nonpuerperal inversions are usually chronic, though occasionally they can be acute.

Diagnosis

Patient may complain of intermittent/irregular vaginal bleeding along with low backache/chronic pelvic pain. Patient may also feel a lump in the vagina, heaviness or bearing down sensation. These complaints might have started following confinement or sometime later, there may be history of postpartum hemorrhage/obstetric shock. Speculum examination reveals a soft pink fleshy mass in the vagina. The inverted fundus is usually infected, congested and ulcerated, and is difficult to distinguish from the infected fibroid polyp. If the inversion is complete, cervical rim may not be seen. Cervical rim may still be seen and felt in cases of incomplete inversion. If it is a submucosal myoma, uterine sound can be passed on the side of the mass all the way into the uterine cavity, right up to the fundus. However, if it is inversion, sound cannot be passed on the side of the mass beyond a short distance. Length of uterine cavity would be reduced in cases of partial inversion, and there would be no cavity at all in cases of complete inversion. If the mass is gently held and pulled down with a vulsellum, upward movement of the cervical rim is highly suggestive of inversion. If the mass in the vagina is a polyp, more of the polyp would be seen, downward traction either does not cause any movement of the cervix, or cervical rim also moves downwards along with the mass.

Chronic inversion can also be mistaken for cervical cancer, however, cancerous growths are friable, bleed on touch, associated with induration, fixity and hard. Other differential diagnosis is retained bits of placenta.

Bimanual and rectal examination confirms absence of palpable fundus or a dimple in the region of the fundus in cases of inversion, whereas fundus will be normally palpable in cases of submucosal myoma. Body of the uterus is usually enlarged in cases of submucus fibroid polyp, which is confirmed by bimanual palpation.

Complete uterine prolapse or procedentia can be mistaken for inversion; however, cervix will be the leading point in procedentia, whereas cervix will be situated normally in its place in cases of inversion.

Chronic inversion associated with a fibroid polyp or a uterine sarcoma can be missed unless this possibility is kept in mind. Before removal of any such polyp, it is better to use the sound to measure the length of uterine cavity. Because if associated inversion is not recognized, surgeon can perforate the uterine fundus in an attempt to transect the pedicle of the polyp, opening directly into the peritoneal cavity, and results can be disastrous.

At times, diagnosis of chronic non-puerperal uterine inversion can be very difficult and possible only with a high index of suspicion.

Abdominal ultrasound done with full bladder helps to differentiate between a fibroid polyp and chronic inversion. When in doubt, MRI should be used as a diagnostic modality and this can be very useful for the diagnosis.[16]

Rarely, laparoscopy may be needed to establish the diagnosis.

Management

First line of management is to give antibiotics, anti-inflammatory drugs and local antiseptic measures (douching or cleansing of the vagina) to reduce infection, congestion and edema. Occasionally, this results in spontaneous cure of the inversion.[1]

If the inversion persists, and the inverted uterus is clean, a special repositor[1] named Aveling's repositor can be placed over the inverted fundus. Continuous pressure is applied using a brace. This and a tight vaginal pack are generally successful in reducing the inversion in a few days. Principle is to lift the uterus high up in the pelvis, so that round ligaments are put under traction, which help in pulling the fundus out of the inversion cup.

However, chronic inversion more often requires surgical approach, either vaginally or abdominally. At laparotomy, above mentioned Huntington's technique is initially tried. If that fails (long standing and resistant cases), principle is to divide the constricting cervicovaginal rim, done either abdominally or vaginally, which can be divided anteriorly or posteriorly taking care to avoid injuring the adjacent viscera, repositioning the uterus back by abdominal and vaginal manipulations, repairing the cut edges of cervix/uterus and vagina at the end.

Abdominal surgeries done are: Haultain's operation where cervicovaginal constriction ring is divided posteriorly. Dobbins described using an anterior incision for the same purpose. By the vaginal route, anterior part of the ring has been divided (Spinelli's technique), posterior part of the ring has been divided (Kustner's technique), uterus replaced and the incision closed.

Above procedures can be done laparoscopically or with a combined laparoscopic and vaginal route, in presence of trained personnel.[17]

The danger inherent to these procedures is the risk of uterine rupture during subsequent pregnancy/labor. Therefore, woman has to be watched carefully for this complication and should be delivered by elective cesarean at/near term.

If it is not desirable to conserve the uterus in a multiparous woman or if it is not possible to conserve the uterus, abdominal/vaginal hysterectomy may be performed rarely.

If chronic inversion is associated with submucosal fibroid polyp, vaginal myomectomy should be done under laparoscopic guidance, to avoid uterine perforation. Tumor should be removed by shelling it out from the capsule, rather than dividing the pedicle.

If the chronic inversion is associated with any other tumor like uterine sarcoma, management depends on the tumor, its size and associated other pathologies. It is better to handle the tumor vaginally followed later by abdominal hysterectomy.[15] It would be better to rule out malignancy before embarking on repositioning surgery.

REFERENCES

1. Kumar P, Malhotra N. Jeffcoat's Principles of Gynecology. 7th edition. New Delhi: Jaypee Brothers, 2008;293-303.
2. Lentz GM. History, physical examination and preventive health care. In: Katz VL, Lobo RA, Lentz GM, Gershenson DM (Eds). Comprehensive Gynecology, 5th edition. Philadelphia: Mosby Elsevier, 2007;137-51.
3. Padubidri VG, Daftary SN. Howkin's and Bourne Shaw's Textbook of Gynaecology, 14th edition. New Delhi: Elsevier, 2008;310-14.
4. Ou CS, Liu YH, Joki JA, Rowbotham R. Laparoscopic uterine suspension by round ligament plication. J Reprod Med. 2002;47(3):211-6.
5. Yen CF, Wang CJ, Lin SL, Lee CL, Soong YK. Combined laparoscopic uterosacral and round ligament procedures for treatment of symptomatic uterine retroversion and mild uterine decensus. J Am Assoc Gynecol Laparosc. 2002;9(3):359-66.
6. Ostrzenski A. Laparoscopic retroperitoneal hysteropexy. a randomized trial. J Reprod Med. 1998;43:361-6.
7. Gottschalk EM, Siedentopf JP, Schoenborn I, Gartenschlaeger S, Dudenhausen JW, Henrich W. Prenatal sonographic and MRI findings in a pregnancy complicated by uterine sacculation: case report and review of the literature. Ultrasound Obstet Gynecol. 2008;32(4):582-6.
8. Newell SD, Crofts JF, Grant SR. The incarcerated gravid uterus: complications and lessons learned. Obstet Gynecol. 2014;123(2 Pt 2 Suppl 2):423-7.
9. Mirza FG, Gaddipati S. Obstetric emergencies. Semin Perinatol. 2009;33:97-103.
10. You WB, Zahn CM. Postpartum hemorrhage: abnormally adherent placenta, uterine inversion, and puerperial hematomas. Clin Obstet Gynecol. 2006;49:184-97.
11. Vijayaraghavan R, Sujatha Y. Acute postpartum uterine inversion with haemorrhagic shock: laparoscopic reduction: a new method of management. BJOG. 2006;113(9):1100-2.
12. Thomson AJ, Greer IA. Non-hemorrhagic obstetric shock. Bailliere's Clin Obstet Gynecol. 2000;14(1):19-41.
13. Matsubara S, Baba Y. MY (Matsubara-Yano) uterine compression suture to prevent acute recurrence of uterine inversion. Acta Obstet Gynecol Scand. 2013;92(6):734-5.
14. Matsubara S. Combination of an intrauterine balloon and the "holding the cervix" technique for hemostasis of postpartum hemorrhage and for prophylaxis of acute recurrent uterine inversion. Acta Obstet Gynecol Scand. 2014;93(3):314-5.
15. Gowri, Vaidyanathan. Uterine inversion and corpus malignancies: A historical review. Obstet Gynecol Surv. 2000;55(11):703-7.
16. Occhionero M, Restaino G, Ciuffreda M, Carbone A, Sallustio G, Ferrandina G. Uterine inversion in association with uterine sarcoma: a case report with MRI findings and review of the literature. Gynecologic and Obstetric Investigation. 2012;73(3):260-4.
17. Auber M, Darwish B, Lefebure A, Ness J, Roman H. Management of non-puerperal uterine inversion using a combined laparoscopic and vaginal approach. Am J Obstet & Gynecol. 2011;204(6):7-9.

CHAPTER 27

Endoscopy in Gynecology

Rajesh Bhakta

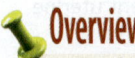
Overview

- Laparoscopy is performed by 2 or 3 small 0.5 cm incision and can be used for both diagnostic as well as operative at the same sitting.
- Laparoscopy gives excellent exposure and visualization of abdominal approach and better postoperative recovery as of vaginal approach.
- Advantages over conventional surgery which includes less postoperative pain hence less pain killer requirement, faster recovery which may be translated into short hospital stay, reduced cost and early return to normal activity and professional work.
- Pneumoperitoneum using CO_2, lifts up the abdominal wall for better visualization of organs and prevents vascular injury by increasing the distance.
- Hysteroscopy is used in patients when ultrasound showing abnormal pathology inside the uterus.
- Hysteroscopy is done at postmenstrually between 7 to 10 days. During this period the endometrium is thin and bleeding will be absent.

INTRODUCTION

The surgical procedures in gynecology performed with the use of either laparoscope or a hysteroscope is termed as endoscopic surgery. Laparoscopy was first performed in animals in the early 1900s, and the Swedish surgeon Jacobaeus coined the term laparoscopy (*laparothorakoskopie*) in 1901. Endoscopy is now an essential part of gynecologic surgery. Historically, gynecologic endoscopy began in the 1930s with the development of diagnostic laparoscopy, but it was not until the 1960s that operative laparoscopy was introduced, primarily for tubal sterilization.[1] By the late 1970s, the role of laparoscopy had expanded to include lysis of adhesions and treatment of endometriosis.[2] Technology and equipment have now advanced to include the use of laparoscopy in hysterectomies, incontinence procedures, and operations for gynecologic malignancies. Latter part of the last century, gynecologic endoscopy, both laparoscopy and hysteroscopy, had become an essential part of gynecologic surgery.

INDICATIONS OF LAPAROSCOPIC SURGERY

- Tubal sterilization
- Infertility: Diagnostic for tubal patency, adhesiolysis, fimbrioplasty (Figs. 27.1 to 27.3)
- Endometriosis: Ovarian cystectomy, drainage of endometriomas, ablation of implants, adhesiolysis (Figs. 27.4 and 27.5)
- Polycystic ovarian disease: Ovarian drilling
- Ectopic pregnancy: Salpingectomy, salpingotomy
- Pelvic inflammatory disease drainage of cyst or abscess
- Fibroid, myomectomy (Fig. 27.6)
- Laparoscopically assisted vaginal hysterectomy
- Total laparoscopic hysterectomy
- Pelvic lymphadenectomy
- Laparoscopically assisted suspension for uterine descent
- Procedures for incontinence.

CONTRAINDICATIONS

- Severe cardiovascular disease: The biochemical changes from CO_2 gas, Trendelenburg position, raised intra-abdominal pressure, anesthetics, pose risk to the patient
- Hemodynamically unstable patient
- Generalized peritonitis
- Hemorrhagic shock
- Bowel obstruction and severe ileus: Distended bowel loops make visualization impossible
- Morbid obesity.

CHAPTER 27 Endoscopy in Gynecology

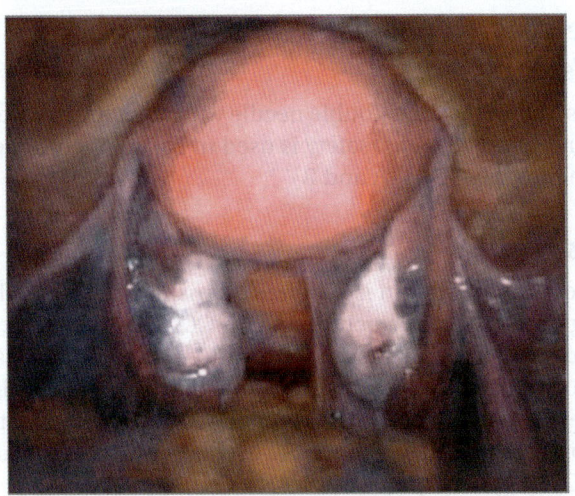

Fig. 27.1: Normal laparoscopy picture.

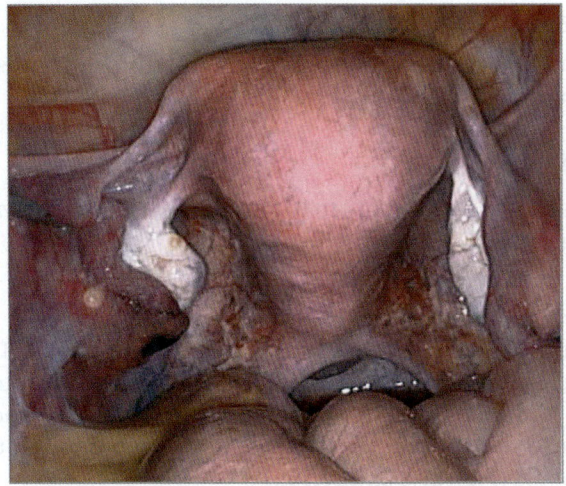

Fig. 27.2: Laparoscopic appearance of dense adhesions.

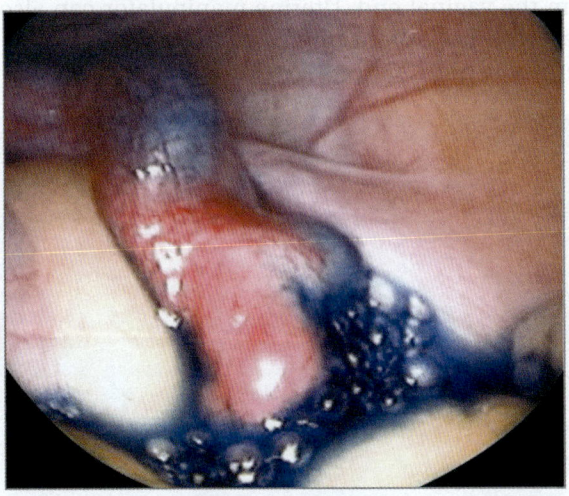

Fig. 27.3: Chromotubation.

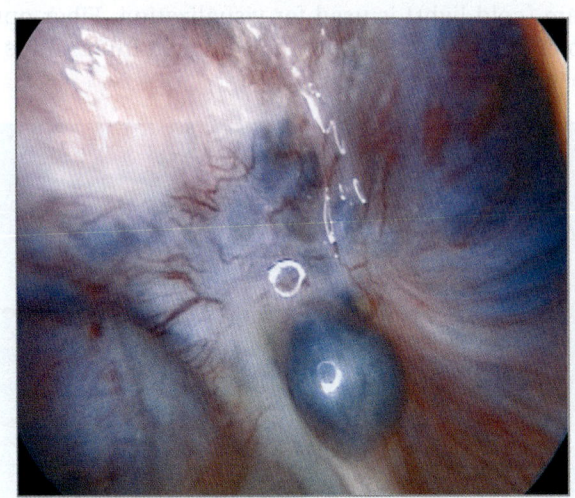

Fig. 27.4: Endometriotic nodule.

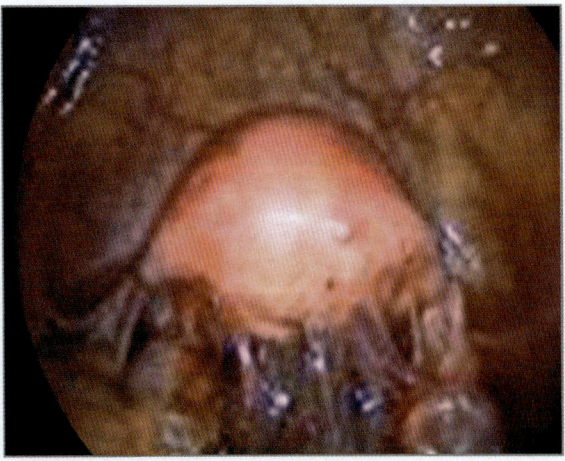

Fig. 27.5: Severe endometriosis.

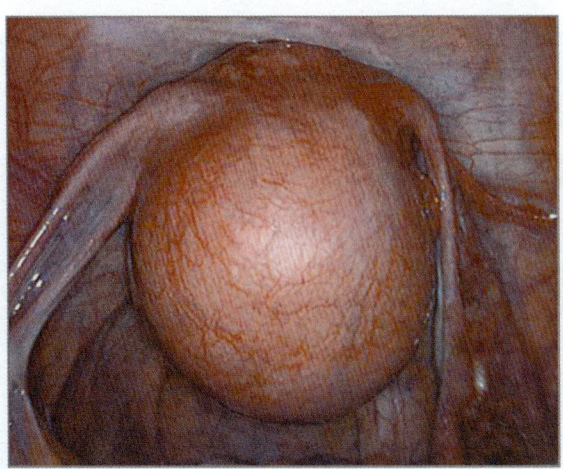

Fig. 27.6: Fibroid.

SECTION 1 General Gynecology

Instruments
Figure 27.7 shows instruments required for diagnostic laparoscopy.

Telescopes
The caliber varies from 4 to 10 mm scopes with 0-30 viewing angle (Fig. 27.8).

Trocar and Cannula
They are different sizes for different telescopes. The trocar tip is conical or pyramidal. It is inserted through the abdominal wall for pneumoperitoneum. The trocar is inserted and the telescope is introduced through the cannula (Figs. 27.9 and 27.10).

Light Source and Cable
A light source with (xenon or halogen) high intensity light beam (cold light) is used for visualization. Fiber optic cables are used to transmit the cold light from source to the telescope.

Needle for Pneumoperitoneum (Veress Needle)
It is a spring loaded double needle with an outer sharp and inner blunt stylet for safety is used to create pneumoperitoneum (Figs. 27.11A and B).

Insufflator
Pneumoperitoneum is required for visualization of pelvic organs. This can be achieved with CO_2 gas, nitrous oxide and air. Electronic pneumo-apparatus (insufflator) is used in operative laparoscopy to maintain the intra-abdominal pressure so as to elevate the abdominal wall for better visualization. Most commonly used gas is carbon dioxide (CO_2) (Fig. 27.12).

Uterine Manipulator
It is used to elevate the uterus and move the uterus from the vaginal end. Uterine manipulator can also be used with or without hollow cannula for injecting the methylene blue.

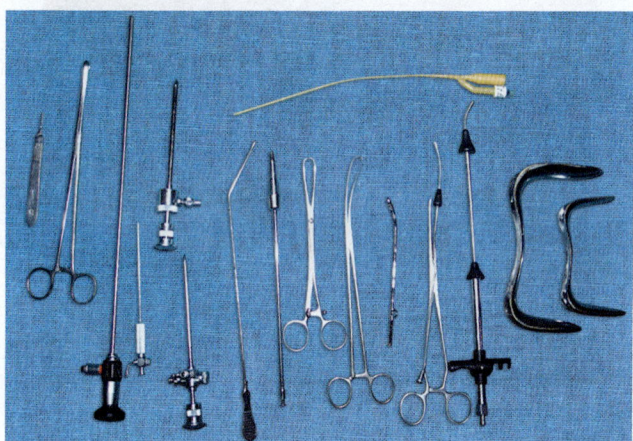

Fig. 27.7: Instruments required for diagnostic laparoscopy.

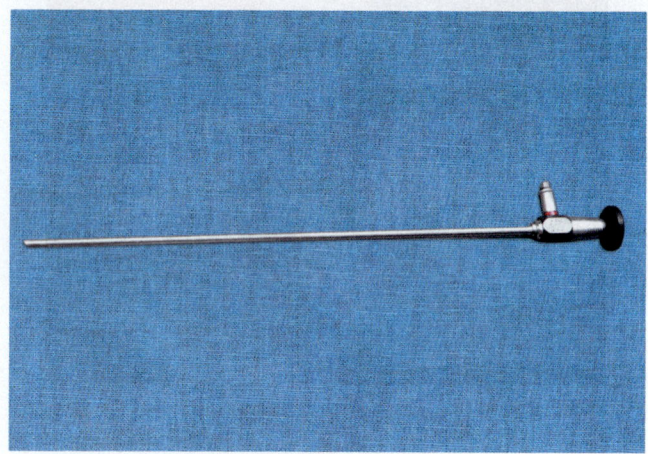

Fig. 27.8: Laparoscope.

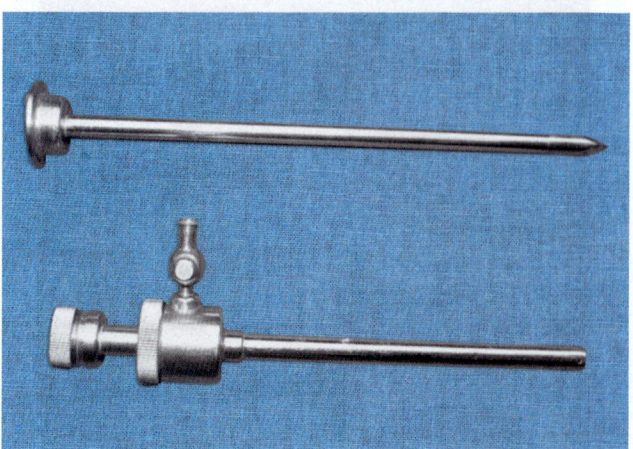

Fig. 27.9: Trocar and cannula.

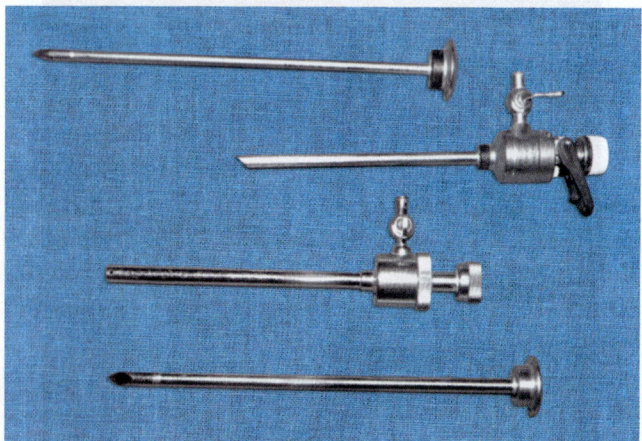

Fig. 27.10: Trocar and cannula 5 and 7 mm.

CHAPTER 27 Endoscopy in Gynecology

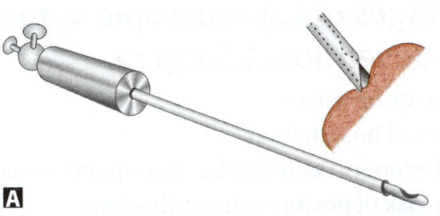
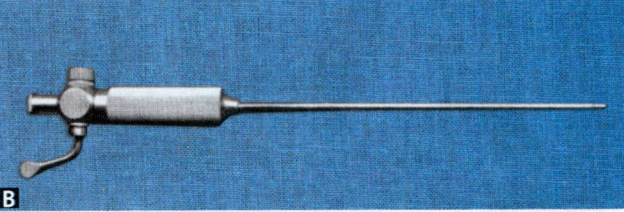

Figs. 27.11A and B: Veress needle.

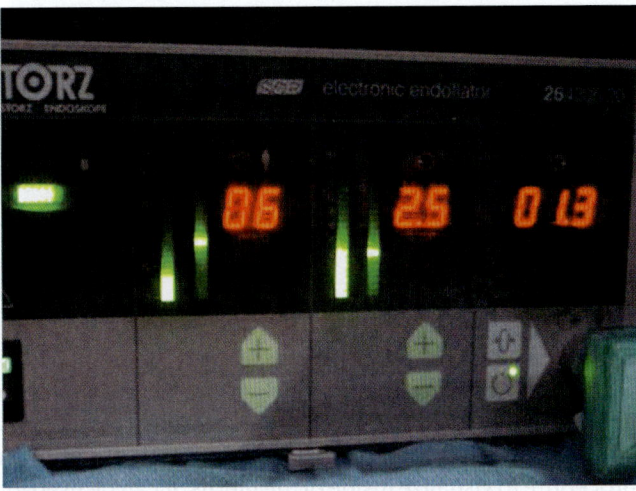

Fig. 27.12: Endoflator.

Video Camera
Telescope is connected with the camera and picture is visualized on the screen. This is necessary for operative laparoscopy.

Ancillary Instruments
Several accessories are used, viz. grasping forceps, biopsy forceps, scissors, suction cannula, ring applicators, bipolar instrument, and morcellator. This may be passed through second and/or third port placed on the abdomen.

Hemostasis
Electrosurgical unit are used for cutting, coagulation of tissues. Two types of current are used namely; monopolar and bipolar. Other modes used are laser and sutures, mechanical clips and staples.

TECHNIQUE OF LAPAROSCOPY
The main steps involved in laparoscopy include:
- Preoperative screening and informed consent
- Anesthesia
- Creating pneumoperitoneum
- Introduction of trocar and cannula
- Introduction of laparoscope
- Creation of accessory ports
- Performing the surgery through laparoscope
- Deflation of the pneumoperitoneum
- Closure of the incision.

Procedure
Patient is placed in dorsal lithotomy position (Fig. 27.13). Abdomen is cleaned with appropriate antiseptic solution and draped. A small incision is made just below the umbilicus. A Veress needle is passed into the abdominal cavity through the umbilicus at 45° angle. After testing, the needle is properly placed pneumoperitoneum is created slowly using carbon dioxide. When the symmetrical distension of abdominal wall or loss of liver dullness is noted after insufflating about 1–4 liters of gas depending upon the patient, suggest adequate pneumoperitoneum. Trocars with cannula are introduced in similar way as Veress needle.

The trocar is removed and telescope is introduced. A systematic inspection of the pelvic organs is carried out (Fig. 27.14). Secondary trocar insertion is done to introduce the accessory instrument (Fig. 27.15). The patient is put in a Trendelenburg position for better visualization of the pelvic organs. The required surgical procedures are carried out. Complete hemostasis should be checked at the end of the procedure. Specimen is removed either by morcellation, or by enlarging the trocar incision or colpotomy incision. At the end the rest of the abdominal cavity is inspected,

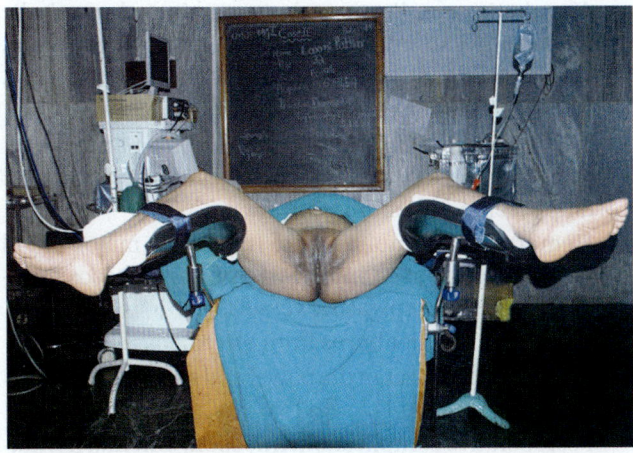

Fig. 27.13: Lithotomy position.

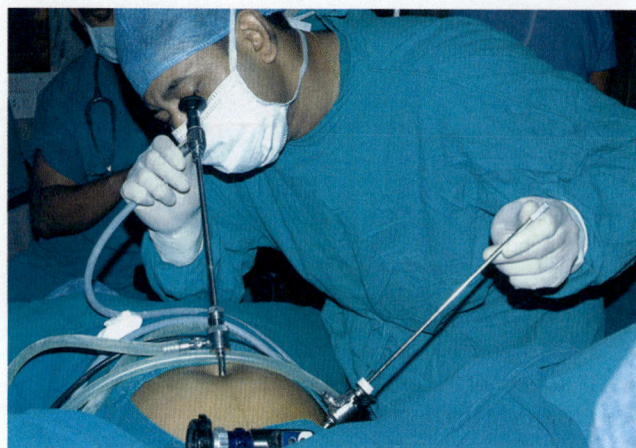

Fig. 27.14: Laparoscopic examination.

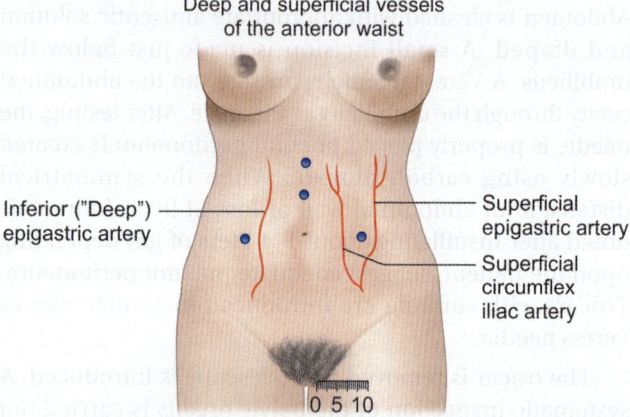

Fig. 27.15: Port site on abdomen.

telescope is retrieved, abdomen is deflated, and cannula removed. The abdominal wound is closed using 1 or 2 sutures.

COMPLICATIONS OF LAPAROSCOPY

- Anesthetic complications; hypercarbia and metabolic acidosis if carbon dioxide is used for peritoneum, cardiac arrhythmias, hypotension, hypoventilation, etc.
- Perforation of the uterus by the manipulator.
- Pneumoperitoneum complications: Pre-peritoneal—leading to surgical emphysema, omental retroperitoneal emphysema, gas embolism, etc.
- Hemorrhagic complications: Injuries to major blood vessels, pelvic or abdominal artery or vein, mesosalpingeal vessels and epigastric vessels.
- Bowel and bladder burns from electrocoagulation.
- Penetrating injuries of the bowel and stomach by Veress or trocar.
- Postoperative complication: Infection, omental herniation.

Advantages of Laparoscopic Surgery Over Conventional Surgery

- Minimally invasive
- Shortened hospital stay
- Less discomfort and quicker postoperative recovery
- Lower-risk of postoperative adhesions
- Smaller scar.

Disadvantages

Depends upon type of case and expertize of the surgeon.
- Operating time may be slightly longer
- High initial cost of the instruments
- Risk of iatrogenic complications.

HYSTEROSCOPY

Introduction

The uterus is an organ with thick muscular walls in apposition with the central triangular virtual uterine cavity lined with an epithelium that bleeds and whose surface constantly changes during the menstrual cycle. Hysteroscopy is a procedure to visualize inside of the uterus. It can be used for diagnostic as well as therapeutic procedures. Hysteroscope is being increasingly used in studying the uterine cavity and in performing intrauterine surgery.

Indications

- Abnormal premenopausal and postmenopausal uterine bleeding.
- Diagnosis and possible transcervical removal of submucus leiomyoma or endometrial polyp (Fig. 27.16).
- Location and retrieval of lost intrauterine contraceptive device.

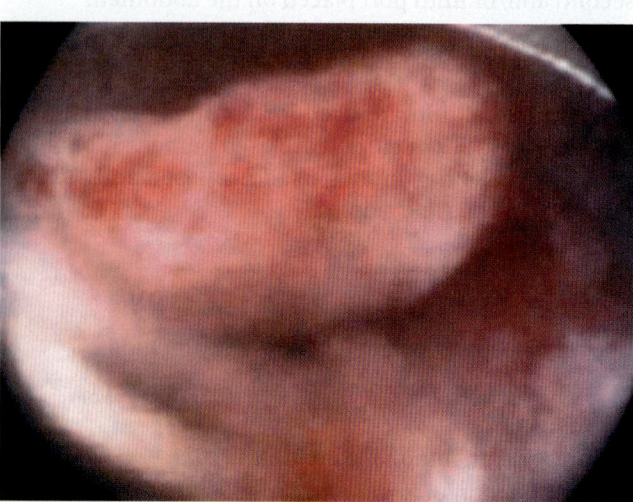

Fig. 27.16: Polyp.

- Evaluation of infertility with abnormal hysterograms.
- Diagnosis and surgical treatment of intrauterine lesion.
- Diagnosis and division of uterine septae (Fig. 27.17).
- Exploration of endocervical canal and uterine cavity in patients with recurrent pregnancy loss.

Instruments in Hysteroscopy (Fig. 27.18)
- Telescope and telescopic sheath
- Camera and light source

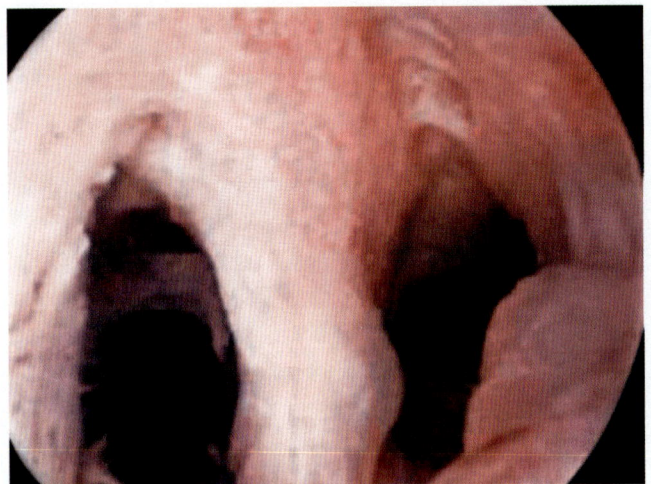

Fig. 27.17: Septum.

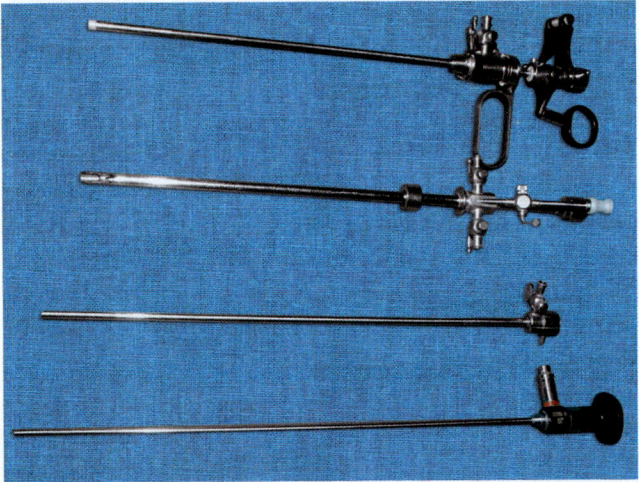

Fig. 27.18: Instruments used in hysteroscopy.

- Distending media—glycine, carbon dioxide, normal saline and mannitol 5%.

Timing of Hysteroscopy
Hysteroscopic procedure should be done in the postmenstrual phase ideally between 7 to 10 days. The endometrium is thin which improved the visualization inside the uterus, bleeding is absent and there is no chance for conception during this part of the menstrual cycle.

Technique
Under anesthesia, patient put on the dorsal lithotomy position, vulva and vagina is cleaned with the appropriate antiseptic solution. The cervix is held with vulsellum/tenaculum. Uterine sound is passed to know the uterocervical length. Dilatation of the internal os is done. Hysteroscope attached with distending media system and light source is introduced into the external cervical os. Insufflation is done to distend the cervical canal and the uterus. By gentle manipulation, the hysteroscopy is advanced slowly, following the small cervical canal to the uterine cavity. Uterine cavity is observed systematically and the findings noted. For operative hysteroscopy, surgery is done as per the needs of the patient.

Complications
- Injury to uterus—perforation
- Pulmonary edema due to fluid overload
- Electrolyte imbalance due to distending media
- Hemorrhage
- Sepsis
- Embolism
- Others: Anesthetic, electrosurgical complications, etc.

Contraindications
- Pregnancy
- Genital tract infection
- Cardiopulmonary disorders
- Severe cervical stenosis
- Heavy uterine bleeding
- Cervical malignancy
- Recent uterine perforation.

REFERENCES
1. Sutton C. A practical approach to surgical laparoscopy. In: Sutton C, Drummond PM (Eds). Endoscopic Surgery for Gynecologists, 2nd edition. London: WB Saunders, 1998;41-53.
2. Redwine DB, Sharpe DR. Laparoscopic segmental resection of the sigmoid colon for endometriosis. J Laparoendosc Surg. 1991;1:217-20.

SECTION 2

Reproductive Endocrinology and Assisted Conception

28. Puberty
29. Disorders of Ovulation
30. Polycystic Ovarian Syndrome
31. Hirsutism
32. Disorders of Sexual Differentiation and Development (Intersex)
33. Infertility
34. Menopause and Hormone Therapy

CHAPTER 28

Puberty

Vani Ramkumar

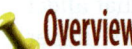 **Overview**

Pubertal Events

The onset of puberty is an evolving sequence of maturational steps. The hypothalamic pituitary gonadal system differentiates and functions during fetal life and early infancy. Thereafter, it is suppressed to low activity levels during childhood by a combination of hypersensitivity of the "gonadostat" to estrogen-negative feedback and an intrinsic CNS inhibitor. At the onset of puberty, GnRH secretion is restored.

The five main physical features of puberty include thelarche, adrenarche, and growth in height, menarche and ovulation. Menarche corresponds to bone age. Psychologic changes are also an important feature.

❑ Follicle stimulating hormone (FSH) and then luteinizing hormone (LH) levels rise moderately before the age of 10 and are followed by a rise in estradiol. An increase in LH pulses is first seen only in sleep but gradually extends throughout the day.

❑ As gonadal estrogen increases (gonadarche), breast development, female fat distribution and vaginal and uterine growth occur. Skeletal growth rapidly increases.

❑ Adrenal androgen (adrenarche) and to a lesser degree, gonadal androgen secretion, cause pubic and axillary hair growth.

❑ At midpuberty, sufficient gonadal estrogen secretion, causes proliferation of the endometrium, and the first menses (menarche) occurs.

❑ Postmenarcheal cycles are initially anovulatory. Sustained, predictable positive LH surge responses to estradiol, with ovulation are late pubertal events.

INTRODUCTION

Adolescence is the span of human growth extending from the immaturity of childhood to the physical and psychological maturity of adulthood. This period extends from 10 to 20 years (WHO, 1977). Puberty marks the beginning of adolescence. During puberty, secondary sexual characteristics appear and mature, adolescent growth spurt takes place, fertility is attained, and significant physical, psychological, and behavioral changes occur, transforming the child into an adult.

In many societies throughout history, puberty has been a time of celebration. Puberty can be a difficult transition for many adolescents, even when it progresses normally, and presents substantially greater challenges when its onset is premature or delayed.

PHYSIOLOGY OF PUBERTY

The hypothalamic-pituitary-ovarian axis is functionally complete during the latter half of fetal life. From 20 weeks, FSH levels are suppressed by the production of estrogen by placenta and fetus. At birth, the fetus is separated from its placenta and therefore the major source of estrogen is removed. Levels of FSH then rise in response to the hypoestrogenic state of the newborn and remain elevated for some 6 to 18 months after birth. During this time, FSH levels are suppressed due to central inhibition of gonadotropin releasing hormone (GnRH), which controls the pituitary production of FSH. The mechanism by which this is achieved remains speculative, but almost certainly is controlled by a gene in the GnRH cell nucleus in the hypothalamus. It is possible that there is a relationship between the production of leptin, a peptide produced by fat cells, and the subsequent control of this gene.

During childhood FSH pulses are almost undetectable, and at around the age of 8 or 9 years a change gradually occurs in the function of the GnRH cell. Levels of FSH and then LH rise moderately before the age of 10 and are followed by a rise in estradiol. An increase in LH pulses is first seen only in sleep but gradually extends throughout the day. In the adult, they occur at roughly 1.5 to 2 hourly intervals. Puberty therefore occurs over a total of 5-10 years.[1]

In general, androgen production and differentiation by the zona reticularis of the adrenal cortex are the initial endocrine changes associated with puberty. Serum concentrations of dehydroepiandrosterone and its sulfate rise between the ages of 8 and 11 years. This rise in adrenal androgens induces the growth of both axillary and pubic hair and is known as adrenarche or pubarche. This increase in adrenal androgen production occurs independent of gonadotropin secretion or gonadal steroid levels, and the mechanism of this initiation is not understood at this time. Recent studies indicate that girls who undergo premature pubarche are more likely to develop polycystic ovarian syndrome as adults.

FACTORS INFLUENCING PUBERTY

Hormonally, puberty involves a change from negative feedback to the establishment of circadian rhythm and positive feedback controls that result in monthly cycles and fertility. Three elements must be present for puberty to progress normally: adequate body mass, adequate sleep, and exposure to light. These factors appear to facilitate or allow the complex hypothalamic, pituitary and ovarian changes that must occur (Box 28.1).

The major determinant of the timing of the onset of puberty is no doubt genetic, but a number of other factors appear to influence both the age at onset and the progression of pubertal development. Among these influences are nutritional state, general health, geographic location, exposure to light and psychological state. The age of menarche is earlier than average in children with moderate obesity and delayed menarche is common in severe malnutrition. Children who live in urban settings, closer to the equator, and at lower altitudes typically begin puberty earlier than those who live in rural areas, farther from the equator and at higher elevations. Other risk factors implicated for precocious puberty include exposure to estrogenic endocrine-disrupting chemicals and the absence of a father in the home. Blind girls apparently undergo an earlier menarche, suggesting some influence of light.

Box 28.1: Factors influencing puberty.

1. Heredity
2. Social class
3. Nutrition
4. Physical and emotional stress
5. Body weight
6. Race and country

Girls of higher socioeconomic status attain menarche earlier. Frisch hypothesized that weight, or more precisely total body fat, plays a critical role in the onset of menses. The girl should attain a critical body weight (47.8 kg) to achieve menarche.[2,3] Indeed a shift in body composition to a greater percent fat (from 16% in the prepubertal state to 23.5%) is required to achieve menarche. Anorexia nervosa is associated with pubertal arrest or delay and is seen in girls from developed nations. Physical illness like diabetes mellitus, inflammatory bowel disease and chronic renal failure can cause pubertal delay. The hypothesis linking menarche to body weight and composition does not always seem valid because menarche is a late event in pubertal development.

Excessive exercise delays puberty due to a change in endogenous opioid peptides. Other factors that affect onset of pubertal hormonal maturation include, hyper or hypothyroid states; growth hormone deficiency and increased sex steroid secretion as occurs in pseudosexual precocity and the congenital adrenal hyperplasias. Thyroid hormone plays a key role in growth and development as illustrated in severe childhood hypothyroidism, which results in a dramatic decrease in the velocity of growth.[4] These effects can be monitored by skeletal age. Onset of puberty in females occurs when bone age is 10.5 to 11 years, whether or not this coincides with chronologic age. Menarche occurs in the average girl at a bone age of about 13 years.

DEFINITIONS

- Adrenarche is the activation of the adrenal cortex for the production of adrenal androgens, and typically occurs before the onset of puberty.
- Gonadarche is the activation of the gonads by FSH and LH.
- Thelarche is the appearance of breast tissue.
- Pubarche is the appearance of pubic hair.
- Menarche is the age of onset of the first menstrual period.
- Spermarche in boys is the age at first ejaculation (heralded by nocturnal sperm emissions and appearance of sperm in the urine).
- Precocious puberty refers to the development of any sign of secondary sexual maturation at an age earlier than 2.5 SD less than the expected age of pubertal onset. In North America, these ages are 8 years for girls and 9 years for boys.
- Delayed puberty exists in girls who fail to develop any secondary sex characteristics by age 13, have not had menarche by age 15 (95th percentile is 14.5 years), or have not attained menarche 5 or more years since the onset of pubertal development.

PHYSICAL CHANGES OF PUBERTY

The changes associated with puberty occur in an orderly sequence over a definite time frame. In girls, pubertal development typically takes place over 4.5 years. The first sign of puberty is accelerated growth, and breast budding is usually the first recognized pubertal change, followed by the appearance of pubic hair, peak growth velocity and menarche. The stages initially described by Marhall and Tanner (1969) are often used to describe breast and pubic hair development.

Breast Development (Thelarche)

Stage 1. Prepubertal, no palpable breast tissue.
Stage 2. Breast and papilla elevated in a small mound, diameter of areola increases.
Stage 3. Breast and areola are further enlarged (small adult breast).
Stage 4. Areola and papilla further enlarge to form a secondary mound.
Stage 5. Secondary mound disappears. Smooth rounded contour; (recession of the areola to match the contour of the breast; the papilla projects beyond the contour of the areola and breast).

Pubic Hair Development (Pubarche)

Stage 1. Prepubertal, no pubic hair.
Stage 2. Sparse growth of long, slightly pigmented hair on labia majora or mons pubis.
Stage 3. An increase in the amount of hair, spread sparsely over the mons pubis, it is considerably darker, coarser and more curly than in Stage 2.
Stage 4. Hair is adult in character but covers a smaller area than in most adults.
Stage 5. Hair is distributed in an inverse triangular pattern, with some spread to the medial surface of the thighs, characteristic of an adult female.

Axillary Hair Development

Stage 1. Prepubertal, no hair.
Stage 2. Intermediate development.
Stage 3. Full development.

Timing and Sequence of Pubertal Phenotypic Changes

Phenotypic changes of puberty begin with acceleration of growth velocity. This somatic landmark is followed by the first visible change in sexual development, thelarche. The appearance of a breast bud occurs between the ages of 9 and 11. It represents the first clinical sign of ovarian estradiol release. It is the initial test of competency of the hypothalamic pituitary ovarian circuit. Adrenarche as evidenced by the initial growth of pubic hair occurs shortly after appearance of the breast bud. In the majority of adolescents, pubarche closely follows thelarche, but in a substantial minority the sequence is reversed and pubarche precedes thelarche. In some instances menstruation occurs prior to axillary hair formation. The appearance of pubic hair shows that the hypothalamus-pituitary-adrenal axis is also intact. Appearance of axillary hair usually follows pubarche by approximately 2 years. Menarche occurs, on average, 2.6 years after the onset of puberty.

The initial growth acceleration in height of approximately 4 cm per year (due to sex steroid induced increase in growth hormone secretion) continues through the early stages of sexual development. An additional increment of 5 cm per year is added to this height velocity during the adolescent growth spurt. This peak velocity of 9 cm per year, occurring at approximately ages 11 to 12, is caused by the production of ovarian steroids. It is an important developmental landmark of puberty. Once the maximum speed of adolescent growth has been attained and the adolescent female begins her deceleration of growth velocity, menarche heralds the closing stage of puberty. The first menses occurs between chronologic ages 11 and 15 for American girls, with a mean age of 12.8 years. With the continued production of ovarian steroids, epiphyses continue to close and growth velocity slows further. As a result, it is rare for the adolescent to grow more than 6 cm in height following her first menses.

Menarche is not the final event of puberty. Rather, it marks the beginning of the last stage of pubertal development. The most important aspect of this entire process is the continued stimulation of ovarian follicles, which eventually results in the maturation of a positive feedback system to the hypothalamus and in ovulation. It takes approximately 20 cycles before this last important function of the ovary begins on a regular basis. The teleological purpose of puberty is to produce an individual capable of reproduction for recapitulation of the species. These events occur at the given chronological ages, which are equal to physiological or bone age (Table 28.1).

Table 28.1: Physical and physiological landmarks of puberty.

Features	Age in years
Breast bud, enlargement of labia minora and physiological vaginal discharge	9–11
Pubic hair	11–12
Growth spurt (peak height velocity of 9 cm per year)	12
Areolar pigmentation, further development of breast and axillary hair	12–13
Menarche	13.5 (9–17)

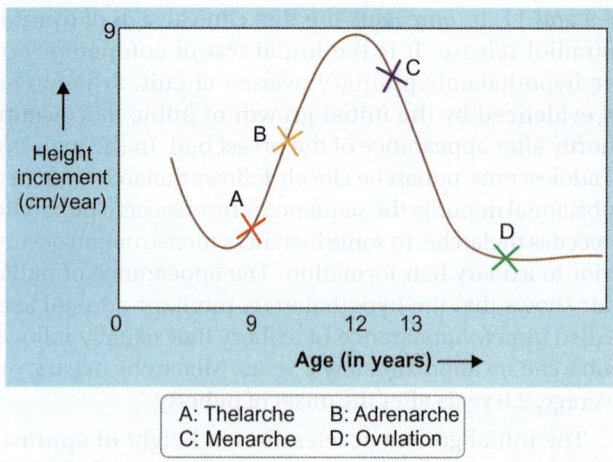

Fig. 28.1: Pubertal development chart showing landmarks of the normal pubertal process, superimposed upon growth velocity.

By plotting height velocity against physiological or bone age, normal pubertal landmarks can be properly anticipated. Figure 28.1 summarizes the developmental landmarks of puberty in the form of a pubertal developmental chart. Thelarche and pubarche are shown to appear during the early growth acceleration. Menarche follows the ensuing peak height velocity, and ovulation begins when epiphyses continue to close and growth slows towards a halt. In the female with pubertal aberrations, genetic, environmental or systemic processes violate this normal temporal relationship of pubertal events. In these patients, bone age (e.g. physiological age) often deviates from chronological age. Pubertal development charts in these individuals often identify these discrepancies. These charts serve as aids for diagnosis and allow therapeutic efforts to be monitored.

The bone or skeletal age of any individual can be estimated closely by comparing X-rays documenting the development of bones in the nondominant hand (most commonly), knee or elbow to standards of maturation in the normal population. The Greulich and Pyle Atlas is one of the most frequently used methods for the assessment of skeletal age around the world.

Boys reach peak height velocity about 2 years later than girls. Boys grow an average of 28 cm during the growth spurt, in comparison to a mean 25 cm for girls. Adult men eventually are an average of 13 cm taller than adult women because they are taller at onset of the growth spurt.

PUBERTY IN BOYS

The earliest stage of male maturation, which has a mean duration of 6 months, is an increase in testicular volume. Almost all boys have an increase in testicular volume (≥ 3 mL) prior to the appearance of penile growth and pubic hair. The appearance of sperm in the urine and the onset of nocturnal sperm emissions occur shortly after the attainment of peak height velocity; many consider these events the male equivalent of menarche.

PSYCHOLOGIC CHANGES OF PUBERTY

The adolescent phase of psychological maturation is a crucial and complex step in a process that continues throughout life. If later psychologic maturation is to proceed, the person must successfully resolve and complete the identity versus role confusion that is an issue in adolescence.[5]

The major characteristics of early adolescent period (12–14 years) include: (1) rebellion, (2) preoccupation with one's body and self, (3) the vital importance of peer group, (4) marked increase in emotional and intellectual capacity and (5) experimentation. The years 15–17 (middle adolescence) is thought to be a period of settling down. The paradox is that this period is usually one in which the teenager most adamantly rebels against parental values. Substance abuse is common. Late adolescence begins at 17 and lasts through the resolution of adolescent struggles. This is a phase of identity formation.

Erikson suggests that we look at adolescence not as a highly disorganized time of turmoil but as a crisis that is a normal phase. Anna Freud has rightly defined it. "It is normal for an adolescent to behave in an inconsistent and unpredictable manner; to deny her impulses and to accept them; to love her parents and to hate them; to be deeply ashamed to acknowledge her mother before others and, unexpectedly, to desire heart to heart talks with her; to thrive on imitation of and identification with others while searching unceasingly for her own identity; to be more idealistic, artistic, generous, and unselfish than she will ever be again, but also the opposite: self-centered, egoistic and calculating. Such fluctuations between extreme opposites would be deemed highly abnormal at any other time of life. At this time, they may signify no more than that an adult structure of personality takes a long time to emerge, that the ego of the individual in question does not cease to experiment and is in no hurry to close down on possibilities."

Those girls who begin menstruating either much earlier or much later than their peers experience stress. Identification with the peer group is important, and girls who are out of step with the group show an increase in anxiety.[5]

PROBLEMS ASSOCIATED WITH ADOLESCENCE

1. Delayed sexual maturation
2. Intersex
3. Abnormal uterine bleeding
4. Dysmenorrhea

5. Pelvic pain
6. Androgens in the adolescent: Hirsutism, obesity and acne
7. Sexually transmitted diseases
8. Contraception
9. Teenage pregnancy
10. Tumors.

RECENT TRENDS

Obesity is the most important predictor of metabolic syndrome. The incidence of obesity is increasing both in childhood and adolescence. Abdominal obesity induces secretion of various cytokines in polycystic ovarian syndrome.[6] A diet low in fat and high in fruits and vegetables along with moderate intensity exercise are recommended for obese adolescents.

Sex education is useful in schools. The risk of pregnancy, sexually transmitted diseases and human immunodeficiency virus should be emphasized and girls guided in personal hygiene.

CONCLUSION

Normal pubertal development occurs in a predictable orderly sequence over a definite time frame. Puberty is the period during which secondary sexual characteristics develop and the capability of sexual reproduction is attained. Hypothalamic maturation with stimulation of sex organs and secretion of sex steroids makes puberty possible. Whereas growth and development of secondary sexual characteristics are the most visible manifestations of the onset of puberty, changes in body composition and cognitive development are no less significant.

The typical "diphasic" pattern of gonadotropin secretion from infancy to puberty results primarily from changing levels of central inhibition of pulsatile GnRH secretion, and to a lesser extent, from high sensitivity to low levels of gonadal steroid feedback.

Kisspeptins are neuropeptides (encoded by the KISS1 gene) that signal via the G-protein coupled receptor, GPR54 (encoded by the KISS1R gene). Kisspeptin signalling via GPR54 might play a major role in the resurgence of pulsatile GnRH secretion at puberty in primates. Leptin is produced by adipocytes and serum concentrations are strongly associated with body fat and changes in body fat content. Leptin plays an important, but only permissive, role in the onset of puberty.

Historically, the trend to an earlier onset of sexual development has been attributed to improved nutrition and less stressful living conditions.

REFERENCES

1. Fritz MA, Speroff L. Clinical gynecologic endocrinology and infertility, 8th edition. Philadelphia: Lippincott Williams and Wilkins, 2011;391-408.
2. Pisarska MD, Alexander CJ, Azziz R, Buyalos Jr RP. Puberty and disorders of pubertal development. In: Hacker NF, Gambone JC, Hobel CJ (Eds): Hacker and Moore's Essentials of Obstetrics and Gynecology, 5th edn. New Delhi: Elsevier, 2010;345.
3. Rebar RW, Paupoo AAV. Puberty. In: Berek JS (Ed). Berek and Novak's Gynecology, 15th edition. Baltimore: Lippincott Williams and Wilkins, 2012;993.
4. Edmonds KD. Dewhurst's Textbook of Obstetrics and Gynaecology, 8th edn. London: Wiley-Blackwell, 2012;472.
5. Lavery JP, Sanfilippo JS. Pediatric and Adolescent Obstetrics and Gynecology. New York: Springer Verlag, 1985.
6. Cirik DA, Dilbaz B. Review: what do we know about metabolic syndrome in adolescents? J Turk Ger Gynecol Assoc. 2014; 1:15(1):49-55.

CHAPTER 29

Disorders of Ovulation

Nuguelis Razali

Overview

- Ovulatory disorder and subsequent infertility is a common gynecology problem. Women with ovulatory disorders commonly present with menstrual disorders such as amenorrhea and irregular, infrequent periods.
- The causes of ovulatory disorders can be categorized into three main categories depending on the site of the lesion and the gonadotropin levels.
- Hypothalamic disorder (hypogonadotrophic hypogonadism) is caused by any lesion affecting the pituitary or hypothalamus and results in inadequate or absent gonadotropin secretion.
- Polycystic ovarian syndrome (PCOS) is a common problem among women of the reproductive age group and contributes to 80–90% of anovulatory infertility. It is characterized by chronic anovulation, clinical and biochemical hyperandrogenism and polycystic ovaries.
- Premature ovarian failure is a rare disorder and is most commonly idiopathic. Identifiable causes include genetic disorder such as Turner's syndrome (XO), autoimmnune disorders, previous chemotherapy or radiotherapy.
- Hyperprolactinemia is the commonest endocrine cause of anovulation and can be effectively treated with dopamine agonist such as bromocriptine and cabergoline.
- Ovulation in patients with PCOS can be successfully achieved medically with clomiphene citrate, letrozole and gonadotropins or surgically with laparoscopic ovarian drilling.

INTRODUCTION

Ovulation, which is the physical release of the oocyte and its cumulus mass of granulosa cells is a crucial step in fertilization. Ovarian follicle development, steroid hormones production and subsequently ovulation are tightly regulated by interplay of hormones from the hypothalamus, anterior pituitary and ovary (HPA axis) and the feedback mechanisms. Therefore, any problems arising from the hypothalamus, pituitary or ovary will cause disruption of this important hormonal axis and lead to menstrual cycle abnormalities and anovulation.

Ovulatory disorders which includes anovulation and oligo-ovulation contribute to about 21% of female infertility.[1] Apart from infertility, it usually presents in menstrual disorders such as amenorrhea and oligomenorrhoea. Regular menstrual cycles of 26–36 days are usually ovulatory, with only 10% of regular menstrual cycles being anovulatory.[2]

CLASSIFICATION

The World Health Organization (WHO) in 1997 has categorized the causes of anovulation into three main categories based on the site of the lesion and the gonadotropin profile.[3]

Group 1 Hypothalamic Pituitary Failure (Hypothalamic amenorrhea or hypogonadotropic hypogonadism)

This group of disorders is caused by any lesion affecting the pituitary or hypothalamus and subsequently causing inadequate or absent gonadotropin release. It is characterized by low gonadotropins, normal prolactin and low oestrogen, and it accounts for about 10% of ovulatory disorders. The low gonadotropin production results in impaired ovarian follicular development and consequently hypo-oestrogenic amenorrhea. The causes for these disorders include:

CHAPTER 29 Disorders of Ovulation

- Idiopathic hypogonadotropic hypogonadism
- Kallmann's syndrome (isolated gonadotropin deficiency and anosmia)
- Functional hypothalamic dysfunction (e.g. excessive weight loss such as in anorexia nervosa, exercise, stress, drugs, iatrogenic)
- Pituitary tumor, pituitary infarct (e.g. Sheehan's syndrome).

Group 2 Hypothalamic Pituitary Dysfunction (Normogonadotropic anovulation)

This group is characterized by gonadotropin disorder and normal estrogen. It accounts for about 85% of ovulatory disorders. Thus, it is the commonest cause of anovulation with 80–90% due to polycystic ovarian syndrome (PCOS).[4] PCOS is one of the most common endocrine disorders, affecting 6–10% of women of the reproductive age group.[5] It is a syndrome including multiple features such menstrual cycle irregularities due to anovulation (60–75%), signs of androgen excess, including hirsutism (65–75%), persistent acne (20–40%) and androgenic alopecia (10%), hyperandrogenemia (70% with elevated free testosterone level) and polycystic ovaries on ultrasound (75–90%).[6]

The etiology of PCOS remains unclear but there is good evidence for a major genetic predisposition to the syndrome.[7] According to the Rotterdam international consensus, the diagnosis of PCOS requires the presence at least two of the following three criteria:

- Oligo- and/or anovulation
- Clinical and/or biochemical hyperandrogenism
- Polycystic ovaries (the presence of at least 12 follicles measuring 2–9 mm in diameter and/or an ovarian volume in excess of 10 cm^3), with the exclusion of other causes of menstrual disturbances and hyperandrogenism.[8] Testosterone is the most frequently measured androgen in diagnosing hyperandrogenism or elevated circulating endogenous testosterone. It is possibly the most important androgen in women. Testosterone (T) is bound to sex hormone binding globulin (SHBG) and other proteins such as albumin in the circulation and only the free or unbound fraction will enter the target tissues. Therefore, free T levels are more sensitive in diagnosing hyperandrogenism compared to total testosterone. Measurement of free T is however limited by highly variable inter and intra laboratory assay. This can be overcome by concomitant measurement of SHBG and free T or free androgen index (FAI) can be calculated from total T and SHBG. Measurements of basal gonadotropin and the reversed ratio of luteinizing hormone (LH) to follicle-stimulating hormone (FSH) are of little value for the routine diagnosis of PCOS.[6]

There is a lot of data available now concerning the long-term health implications of PCOS. Women with a history of PCOS have a higher risk of endometrial cancer and Type 2 diabetes (increased 3–4-fold) women in the general population. Cardiovascular risk markers are also more common in women with PCOS. Management of these anovulatory women should extend beyond induction of ovulation with lifelong screening with respect to long-term health.[9]

Group 3 Hypergonadotropic Hypogonadism (Ovarian Failure)

Women in this group will be amenorrheic, with elevated levels of FSH and LH (hypergonadotropic hypogonadism) and no (or low) endogenous estrogen. The causes for ovarian failure could be due to genetic (e.g. Turner's syndrome), autoimmune disease, infection of the ovaries (e.g. mumps oophoritis), iatrogenic (e.g. surgical menopause, post-radiotherapy or chemotherapy) and most commonly idiopathic.

Other causes of anovulation are endocrine disorders such as hyperprolactinemia, thyroid dysfunction, other conditions of hyperandrogenemia such as congenital adrenal hyperplasia and androgen-secreting adrenal and ovarian tumors. Among these, hyperprolactinemia is the commonest.

Hyperprolactinemia

Hyperprolactinemia contributes to 5% of anovulatory infertility and is also noted in 20% of patients with menstrual disturbances.[10] Prolactin is secreted by the anterior pituitary gland and is controlled by negative inhibition by dopamine on the hypothalamus. Elevated prolactin level interferes with the pulsatile secretion of GnRH and consequently ovarian function and ovulation.

Hyperprolactinemia is associated with a pituitary tumor (mainly adenoma) in 30–50% of patients.[11] The tumors are divided into macro- (≥10 mm) and micro (<10 mm) adenomas. In others, there is no evidence of a space occupying lesion. The pathological causes of hyperprolactinemia are summarized in Box 29.1.

Box 29.1: Pathological causes of hyperprolactinemia.

1. Prolactin secreting adenoma
2. Other pituitary tumors that block the inhibitory signal of the hypothamus
3. Primary hypothyroidism
4. Drugs such as estrogens (oral contraceptive pills), dopamine-depleting agents (reserpine, methyldopa) and dopamine receptor blocking agents (phenothiazines, metoclopramide).
5. Chronic renal failure

HISTORY

Detailed menstrual, medical, surgical and drug history should be elicited. Other associated symptoms such as symptoms suggestive of hyperprolactinemia (e.g. galactorrhea, headache, visual disturbances), thyroid disturbances and climacteric symptoms should also be taken. Patients with PCOS and other causes of androgen excess might present with hirsutism, increased acne, and male pattern baldness. Other important history to note would be any recent weight changes, diet, stress and exercise patterns. During physical examination, chromosomal abnormalities, secondary sexual characteristics, body mass index, signs of androgen excess, galactorhea, and goiter should be noted.

INVESTIGATIONS

The recommended investigation to confirm ovulation in a regularly menstruating woman is mid-luteal phase serum progesterone and level of 30 nmol/L or above confirms ovulation occurred. Progesterone is secreted by the corpus luteum formed after ovulation and the level will peak at the mid-luteal phase (a week before the expected period). The timing for this test need to be accurate and the accuracy can be assessed by noting the menstrual date after the blood test.

For women with irregular menstruation, a more detailed hormonal profile should be taken. This will include measurement of FSH, LH, prolactin (PRL), testosterone (T), thyroid-Stimulating hormones (TSH) and sex hormone binding globulin (SHBG) if suspicious of PCOS. Other tests such as 17-hydroxyprogesterone measurement must be done in patients with markedly elevated testosterone levels or signs of marked hirsutism and virilization to exclude late-onset congenital adrenal hyperplasia and an overnight dexamethasone suppression test to exclude Cushing's syndrome.

Pelvic ultrasonography is required to look for polycystic ovaries in patients with PCOS (Fig. 29.1) and to confirm the presence of genital organs in patients with primary ovarian failure. Imaging studies such as CT scan of the skull might be required in cases of hyperprolactinemia (Figs. 29.2A and B) and the adrenals in cases of suspected adrenal tumors.

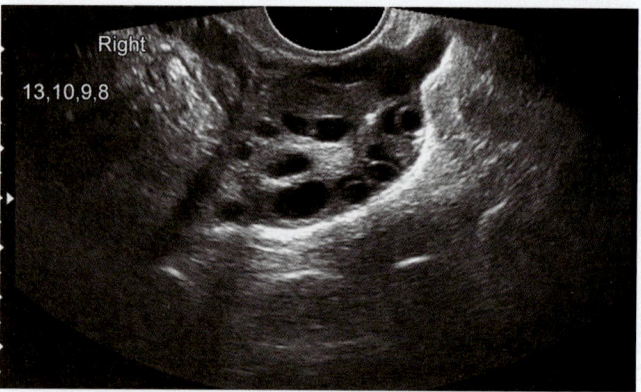

Fig. 29.1: Transvaginal ultrasound of a polycystic ovary.

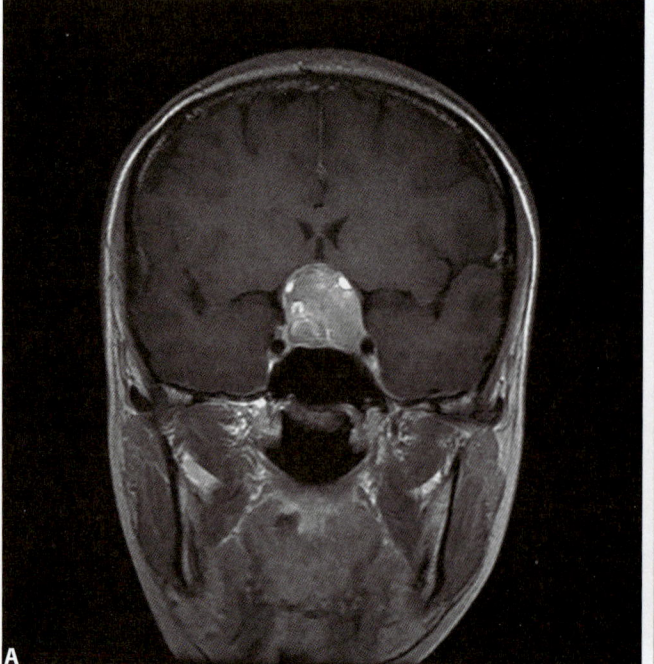
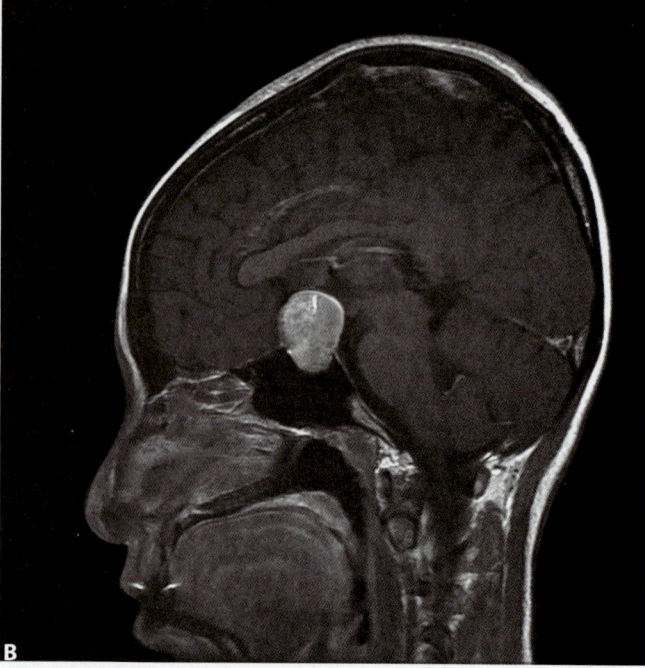

Figs. 29.2A and B: CT scan showing pituitary macroadenoma. Note the well-defined heterogenously enhancing sellar mass extending superiorly and compressing the optic chiasm. This mass measures 2.9 cm (H) x 2.4 cm (AP) x 2.7 cm (WT).

MANAGEMENT

WHO Group 1 (Hypogonadotropic hypogonadism)

Treatment for this group of patients should initially address the underlying cause. For example, weight optimization for patients with severe weight loss or those with anorexia nervosa and surgery for patients with intracranial tumor.

However, even after they have regained their ideal body weight many women remain amenorrheic for several months.[12] Ovulation can be successfully induced in these women and those with no obvious cause for hypothalamic dysfunction by pulsatile gonadotropin-releasing hormone therapy (GnRH) administered subcutaneously by an infusion pump. The injections are given at intervals of 90 minutes at a dose of 15 mg. Gonadotropin injection containing both FSH and LH (human menopausal gonadotropin as opposed to purified recombinant follicular-stimulating hormone) is the alternative for this purpose.

WHO Group 2 (Normogonadotropic anovulation)

Management for this group which mainly consists of patients with PCOS is ovulation induction (which will be discussed in detail later). Patients with other causes of androgen excess should be managed accordingly. Lifestyle management targeting weight loss in overweight and obese patients with PCOS should include both reduced dietary (caloric) intake and exercise, and should be the first-line therapy for all women with PCOS. Modest reduction in body weight (5–10%) is often sufficient to restore ovulation and decrease markers for metabolic disease. Response to ovulation induction agents and pregnancy rates are also improved by weight reduction.

WHO Group 3 (Hypogonadotropic hypogonadism)

Patients in this group generally will not respond to any form of ovulation induction and thus, should be counseled for assisted reproduction using donor eggs.

Hyperprolactinemia

Dopamine agonist (bromocriptine and cabergoline) is the first line treatment for anovulatory women with elevated prolactin levels. It effectively reduces prolactin level and shrink pituitary adenoma. The dose for bromocriptine is 2.5–20 mg daily in two to three divided doses. Cabergoline has a longer half-life that bromocriptine and thus is given once or twice weekly.

Treatment with dopamine agonist results in ovulation in 90% of women with anovulation due to hyperprolactinemia.

It is also effective in regulating menstrual cycles, suppressing galactorhea and achieving pregnancy. For women who failed to ovulate despite normalization of prolactin level, other ovulation induction agents such as antiestrogen and gonadotropins can be added to the dopamine agonist.

Side effects of bromocriptine are nausea, vomiting, abdominal cramps, vertigo, postural hypotension, headaches and drowsiness. These side effects may be minimized by taking medication before bedtime in a smaller dose and gradually increase to the required dosage. The response to treatment can be monitored by measuring serum prolactin level and observing menstrual patterns. Treatment with dopamine agonist maybe discontinued once the patient is pregnant with no further monitoring required if she has microprolactinemia or idiopathic hyperprolactinemia as the likelihood of significant tumor expansion is very small (less than 2%). Patient with a macroprolactinoma will need to continue treatment as the tumor has a 25% risk of expanding during pregnancy.[10]

Women with macroadenoma should conceive after their serum prolactin has normalized and tumor volume has significantly reduced. This is to reduce the neurological risk of optic chiasm compression during pregnancy.[11] These women should be jointly managed with the neurosurgeon. Surgery such as transphenoidal pituitary adenectomy and rarely radiotherapy might be indicated if medical treatment fails to shrink a macroadenoma.

OVULATION INDUCTION

Ovulation induction is mainly achieved by medical treatment. Surgery such as laparoscopic ovarian drilling can be considered in a selective group of patients. It is important to rule out other causes of infertility such as male factor and tubal factors before commencing on ovulation induction agents (Flowchart 29.1).

Medical Induction of Ovulation

Clomiphene Citrate

Clomiphene citrate (CC) is a commonly used selective estrogen receptor modulator in the treatment of WHO group II anovulation. It occupies the estrogen receptors in the hypothalamic-pituitary axis thus blocking the negative feedback effect of the circulating estrogens and leads to increased secretion of endogenous gonadotropin releasing hormone. The resultant increases in gonadotropins stimulate the growth of ovarian follicles and induces ovulation.

Clomiphene citrate is administered on day three to five of a menstrual cycle following spontaneous or induced withdrawal bleed. The initial daily dose is 50 mg for 5 days, increasing to the recommended maximum daily dose of 150 mg if patient remains anovulatory. Mid-luteal phase

SECTION 2: Reproductive Endocrinology and Assisted Conception

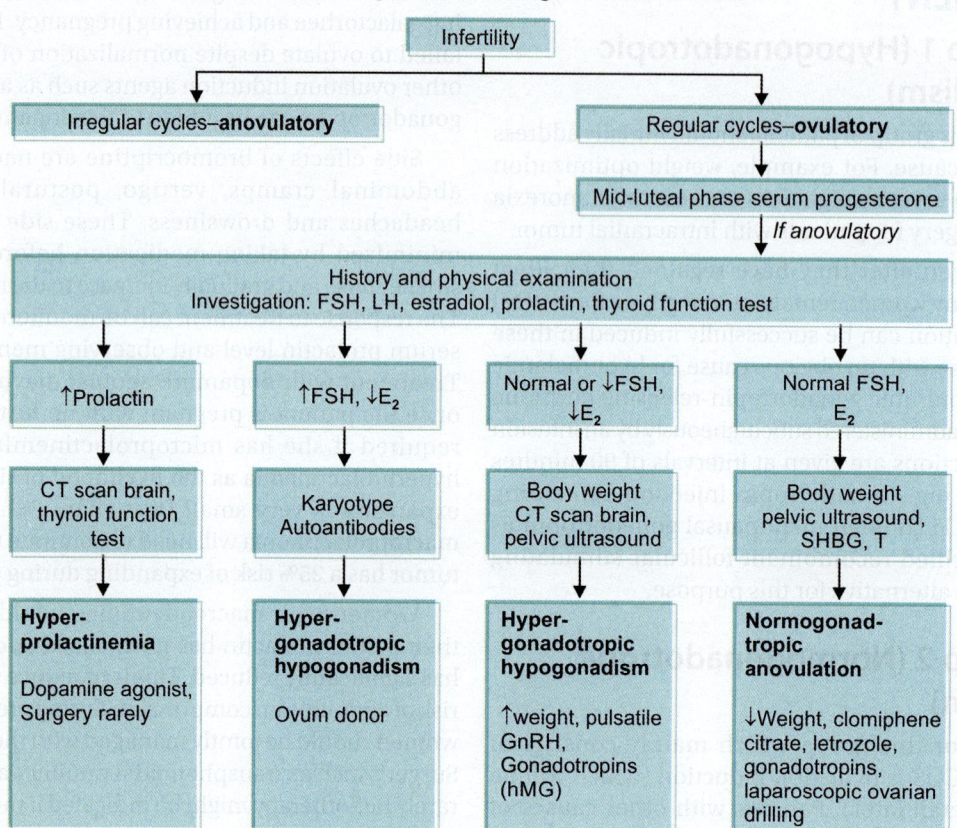

Flowchart 29.1: Diagnosis and management of anovulation.[18]

(FSH: follicle stimulating hormone; CT: computerized tomography; hMG: human menopausal gonadotropin; GnRH: gonadotropin-releasing hormone; E2: estradiol; LH: luteinizing hormone; SHBG: sex hormone-binding globulin; T: testosterone)

progesterone level should be checked during the first cycle to assess ovulation. Patients who failed to ovulate with CC at doses of 150 mg/day are considered to be CC resistant and should be offered second line treatment with gonadotropin or laparoscopic ovarian drilling. Majority of patients will conceive in the first 3 months, therefore other treatments such as above should be considered in those who do not conceive after 6 months of therapy.

Treatment with clomiphene citrate has been shown to result in an ovulation rate of 60–85% and a pregnancy rate of 30–50% after six ovulatory cycles, with an increased risk of multiple pregnancy (5–7%).[12] Side effects of CC include hot flushes, breast discomfort, abdominal distension, nausea, vomiting, nervousness, mood swing, dizziness, hair loss and disturbed vision. These side effects are however, transient.

Letrozole

Letrozole, an aromatase inhibitor (AI) is an alternative to clomiphene citrate. It suppresses estrogen production by blocking the action of aromatase, an enzyme that converts androgens to estrogens. The hypothalamus will be released from the negative feedback effect of estrogens and this leads to an increased secretion of FSH.[13]

Letrozole is given in a dose of 2.5–5 mg/day for 5 days starting on days 2–5 of the cycle, similar to clomiphene citrate.[9] There was no significant difference noted between letrozole and CC in the ovulation rate and pregnancy rate in a meta-analysis. However, letrozole has a shorter half-life than CC that leads to preservation of the central nervous system. It therefore, has the advantage of producing monofollicular development rather than multifollicular.[13] It should be noted that letrozole is not licensed for treatment of infertility. Concerns regarding the potential teratogenic effect of letrozole for infertility treatment such as higher risk of congenital cardiac and bone malformations in newborns have been raised.[14] but two subsequent publications did not find an increased risk of fetal anomaly.[15,16]

Gonadotropins

Exogenous gonadotropin is used to overcome the FSH threshold required for follicular development. Gonadotropins are used as a second line treatment in patients with CC resistance or for those who fail to conceive despite ovulating with CC for 6 cycles.

Serious complications of gonadotropin treatment are ovarian hyperstimulation syndrome and multiple pregnancies due to multifollicular development.

Patients with PCOS who are given gonadotropins have a higher risk of ovarian hyperstimulation syndrome because they have an increased FSH threshold that is the critical "threshold" level needed for to stimulate follicle recruitment. Secondly, they also have an increased sensitivity to exogenous gonadotropins. Gentle stimulation regimen such as a low dose step up regimen is recommended and follicular development must be monitored with serial ultrasound scan to minimize this risk. The cumulative ovulation rates are as high as 90%, with pregnancy rates of 50–70%, multiple pregnancy rates up to 15% and OHSS 2% with the low dose regimens.[17]

Surgical Induction of Ovulation

Laparoscopic Ovarian Drilling

Ovarian drilling is an alternative second line treatment for patients with CC resistance or failure.

Historically, the procedure follows on from the earliest surgical procedure to induce ovulation in women with PCOS involving laparotomy and wedge resection of the ovary. However, laparotomy and bilateral ovarian wedge resection is associated with a higher risk of postoperative adhesion formation. This procedure has now been abandoned and laparoscopic ovarian drilling (LOD) is the preferred surgical method of ovulation induction. During laparoscopy, multiple ovarian punctures (7–8 mm depth) using monopolar diathermy are performed. Alternatively, laparoscopic laser delivery systems can be used. The exact mechanism of action is unknown but it is believed to be due to destruction of androgen-producing tissue in the ovary. LOD usually results in ovulatory cycles in around 50% of women, and the rest of the women will require additional ovulation-induction agents to ovulate. LOD has several advantages when compared to gonadotropins such as:

1. Less costly
2. It enables laparoscopic tubal and pelvic assessment
3. Achieve monofollicular ovulation without the need for intensive monitoring.

However, there is still risk associated with general anaesthesia and surgery involved with possibility of adhesion formation and damage to ovarian reserve.

REFERENCES

1. Hull MG, Glazener CM, Kelly NJ, Conway DI, Foster PA, Hinton RA, et al. Population study of causes, treatment, and outcome of infertility. BMJ. 1985; 291:1693-7.
2. Collins JA. Diagnostic Assessment of the infertile female partner. Curr Probl Obstet Gynecol Fertil. 1988;11:6-42.
3. Rowe PJ, Comhaire FH, Hargreave TB, Mellows HJ. WHO manual for the standardized investigation and diagnosis of the infertile couple. Cambridge: Cambridge University Press; 1997.
4. Morin-Papunen L, Rantala AS, Unkila-Kallio L, et al. Metformin improves pregnancy and live-birth rates in women with polycystic ovary syndrome (PCOS): a multicenter, double-blind, placebo-controlled randomized trial. J Clin Endocrinol Metab. 2012;97:1492-500.
5. Diamanti-Kandarakis E, Kouli CR, Bergiele AT, et al. A survey of the polycystic ovary syndrome in the Greek island of Lesbos: hormonal and metabolic profile. J Clin Endocrinol Metab. 1999;84:4006-11.
6. The Androgen Excess and PCOS Society criteria for the polycystic ovary syndrome: the complete task force report. Azziz R, Carmina E, Dewailly D, Diamanti-Kandarakis E, Escobar-Morreale HF, Janssen OE, et al. Fertility and Sterility. 2009;91:(2);456-88.
7. Escobar-Morreale HF, Luque-Ramirez M, San Millan JL. The molecular-genetic basis of functional hyperandrogenism and the polycystic ovary syndrome. Endocr Rev. 2005a;26:251-82.
8. The Rotterdam ESHRE/ASRM-sponsored PCOS consensus workshop group. Revised 2003 consensus on diagnostic criteria and long-term health risks related to polycystic ovary syndrome (PCOS). Hum Reprod. 2004;19;41-7.
9. ESHRE Capri Workshop Group. Health and fertility in World Health Organization group 2 anovulatory women. Hum Reprod Update. 2012;18(5):586-99.
10. Balen A. Ovulation Induction. Current Obstetrics & Gynaecology. 2004;14:261-8.
11. Sharif K, Afnan M. Ovarian function and ovulation induction. Gynaecology (2nd ed). 1997;223-46.
12. ESHRE Capri Workshop Group. Nutrition and reproduction in women. Hum Reprod Update. 2006;12:193-207.
13. Requena A, Herrero J, Landeras J et al. Use of Letrozole in assisted reproduction: a systematic review and meta-analysis. Hum Reprod Update. 2008:14;571-82.
14. Biljan MM, Hemmings R, Brassard N. The outcome of 150 babies following the treatment with letrozole or letrozole and gonadotropins. Fertil Steril. 2005; 84 (Suppl 1); 0-231, Abstract 1033.
15. Tulandi T, Martin J, Al-Fadhli R, et al. Congenital malformations among 911 newborns conceived after infertility treatment with letrozole or clomiphene citrate. Fertil Steril. 2006; 85:1761-5.
16. Forman R, Gill S, Moretti M, et al. Fetal safety of letrozole and clomiphene citrate for ovulation induction. J Obstet Gynaecol Can. 2007;29: 668-71.
17. The Thessaloniki ESHRE/ASRM sponsored PCOS consensus workshop group. Consensus on inferirilty treatment related to PCOS. Hum Reprod. 2008; 23:462-77.
18. Li RHW, Ng EHY. Management of anovulatory infertility. Best practice and research. Clinical Obstetrics and Gynaecology. 2012;26:757-68.

CHAPTER 30

Polycystic Ovarian Syndrome

Pratap Kumar, Alok Sharma

Overview

- Polycystic ovarian syndrome (PCOS) is the most common endocrine disorder in women of reproductive age group, affecting 5 to 10% of women exhibiting the full blown syndrome of hyperandrogenism, chronic anovulation and polycystic ovaries.
- The elevated LH levels are partly due to increased sensitivity of the pituitary to gonadotropic releasing hormone stimulation.
- The onset of pulsatile growth hormone (GH) secretion during early puberty induces the release of IGF-1 (Insulin like growth factor-1) by the liver and most other tissues. GH also provokes insulin resistance, which selectively affects peripheral glucose.
- There is growing evidence that hyperinsulinemia may stimulate P 450c 17 enzyme resulting in hyperandrogenism. P 450c 17 is the key enzyme that regulates androgen synthesis.
- The characteristic feature of anovulation in PCOS is the arrest of growth of antral follicles after reaching a diameter between 5 and 8 mm.
- The diagnosis of PCOS is usually made on the basis of a combination of clinical, ultrasonographic and biochemical criteria. Almost 50% of women with PCOS have an android type of phenotype characterized by waist: hip ratio greater than 0.85(9). Hence, weight loss is very essential for better results.
- Metformin therapy improves insulin sensitivity shown by a reduction in fasting plasma glucose and insulin concentrations. It is not effective in the absence of insulin. It decreases basal hepatic glucose output in patients.
- Ovulation induction is the main choice of treatment.

INTRODUCTION

Polycystic ovarian syndrome (PCOS) is the most common endocrine disorder in women of reproductive age group, affecting 5–10% of women exhibiting the full blown syndrome of hyperandrogenism, chronic anovulation and polycystic ovaries.[1] We now know that approximately 75% of anovulatory women of any cause have polycystic ovaries and 20–25% of women with normal ovulation demonstrate ultrasound findings typical of polycystic ovaries.[2] Chronic anovulation accompanied by hyperandrogenism and clinical manifestations including hirsutism, acne, elevated testosterone and androstenedione, and frequently but not always obesity is seen in PCOS.[3]

PATHOPHYSIOLOGY

The major features of PCOS include menstrual dysfunction, anovulation, and signs of hyperandrogenism. Although, the exact etiopathophysiology of this condition is unclear, PCOS can result from abnormal function of the hypothalamic-pituitary-ovarian (HPO) axis. In addition, one of the most consistent biochemical features of PCOS is a raised plasma testosterone level.

When compared with levels found in normal women, patients with persistent anovulation have higher mean concentration of Luteinizing hormone (LH), but low or low normal levels of FSH. The elevated LH levels are partly due to increased sensitivity of the pituitary to gonadotropic releasing hormone stimulation. Because the FSH levels are not totally depressed, new follicular growth is continuously stimulated, but not to the point of full maturation and ovulation, and they are in the form of multiple follicular cysts 2–10 mm in diameter. These follicles are surrounded by hyperplastic theca cells, often luteinized in response to high LH levels. As various follicles undergo atresia, they are immediately replaced by new follicles of similar limited growth potential.

Stein and Leventhal were the first to recognize an association between the presence of polycystic ovaries and signs of hirsutism and amenorrhea (e.g. oligomenorrhea, obesity). After women diagnosed with Stein-Leventhal syndrome underwent successful wedge resection of the ovaries, their menstrual cycles became regular, and they were able to conceive.[4] As a consequence, a primary ovarian defect was thought to be the main culprit, and the disorder came to be known as polycystic ovarian disease.

PUBERTY AND PCOS

Polycystic ovary syndrome originates in puberty. Clinical observation teaches that PCOS often develops during adolescence. Excessive hair growth usually originates from before the onset of menstrual cycles. Menarche tends to be delayed. Irregular cycles, although considered a normal phenomenon during the first gynecological years, frequently continues into adulthood.

Mechanism of Onset of PCOS During Puberty (Flowchart 30.1)

Taking into account the above remarks, the following hypothesis is postulated.[4,5]

The onset of pulsatile growth hormone (GH) secretion during early puberty induces the release of IGF-1 (Insulin like growth factor-1) by the liver and most other tissues. GH also provokes insulin resistance, which selectively affects peripheral glucose. The resulting hyperinsulinemia acting on IGF-1 causes ovarian hyperstimulation inducing thecal cell hyperplasia and excessive androgen production. The increased androgens cause follicular atresia and increased circulating estrone levels because of peripheral conversion in adipose tissues.[5] The altered endocrine milieu provokes increased pituitary LH secretion, which aggravates the theca cell stimulation.

After puberty, the insulin and IGF-1 levels progressively decline in most patients, resulting in normalization of clinical and morphological picture. Only in a few cases PCOS persists.

Insulin and the Mechanism of Anovulation in PCOS

There is growing evidence that hyperinsulinemia may stimulate P 450c 17 enzyme resulting in hyperandrogenism.

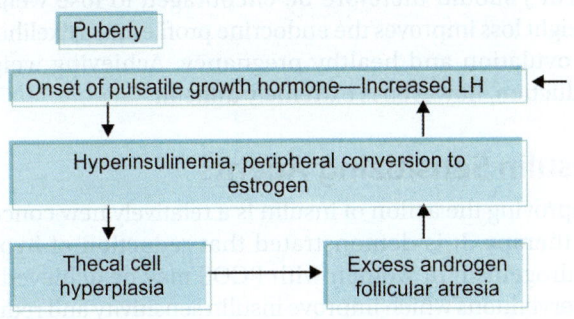

Flowchart 30.1: Mechanism of onset of PCOS.

P 450c 17 is the key enzyme that regulates androgen synthesis.

The characteristic feature of anovulation in PCOS is the arrest of growth of antral follicles after reaching a diameter between 5 mm and 8 mm. This may be caused by premature activation of LH. It is well-known that the syndrome is clustered in families. The sister of a woman with PCOS in such a family has a 50% risk of PCOS compared with a population prevalence of only 5–10%. There is evidence from family studies to support a genetic predisposition to develop PCOS[6] and insulin resistance that seems to coexist in this syndrome.

Role of Hyperinsulinemia in the Pathogenesis of PCOS (Flowchart 30.2)

Obesity, genetic predisposition and insulin receptor disorders lead to insulin resistance. Insulin resistance leads to abnormal glucose tolerance raising the blood sugar, and hyperinsulinemia. This hyperinsulinemia acts on the liver and reduces sex hormone binding globulin (SHBG) and also increases IGF-1(Insulin-like growth factor-1). Reduction of SHBG increases the testosterone, whereas the increased IGF-1 will cause increased androgen production from ovaries. Hyperinsulinemia itself causes the theca cell hyperplasia and increased androgens.

Considering these clinical observations and in vivo/in vitro studies, it was proposed that hyperinsulinemia and hyperandrogenism, regardless of which is the primary event, is connected to PCOS.

DIAGNOSIS

The diagnosis of PCOS is usually made on the basis of a combination of clinical, ultrasonographic and biochemical criteria. A woman presenting with oligomenorrhea is likely to have the problem of PCOS if she has one or more of these three features: Polycystic ovaries on ultrasound, hirsutism and hyperandrogenemia. Many women have high LH, although normal LH do not rule out the diagnosis.

In its fully developed form, PCOS is characterized by menstrual abnormalities, hirsutism, obesity, hyperandrogenemia, elevated plasma LH and ultrasonographic evidence of polycystic ovaries. However, thin women can also have the problem. Ultrasonographically, there should be more than 10 cysts 2–8 mm in diameter, scattered either around or through an echodense, thickened central stroma.[6] Indeed many women with polycystic ovaries detected by sonography do not have symptoms of the PCOS. Ovarian morphology appears to be the most sensitive marker for the PCOS compared with the classic endocrine features of a raised serum LH and/or testosterone concentration. Currently, if two of the three features of polycystic ovaries, biochemical endocrine aspects described with PCO or

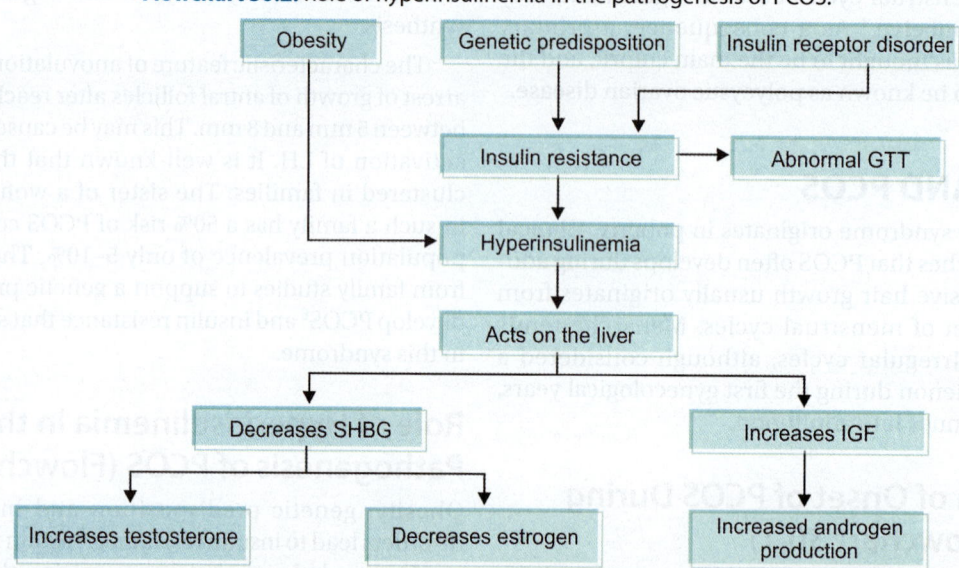

Flowchart 30.2: Role of hyperinsulinemia in the pathogenesis of PCOS.

(GTT: glucose tolerance test; SHBG: Sex hormone-binding globulin; IGF: insulin-like growth factor)

clinical features (of hyperandrogenesis) that are described are present. Exclusion of other disorders that can result in menstrual irregularity and hyperandrogenism then the diagnosis of PCOS is made.

Important Clinical Features

- Hirsutism
- Oligomenorrhea
- Obesity
- USG showing
- Subcapsular cysts.

APPROACH TO INFERTILITY IN A PATIENT WITH PCOS

Women with PCOS often present to gynecologists and reproductive endocrinologists for treatment of infertility caused by anovulation. The approach to the patient with PCOS should involve the use of progressively more aggressive treatment strategies until ovulation is established and pregnancy can be achieved. Barbieri et al.[7] suggested a step-by-step approach to ovulation induction in women with PCOS (Table 30.1).

Weight Loss

Although, obesity is not a prerequisite for the diagnosis of PCOS, it is a common feature. Almost 50% of women with PCOS have an android type of phenotype characterized by waist: hip ratio greater than 0.85.[8] Obesity may induce hyperandrogenism by increasing the production of androgens, reducing sex hormone-binding globulin levels (SHBG), thereby increasing free testosterone

Table 30.1: Stepwise approach to ovulation induction in PCOS.

Step	Approach
1.	If BMI is elevated: loss of at least 5% of current body weight
2.	Ovulation induction with clomiphene citrate
3.	Insulin sensitizer as a single agent (Metformin)
4.	Insulin sensitizer in combination with clomiphene citrate
5.	Gonadotrophin therapy
6.	Insulin sensitizer in combination with gonadotropin therapy
7.	Ovarian surgery—Laparoscopic ovarian puncture
8.	In vitro fertilization

levels[9] causing hyperestrogenemia. This causes pulsatile LH secretion and/or insulin resistance and therefore, insulin secretion which could amplify the LH dependent regulatory mechanisms that regulate ovarian androgen secretion.

Increase of LH can cause a vicious cycle of hyperandrogenemia and follicular atresia. Even moderate obesity (BMI >27 kg/m²) is associated with a reduced chance of ovulation. Obese women with PCOS (BMI >30 kg/m²) should therefore be encouraged to lose weight. Weight loss improves the endocrine profile and a likelihood of ovulation and healthy pregnancy. Achieving weight reduction, however, is extremely difficult.

Insulin Sensitizing Agents

Improving the action of insulin is a relatively new concept in therapy. It is demonstrated that reduction of hyperandrogenism in women with PCOS may be achieved by interventions which improve insulin sensitivity and reduce circulating insulin.[10] Such measures might include, but are not limited to weight loss, dietary modifications and insulin sensitizing agents like metformin.

Metformin[11]
Metformin (dimethyl biguanide) is an orally administered drug used to lower blood glucose concentrations in patients with noninsulin dependent diabetes mellitus (NIDDM) and is now also being used for infertile patients with PCOS.

Mechanism of Action of Metformin
Metformin therapy improves insulin sensitivity shown by a reduction in fasting plasma glucose and insulin concentrations. It is not effective in the absence of insulin. It decreases basal hepatic glucose output in patients.

Ovulation Induction Methods

Clomiphene Citrate[12]
It acts by binding with the estrogen receptor, thus modifying the hypothalamic pituitary activity by an antiestrogen effect. This in turn diminishes the negative feedback of estrogen, activates GnRH secretion and raises the amplitude of gonadotrophin pulses.

The first-line drug for the treatment of PCOS-induced anovulation is clomiphene citrate. After spontaneous or progesterone-induced withdrawal bleeding, the starting dose of 50 mg is given for 5 days starting on day 2, 3, 4, or 5. The patient's ovulation is usually monitored by transvaginal ultrasound from day 11, but may also be documented by basal body temperature charts, midluteal progesterone levels or ovulation detection kits. If there is a mature follicle (>18 mm) as seen by ultrasound, the patient can either ovulate spontaneously or it can be triggered by 5000/10,000 IU of hCG. The maximum dose of clomiphene citrate should not exceed 150 mg/day. If the dose required is more than this, it is generally considered as a clomiphene nonresponder.

Human Menopausal Gonadotrophin[13]
This is the second line of treatment. Purified FSH has a theoretical advantage of avoiding additional LH in PCOS, which often have elevated LH levels. The complications of ovarian hyperstimulation syndrome has to be borne in mind when gonadotrophins are used which could lead to enlargement of ovaries with ascites, vomiting and electrolyte imbalance and may progress to severe problems. The dose of 75 IU per day is used for about a week, which also requires monitoring, by ultrasound for the response.

GnRH Therapy
Women with elevated baseline or mid-follicular LH levels have higher rates of anovulation, ovulation without conception, and early pregnancy loss than normal controls.[14] It has been hypothesized that by suppressing the pituitary with a GnRH analogue before ovulation induction will reduce the LH. But both LH and FSH will get reduced. Hence, more[7] of gonadotropins have to be given for ovulation induction later.

Surgical Induction of Ovulation
In 1939, after removing wedges of ovarian tissue for pathologic analysis, Stein and Cohen observed that ovulatory function and regular menses were restored. For years, ovarian wedge resection via laparotomy was standard therapy for infertile women with PCOS until it was observed that, although ovulation was restored, postoperative adhesions were high and this caused mechanical infertility. Medical treatments replaced surgery for PCOS-induced infertility. With the development of laparoscopic and microsurgical techniques, the possibility of a single minimally invasive operation as a potential treatment for PCOS, restored interest in surgical operations. Techniques, such as multiple biopsies and ovarian "drilling" by laparoscopic cautery or laser vaporization on one or both ovaries have been used to restore ovulation and a more normal hormonal environment. Other potential benefits of surgical treatment are lower cost, avoidance of risk of ovarian hyperstimulation and lower rates of pregnancy loss (~15%) and multiple gestation (~2% twin pregnancies) in comparison with pharmacologic treatment.[15] The rates of ovulation and pregnancy with surgical treatment are at least comparable with the rates achieved medically (approximately 80% and 50%, respectively). Surgical treatment is probably most effective in the first year after operation when conception rates are highest.

Assisted Reproductive Technology (ART)
Anovulation alone, in principle, is not an indication for IVF/intracytoplasmic sperm injection (ICSI) and therefore IVF/ICSI treatment in women with PCOS is recommended either as a third-line treatment (after failed first- or second-line therapies including clomifene citrate, gonadotropin or LOD ovulation induction) or in the presence of other infertility factors, such as tubal damage, severe endometriosis or male factor infertility.

IVF/ICSI treatment in women with PCOS poses a number of clinical challenges, in particular that of moderate-to-severe ovarian hyperstimulation syndrome (OHSS), with a risk of approximately 10% compared with a risk of 0.5–4.0% observed in the general IVF population.

Long-term Effects
Women with PCOS may be at increased risk for cardiovascular and cerebrovascular disease.[17-19] Approximately 40% of patients with PCOS have insulin resistance. These women are at increased risk for type 2 diabetes mellitus and

consequent cardiovascular complications. Patients who initially test negative for diabetes should be periodically reassessed throughout their lifetime. Patients with PCOS are also at an increased risk for endometrial hyperplasia and carcinoma.[20,21] The chronic anovulation in PCOS leads to constant endometrial stimulation with estrogen without progesterone, and this increases the risk of endometrial hyperplasia and carcinoma. No known association with breast or ovarian cancer has been found.[20]

SUMMARY

Polycystic ovarian syndrome is a disorder of unknown cause characterized by anovulation, hyperandrogenism, hyperinsulinemia and/or obesity. There is a great individual variation. Restoring fertility can be challenging since not all patients with this problem respond satisfactorily to ovulation induction. Weight loss and the use of insulin sensitizers may benefit the individuals. The Endocrine Society in October 2013 released practice guidelines for the diagnosis and treatment of PCOS.[22] Some of the guidelines are here to summarize:

- Use the Rotterdam criteria for diagnosing PCOS (Presence of 2 of the following: androgen excess, ovulatory dysfunction, or polycystic ovaries)
- In adolescents with PCOS, hyperandrogenism is central to the presentation; hormonal contraceptives and metformin are treatment options in this population
- Exclude alternate androgen-excess disorders and risk factors for cardiovascular disease, diabetes, endometrial cancer, mood disorders, and obstructive sleep apnea
- For menstrual abnormalities and hirsutism/acne, hormonal contraceptives are first-line treatment
- For infertility, clomiphene is first-line treatment
- For metabolic/glycemic abnormalities and for improving menstrual irregularities, metformin is beneficial
- Metformin is of limited or no benefit for managing hirsutism, acne, or infertility.

REFERENCES

1. Dunaif A. Hyperandrogenic anovulation (PCOS): A unique disorder of insulin action associated with an increased risk of noninsulin-dependent diabetes mellitus. Am J Med. 1995; 98(IA):33S-9S.
2. Polson DW, Adams J, Wadsworth J, Franks S. Polycystic ovaries—a common finding in normal women. Lancet. 1988;16:1(8590):870-2.
3. Franks S. Polycystic ovary syndrome. N Engl J Med. 1995; 333:853-61.
4. Nobels F, Dewailly D. Puberty and polycystic ovarian syndrome. The insulin/insulin-like growth factor I hypothesis. Fertil Steril. 1992;58:655-66.
5. McKenna JT. Current concepts: Pathogenesis and treatment of polycystic ovary syndrome. N Eng J Med. 1988;318(9):558-62.
6. Krook A, Kumar S, Laing I, Andrew JM, Boulton M, John AH. Wass and Stephen O'Rahilly. Molecular scanning of the insulin receptor gene in syndromes of insulin resistance. Diabetes. 1994;43:357-68.
7. Lena H Kim, Ann E Taylor, Robert L Barbieri. Insulin sensitizers and polycystic ovary syndrome: Can a diabetes medication treat infertility? Fertil and Steril. 2000;73(6):1097-98.
8. Lefebvre P, J Bringer, E Renard, F Boulet, S Clouet, C Jaffiol. Influences of weight, body fat patterning and nutrition on the management of PCOS. Hum Reprod. 1997;12 Suppl 1:73-81.
9. Plymate SR, Fariss BL, Bassett ML, Matej L. Obesity and its role in polycystic ovary syndrome. J Clin Endocrinol Metab. 1981;52:1246.
10. Nestler JE. Insulin regulation of human ovarian androgens. Hum Reprod. 1997;12 Suppl 1:53-61.
11. Bailey CJ, Turner RC. Metformin. N Eng J Med. 1996;334(9):574-78.
12. Isaacs JD Jr, Lincoln SR, Cowan BD. Extended clomiphene citrate (CC) and prednisone for the treatment of chronic anovulation resistant to CC alone. Fertil Steril. 1997;67:641-3.
13. Loughlin T, Cunningham S, Moore A, Culliton M, Smyth PPA, Mckenna TJ. Adrenal abnormalities in polycystic ovary syndrome. J Clin Endocrinol Metab. 1996;62:142-7.
14. Venturoli S, Paradisi R, Fabbri R, Magrini O, Porcu E, Flamigni C. Comparison between human urinary follicle-stimulating hormone and human menopausal gonadotropin treatment in polycystic ovary. Obstet Gynecol. 1984;63:6.
15. Adams J, Franks S, Polson DW, et al. Multifollicular ovaries: Clinical and endocrine features and response to pulsatile gonadotrophin-releasing hormone. Lancet. 1985;ii:375-84.
16. Damario MA, Barmat L, Liu HC, Davis OK, Rosenwaks Z. Dual suppression with oral contraceptives and gonadotrophin releasing-hormone agonists improves in vitro fertilization outcome in high responder patients. Hum Reprod. 1997;12(11): 2359-65.
17. Christian RC, Dumesic DA, Behrenbeck T, et al. Prevalence and predictors of coronary artery calcification in women with polycystic ovary syndrome. J Clin Endocrinol Metab. 2003;88(6):2562-8.
18. Dokras A. Cardiovascular disease risk factors in polycystic ovary syndrome. Semin Reprod Med. 2008;26(1):39-44.
19. American Association of Clinical Endocrinologists. American Association of Clinical Endocrinologists position statement on metabolic and cardiovascular consequences of polycystic ovary syndrome. National Guideline Clearinghouse. Available at http://guideline.gov/summary/summary.aspx?doc_id=7108. Accessed August 28, 2009.
20. Hardiman P, Pillay OC, Atiomo W. Polycystic ovary syndrome and endometrial carcinoma. Lancet. 2003;361(9371):1810-2.
21. Royal College of Obstetricians and Gynaecologists. Long-term consequences of polycystic ovary syndrome. London, UK: Royal College of Obstetricians and Gynaecologists; 2007. Green-top guideline; no. 33.
22. Legro RS, Arslanian SA, Ehrmann DA, et al. Diagnosis and treatment of polycystic ovary syndrome: an Endocrine Society clinical practice guideline. J Clin Endocrinol Metab. 2013.

CHAPTER 31

Hirsutism

Muralidhar V Pai

Overview

- Hirsutism is conversion of villus hair to terminal hair in a masculine pattern.
- Hirsutism in itself is not a disease but rather a cutaneous manifestation of hyperandrogenism.
- Hyperandrogenism may result from multiple causes. They may be divided into endocrine and nonendocrine causes.
- The major androgens of biological importance are testosterone (T) and its metabolite dihydrotestosterone (DHT); latter is more potent and is produced in the skin by conversion of T by the enzyme 5α-reductase.
- The severity of hirsutism is determined according to modified Ferriman and Gallwey scoring system.
- Estimation of FSH, LH, PRL, Testosterone (T) and TSH are advocated routinely in all cases of hirsutism.
- Pharmacological intervention slows the growth of new hair but does not lead to loss of established hair.
- Established hair has to be removed using one of the mechanical methods.
- The selection of a pharmacological agent depends on the severity of the hirsutism, patient preference and need to treat other associated conditions.
- The dosage of drugs used to treat hirsutism should be the lowest, which is effective.
- Most pharmacological therapies fall into two major categories: (1) Suppression of androgen secretion, (2) Antiandrogen.

DEFINITION

Hirsutism is defined as conversion of villus hair to terminal hair in a masculine pattern (on the upper lip, chin, chest, back and/or thighs) of female.

Androgens stimulate hair follicles to promote the conversion of villus hair, which is fine and lightly pigmented to terminal hair, which is coarse and darkly pigmented.

Nonsexual terminal hair occurs in both men and women in the scalp, eyebrows and eyelashes. During puberty in both sexes, villus hair is converted to terminal hair in the axilla, legs, forearms and lower pubic triangle (ambo-sexual hair). In adult men, androgens cause terminal hair growth in other areas, such as the upper lip, chin and intergluteal region.

HYPERTRICHOSIS

Hypertrichosis is the term reserved to describe androgen-independent growth of hair, which is villus, prominent in areas, such as the forehead, forearms or legs, and does not grow in a male pattern of distribution. It is most commonly congenital or caused by metabolic disorders (e.g. hypothyroidism, anorexia nervosa, porphyria cutanea tarda), or medications (e.g. phenytoin, minoxidil, cyclosporine, diazoxide, excess of glucocoticoids) or by starvation. Excess hair in a nonandrogen dependent distribution may have an ethnic or racial basis for which medical treatment is inappropriate.

PATHOPHYSIOLOGY

The pathophysiology of hirsutism is best understood in the context of the physiology of normal hair growth. The number of hair follicles is fixed before birth. They cover the entire body except for the palms, lips, and the soles.

Normal women rarely have terminal hair on the upper back or upper abdomen. Thus, the type and distribution of the excess hair is important in the diagnosis of hirsutism. The amount of terminal hair increases with age. Women gradually develop more facial and body hair with age.

Hirsutism in itself is not a disease but rather a cutaneous manifestation of hyperandrogenism. It may rarely be a manifestation of a serious underlying disorder, most often resulting from a combination of increased androgen production (compared to non-hirsute women) and increased sensitivity to androgens.

Hirsutism is usually associated with other hyperandrogenic conditions like alopecia, seborrhea and acne. Obesity is common but not universal finding in women with hirsutism caused by the polycystic ovary syndrome (PCOS). It may be associated with **acanthosis nigricans**, a consequence of marked insulin resistance. In this condition, the skin is thickened and hyperpigmented, characteristically in the neck and axilla and also in flexures, over the knees, elbows and vulva. Hyperandrogenism (HA), insulin resistance (IR), and acanthosis nigricans (AN) is together termed as **HAIR-AN syndrome**.

The major androgens of biological importance are testosterone (T) and its metabolite dihydrotestosterone (DHT); this metabolite is more potent and is produced in the skin by conversion of T by the enzyme 5α-reductase. Dihydrotestosterone is more potent than T primarily because of its higher affinity for and slower dissociation from the androgen receptor.

Most hirsute patients have elevated androgen levels upon thorough evaluation. If only urinary 17-ketosteroids are measured; only 15% of hirsute women will have elevated values. If total plasma testosterone is measured, about 40% of hirsute patients are found to have an elevated level. If total plasma levels of several androgenic hormones and prehormones—testosterone, DHT, DHEAS, androstenedione, and 17-hydroxyprogesterone are measured, approximately 90% of hirsute women will have elevated value of one or more. Free testosterone is elevated in about 50% cases.

Hirsute women with PCOS have higher insulin levels than those with PCOS alone, and there is a significant correlation between plasma insulin concentration and plasma testosterone or androstenedione levels.[1]

Prolactin (PRL) may increase adrenal androgen secretion. Hirsutism and acne have been reported in about 20% of women with prolactin-secreting microadenomas. Hyperprolactinemia also affects androgen metabolism.[2]

Hirsutism and virilization occurring during menopause or pregnancy involve a somewhat different differential diagnosis. Androgen levels generally fall during the menopause, so estrogen deficiency may play a role in these cases. Postmenopausal virilization may be due to hyperthecosis or hilar cell hyperplasia. Virilization during pregnancy is usually due to various manifestations of ovarian over-stimulation by hCG.[3]

ETIOLOGY

Hyperandrogenism may result from multiple causes. They may be divided into endocrine and nonendocrine causes as follows (Tables 31.1 and 31.2):

Table 31.1: Endocrine causes.

	Functional	Neoplastic
Ovarian	Polycystic ovary syndrome (PCOS)	• Sex cord stromal tumor Arrhenoblastoma • Lipoid cell tumor • Luteoma
Adrenal	• Congenital adrenal hyperplasia • Idiopathic adrenal hyperandrogenism	• Adrenal adenoma • Adrenal carcinoma
Pituitary		• Cushing's disease • Acromegaly • Hyperprolactinemia

Table 31.2: Nonendocrine causes.

Functional hirsutism	Cause hypertrichosis
• Racial • Familial • Idiopathic	• Iatrogenic (drugs): – Phenytoin – Diazoxide – Minoxidil – Cyclosporin

Androgenic progestins, e.g. norethisterone, levonorgestrel, danazol, corticosteroids

The most common cause of hirsutism is idiopathic or PCOS. Androgen producing ovarian tumors are an uncommon cause of hirsutism and virilization. The underlying defect leading to hyperandrogenism in idiopathic hirsutism remains to be identified.

DIAGNOSIS

The medical evaluation should be directed at ruling out serious underlying disorder. This can often be accomplished by evaluating patient's history, clinical examination and few basic hormonal investigations.

History of familial hirsutism, oligomenorrhea or amenorrhea, galactorrhea or symptoms of thyroid dysfunction, intake of drugs, such as androgens, anabolic agents and Danazol or 19-nortestosterone derivatives should be elicited.

The **severity of hirsutism is** determined according to modified Ferriman and Gallwey scoring system (Fig. 31.1).[4] With this system 9 body areas that contain hormone-sensitive hair are graded from 0 (no terminal hair) to 4 (frank virilization). The grade for each area is added (maximum possible score = 36). A score of 8 or more was established as the threshold for hirsutism. A total score of 8 or more is seen in only 5% of premenopausal women.

Other signs of hyperandrogenism like acne, alopecia, seborrhea or acanthosis nigricans should be looked for.

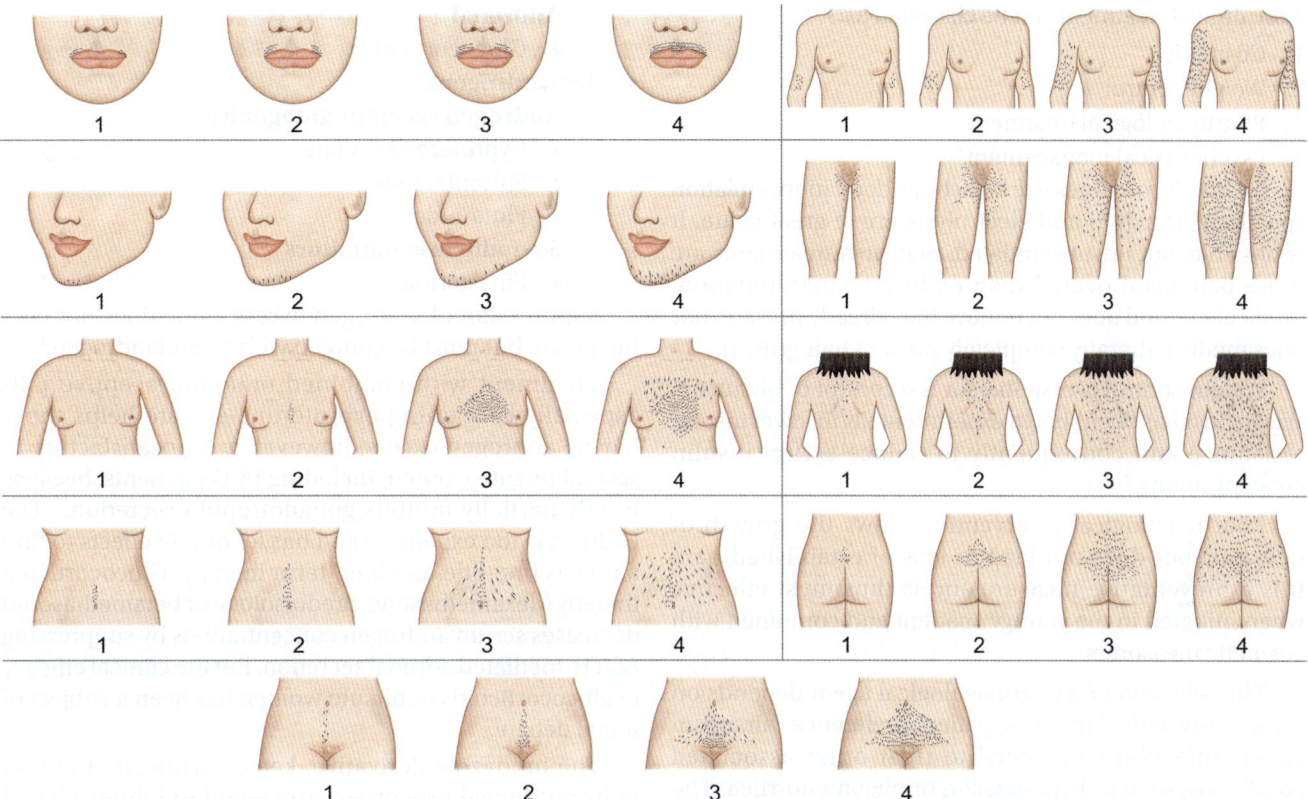

Fig. 31.1: Ferriman and Gallwey scoring system.

The **presence of virilization**, which may include clitoromegaly, temporal baldness, breast involution, hoarseness of voice and male-pattern muscular development, alerts the clinician to the possibility of a neoplastic etiology. In general, neoplasm can be excluded when masculinization is absent.

Hyperprolactinemia may be suspected by demonstrating galactorrhea.

Drug-induced hirsutism (other than that caused by androgens) consists of an increase in lanugo-like hair that is not restricted to androgen-dependent areas of the body.

Other signs on physical examination may indicate a specific endocrine disorder, such as **Cushing's syndrome**.

An abdomino-pelvic examination should be done to look for any palpable ovarian or adrenal tumor. Although adrenal adenomas can be quite small, most adrenal carcinomas are large by the time they cause symptoms; half are palpable abdominally. About half of ovarian tumours are palpable on pelvic examination. **Functioning ovarian tumors** are almost always palpable.[5]

Abdomino-pelvic ultrasound is the key investigation when PCOS is suspected. Routine MRI, selective venous catheterization, or extensive hormonal analysis is not required. More extensive investigation is required only if an androgen secreting tumor is suspected by history or basic investigations.

Estimation of FSH, LH, PRL, testosterone (T) and TSH are advocated routinely in all cases of hirsutism. Measurement of serum DHEAS is not required, because its concentration does not change the therapeutic approach as long as T levels are within 2 ng/mL.[6] Urinary 17-ketosteroids (KS) are of little or no use in the evaluation. Although, DHEAS is its major contributor, nonandrogen steroids and nonsteroid chromogens also contribute significantly to urinary 17-KS production. Only gross elevations of 17-KS (>30 ng/24 hours) reliably reflect pathology.

Urinary-free cortisol level is measured only if Cushing's disease is suspected. If elevated, an overnight dexamethasone suppression test is indicated. Basal insulin level and the insulin response to a glucose load should be measured if insulin resistance is suspected.

TREATMENT

Patients' distress is the prime indication for therapy. Apart from the rare circumstance when a tumor is present, surgery does not play a role in the management of hirsutism. Most women respond to medical therapy, it is easier to prevent hair growth than to treat established hirsutism. Adolescent girls who are beginning to develop hirsutism and who have a family history of excessive hair growth are excellent candidates for medical therapy.

Nonsurgical treatment can be classified as:
1. Cosmetic
2. Weight control
3. Pharmacological treatment
4. Psychological management.

Cosmetic measures like bleaching, depilation, epilation (plucking, shaving) and electrolysis are of great value. It is possible, but unsubstantiated, that such treatments are more beneficial overall than endocrine manipulation. Medical method does not remove hair already present, nor does medical therapy completely prevent hair growth.

Weight control is essential for the control of hirsutism. Weight loss has been shown experimentally to lower insulin resistance and consequently to reduce serum insulin concentrations.[7]

Pharmacological intervention slows the growth of new hair but does not lead to loss of established hair. It is a preventative measure and is thus most effective when initiated in the younger patient and combined with cosmetic measurers.

The selection of a pharmacological agent depends on the severity of the hirsutism, patient preference (hirsutism versus infertility) and need to treat other associated conditions, such as hypertension or oligomenorrhea. The dosage of drugs used to treat hirsutism should be the lowest, which is effective, although high doses of medication may be required initially to induce remission of hair growth. Most drugs, nevertheless, have a shallow dose-response relationship, and maximal doses are often only slightly more effective than midrange doses.

Women must have a clear understanding that medication does not offer a permanent cure and benefit may be lost when treatment is stopped. Women should also be aware that antiandrogen medication could not be used while fertility is being pursued.

Typically, long-standing facial hirsutism responds slowly to medical treatment even if androgens are suppressed to undetectable levels. When starting a medication, it may take as long as 6 months for a woman to note an improvement, especially if she is not mechanically removing hair at the same time. If after 6 months of medical therapy, no improvement is seen or unacceptable hirsutism remains, either a higher dose or a second medication should be used.

Most pharmacological therapies fall into two major categories:
- **Suppression of androgen secretion**
  - **Ovarian**
    - Combined oral contraceptive pills (especially those containing cyproterone acetate)
    - GnRH analogues
    - Ketaconazole.
  - **Andrenal**
    - Glucocorticoids
- **Antiandrogens**
  - **Androgen receptor antagonists**
    - Cyproterone acetate
    - Spironlactone
    - Flutamide.
  - **5α-reductase inhibitors**
    - Finasteride.

Suppression of androgen excess alone does not cure hirsutism, but must be coupled with an antiandrogen.[8]

Treatment with combined oral contraceptive pills especially containing cyproterone acetate helps those having androgen excess, however, it is unsatisfactory in several hirsute women, including PCOS patients, because it only partially inhibits gonadotrophin secretion.[9] The GnRH-a is too expensive and has lot of side effects to find a role as first-line and long-term therapy. Glucocorticoid therapy (dexamethasone, prednisolone or betamethasone) decreases serum androgen concentrations by suppressing ACTH-mediated adrenal secretion. But the clinical efficacy of glucocorticoids in hirsute women has been a subject of much debate.

The imidazole derivative, ketoconazole, in addition to its antifungal properties, was found to inhibit several enzymes involved in adrenal and gonadal steroid synthesis. This causes a fall in gonadal androgen synthesis without an associated fall in adrenal cortisol. There is also serum testosterone fall along with SHBG rise. On this basis, ketoconazole would seem a rational choice of drug to use for the treatment of hirsutism. Doses of ketoconazole ranging from 400 to 1200 mg/day were used. Although, antiandrogen effects are dose dependent, starting with a low dose is recommended because of side effects.[10]

Spironolactone is a steroid and its use is widespread in North America. The clinical efficacy of spironolactone is dose dependent.[11] It is generally used in doses of between 25 and 200 mg daily with treatment being commenced at 25–50 mg. Most patients require at least 100 mg to achieve a satisfactory response. Spironolactone works best in ovulatory women with normal testosterone levels. In women with PCOS, the addition of an oral contraceptive improves response rates. Side effects are also dose-related.

Cyproterone acetate is one of the most commonly used antiandrogen in European countries. Cyproterone acetate is a potent progestogen that is derived from 17α-hydroxyprogesterone and has moderately potent antiandrogenic peripheral activity and is a weak glucocorticoid.[12] It is generally well-tolerated, but can be associated with gastrointestinal upset and breast engorgement.

Flutamide (4'-nitro-3'-trifluoromethylisobutyranilide) is a potent, nonsteroidal antiandrogen devoid of hormone agonist activity,[13] which compete with the binding of testosterone and dihydrotestosterone to the target tissues.

Because of its antiandrogen activity, Flutamide recently has been proposed for women as a therapeutic approach to hirsutism.

Motta et al.[14] were among the first one to suggest that **250 mg of Flutamide once a day** for 6 months could be effective for most patients with hirsutism. They found a reduction up to 50% in hair growth. No side effects were noted, and there were no abnormalities in hepatic, renal, or hematological function.

Finasteride inhibits 5α-reductase activities, blocking dihydrotestosterone production, thus peripherally decreasing the amount of hormone available for interaction with androgen receptors without altering ovarian and adrenal testosterone secretion. The drug has a good safety profile. Doses of up to 400 mg daily have been given to men without serious adverse effects, but also with no greater reduction in serum dihydrotestosterone levels.

The educational and psychotherapeutic aspects of treating hirsutism should not be under valued. The presence of unwanted hair in a masculine distribution may conflict with a woman's concept of her femininity and so distort her self-image. Fears regarding gender identity may need to be addressed and dispelled.

The patient's perception of the verity of her hirsutism should be assessed. Even mild degree of hirsutism can undermine confidence and led to disproportionate self-consciousness. This may lead to social withdrawal and interfere with interpersonal relationships to such an extent that psychotherapeutic intervention is warranted. It has been documented that anxiety and depression are common in the PCOS. Associated fears regarding potential fertility may remain unexpressed and it is important to address this issue if appropriate to the clinical context.

REFERENCES

1. Barbieri RL, Makris A, Randall RW, Daniels G, Kistner RW, Ryan KJ. Insulin stimulates androgen accumulation in incubations of ovarian stroma obtained from women with hyperandrogenism. J Clin Endocrinol Metab. 1985;62:904.
2. Barnes RB. Adrenal dysfunction and hirsutism. Clin Obstet Gynecol. 1991;4:827.
3. Braithwaite SS, Erkman-Balis B, Avila TD. Postmenopausal virilaization due to ovarian stromal hyperthecosis. J Clin Endocrinol Metab. 1978;46:295.
4. Ferriman D, Gallwey JD. Clinical assessment of hair growth in women. J Clin Endocrinol Metab. 1961;21:1440.
5. Speroff L, Glass RH, Kase NG. Hirsutism. In: Mitchell C (Edi). Clinical Gynecologic Endocrinology and Infertility (5th edition)., Williams & Wilkens; 1994. p. 501.
6. Rittmaster RS. Medical treatment of androgen-dependent hirsutism. J Clin Endocrinol Metab. 1995;80:2559.
7. Franks S. Polycystic ovary syndrome: a changing perspective. Clin Endocrinol. 1989;31:87.
8. Eden JA. Hirsutism. In: John Studd (Ed). Progress in Obstetrics and Gynaecology. Churchill Livingstone;1991. p. 319.
9. Hancock KW, Levell MJ. Use of ooestrogen/progestogen preparation in the treatment of hirsutism in female. J Obstet Gynaecol Br Commonwealth. 1974;81:804.
10. Schriock EA, Schriock ED. Treatment of hirsutism. Clin Obstet Gynecol.1991;4:852.
11. Lobo RA, Shoupe D, Seafini P, Brinton D, Horton R. The effects of two doses of spironolactone on serum androgens and anagen hair in hirsute women. Fertil Steril. 1985;43:200.
12. Belisle S, Love EJ. Clinical efficacy and safety of cyproterone acetate in severe hirsutism: results of a multicentric Canadian study. Fertil Steril. 1986;46:1015.
13. Sogani PC, Vagaiwala MR, Withmore WF. Experience with Flutamide in patients with advanced prostatic cancer without prior endocrine therapy. Cancer. 1984;54:744.
14. Motta T, Maggi G, Perra M, Azzolari E, Casazza S, D'Alberton A. Flutamide in the treatment of hirsutism. Int J Gynecol Obstet. 1991;36:155.

CHAPTER 32

Disorders of Sexual Differentiation and Development (Intersex)

Muralidhar V Pai

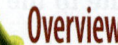

Overview

- Genetic sex is determined by the presence or absence of the Y chromosome.
- Phenotypic sex is genital sex whether apparent female or apparent male.
- Gonadal sex is determined by the presence of normal ovaries or testes.
- Sex differentiation in the embryo usually harmonises with the sex genotype, but hormonal disturbances can lead to abnormalities.
- Disorders of sexual differentiation - DSD (old term – Intersex) is defined as the presence of both male and female external and/or internal genital organs in the same individual causing confusion in the diagnosis of true sex.
- DSD is classified as follows: 1. Disorders of gonadal differentiation; 2. Ovotesticular DSD (True hermaphrodite); 3. Masculinized female; 4. Under-masculinized male; 5. Unclassified.
- Most cases of ambiguity of sex detected at birth are due to either congenital adrenal hyperplasia or to androgenic drugs administered to the mother in early pregnancy.
- The diagnosis is made on careful physical examination, chromosomal studies, hormonal evaluation, pelvic/abdominal ultrasound or MRI. Laparoscopy and gonadal biopsy may be necessary to confirm true hermaphroditism.
- It is always better to diagnose the correct nature of intersex at birth or as early as possible not only to correct the underlying disorders promptly but to avoid the adverse psychological effect on the child and the family.
- After the diagnosis is made, a detailed and frank discussion with the parents regarding gender assignment should be done. Issues related to sexual function, fertility and malignancy should be addressed.
- If karyotyping shows presence of Y chromosome removal of gonads is necessary. After gonadectomy long-term estrogen replacement therapy should be considered.
- Surgical care generally is limited to reconstruction of ambiguous genitalia in female patients and usually involves both clitoroplasty and vaginoplasty.

INTRODUCTION

One of the greatest responsibilities of the obstetrician is the assignment of sex to the newborn. Sexual differentiation and normal subsequent development are fundamental to the continuation of the human species. If the external genitalia of the newborn are ambiguous (with respect to complete male or female development), a profound dilemma is faced. An incorrect assignment of sex threatens and create grave psychological and social problems for the baby and family. So every obstetrician must be well-versed with the problem and be able to establish the diagnosis.

To have uniform and correct communication among colleagues and keeping sensitivity of patients in mind by eliminating terms, such as pseudohermaphroditism, the term intersex disorders has been replaced by disorders of sex differentiation/development (DSDs). Consequent to better understanding of the etiologic mechanisms of normal and abnormal sexual differentiation there has been change in classification also.

SEXUAL DIFFERENTIATION OF THE FETUS

Genetic sex is determined by the presence or absence of the Y chromosome. The Y chromosome determines the development of testes and maleness (Fig. 32.1). The Y chromosome contains a *sex-determining region* (the SRY gene), which encodes the *testis-determining factor* (TDF). The genetic sex is independent of the ovum. If the ovum is fertilized by an X spermatozoa (22 + X-chromosomes) the offspring is XX, a female and if it is fertilized by a Y spermatozoa (22 + Y-chromosomes) the offspring is XY, a male.

CHAPTER 32   Disorders of Sexual Differentiation and Development (Intersex)

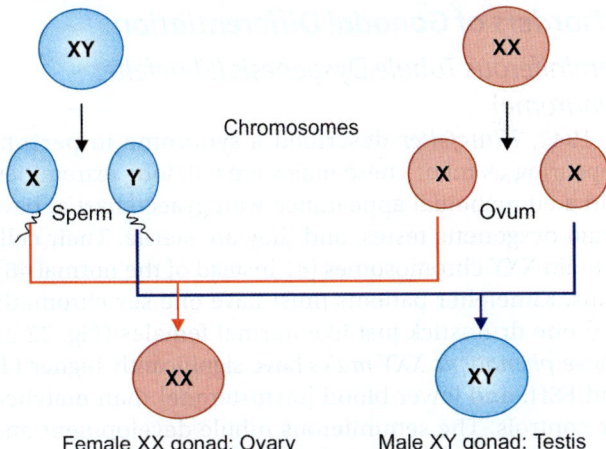

Fig. 32.1: Sperms decides the genetic sex.

Phenotypic sex is genital sex whether apparent female or apparent male.

Gonadal sex is determined by the presence of normal *ovaries* or *testes*. It is clear that male phenotype sexual differentiation is directed by the function of the fetal testis. In the absence of the testis, female differentiation ensues irrespective of the genital sex.

Sex differentiation in the embryo usually harmonises with the *sex genotype*, but hormonal disturbances can lead to abnormalities. Proliferation of nongerminal and germinal cells in the *genital ridge* creates the gonadal *primordia*, which develops into a cortex surrounding the medulla. Until the 7th week of gestation, each sex has a bipotential system (the sexual indifferent stage) with both Wolffian and Müllerian ducts. The *urogenital sinus* develops into the external genitals in both females and males.

Around the 7th week, the medulla of the primitive gonad begins to differentiate into a *testis*, if a *Y chromosome* is present. As the testes grow and their Leydig cells start to produce testosterone, the *Wolffian ducts* develop into the male reproductive tract (epididymis, vas deferens, seminal vesicles and the ejaculatory ducts), whereas the *Müllerian ducts* regress. Testosterone stimulates the growth and differentiation of the Wolffian ducts in the male. The regression of the Müllerian ducts is caused by the *anti-Müllerian hormone* from the Sertoli cells.

Conversely, in the female, the cortex of the indifferent gonads differentiate into *ovaries*, if only two X chromosomes are present and no Y. In the female fetus, where there is a developing ovary and no anti-Müllerian hormone, the Müllerian ducts develop into the female reproductive tract (the uterine tubes, uterus and the upper vagina), and the Wolffian ducts degenerate because the ovary does not secrete testosterone. When a normal female fetus is exposed to androgens during the period of differentiation of the external genitalia, an *apparent male* can result.

Visible differentiation of the gross anatomy does not appear until late in the second month of embryonic life. Testosterone causes the *differentiation* of the fetus to a male. The fetal genital tract will always develop into female genitals, if unexposed to embryonic testicular secretion. The *genital sex* is a phenotypic female. If testosterone is present, male external sex organs develop and the *genital tubercle* elongates to form the male phallus. If testosterone is absent, female organs develop instead. It is the action of *testosterone* and *5-α-dihydrotestosterone* on the urogenital sinus that is behind the normal development of the male external genitalia. In the last months of gestation, the growth of the external genitalia depends upon fetal pituitary luteinizing hormone (LH).

Definition of Disorders of Sexual Differentiation/Development

Disorders of sexual differentiation/development (old term – Intersex) may be defined as the presence of both male and female external and or internal genital organs in the same individual causing confusion in the diagnosis of true sex. The incidence is about 2 per 1000.

Classification of Disorders of Sexual Differentiation

- **Disorders of gonadal differentiation**
  - Seminiferous tubule dysgenesis
    * Klinefelter syndrome.
    * 46,XX male
  - Syndromes of gonadal dysgenesis
    * Turner syndrome
    * Pure gonadal dysgenesis
    * Mixed gonadal dysgenesis
    * Partial gonadal dysgenesis (dysgenetic male pseudohermaphroditism).
  - Bilateral vanishing testis/testicular regression syndromes.
- **Ovotesticular DSD (True hermaphroditism)**
- **46,XX DSD (Masculinized female)**
  - Congenital adrenal hyperplasia (21-hydroxylase, 11β-hydroxylase, 3β-hydroxysteroid dehydrogenase deficiencies)
  - Maternal androgens.
- **46,XY DSD (Undermasculinized male)**
  - Leydig cell agenesis, unresponsiveness
  - Disorders of testosterone biosynthesis
  - Variants of congenital adrenal hyperplasia affecting corticosteroid and testosterone synthesis
    * StAR deficiency (congenital lipoid adrenal hyperplasia)

SECTION 2 Reproductive Endocrinology and Assisted Conception

- Cytochrome P450 oxidoreductase (POR) deficiency
- 3β-Hydroxysteroid dehydrogenase deficiency
- 17β-Hydroxylase deficiency.
  - Disorders of testosterone biosynthesis
    - 17,20-Lyase deficiency
    - 17β-Hydroxysteroid oxidoreductase deficiency.
  - Disorders of androgen-dependent target tissue
    - Androgen receptor and postreceptor defects
    - Syndrome of complete (severe) androgen insensitivity
    - Syndrome of partial androgen insensitivity
    - Mild androgen insensitivity syndrome (MAIS)
  - Disorders of testosterone metabolism by peripheral tissues
    - 5α-reductase deficiency
    - Disorders of synthesis, secretion, or response to Müllerian-inhibiting substance.
  - Persistent Müllerian duct syndrome.
- **Unclassified Forms**

In females—Mayer-Rokitansky-Küster-Hauser syndrome (from Grumbach MM, Conte FA: Disorders of sex differentiation. In: Wilson JD, Foster DW, Kronenberg HM, Larsen PR (Ed). Williams textbook of endocrinology, 9th editon. Philadelphia: WB Saunders; 1998:1303-426).

Descriptions of only common disorders are given below in each category.

Disorders of Gonadal Differentiation

Seminiferous Tubule Dysgenesis (Klinefelter Syndrome)

In 1942, *Klinefelter* described a syndrome in persons appearing as men. These males are tall, long extremities, and a eunuchoidal appearance with gyaecomastia, have small dysgenetic testes, and they are sterile. Their cells contain XXY chromosomes (47 instead of the normal 46). Thus, Klinefelter patients must have one sex chromatin and one drumstick just like normal females (Fig. 32.2). These *phenotypic XXY-males* have significantly higher LH and FSH, and lower blood [testosterone] than matched XY controls. The seminiferous tubule development and spermatogenesis are deficient in Klinefelter males. The XXY-males did not show more feminine behavior than matched controls. A similar group of tall males with *XYY chromosomes* were not extraordinarily masculine. Some XYY-males have significantly higher (testosterone) in their blood than matched XY controls.

46 XX Male

This occurs in 1 of every 20,000 males, closely related to Klinefelter syndrome. XX maleness, was first described by de la Chappelle and coworkers in 1964, is characterized by testicular development in subjects having two X chromosomes and lack a normal Y chromosome. Most of them have normal male external genitalia, but 10% have hypospadias and all are infertile. These patients are shorter

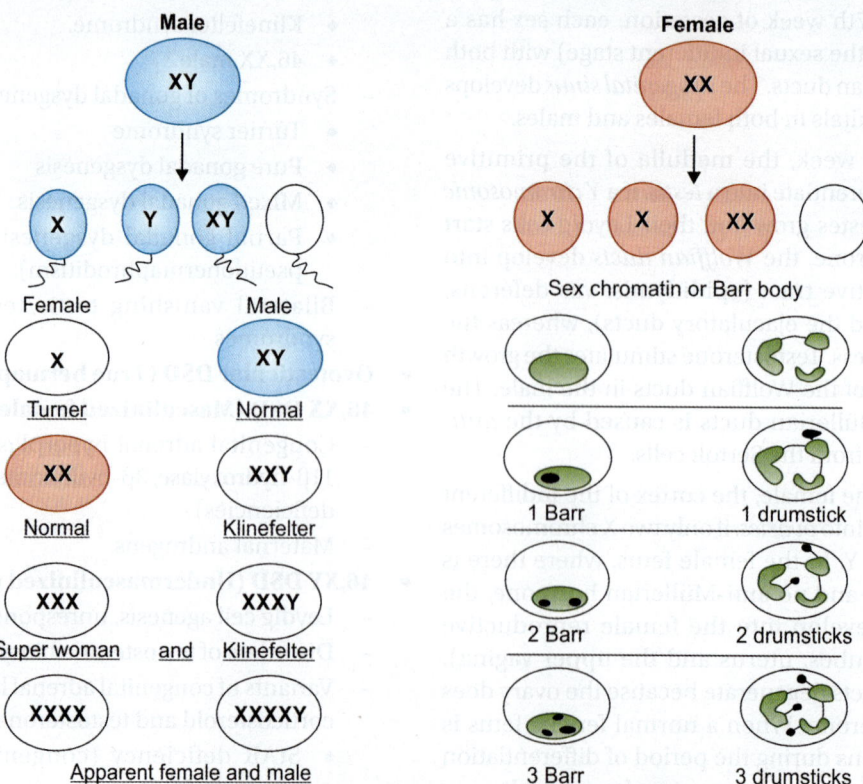

Fig. 32.2: Syndromes of disorders of sexual differentiation.

CHAPTER 32 Disorders of Sexual Differentiation and Development (Intersex)

(mean height 168 cm) than those with Klinefelter syndrome and have normal skeletal proportions.

Syndromes of Gonadal Dysgenesis

Turner's syndrome: In 1938, Turner described a syndrome in small persons, retarded in growth and in sexual development. They are apparent females with small or no ovaries and a *XO chromosomal karyotype*. Since they have only one sex chromosome (X), their total chromosome number is 45. The *Turner patient* lacks the inputs from two active X chromosomes and from an Y chromosome. The lack of anti-mullerian hormone and testosterone leads to Mullerian duct development and female genitals, but the ovary is just a fibrous streak devoid of germ cells. The Turner patients have no sex chromatin and no drumstick (Fig. 32.2).

The syndrome is characterized by short stature (mean adult height 141 + 0.6 cm) and poor development of secondary sex characters. They are mentally retarded. Other physical findings associated with classical forms of gonadal dysgenesis include: Epicanthal folds, high-arched palate, low nuchal hairline, webbed neck, shield chest, coarctation of the aorta, ventricular septal defect, renal anomalies, pigmented nevi, nail hypoplasia, cubitus valgus, and short fourth metacarpal. These patients usually will have primary amenorrhea. Hypertension is relatively common in adults with the disorder. They also frequently have autoimmune thyroid disorders (Hashimotos thyroiditis).

The disorder is a result of accelerated oocyte atresia in which these women undergo menopause before they enter puberty. Both X chromosomes are required for female germ cell survival. Because of oocyte atresia ovarian development is altered and sex steroid secretion is deficient resulting in elevated FSH levels consistent with menopause. Additionally, the deficiency of the X chromosome results in abnormalities of skeletal structures; epiphyses, teeth, and skull. These patients also have an unusual cognitive defect, which renders them unable to appreciate the shapes and relationships of objects to each other (space-form blindness). While Turner's syndrome (45, X) is the sine quo non of gonadal dysgenesis and is the chromosomal-complement found by pediatricians in 80% of young women manifesting these signs and symptoms, only 40% of women presenting with primary amenorrhea have the 45,X complement. The remainders are divided between 46,XX or 46,XY (40%) or X-chromosome structural abnormalities or mosaicism (20%). Approximately 20–30% of patients with 46,XY gonadal dysgenesis develop a dysgerminoma or gonadoblastoma; therefore gonads should be removed from individuals with 46,XY gonadal dysgenesis.

46, XX "Pure" Gonadal Dysgenesis

Patients with 46,XX "pure" gonadal dysgenesis are similar to Turner syndrome except that they have normal height, female external genitalia, Müllerian ducts but absence of Wolffian duct structures. They have bilateral streak gonads, sexual infantilism, with a normal 46,XX karyotype. Their serum gonadotropins are elevated. Management involves cyclic hormone replacement with estrogen and progesterone. Growth hormone is not required. Since they do not have Y chromosome gonadectomy is also not required.

46, XY Complete (Pure) Gonadal Dysgenesis (Swyer Syndrome)

They are characterized by normal female genitalia, well-developed Müllerian structures, bilateral streak gonads, and a nonmosaic karyotype. Because there is complete absence of testicular determination in this condition, ambiguity of genitalia is not an issue but sexual infantilism is the primary clinical problem. The majority of individuals present in their teens with delayed puberty. In addition to amenorrhea, breast development is usually absent. The serum concentration of gonadotropins is abnormally elevated, which leads the clinician to the determination of karyotype and the subsequent diagnosis. Management is removal of both streak gonads and proper cyclic hormone replacement with estrogen and progesterone.

Mixed Gonadal Dysgenesis

This is characterized by a unilateral, often intra-abdominal testis, a contralateral streak gonad, and persistent Mullerian structures associated with varying degrees of inadequate masculinization. Most patients have a 45,XO/46,XY karyotype. The phenotypic spectrum of patients with XO/XY mosaicism extends from phenotypic females with Turner syndrome (25%), to those with ambiguous genitalia, to rarely those appearing as normal males. The majority of these patients present with varying degrees of phallic development, a urogenital sinus with labioscrotal fusion, and an undescended testis. In the neonatal period, mixed gonadal dysgenesis is the second most common cause of ambiguous genitalia (after CAH) and must be in the differential diagnosis. The risk of developing a gonadal tumor (gonadoblastoma, dysgerminoma) is increased in mixed gonadal dysgenesis. Patients with mixed gonadal dysgenesis are also at increased risk for Wilms tumor. The management of mixed gonadal dysgenesis entails gender assignment, appropriate gonadectomy with androgen replacemnt, and proper screening for Wilms tumor.

Partial Gonadal Dysgenesis (Dysgenetic Male Pseudohermaphroditism)

In this condition, patients have two dysgenetic testes rather than one dysgenetic testis and a streak gonad. As with mixed gonadal dysgenesis, these individuals have a 45,X/46,XY or 46,XY karyotype. They may present with a variety of external genital abnormalities, depending on the capability of the dysgenetic gonads to produce testosterone.

Similarly, persistent Müllerian structures are present. The management of this condition is similar to that for patients with mixed gonadal dysgenesis.

Ovotesticular DSD (True Hermaphroditism)

A very small number of individuals end up being of *indeterminate gonadal sex* (i.e. has both ovarian and testicular tissues present). Some persons have an ovary on one side and a testis on the other—a *true hermaphrodite*. In the Greek mythology, *Hermaphrodites* was the child of Hermes and the beautiful Aphrodite. *Pseudohermaphrodites* have external genitals from both sexes, but only one gonadal sex. Males have normal XY chromosomes, but small testes with poor sperms (poor spermatogenesis). An enzyme defect that blocks the conversion of testosterone to *5-α-dihydrotestosterone* disturbs the development of the external genitals. Female hermaphrodites have ovaries, female ducts, XX chromosomes, and varying degrees of masculine differentiation of the external genitals. Any XY individual with a genetic defect in testosterone synthesis develops testes due to the presence of the Y chromosome, and Müllerian duct regression due to the presence of anti-mullerian hormone. The Wolffian duct does not develop normally, because of the testosterone deficiency.

True hermaphroditism is a rare condition and makes up less than 10% of all intersex cases. More than 400 cases have been reported worldwide.

True hermaphrodites have ambiguous genitalia at birth. The majority of affected individuals have been reared as males. However, because of functioning, normal ovarian tissue, most true hermaphrodites experience breast development at puberty, and 40% with a 46,XX peripheral karyotype menstruate. Some of these genetic (XY) boys are born as apparent girls, but they may change from female to male at puberty if the penis grows.

Aside from the physical and emotional consequences associated with genital ambiguity, patients with true hermaphroditism usually do not possess other developmental malformations. These individuals usually possess average intelligence and in general have a normal life expectancy.

Gonadal tumors with malignant potential occur in 2.6% of all true hermaphrodites. Dysgerminomas, seminomas, gonadoblastomas, and yolk sac carcinomas have been reported. Benign tumors including mucinous cystadenomas, benign teratomas, and Brenner tumors have also been reported.

Cryptomenorrhea, hematometra, and lower abdominal pain associated with endometriosis may occur in those individuals with cervical atresia or other forms of Müllerian duct anomalies.

Because of malposition of the gonads, gonadal torsion, and associated duct structures, a variety of organs have been encountered within the inguinal canal, and inguinal hernias are a common complaint. Complications associated with undescended or partial testicular descent may also be encountered.

46,XX DSD (Masculinized Female)

Congenital Adrenal Hyperplasia

Congenital adrenal hyperplasia (CAH) actually describes a group of enzyme defects, which are inherited in an autosomal recessive fashion. The 21hydroxylase deficiency is the most common cause (95%). Because patients with this disorder cannot form cortisol in normal amounts, there is a compensatory increase in ACTH, leading to hyperplasia of the adrenal gland. The excess ACTH drives steroid production to the point of the enzymatic block, with a resultant increase in 17-hydroxyprogesterone production and testosterone. This results in virilization of female neonates and/or salt-wasting secondary to a lack of aldosterone production (salt-wasting CAH).

Affected girls are born with some degree of virilization of their external genitalia, while the internal genital structures derived from the Müllerian ducts (fallopian tubes, uterus and cervix) are unaffected. Postnatally, both sexes may experience rapid somatic growth, accelerated skeletal maturation and premature development of sexual and body hair. Affected boys present with premature sexual maturation.

A third form of the 21 hydroylase deficiency is referred to as "nonclassic" or "late onset" and results in virilization in childhood or adolescence and in females subsequent hirsutism, acne and infertility. Most of the patients with the nonclassic form do not demonstrate over activation of the hypothalamic pituitary axis, as do the other forms. Glucocorticoid therapy suppresses the overactivity of the HPO axis in the severe forms and mineralocorticoid replacement is necessary in the salt-wasting form.

About two-thirds of patients with the severe classic variant of 11-beta-hydroxylase deficiencies have early-onset hypertension. This hypertension generally is mild to moderate but, in as many as one-third of cases, is associated ultimately with left ventricular hypertrophy, retinopathy, and macrovascular events. The exact cause of the hypertension is unclear and is presumed to be due to excessive secretion of DOC, a mineralocorticoid.

Rarely, patients with 11-beta-hydroxylase deficiencies may have salt wasting, especially during infancy. The exact pathophysiology of this is unclear. In some cases, excess glucocorticoid administration appears to play a role through suppression of DOC secretion.

Congenital adrenal hyperplasia is estimated to occur in 1/14,000 births, and is much higher in the Ashknazic Jewish and Eskimo population. The other enzyme defects, which can result in virilization of the female in utero, are 11-beta hydroylase deficiency, and 3-beta hydroxysteroid dehydrogenase deficiency.

Polycystic ovary syndrome is one of the most important differential diagnoses of late-onset or nonclassic variants of virilizing CAH. CAH is far less common than PCOS.

46,XX DSD (Masculinized Female) Secondary to Maternal Androgens and Progestins and Maternal Tumor

The masculinization of a female fetus as a result of maternal administration of synthetic progestational agents or androgens is a rare occurrence. The degree to which any androgen or progestational agent affects female fetal development is a function of the strength of the agent, its maternal dosage, and timing and duration of administration. Very rarely, a maternal ovarian or adrenal tumor has virilizing effects on a female fetus. In any case of exogenous androgen effect on a female fetus, normal endocrine status is recognized postnatally and management is confined to external genital reconstruction, as required.

46,XY DSD (Undermasculinized Male)

The term 46,XY DSD (undermasculinized male) refers to 46,XY individuals with differentiated testes who exhibit varying degrees of feminization phenotypically. Impaired male differentiation in these patients is secondary to inadequate secretion of testosterone by the testes at the necessary period in development, inability of target tissue to respond to androgen appropriately, or impaired production.

Leydig Cell Aplasia (Luteinizing Hormone Receptor Abnormality)

In its pure form, this rare disorder is characterized by a normal 46,XY male karyotype associated with a normal-appearing female phenotype. Typically, testes are palpable in the inguinal canals or labia majora. On investigation, there are no Müllerian structures and the vagina is short. A low testosterone level is noted in conjunction with an elevated LH concentration. The differential diagnosis includes androgen insensitivity syndrome.

Variant of CAH

The rare variant of congenital adrenal hyperplasia (CAH) known as 17-hydroxylase deficiency was first described in the 1960s in patients with sexual infantilizm and hypertension. The disorder reportedly is very rare. It comprises less than 1% of all patients with CAH.

Patients with 17-hydroxylase deficiencies have reduced secretion of cortisol, androgen, and estrogen, with both adrenal and gonadal steroidogenesis impairment. Although patients with 17-hydroxylase deficiencies have decreased cortisol production, they do not have signs or symptoms of adrenal insufficiency due to elevations of corticosterone and glucocorticoids.

Congenital adrenal hyperplasia due to 17-hydroxylase deficiencies is associated with hypertension and an excess of deoxycorticosterone (DOC), which is the second most common naturally occurring mineralocorticoid after aldosterone.

The major morbidities and mortality associated with the condition mainly stem from delayed or non-recognition of hypertension. The long-term sequelae of myocardial infarction, cerebrovascular accident, renal failure, heart failure, and peripheral vascular disease may occur if blood pressure is not well-controlled.

Testicular Feminization Syndrome

In this XY individuals lack the androgen receptor. They develop testes (Y chromosome presence) and the so-called *X-linked testicular feminization syndrome*. These XY persons show Müllerian duct regression because the anti-mullerian hormone is present. The lack of androgen receptors and the effects of androgens on the Wolffian ducts prevent masculinization and the external genitals are feminine.

Androgen Insensitivity

Patients have an XY chromosomal complement, lack of Mullerian structures and a blind vaginal pouch and absence of sexual hair. The syndrome is a result of an inability to respond to testosterone through a target organ androgen receptor defect (60–70%) or a postreceptor signaling defect (30–40%).

Mullerian structures are absent because the gonads secrete Mullerian inhibiting substance.

The gonads may be located in the abdomen, inguinal canal, or labia. The development of gonadal neoplasia is thought to be increased to approximately 5%, however, the incidence is very low before the age of 30. Routinely, orchiectomy is performed after puberty, to allow full pubertal development. Some of these patients show clitoral enlargement and labioscrotal fusion. Their condition is referred to as incomplete (partial) androgen insensitivity. These entities (complete and incomplete androgen insensitivity) are a result of mutations of genes located on the long arm of the X chromosome.

5α-reductase Deficiency

5α-reductase is a microsomal enzyme that catalyzes the conversion of testosterone to DHT. Individuals with this disorder present as neonates with a 46,XY karyotype and a phenotype that may vary from penoscrotal hypospadias to, more commonly, markedly ambiguous genitalia. Typically, the phallus is quite small, appearing as a normal or enlarged clitoris. On endocrine evaluation, these individuals have elevated mean plasma testosterone but low DHT levels. Exogenous DHT could be used at puberty in an attempt to promote phallic growth, but it would be likely to impair spermatogenesis. For these patients, gonadectomy should be performed as early as possible and certainly well before puberty to prevent virilization. Estrogen/progestin should be administered at the expected time of puberty.

Vaginoplasty and clitoral reduction may be performed within the first year of life in those with a severe defect to provide for normal appearance of the external genitalia and to allay parental anxiety.

Persistent Müllerian Duct syndrome

Persistent Müllerian duct syndrome (PMDS), or hernia uteri inguinale, characteristically describes a group of patients with a 46,XY karyotype and normal male external genitalia but internal müllerian duct structures. Typically, these phenotypic males have unilateral or bilateral undescended testes, bilateral fallopian tubes, a uterus, and an upper vagina draining into a prostatic utricle. The treatment of persistent müllerian duct syndrome is relatively straightforward, in that all patients are phenotypic males who require orchidopexy.

Unclassified Forms

Mayer-Rokitansky-Küster-Hauser Syndrome

It is a rare disorder (1 in 4000) characterized by congenital absence of the uterus and vagina. They have a 46,XX karyotype and are normal-appearing females with normal secondary sex characteristics. The external genitalia appear normal, but only a shallow vaginal pouch is present. In the typical form of the syndrome there is symmetrical anatomy with absence of both vagina and uterus. Normal ovaries and fallopian tubes are present, and ovarian function is normal, but only symmetrical uterine remnants are found.

The most common clinical presentation for MRKH syndrome is primary amenorrhea, but patients may present with infertility or dyspareunia. Upper urinary tract anomalies occur in approximately one-third of patients and include renal agenesis, pelvic kidney, and horseshoe kidney.

Atypical forms of MRKH syndrome have been described in up to 10% of cases, in which asymmetrical uterine remnants and/or aplasia of one or both fallopian tubes is discovered.

A radiologic evaluation with ultrasonography and magnetic resonance imaging may define Müllerian anatomy accurately in MRKH and distinguish between typical and atypical forms of the disorder.

Treatment entails creation of a neovagina, surgically or by means of dilation, to allow for sexual function. Surrogacy is an option to have children.

OTHER INTERSEX SYNDROMES

Some small *super women* have an extra X chromosome: XXX, making a total of 47 chromosomes. They have two sex chromatin and two drumsticks. The XXX females have deficient germ cell development and often a short reproductive life.

Apparent men with XXXY (48) chromosomes have Klinefelter *characteristics* with testes, and also two sex chromatin and two drumsticks (Fig. 32.2).

Individuals with *four* X-chromosomes are extremely rare. They are *apparent females* with XXXX (48), and *apparent males* with XXXXY (49). Cells with 4 X-chromosomes contain a maximum of 3 sex chromatin (Barr bodies) and 3 drumsticks, regardless of whether the cells come from apparent females or males (Fig. 32.2).

Hormonal Differentiation Disturbances

The virilizing effect of testosterone on the *urogenital sinus* in early life causes the *adrenogenital syndrome* in XX individuals. They have ovaries (XX chromosome presence) and the Mullerian duct develops normally, because of the absence of anti-mullerian hormone. The androgen hypersecretion results in variable development of male external genitalia. The *adrenal hyperplasia* is caused by enzyme defects.

XY individuals with deficient testosterone synthesis ability to convert testosterone to dihydrotestosterone develop testes, but the Wolffian duct structure are underdeveloped to a varying degree ranging from a partial to a complete female pattern.

XY individuals who lack estrogen receptors or have a mutant gene for aromatase, lack estrogen effects. The functional lack of estrogen results in unfused epiphyseal zones, so these males are tall, and they have high plasma concentrations of LH although testosterone is normal.

Kallman's Syndrome

Hypogonadotropin eunuchoidism or Kallman's syndrome is the most common form of isolated gonadotropin deficiency. Recent studies demonstrate that GnRH neurons originate in olfactory tissues and migrate to the hypothalamus. Thus, hypogonadism and anosmia are classic presentations for this disorder.

This disorder of sexual differentiation results in delayed puberty and primary amenorrhea. Deletions of the Kallman's gene (KALIG-1) on the short arm of X have been identified with subjects demonstrating an X-linked form of Kallman's syndrome. This gene encodes a cell adhesion protein, which participates in the migration of the GnRH neurons from the medial olfactory placode to the hypothalamus.

Psychosocial Sex-Deviations

Sex identity is the individual *perception* of herself or himself as a female or a male. Sex identity is established early, and is not lost by castration. Both psychological and social factors can interfere with normal sexual development on the psychological plane. An imminent urge to change sex (operative sex shifts) characterises *transsexual persons*.

The *sex role* is the social behavior or cultural role played by or forced upon each individual. Some male homosexuals wish to express their femininity while other males clearly signal that they are men. *Transvestites* love to dress like the opposite sex. Transvestites are heterosexual, homosexual or asexual just as others.

Cryptorchidism

Cryptorchidism is the most common genital problem encountered in pediatrics. Cryptorchidism literally means hidden or obscure testis and generally refers to an undescended or maldescended testis. Despite over 100 years of research, many aspects of cryptorchidism are not well-defined and remain controversial. If the testes do not descend from the abdominal cavity to the scrotum, heat destroys the sperm-producing seminiferous tubule cells. Heat does not harm the Leydig (testosterone-producing) interstitial cells. Untreated cryptorchidism clearly has deleterious effects on the testis over time.

Understanding the abnormalities of morphogenesis and the molecular and hormonal milieu associated with cryptorchidism is critical to contemporary diagnosis and treatment of this extremely common entity.

Overall, cryptorchidism is seen in 3% of full term newborn boys, decreasing to 1% at 1 year of age. Prevalence is 30% in premature boys. Predisposing factors include prematurity, low birth weight, small size for gestational age, twinning, and maternal exposure to estrogen during first trimester. A 7% incidence is seen in siblings of boys with undescended testes. Spontaneous descent after the first year of life is uncommon.

Clinically, the most useful classification is whether testes are palpable upon physical examination. Accordingly, there may be:

Nonpalpable testes
- Intra-abdominal
- Absent

Palpable testes
- Undescended
- Ectopic and retractile

Nonpalpable testes occur in about 20–30% of the cryptorchid population. The absent testis is thought to occur from an intrauterine or perinatal vascular event. It is likely a late gestational event since most of these testicular nubbins are found below the internal inguinal ring. Only 20–40% of nonpalpable testes will be absent at surgical exploration.

Ectopic testes exit the external inguinal ring and then are misdirected along the normal course of the testis. Retractile testes may be palpated anywhere along the natural course of the testis, although most are inguinal. Though not truly undescended, these testes may be suprascrotal due to an active cremasteric reflex. This reflex is usually weak during infancy and most active at 5 years. These testes can be manipulated into the scrotum where they will remain without tension.

Castration

Certain cultures castrate boys to preserve their tenor voices. Puberty and natural sex development does not take place. Adult males retain their *secondary* sex characteristics and *erection* but they often lose libido. The effects of castration of adult females are surprisingly trivial, as long as the pituitary is working well. Castration, of course, stops their menstrual periodicity (*artificial menopause*), and they are *sterile*.

DIAGNOSIS OF INTERSEX (DISORDERS OF SEXUAL DEVELOPMENT)

Most cases of ambiguity of sex detected at birth are due to either congenital adrenal hyperplasia or to androgenic drugs administered to the mother in early pregnancy. Cases presented at puberty are late manifestations of congenital adrenal hyperplasia, those of gonadal dysgenesis and rarely male intersex (testicular feminization syndrome). In these conditions, the child is reared up as girl and she is brought either for poor development of secondary sex characters or for primary amenorrhea with or without hirsutism.

The diagnosis is made on careful general physical, abdominopelvic examination of clinical presentations. Chromosomal studies to find out genetic defects and karyotyping are essential to confirm genetic disorders. Hormonal evaluation is essential in diagnosing hormonal differentiating disturbances. Pelvic/abdominal ultrasound may aid in the identification of gonads and duct structures. A scrotal ultrasound may pick up occult gonads. A genitogram is used to evaluate the structure of the urethra and to confirm the presence of a vagina. An intravenous pyelogram is important to rule out any associated urinary tract anomalies. Cystoscopy may be used to determine the position of entry of the vagina into the urethra or urogenital sinus. Laparoscopy and gonadal biopsy may be necessary to confirm true hermaphroditism.

MANAGEMENT OF INTERSEX

It's always better to diagnose the correct nature of intersex at birth or as early as possible not only to correct the underlying disorders promptly but to avoid the adverse psychological effect on the child and the family. If the diagnosis remains uncertain or the corrective surgery is deferred for the future, the baby is to be reared up as female.

Gonadal Dysgenesis

If karyotyping shows presence of Y chromosome removal of gonads is necessary as there is chance of dysgerminomas or gonadoblastoma in such ovaries. Substitution therapy with estrogen and progesterone will help develop secondary sex characters.

Testicular Feminization

The individual should be reared up as girl. The ectopic gonads are to be removed, for fear of malignancy, along with vaginoplasty after the growth is completed with development of secondary sexual characters. After gonadectomy long-term estrogen replacement therapy should be considered.

Hermaphrodite

With the exception of 46,XX individuals with congenital adrenal hyperplasia or documented maternal androgen excess, most patients with genital ambiguity will require surgical exploration for diagnostic confirmation and removal of contradictory gonadal tissue. This should be done to allow for maximal gender specific development and to increase fertility potential. True hermaphroditism can only be confirmed with gonadal biopsy. Clitoral recession, vaginoplasty, and labioscrotal reduction will be necessary for true hermaphrodites given a female sex assignment. Ideally, this should occur at 3–6 months of age.

Congenital Adrenal Hyperplasia

This can be life-threatening in the neonatal period secondary to sodium depletion, hyperkalemia, and dehydration. Newborn female babies with ambiguous genitalia and males with dehydration must be evaluated for CAH immediately and treated with corticosteroids, mineralocorticoids, and sodium chloride if the salt-wasting form is diagnosed. Treatment of the 17-hydroxylase deficiencies is also on similar lines.

Glucocorticoid replacement is vital because it reduces ACTH secretion and thus reduces the production of ACTH-dependent androgens and mineralocorticoids. Oral hydrocortisone is the ideal glucocorticoid for replacement therapy in children. A typical dose is 12–25 mg/m^2/d in 2–3 divided doses. If the response to hydrocortisone is poor, dexamethasone may be used in adults.

Antihypertensive therapy often is needed. Potassium-sparing diuretics, such as spironolactone or amiloride, with or without a calcium channel blocker, such as nifedipine, often are used.

Prenatal treatment is an option for fetuses known to be at risk for classic 11-beta-hydroxylase deficiency. The only setting in which this therapy should be considered is if both parents are known carriers of virilizing CAH. Dexamethasone may be used in mothers during pregnancy at a dose of 20 mcg/kg initiated as soon as the pregnancy is confirmed, starting at 4–5 weeks' gestation. However, the long-term effects on the child are unknown. Genetic testing is performed on the fetus, typically via chorionic villus sampling. Dexamethasone is discontinued if the fetus is XY or unaffected XX.

Surgical care generally is limited to reconstruction of ambiguous genitalia in female patients and this is the subject of continuing debate. The surgical procedure usually involves both clitoroplasty and vaginoplasty in infancy or clitoroplasty in infancy with vaginoplasty in late adolescence. Use of vaginal dilators sometimes is necessary to prevent restenosis.

Cryptorchidism

Indications for hormonal or surgical correction of cryptorchidism are possible improved fertility, self-examination for testis mass (cancer), correction of associated hernia, prevention of testicular torsion and psychological effects of empty scrotum.

The appropriate time for treatment is approximately 1 year of age. This age has decreased over the recent decades and is based on (1) the rarity of spontaneous descent after 1 year of age and (2) the possible salvage of improved fertility by earlier intervention. The choice of initial treatment is a reflection of both physician and patient preference.

Primary hormonal therapy with hCG or gonadotropin-releasing hormone has been used for many years, especially in Europe. The action of hCG is virtually identical to that of pituitary LH although hCG appears to have a small degree of FSH activity as well. It stimulates production of gonadal steroid hormones by stimulating the Leydig cells to produce androgens. The exact mechanism of action of the increased androgens in testicular descent is not known but may involve effects on the testicular cord or cremaster muscle. This medication is administered by intramuscular injection.

Successful placement of the testis in the scrotum by surgery is based on the principles originally described by Bevan in 1899. These include adequate mobilization of the testis and spermatic vessels, ligation of the associated hernia sac, and adequate fixation of the testis in a dependent portion of the scrotum. Many different techniques have been described and are highlighted in the following intraoperative details section.

GENDER ASSIGNMENT

After the diagnosis is made, a detailed and frank discussion with the parents regarding gender assignment should be done. Issues related to sexual function, fertility and malignancy should be addressed.

CHAPTER 33

Infertility

Prashant Nadkarni

Overview

- Infertility is defined as the inability to conceive a pregnancy after two years of unprotected intercourse (i.e. without contraceptive precautions). It can either be primary, where no previous pregnancy has occurred, or secondary where there has been a previous documented pregnancy.
- In general, 40% are due to the male partner and 40% the female, the remaining being unexplained infertility.
- Any dysfunction of this regular ovulatory mechanism compromises fertility potential and this occurs in approximately 20% of couples. These disorders are among the easiest to diagnose and have the best prognosis for fertility, as they are often the easiest to treat.
- Ascending infection from the cervix, commonly chlamydial or gonococcal, results in pelvic inflammatory disease, which damages the delicate ciliated columnar epithelial cells of the fallopian tube as well as resulting in the formation of peritubal adhesions. Other causes of adhesions include peritonitis (e.g. after a ruptured appendix), endometriosis and postpelvic surgery (e.g. for an ovarian cyst or uterine myoma).
- Investigations should include assessment of the sperm, the oocyte, the fallopian tubes and uterus.
- Treatment varies according to the problems.

INTRODUCTION

Infertility is a worldwide phenomenon and is prevalent in every community. The psychological trauma of prolonged infertility on the couple is enormous. This Chapter will explain some of the mechanisms involved in establishment of a pregnancy, and the investigation of the infertile couple. Common treatment modalities are discussed.

Infertility is defined as the inability to conceive a pregnancy after two years of unprotected intercourse (i.e. without contraceptive precautions). It can either be primary, where no previous pregnancy has occurred, or secondary where there has been a previous documented pregnancy. The previous pregnancy may be a live birth, or even a failed pregnancy, e.g. miscarriage or ectopic pregnancy.

Infertility is a common condition, occurring in approximately 10–15% of couples worldwide. The prevalence is similar across racial and ethnic groups and, apart from certain parts of sub-Saharan Africa, is the same worldwide.

CAUSES OF INFERTILITY

The main causes of infertility can be subdivided as shown in the pie chart (Fig. 33.1):

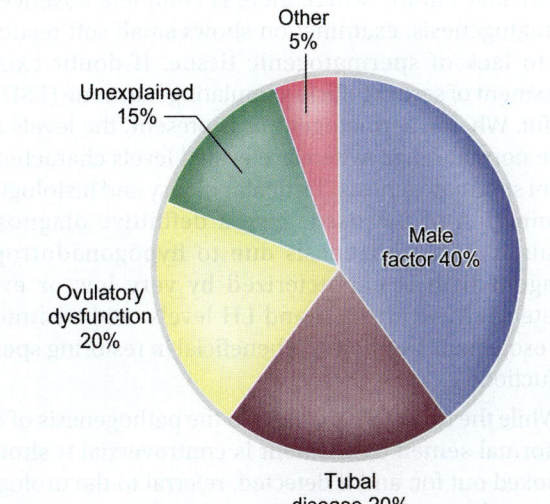

Fig. 33.1: Causes of infertility.

Male Factor Infertility

This is an often underestimated cause of infertility. Current statistics show that abnormalities of seminal parameters represent the single most important cause of infertility, accounting for approximately 40% of infertility in couples. There has recently been controversy regarding whether sperm parameters (especially sperm counts) have been deteriorating in recent years due to environmental pollutants commonly referred to as endocrine disrupters (ED).[1] If this is proven, the contribution of the male factor to infertility may be even greater in years to come.

Spermatozoa are produced in the testicles under the influence of the anterior pituitary hormones, luteinizing hormone (LH) and follicle-stimulating hormone (FSH). The former acts on Leydig cells in the testicle to stimulate production of testosterone, which in conjunction with FSH, stimulates spermatogenesis in the seminiferous tubules. It takes an average of 74 days for the functionally competent spermatozoa to develop and when mature, they are stored in the epididymis prior to ejaculation. Any insult to the developing spermatozoa during this relatively long development time can potentially damage the spermatozoa. Damage from excessive cigarette smoking, alcohol intake or high local temperature is thought to work in this way.[2]

While up to 70% of men with subnormal semen may have no demonstrable cause, a detailed history, physical and genital examination of the male partner is mandatory as clues to the diagnosis may be evident.

In congenital absence of the vas deferens (CAVD) linked to cystic fibrosis, or occlusion due to previous infection and scarring by gonorrhea, spermatogenesis is present but the obstruction of vas deferens prevents sperm from being released in the ejaculate. These men have normal sized testes but the vas may be absent (CAVD). Conversely, in testicular failure, where there is complete absence of spermatogenesis, examination shows small soft testicles due to lack of spermatogenic tissue. If doubt exists, assessment of serum follicle stimulating hormone (FSH) is helpful. Where spermatogenesis is present, the levels are in the normal range, whereas elevated levels characterize absent spermatogenesis. Testicular biopsy and histological examination of the tissue give a definitive diagnosis. Impaired spermatogenesis due to hypogonadotropic hypogonadism is characterized by very low or even undetectable serum FSH and LH levels, and treatment with exogenous hormones is beneficial in restoring sperm production.

While the role of a varicocele in the pathogenesis of the subnormal semen assessment is controversial it should be looked out for, and if detected, referral to the urologist sought to discuss the potential benefits of correction of the anomaly.

Tubal Factor

The fallopian tube retrieves the oocyte either from the ovulatory follicle or from the peritoneal fluid postovulation. It then nourishes the oocyte and spermatozoa, facilitates fertilization and subsequently transports the embryo into the uterus, where it reaches approximately 96 to 120 hours postovulation (4–5 days). It is thus easy to imagine that any disease process, which interferes with the structure or function of this vital organ, would seriously compromise fertility.

Ascending infection from the cervix, commonly chlamydial or gonococcal, results in pelvic inflammatory disease, which damages the delicate ciliated columnar epithelial cells of the fallopian tube as well as resulting in the formation of peritubal adhesions. These sequelae prevent both the retrieval and transport of the oocyte.

Other causes of adhesions include peritonitis (e.g. after a ruptured appendix), endometriosis and postpelvic surgery (e.g. for an ovarian cyst or uterine myoma).

Ovulatory Dysfunction

The normal menstrual cycle results in the ovulation of usually a single mature oocyte approximately once a month. On average, therefore, a woman releases only twelve oocytes a year.

Any dysfunction of this regular ovulatory mechanism compromises fertility potential and this occurs in approximately 20% of couples. These disorders are among the easiest to diagnose and have the best prognosis for fertility, as they are often the easiest to treat.

The disorders of ovulation are discussed in another Chapter.

Unexplained Infertility

Sometimes called idiopathic infertility, this is a diagnosis of exclusion after full assessment of the infertile couple. Despite the lack of a definite diagnosis of cause, they often have a good prognosis with treatment.

Other Causes

This heterogenous group of causes includes sexual dysfunction, immunological or anatomical disorders, chronic illness, etc. A good history from the couple will often reveal the root cause.

ASSESSMENT OF THE INFERTILE COUPLE

It is often the case that only the female partner attends a consultation, but as the problem of infertility involves the couple, the presence of both the partners is essential. Not only is the male partner a significant cause of infertility, he is also involved in the treatment. The psychological impact of infertility and its treatment on the couple may also be readily assessed if the couple are together. A joint consultation with both partners also allows discussion of diagnosis, further evaluation necessary and the planned treatment so that any questions from the husband can be addressed. Treatment of infertility can sometimes be a long process and getting the male partner's cooperation and trust at the outset is of great benefit.

A full history from both partners is imperative. Each partner's age, general health, duration of the union (including previous unions) and previous pregnancy is elucidated. Frequency of coitus and any difficulty thereof may also be gently questioned.

Important information from the woman includes a detailed menstrual history encompassing premenstrual and menstrual symptoms, previous pelvic infections, usage of an intrauterine contraceptive device and previous pelvic surgery. A full general and pelvic examination, including a cervical smear is undertaken. Ultrasonography of the pelvic organs may also be helpful.

Similarly, a detailed history and examination of the male partner is obtained, including any previous history of genital injury or sexually transmitted disease. Genital examination includes the assessment of testicular size, the presence of vas deferens and the absence of a palpable varicocele or hernia.

INVESTIGATION OF THE INFERTILE COUPLE

This should include assessment of:
- The sperm
- The oocyte
- The fallopian tubes and uterus.

Investigation of the Sperm Factor

The basic laboratory assessment of the male factor is the semen analysis. As it is easily obtained and assessed, this should be done early in the investigative process. The man should be asked to abstain from ejaculation for two to three days prior to the test, as recent ejaculation gives falsely low sperm counts. Additionally, he should be advised to collect the semen by masturbation and into a clean, sterile container. The specimen should be taken to the laboratory within an hour of collection.

The WHO criteria for assessment are most commonly used in assessing normality.[3] Normal parameters are as follows:

- Volume   : >1.5 mL
- Viscosity   : Liquefaction within 1 hour
- pH   : >7.2
- Count   : 15 million/mL or more
- Motility   : 40% or more
- Morphology   : 4% normal forms or greater

Investigation of the Egg Factor (Ovulation)

A good history will invariably identify the woman with ovulatory dysfunction. Ovulation is characterized by regular cycles and premenstrual symptoms such as breast tenderness and low abdominal bloating as well as primary dysmenorrhea. Nevertheless, as ovulation is essential to conception, it is important to confirm its occurrence objectively. Many means are available to do so, and are described below:

Basal Body Temperature

This is an easy and inexpensive method, which the patient performs at home. On waking, a specially graduated thermometer is used to determine her body temperature and the reading recorded on a graph. This is done daily over the whole menstrual cycle. As progesterone is a thermogenic hormone, the postovulatory half of the cycle (luteal phase) is characterized by an elevated basal temperature of about 0.2–0.4°C in the last twelve to fourteen days of the cycle. A biphasic graph with a lower temperature in the first half and an elevated temperature in the second half of the cycle indicates ovulation. The patient is also asked to mark coital encounters and this also serves to objectively assess coital frequency.

Luteinizing Hormone Monitoring

Commercially available home testing kits now make it easy to determine the presence of the LH surge, which triggers ovulation. The early morning urine is tested in the days leading to ovulation and a positive test is an indicator of impending ovulation.

Midluteal Serum Progesterone

After ovulation, a corpus luteum is formed from the ovulatory follicle and this secretes progesterone. The level peaks between seven and nine days after ovulation and the finding of an elevated serum level at this time confirms ovulation. However, the timing of the test can be difficult given that menstrual cycle length can vary month to month, and a negative test may be a signal that the test was mistimed.

Ultrasound Monitoring

The developing ovarian follicle can be monitored over a period of days until evidence of ovulation is seen. However, one drawback is that the patient needs to attend the doctor's surgery repeatedly as the developing follicle is ultrasonically tracked over the days leading to ovulation.

Endometrial Biopsy

Progesterone causes the development of a secretory endometrium and accurate histological confirmation is possible with an endometrial biopsy. However, as this is an invasive test and may also disrupt an early implanted pregnancy. It is seldom used.

Investigation of the Uterus and Fallopian Tubes

As discussed previously, tubal damage results in mechanical disruption of the process of fertilization and embryo transport. Similarly, a space occupying lesion in the uterus (e.g. fibroid or endometrial polyp) disrupts the process of implantation of the embryo. There are currently two commonly performed investigations to assess normality:

Hysterosalpingography (HSG)

This is a radiological procedure, which involves the injection of a radiopaque dye through the cervix. The dye courses through the uterus and tubes and into the peritoneal cavity. Blocked tubes are characterized by obstruction to this flow into the peritoneum. Additionally, filling defects in the uterus may delineate intrauterine lesions discussed above. To reduce X-ray exposure to the ovaries, the procedure is performed under continuous fluoroscopy and two or three X-rays are taken as a permanent record of the outcome. It is performed prior to ovulation to prevent accidental irradiation of an embryo.

Laparoscopy

This is the gold standard in tubal and peritoneal assessment. A telescope is inserted into the peritoneal cavity to allow direct visualization of the pelvic organs. Any abnormality, including endometriosis and pelvic adhesions which would not be visualized by ultrasonography or hysterosalpingography, would be readily diagnosed. An inert colored dye such as methylene blue is injected into the cervix and its passage freely through the fimbrial ends of the fallopian tubes confirms patency.

Occasionally, a hysteroscopy may also be performed at the same time. In this procedure, a telescope is inserted intracervically into the uterus to assess the uterine cavity.

Disadvantage of this method of assessment are the need for a surgical incision to insert the laparoscope, as well as the need for general anesthesia.

TREATMENT OPTIONS

Once the tests are completed, the physician is in a better position to make a diagnosis and plan treatment. Even in unexplained infertility, good pregnancy rates can be achieved with available treatment. It is important to remember that apart from total bilateral tubal obstruction or azoospermia, pregnancies occur in the infertile even without treatment, although with a lowered frequency. While treatment increases the chance of pregnancy in any one cycle, it does not guarantee success.

Induction of Ovulation

This is beneficial in ovulatory dysfunction and unexplained infertility with high odds ratios for pregnancy.[4,5]

The commonest agent used is clomiphene citrate, an antiestrogen agent which acts as a competitive inhibitor at the hypothalamic level. In anovulatory women, ovulation rates of up to 80% have been reported with its usage. It is taken usually from days 2 to 6 of the menstrual cycle and results in an increased secretion of pituitary FSH resulting in ovulation. Occasionally, multiple ovulation may occur, resulting in multiple pregnancy, generally twins (5–8% of conceptions).

Where clomiphene citrate has failed, in hypogonadotropic hypogonadism and in assisted reproductive technology (e.g. in vitro fertilization), more potent agents are required. Gonadotropins are the agent of choice. They may either be derived from the urine of postmenopausal women or more recently, synthetically derived from recombinant technology. They are administered parenterally and as they contain FSH, act directly on the ovary to recruit multiple ovarian follicles for ovulation. They are potent stimulators of folliculogenesis, and their use must be combined with strict patient monitoring if complications are to be avoided. The two most common adverse effects are multiple gestation and the ovarian hyperstimulation syndrome.

The reported incidence of multiple gestation can be up to 30%, and while most of these are twins, higher order gestations such as triplets and quadruplets (quintuplets, sextuplets) are reported.

The ovarian hyperstimulation syndrome is a consequence of ovulation following gonadotropin usage, especially if pregnancy occurs. It is directly related to the number of follicles stimulated; the greater the number of follicles, the higher the risk. It is characterized by ovarian enlargement, ascites, hemoconcentration, hypercoagulability, and in severe cases, even pleural and pericardial effusion. Death can occur in the severe case.

Intrauterine Insemination

This involves the injection of a small volume of concentrated spermatozoa into the uterine cavity at the time of ovulation, thus optimizing the process of natural fertilization. Ovulation is usually stimulated with clomiphene citrate, gonadotropin therapy or a combination of the two, and the semen has been previously prepared in the laboratory to yield highly active spermatozoa and to remove dead cells, debris and prostinoid substances found in the raw semen. This method is widely practiced and has good results in unexplained infertility, ovulatory dysfunction and mild male factor infertility. Pregnancy rates are approximately 15% per cycle.[6]

In Vitro Fertilization (IVF, "Test Tube Treatment")

Fertilization takes place outside the human body, in the laboratory environment. This process allows the fallopian tubes to be bypassed and is especially useful in tubal infertility although, it is increasingly being used for all forms of infertility. Once again, multiple oocytes development is induced, but just prior to ovulation, the ovarian follicles are punctured and the oocytes retrieved. These are then inseminated with the spermatozoa in the laboratory, where the embryos are nurtured before transfer into the uterus at 48–72 hours usually. At this time, the embryo is at the 4–8 cell stage of division. More recently, embryos are being transferred at day 5 or 6 (blastocyst stage) where a small but significant increase in pregnancy rates has been demonstrated.[7] The delivery rate per treatment cycle (i.e. the chance of having a live delivery after each completed treatment cycle) is almost 30%.[8]

Intracytoplasmic Sperm Injection

Until very recently, the majority of men with severe male factor infertility were virtually untreatable and even with in vitro fertilization, embryos could not be generated because of the inability of the spermatozoa to penetrate the oocytes. With the advent of ICSI, single spermatozoa can now be introduced directly into the oocytes resulting in fertilization in the majority of patients. This has opened a whole new avenue of treatment for couples previously considered untreatable except by donor sperm insemination of the female partner. ICSI is an offshoot of in vitro fertilization, and the procedure is very similar to IVF, except for the laboratory aspects. Pregnancy rates and delivery rates are similar to IVF.

FUTURE DIRECTIONS

Cryopreservation

In recent years freezing of gametes and embryos has become an important part of fertility medicine due to the development of vitrification techniques which have substantially improved cellular survival.[9] Because these embryos can be used at a later stage, significantly less embryos are being transferred during IVF and ICSI, resulting in a decrease of multiple pregnancy which is the leading complication of these techniques. Frozen embryos have similar pregnancy rates compared to fresh embryos.[8]

At the same time more patients are seeking gamete cryopreservation. The gonadotoxicity of some chemotherapeutic agents and radiotherapy used in cancer treatment can cause permanent sterility. These patients are increasingly being encouraged to store their eggs and sperm prior to such treatments so that there is an option for the stored gametes to be used when a child is desired.

Women trying to preserve their fertility are also increasingly turning to oocyte cryopreservation in an attempt to address the decline in fertility associated with female age. Thus, women in their thirties who are not contemplating pregnancy are going through what is termed social egg freezing.

CONCLUSION

As the fields of medicine and embryology develop, newer and more sophisticated treatment modalities become available to the infertile couple. However, the principles of management remain the same as in any other field of medicine: A good history and physical examination from both partners, relevant investigations and proper diagnosis are essential for treatment and counseling. Infertility is a complex problem and despite advances in treatment, not all couples will achieve their desired family size. In managing these couples, the clinician needs to bear in mind the emotional pressures that they face and try to minimize further stresses. A sympathetic and caring attitude helps to ease the pressures of treatment, given that even with the most advanced treatment modalities, there is a high failure rate.

REFERENCES

1. Skakkebaek NE, Rajpert-De Meyts E, Main KM. Testicular dysgenesis syndrome: an increasingly common developmental disorder with environmental aspects. Human Reproduction. 2001; 16(5):972-8.
2. Hruska KS, Furth PA, Seifer DB, Sharara FI, Flaws JA. Environmental factors in infertility. Clinical Obstetrics and Gynecology. 2000;43(4):821-29.
3. World Health Organization. Laboratory Manual for the examination and processing of human semen. Fifth edition. Cambridge University Press; 2010.
4. Hughes E, Collins J, Vandekerckhove P. Clomiphene citrate for ovulation induction in women with oligoamenorrhea. Cochrane Database of Systematic Reviews. Issue 3, 2002.
5. Hughes E, Collins J, Vandekerckhove P. Clomiphene citrate for unexplained subfertility in women. Cochrane Database of Systematic Reviews. Issue 3, 2002.
6. Hughes EG. The effectiveness of ovulation induction and intrauterine insemination in the treatment of persistent infertility: A meta-analysis. Human Reproduction. 1997;12:1865-72.
7. Glujovski D, et al. Cleavage stage versus blastocyst stage embryo transfer in assisted conception. Cochrane Database of Systematic Reviews. 2012.
8. 2012 ART National Summary Report. Center for Disease Control. USA.
9. Kuwayama M, Vajta G, Kato O, Leibo SP. Highly efficient vitrification method for cryopreservation of human oocytes. Reprod Biomed Online. 2005;11:300-8.

CHAPTER 34

Menopause and Hormone Therapy

Premitha Damodaran

Overview

- The staging of reproductive aging has been clearly defined using criteria such as the menstrual cycle length, serum levels of follicular stimulating hormone (FSH), Anti-Müllerian hormone (AMH) and Inhibin, antral follicle count and symptoms.
- Vasomotor symptoms can affect quality of life in up to 25% of women with 15% of women continuing to flush for 15 years or more. Hormone therapy (HT) remains the ideal treatment for symptomatic menopausal women when quality of life is affected.
- Genitourinary symptoms of the menopause (GSM) is now recognized as a significant problem with the menopause which worsens with time. Vaginal estrogen therapy and vaginal moisturizers is the treatment of choice.
- HT should not be used for the sole prevention of cardiovascular disease (CVD). Women who initiate HT around the time of menopause are at a low risk for CVD events whilst those who imitate late (after 10 years) have a higher risk especially in the first 2 years of use.
- The risk of venous thromboembolism (VTE) and ischemic stroke increases with oral HT but the absolute risk is rare below the age of 60 years.
- Though HT is recommended for prevention of osteoporosis in women "at risk", it is not initiated after the age of 60 years as long term complications may outweigh the potential benefits in these women.
- Though the oral route of HT is more common, the non-oral route avoids the first pass effect of the liver thus, suitable for women with hypertriglyceridemia, liver diseases and migraines.
- Breast cancer risk remains controversial, however seems more associated with combined estrogen progestin users (combined therapy > sequential therapy) with an increased risk in long-term HT users.
- Available data does not support HT for cognitive decline or dementia.
- There is presently no time limit for the duration of HT use. Every woman on HT should be regularly followed up and should have a risk/assessment carried out yearly.

INTRODUCTION

Menopause marks the end of the reproductive phase of the woman. It is not an abrupt event but a gradual process that lasts many years. A woman is said to be in the menopause when she does not get her periods for more than one year. She may face problems such as irregular periods, vasomotor symptoms such as hot flushes and night sweats, joint pains, mood swings, insomnia, tiredness, urinary disturbances and vaginal dryness. More importantly are long-term problems such as cardiovascular disease, osteoporosis, cognitive aging and dementia.

Hormone therapy (HT) remains the ideal treatment for symptomatic postmenopausal women when these symptoms interfere with quality of life. When started around the time menopause, HT does not increase the risk of cardiovascular disease, stroke and venous thromboembolism. HT has also been shown to increase bone mineral density and decrease osteoporotic fracture risk.

An individual risk profile is essential for every woman contemplating HT. There is presently no time limit for the use of HT; however, a risk/benefit assessment should be carried out on a yearly basis.

Definition

The reproductive life of a woman begins at puberty and ends at menopause. Her levels of estrogen and progesterone are dependent upon the oocytes that are recruited at the start of every menstrual cycle. Declining oocytes contribute to irregular periods and eventually menopause. The decrease in oocytes is reflected in decrease in serum concentration of inhibin B and a rise in follicular stimulating hormone (FSH)[1]

SECTION 2 Reproductive Endocrinology and Assisted Conception

Stage	−5	−4	−3b	−3a	−2	−1	+1a	+1b	+1c	+2
Terminology	Reproductive				Menopausal Transition		Postmenopause			
	Early	Peak	Late		Early	Late	Early			Late
					Perimenopause					
Duration	Variable				Variable	1–3 years	2 years (1+1)	3–6 years		Remaining lifespan
Principal criteria										
Menstrual cycle	Variable to regular	Regular	Regular	Subtle changes in flow/length	Variable length persistent ≥7 day difference in length of consecutive cycles	Interval of amemorrhea of >= 60 days				
Supportive criteria										
Endocrine FSH AMH Inhibin B				Low Low	↑Variable* Low Low	↑Variable* Low Low	↑>25 IU/L* Low Low	↑Variable Low Low	Stabilizes Very low Very low	
Antral follicle count				Low	Low	Low	Low	Very low	Very low	
Descriptive characteristics										
Symptoms							Vasomotor symptoms Likely	Vasomotor symptoms Most likely		Increasing symptoms of urogenital atrophy

(↑: elevated; FMP: final menstrual period; FSH: follicle-stimulating hormone; AMH: anti-Müllerian hormone)
* Blood draw on cycle days 2 to 5.
• Approximate expected level based on assays using current international pituitary standard.

Fig. 34.1: The STRAW + 10 Classification.[2]

The STRAW + 10 (2012) (Fig. 34.1) has replaced the original STRAW classification (2001) in an attempt to correctly identify the various stages of reproductive aging.[2]

Menopause Transition
The period of time when there is a variation in the menstrual cycle till the last period. The menopause transition is divided into:
- *Early (Stage -2):* Variable cycles with a ± 7 days change in intervals of amenorrhea. The FSH levels may be variable, however the Anti Müllerian Hormone (AMH) and inhibin B levels are low.
- *Late (Stage-1):* Lasts for 1–3 years with intervals of amenorrhea of ≥ 60 days. The FSH levels are >25 IU/L along with low AMH and inhibin B.

Perimenopause
The period of the time from the start of the variable periods till 1 year after the last period.

Menopause
One full year after the last period or any form of staining.

Postmenopause
The period of time from the last menstrual period till the end of her lifespan. The post menopause is divided into:
- *Early postmenopause:* The first 5–6 years since the last menstrual period. This can be further divided into the first 1–2 years (*Stage +1a*) and later 3–6 years (*Stage +1b*).
- *Late postmenopause (Stage +2):* The time frame till the end of her lifespan.

CHAPTER 34   Menopause and Hormone Therapy

The average of menopause is 51 years.[3] In Malaysia, two separate studies have confirmed the average age of menopause to be 50.7 and 49.6 years.[4,5] Factors that affect the age of menopause are:

- Current and past history of cigarette smoking. Smoking makes menopause earlier by 2 years. The age of menopause is also affected by passive smoking[6]
- Family history of early menopause[7]
- Ethnicity: Menopause occurs earlier in Japanese-American women and Hispanic women when compared to Caucasian women[8]
- Low body weight
- Living in high altitudes
- Vegetarianism
- Malnourishment in women.[9]

ENDOCRINOLOGY

The basis of reproductive aging in a woman is the loss of oocytes from her ovary. As a female fetus, germ cell differentiation start soon after the two cell zygote stage. Five to seven million germ cells are found five months after conception. Subsequent follicular growth and atresia result in one to two million oocytes being present at birth. A further depletion to 500,000 follicles occur by menarche followed by a steady exponential decline in follicles throughout the reproductive years. The rate of uptake and loss of follicles vary with time and in different women. In addition to providing the oocyte, the follicles secrete sex hormones. At menopause, the number of ovarian follicles fall below a certain threshold resulting in lower levels of estrogen, progesterone and to a lesser extent testosterone.[10,11]

The viability of the oocytes declines even before the corresponding increase in FSH which explains the gradual decrease in fecundity even from 30–35 years in normal women.

The **climacteric** is the phase from the sharp decline of the reproductive capacity which is signified by the drop in the number of ovarian follicles around 37.5 years of age, about 10 years before menopause.[10]

The increase in FSH levels is the cause of irregular cycles in the perimenopause. Estrogen levels which are higher than normal can be seen during the perimenopause, however, this is transient and due to episodic bursts of ovarian activity. The increase in serum luteinizing hormone (LH) only occurs when both the estrogen and progesterone levels drop due to disruption of the LH feedback mechanism.

The levels of testosterone also start declining, however, this is not in tandem with estrogen and progesterone. This imbalance between the estrogen and testosterone levels lead to hirsutism (over the face and chin) and loss of scalp hair in the woman.

SIGNS AND SYMPTOMS OF MENOPAUSE

The symptoms of menopause may start even before the last period. Many women start experiencing premenstrual symptoms (PMS) in the early 40's, even ten years before menopause. Women with history of severe PMS changes and postnatal depression are more likely to have a bad symptomatic menopause.

The signs and symptoms of menopause are classified into early menopausal, medium-term and late menopausal problems.

EARLY MENOPAUSAL PROBLEMS

Irregular Periods

Due to the rise in FSH levels, periods cycles may vary. The cycles may initially get shorter, and then longer. Due to estrogen dominance in the hormonal milieu, some women experience heavier flow, with clots and more painful periods during this time. Pelvic pathology such as fibroids, adenomyosis, uterine hyperplasia, cancer and ovarian cysts should always be ruled out. Changes in the breasts can occur simultaneously.

Vasomotor Symptoms

Vasomotor symptoms (VMS) affects 60–80% of women entering the menopause. They are common in the luteal phase of women with PMS and in the perimenopausal state. Low estrogen levels lead to a disturbance of the temperature regulating mechanism in the hypothalamus resulting in hot flushes.[12]

The community based SWAN study in the US showed a lesser incidence of hot flushes in the Asian women.[13] However, local Malaysian studies have shown the incidence of hot flushes to be about 57%.[14]

In up to 25% of women, physical discomfort and social embarrassment due to VMS can affect quality of life.[15] Although, most postmenopausal women experience hot flashes for less than 7 years, 15% of women continue having hot flushes for 15 years and more.[16]

Other vasomotor symptoms are sweating (night sweats), headaches, palpitations, tiredness and general lethargy, joint pains and sleep disturbances. The differential diagnosis for this group of symptoms include hyperthyroidism, hypertension, carcinoid tumors and neurological flushing.[13]

Treatment modalities can be divided into:

- Lifestyle modifications: Regular exercise, cessation of smoking and avoidance of known triggers such as hot drinks and alcohol.

- Hormone therapy:
  - Either estrogen alone (in women without a uterus) or an estrogen—progestogen combination (for women with intact uterus) have shown to decrease both frequency and severity by 75%[17,18]
  - Progestogen alone oral tablets (20 mg) or intramuscular injections (150 mg) can be given. The risk of breast cancer with progestogen alone therapy is still unanswered.[19]
- Non-hormonal therapy:
  - Antidepressants such as selective serotonin reuptake inhibitors (SSRIs) and selective serotonin and norepinephrine reuptake inhibitors (SNRIs) show a modest effect on hot flashes. Key points to their use include a more rapid response (in days) to hot flushes (in comparison to their response to depression) and their safe use in women with estrogen-related cancers.
    SSRIs such as venflaxine have been shown to have similar efficacy to low dose estradiol. However, these drugs have side effects such as dry mouth, reduced libido, constipation, headaches and vomiting. SSRIs cannot be taken in women on tamoxifen.[20,21]
  - Gabapentin, a known anti-epileptic and neuropathic drug has been shown to be affective mainly for night sweats, reducing it by 40–50%.[22]
- Complementary therapy: Acupuncture, paced respiration, hypnosis.[23]

Psychological Symptoms

The psychological symptoms associated with the menopause are insomnia, memory loss, mood swings, anxiety, loss of libido, difficulty in concentration and irritability. Though, the prevalence of depression is similar before and after menopause, depression was 2.5 times more likely to happen during the menopause transition than at any other time.[24]

Serotonin levels (which have a positive effect on mood) decrease when the estrogen levels drop leading to the emotional disturbances during the transition.

Treatment would consist of:

- Hormone therapy: Short-term HT has been shown to be useful for depression in the perimenopausal and early menopause, but not late into menopause[25]
- Antidepressants such as serotonin selective uptake inhibitors (SSRIs) are effective for perimenopausal depression
- SSRIs in combination with HT is given in women with both vasomotor symptoms and depression
- Counseling
- Behavioral therapy.

MEDIUM-TERM PROBLEMS

Genitourinary Symptoms of the Menopause (GSM)

The vagina and lower urinary tract are estrogen dependent tissues and estrogen deficiency leads to thinning of the vaginal epithelium. There is loss of glycogen content which causes a change in the vaginal ecosystem. There is loss of tone and contractility resulting in the vagina becoming narrower and shorter with a surface which is vulnerable to infections and ulcerations. Vaginal dryness, burning, pruritus, vaginal discharge and dyspareunia are common.[26]

The urethra and bladder trigone undergo similar atrophy. As the vagina shrinks, the urethral meatus becomes anatomically closer to the vagina. Infections in the vagina can lead to urinary tract infections and vice versa. Estrogen deprivations also leads to weakening of the connective tissue and muscles supporting the uterus, bladder and rectum which can result in uterine prolapse, cystocele, rectocele and enterocele. All this contributes to incontinence and pelvic pressure. Urinary tract infections become more prevalent.[27]

Menopause affects a woman's sexuality. The shortening and loss of elasticity of the vagina, along with vaginal dryness can cause dyspareunia. There is decreased blood flow to the vulva and other reproductive organs such as breast and skin resulting in reduced sexual arousal. A concomitant fall in androgen levels results in loss of libido as testosterone is important for desire, motivation and fantasies in both men and women.

Treatment

1. Moisturizers and lubricants: Vaginal moisturizers are intended for use one or more times a week and not just during sexual activity. Lubricants are added to decrease irritation during sexual activity. Together they improve vaginal moisture content and improve coital comfort but do not reverse most atrophic vaginal changes. They are ideal for mild vaginal atrophy.[28]
2. Vaginal estrogen therapy: Estrogen therapy is the most effective treatment for moderate to severe vaginal atrophy. Adequate estrogen therapy leads to restoration of the normal vaginal acidic pH and microflora, thickening of the epithelium, increased vaginal secretions and decreased vaginal dryness. Urinary tract infections and symptoms of overactive bladder is reduced. Stress incontinence and urgency do not improve with estrogen therapy alone.[29,30]

    Low dose vaginal estrogen therapy appears to be more effective than systemic therapy for treatment of vaginal atrophy; however, it is insufficient for the

relief of vasomotor symptoms or preservation of bone density.[31,32]
3. Selective estrogen receptor modulators such as ospemifene has been approved for treating moderate to severe dyspareunia. It appears to have a safe endometrial safety profile; however, hot flushes are common and the risk of thrombosis is present.[33,34]

Skin Changes

Type 1 collagen which is predominant in both the skin and bone decrease with menopause. About 30% of collagen is lost in the first 5 years of menopause after which there is a 2% decrease yearly. Decreased cutaneous collagen leads to increased aging and wrinkling of skin. External factors such as the sun and toxins cause further damage to the skin.[35]

Treatment

1. Hormonal therapy effect on skin has been controversial. Estrogen has been widely thought to increase the thickness and collagen content of the skin; however, the increase in skin thickness and elasticity is not statistically significant.[36-38]
2. Topical administration of all-trans-retinoic acid (tretinoin) appears to reverse many of the age-related changes in sun-protected skin.[39]

LATE MENOPAUSAL PROBLEMS

Cardiovascular Disease

Cardiovascular disease (CVD) is the principal cause of morbidity and mortality in postmenopausal women. The frequency of myocardial infarction (MI) begins to rise in the perimenopausal period and is approximately similar to the man by 70 years. However, women present differently, have atypical symptoms, remain undiagnosed till late which then increases morbidity.

The lipid profile alters drastically with the menopause. In women, an increase in triglyceride levels is seen as the main risk factor for CVD (Table 34.1). However, an increase in total cholesterol levels (even by 1%) is equally dangerous. Reversal of HDL/LDL ratios leads to formation of atheromatous plaques which then cause thrombus formation and strokes.[40]

Treatment

- Lifestyle changes: Modification in diet and exercise regimes to achieve a healthy normal body weight.
- Cessation of smoking.
- Active treatment of blood pressure, diabetes mellitus and hypercholestrolemia
- Hormone therapy.

Table 34.1: Risk factors for coronary heart disease in women.[41]

Unmodifiable risks	Modifiable risks
• Family history of MI or sudden death in male relative before the age of 55 years or female relative before the age of 65 years	• Sedentary lifestyle • Obese/overweight • Smoking or using any tobacco-related products • High blood pressure + diabetes mellitus

• Female >55 years
• Premature menopause < 40 years
• Preeclampsia or gestational diabetes during pregnancy or delivery of an IUGR (growth restricted baby)
• History of bilateral oophorectomy prior to menopause
	• Altered lipid profile
	  − Elevated serum cholesterol levels (> 6.2 mmol/L)
	  − Low plasma HDL levels (<0.9 mmol/L)
	  − Raised triglycerides
	• Excessive alcohol intake
	• Use of oral contraceptives
	• Metabolic syndrome
	• Increased levels of C reactive protein (CRP)
	• Stress

(BMI: Body mass index)

Effect of Hormonal Therapy

- Irrespective of age, oral estrogens effect lipid profile by:
    - decreasing low-density lipoprotein (LDL) levels up to 15%
    - increasing high-density lipoproteins (HDL) up to 16%
    - increasing triglyceride levels up to 24%.

    Transdermal estrogen preparations have a lesser effect.[42,43]
- Estrogens enhance endothelial function in young healthy women but not older postmenopausal women with established coronary disease[44]
- Estrogens improve insulin sensitivity; however, the data still remain inconsistent
- Oral estrogens cause a reduction in serum fibrinogen, factor VII and antithrombin III levels leading to increase in thrombosis. This is less affected by transdermal estrogen[45]
- Estrogens play a role as an antioxidant and as an anti-inflammatory. Estrogens cause an increase in hepatic synthesis of vascular inflammatory markers such as C reactive protein (CRP).[46] This increase in CRP correlates with changes in IL-6 through a non-inflammatory pathway with the estrogen only therapy and an inflammatory pathway for the combined therapy[47]
- Some synthetic progestogens such as medroxyprogesterone acetate (MPA) may negate some of the effects of estrogen on lipids and endothelial function.[44]

The effects of menopausal hormone therapy on cardiovascular disease have been confusing. The landmark studies that have helped clarify the role of HT and CVD are as follows.

The Heart and Estrogen Replacement Study

The Heart and Estrogen Replacement Study (HERS) was a randomized, blinded placebo controlled trial of continuous combined estrogen—progestogen use in post-menopausal women with documented coronary heart disease (CHD). HERS I ended at 4.1 years[48] when the study showed no significant decrease in CHD events (non-fatal myocardial infarction plus CHD related death) or in any secondary cardiovascular outcomes when compared to placebo group. The first year of HERS I actually showed an increase in coronary events, however post hoc analyses suggested a significant time trend decrease in CHD. There was also a 35% reduction in the risk of developing type 2 diabetes mellitus.

About 93% of the initial HERS I participants then continued treatment for an additional 2.7 years (HERS II).[49] Unfortunately, despite the additional years, HERS II failed to show a significant decrease in cardiovascular events in postmenopausal women with established heart disease. There were no differences in CHD events in women taking statins or aspirin simultaneously.

The Women's Health Initiative Study

The Women's Health Initiative Study (WHI) divided 27,000 apparently healthy postmenopausal women aged 50–79 years into 2 groups based on their estrogen only use (women without a uterus) or combined HT (estrogen/progestogen) use. The combined HT arm was terminated at 5.2 years whilst the estrogen only arm was stopped at 6.8 years.[50,51]

The combined HT arm of the WHI showed an increase in coronary heart disease by 29% (RR1.29, 95% CI 1.02-1.63) and stroke by 41% (RR 1.41, 95% CI 1.07–1.85), despite significantly improved lipid profiles.

The 'estrogen only' arm however, did show a decrease in CHD events, which unfortunately did not reach clinical significance (RR 0.91, 95% CI 0.75–1.12). The increase in stroke was similar in both arms (RR 1.39, 95% CI 1.10–1.77).

Post WHI analysis has shown that timing of exposure to HT as an important factor in determining cardiovascular risk. In the further combined analysis of the WHI trials, women who started HT closer to menopause appear to have a lower risk of CHD compared to women further away from the menopause.[52]

The Women's Health Initiative-Coronary Artery Calcium Study (WHI)-(CACS), an ancillary sub study performed in younger women between 50-59 years showed lowered evidence of subclinical atherosclerosis measured by coronary artery calcium scores on electron beam computed tomography (CT) in those on estrogen only therapy.[53]

The Danish Osteoporosis Prevention Study

The Danish Osteoporosis Prevention Study (DOPS) randomly assigned 1,006 women between the ages of 45–58 years to either combined hormone therapy or no treatment. After 10 years (and with a 16 year follow-up), women who were on combined hormone therapy had a significantly decreased risk of heart disease (HR 0.48; CI 0.26–0.87). There was no increased risk of cancer or stroke.[54]

The Kronos Early Estrogen Prevention Study

Kronos Early Estrogen Prevention Study (KEEPS) randomized 4 year double blinded placebo controlled trial in 727 women aged between 45–54 years showed that HT either in the form of cyclical hormone therapy, oral conjugated estrogen (0.45 mg daily) or transdermal estradiol (50 mcg daily) reduced menopausal symptoms and improved markers of cardiovascular disease such as HDL (increased), LDL (decreased with oral estrogen) and decreased insulin resistance (only with transdermal estrogen). There were no changes in surrogate markers of atherosclerosis progression.[55,56]

In view of the above data, the present stand on the use of HT and for cardiovascular protection is as follows:[57,58]

- HT should not be used for sole prevention of primary or secondary prevention of CVD
- Women who initiate HT shortly after menopause are at a low-risk for CVD events
- Women who initiate HT 10 years or more after menopause are at an increased risk of adverse cardiac events, especially in the first two years of use. The use of statins may mitigate the risks of coronary events with HT use.

Hormone Therapy, Cerebrovascular Events and Venous Thromboembolism

The association of estrogen with stroke has been conflicting over the years. The HERS study showed an increased risk in fatal stroke (RR 1.61, 95% CI 0.97–3.55).[59]

Both arms of the WHI trial was discontinued due to increased risk of stroke. The combined hormone therapy arm was stopped at 5.2 years due to a 31% increase in stroke risk (HR 1.31, 95% CI 1.02–1.9).[50] The estrogen arm was stopped at 6.8 years due to a 30% increased risk (HR 1.3, 95% CI 1.1–1.77).[51] There was an increase in ischemic stroke (HR 1.4, 95% CI 1.09–1.90) compared to hemorrhagic stroke (HR 0.82, 95% CI 0.43–1.56).

The Women's Estrogen for Stroke Trial (WEST) further reiterated the increased risk of ischemic stroke with a tendency towards a more fatal stroke.[60]

The baseline risk of stroke is correlated with age and is rare in the 50-59 years age group. The increased risk with

HT only becomes apparent 1-2 years after randomization and is further apparent after 60 years of age.

Venous thromboembolism (VTE) risk was noted to be increased in both arms of the WHI; the combined HT arm carried an increased risk of almost 2 fold (HR 2.06, 95% CI 1.6-2.7) and the estrogen only arm having a slightly lower risk in comparison (HR 1.32, 95% CI 0.99-1.75).[50,51]

The increase in risk was similar for both deep vein thrombosis (DVT) and pulmonary embolism and was particularly high in women with a previous event. This increased risk was also highest in the first year of therapy but persisted in the 5 years of follow-up.

Factors that increase the risk of VTE include the presence of factor V Leiden, a high dose of estrogen, older age, and obesity. Progestogens such as medroxyprogesterone acetate have also been associated with a higher risk of VTE.[61]

Further analysis of all data have now concluded:[57,58,62]

- VTE is higher in the older obese women, smokers and those with a family history of clotting problems. Avoidance of HT in these women is advised
- The risk of VTE and ischemic stroke increases with oral HT but the absolute risk is rare below the age of 60 years
- The incidence of venous thromboembolism with HT is very low amongst Asian women
- Observational studies point to a lower risk with low dose transdermal therapies.

Osteoporosis

Osteoporosis is a progressive bone disease that is characterized by a decrease in bone mass and density and structural deterioration of bone tissue which then leads to fragile bones and an increased risk of fracture of the spine, wrist and hip. Bone loss is exaggerated by menopause and estrogen deprivation. In the first 5-7 years after menopause, a woman might lose about 20% of her bone, while an average woman loses half her bone by the age of 70 years. Osteoporosis is twice more common in females as compared to males.[63]

Peak bone mass is achieved in men and women by the age of 25-30 years. Factors that determine the peak bone mass are genetics, physical activity and diet (Table 34.2). Bone loss is highest in small built, fair skinned women. In 1997 alone, the Chinese women in Malaysia accounted for 44.8% of hip fractures in Malaysia.[64,65]

Treatment

1. Lifestyle changes which include a healthy weight maintaining diet, weight bearing exercises to increase bone density, cutting down excessive coffee and alcohol intake along with stopping smoking.
2. Prevention of falls by organizing the house and work environment. Muscle and balance training exercises are important.
3. Adequate supplementation of calcium (1,000 mg to 1,200 mg) and Vitamin D (600 to 800 IU) daily. Optimal intake can be achieved with both diet and supplements, although ideally half of the calcium intake should be dietary.

Calcium carbonate (best taken with meals) and calcium citrate (can be taken in the fasting state) are among the common calcium supplements. Calcium citrate is advised for patients on proton pump inhibitors or H_2 blockers or who have achlorhydria.

The total dose of calcium (dietary plus supplements) should not exceed 2,000 mg/day as higher doses may be associated with nephrolithiasis. There is no proven increase in cardiovascular morbidity or all-cause mortality with regular calcium intake.[67]

In established osteoporosis, calcium supplementation alone is not adequate for fracture prevention, however is necessary for optimal response to other treatment modalities.[65]

Elderly who are institutionalized, immobile, lack outdoor activities and have a poor diet will benefit from 800 IU vitamin D supplementation daily. Vitamin D3 (cholecalciferol) is recommended over Vitamin D2 (ergocalciferol). Calcitriol, the most active metabolite of vitamin D is not recommended as it can frequently cause hypercalcemia and or hypercalciuria, necessitating close monitoring of its intake.[67]

Vitamin D supplementation has also shown improvement in muscle strength, balance, and risk of falling as well as improvement in survival.[68]

Vitamin D supplementation at 800 IU/day in combination with calcium, reduces fractures in elderly populations with vitamin D insufficiency.[69]

Table 34.2: Risk factors for osteoporosis.[66]

Nonmodifiable	Modifiable
- Advancing age - Ethnic group (Oriental/Caucasian) - Female gender - Premature menopause (< 40 years), early menopause (< 45 years) or surgical menopause - Fair skinned - Family history of osteoporosis in first degree relative - Personal history of fracture as an adult	- Low calcium and/or Vit D intake - Cigarette smoking - Sedentary lifestyle - Excessive alcohol intake (>3 units/day) - Excessive caffeine intake (>3 drinks/day) - Low BMI (<19 kg/m^2) - Impaired vision - Recurrent falls

(BMI: Body mass index)

In most of the recent osteoporosis trials, active therapies have demonstrated significantly increased bone density and greater fracture reduction when calcium and vitamin D is added to the main trial drug.[65]

4. Hormone therapy: Hormone therapy is effective in preventing the acceleration of bone turn over and bone loss associated with menopause. It also decreases the incidence of all osteoporosis related fractures even in women (of all ages) who are not at risk.

In the WHI study, there were 5 fewer hip fractures in the combined estrogen/progestogen arm (HR 0.67, 95% CI 0.4–0.9) while the estrogen arm showed a reduction of 6 fewer hip fractures (HR 0.61, 95% CI 0.41–0.91). Vertebral and other osteoporotic fractures were also reduced.[50,51]

Hormone therapy is the recommended treatment for the prevention of fracture in 'at risk' women before the age of 60 years or within 10 years of menopause. This reduction in fractures is present only if sufficient supplementation with calcium and vitamin D is present.

The initiation of HT after the age of 60 for prevention of fractures is not recommended since the long-term complications may outweigh the potential benefits.[58] Alternate osteoporosis therapies are available for the older osteoporotic woman.

Low and ultra-low doses of HT have been shown to be bone sparing and prevent postmenopausal bone loss though fracture prevention data is unavailable.[70]

HT does not have a long-term effect on bone. Its protective effect on bone mineral density may decline after cessation of therapy at an unpredictable rate and only some fracture protection may remain. In the WHI study, within a few years of discontinuation of estrogen, the cumulative incidence of hip fracture was the same in the estrogen and placebo arms.[71]

5. Selective estrogen receptor modulators (SERMs): Raloxifene can be used as therapy for the prevention and treatment of osteoporosis especially for women with an increased risk of breast cancer. It improves and preserve bone density at both the spine and hip after 4 years of use along with a simultaneous reduction in the risk of invasive breast cancer by 76%.

Raloxifene and estrogen are associated with a similar increased risk of VTE.[72,73]

6. Other treatment for osteoporosis would include bisphosphonates, parathyroid hormone, denosumab, teriparatide, calcitonin and strontium ranelate. Whilst bisphosphonates are used for both prevention and treatment of osteoporosis, the others are used purely for treatment.

Management of a Postmenopausal Woman

As menopause brings in a wide variety of changes both physically and mentally, awareness and preparation towards menopause become essential for every woman. A woman's health and well-being should be optimized for this transition and life beyond the menopause. Primary prevention becomes important and simple lifestyle measures should be emphasized.

Key lifestyle changes for a menopausal woman are:
- to normalize weight
- to initiate healthy dietary interventions
- to carry out regular exercises (preferably stretching and weight bearing variety)
- to avoid active or passive smoking
- to control excessive alcohol intake
- to control/delay medical disorders such as hypertension, diabetes and cholesterol
- regular physician reviews which would include relevant blood tests, gynecological examinations, risk factor scoring for gynecological and non gynecological cancers, and imaging such as regular mammograms and bone mineral density.

Hormone Therapy

The declining estrogen levels during the menopause lead to varying symptoms in women. Replacing their estrogen levels help restore normalcy, allowing them to cope with these changes better. Estrogen replacement was first introduced in the 1950s to women, without any deference to the presence of an intact uterus. Unfortunately non hysterectomized women then developed a higher incidence of hyperplasia and endometrial cancer; which led to the addition of progestogens to reduce this risk.

The present treatment modalities of HT are:

Estrogen Only Hormone Therapy

This is given for women who have had a hysterectomy. If she is still premenopausal and her ovaries (or ovary) is still intact, HT is not needed until the menopausal symptoms start. A blood test for follicular-stimulating hormone (FSH) would help confirm menopause.[74,75]

The types of oral estrogen available are:
- Estradiol valerate: A synthetic natural estrogen given at a dose of 2 mg/day. Low dose 1 mg tablets are available.
- Estradiol; a micronized version of natural estrogen given at doses of 2 mg/day. Low dose 1 mg tablets are available.
- Conjugated equine estrogens: estrogens distilled from the urine of pregnant mares given at the dose of 0.625 µg/day. Low dose 0.3 µg tablets are available.[76]

Combined HT (Estrogen and Progestogen)

Women with intact uterus need both estrogen and progestogens as the latter reduces the risk of endometrial hyperplasia and endometrial carcinoma. Progestogens given for ten days or more, offers endometrial protective effect with an odds ratio of less than 1.0.[50]

Progestogens (progestins) refer to all steroids used as a substitute for endogenous progesterone. Natural progesterones can be either micronized or in the form of dydrogesterone. Unfortunately, natural progesterones have low bioavailability and increasing its dose may lead to unpleasant side effects. The progestogens available are either derivatives of the 17α hydroxyl progesterone or the 19-nortestosterone.[77]

Multiple progestogen dosing regimen options are available for endometrial safety. The doses vary based on the type of progestogen used, starting at the lowest effective dose of 1.5 mg medroxyprogesterone acetate, 0.1 mg norethindrone acetate, 0.5 mg drospirinone or 100 mg micronized progesterone.[78]

There are two types of combined HT available:

Sequential HT
Progestogens are added for at least 10–12 days of every cycle. This causes a withdrawal bleed every month. Sequential HT is recommended for women who are in the perimenopause phase when bleeding irregularities are more common.

Continuous combined HT
Progestogens and estrogens are taken daily. It is recommended for women 1 year after their last period. There is continuous suppression of the endometrial lining of the uterus and if taken correctly this regime does not cause any bleeding after the initial adjustment period of 4 months when irregular bleeding is common. For long-term use, the continuous combined HT regime is preferred to the sequential regime. Though, a higher rate of endometrial cancer was found in the sequential group after 5 years of use, the addition of 10–12 days of progestogens every month appears to be adequate.[79]

HORMONE THERAPY DELIVERY SYSTEMS

There are varied delivery systems available for hormone therapy. The main differences in these delivery methods are in the hepatic by pass effect, achievable concentrations in the blood, and the biological activity of the active ingredient.

- Oral route: This remains the most common route. Both estrogen only and estrogen/progestogen combinations are available. There is a first pass effect through the liver which may contribute to increased triglycerides, thrombosis and pigmentation.
- Nonoral route: Patches (estrogen or estrogen/progestogen), gel (estrogen only), implants (estrogen, testosterone).

The nonoral route avoids the first pass effect of the liver and is thus, suitable for women with hypertriglyceridemia, liver diseases and migraines. There is no increase in VTE even in women with risk factors such as obesity and thrombophilias. C reactive proteins and sex hormone binding globulin levels are not raised with little effect on blood pressure. Transdermal ET may also be associated with lowered risk of deep vein thrombosis (DVT), stroke and myocardial infarction (MI).

A significant side effect in Asia to the patch is the irritation around the edge of the patch and premature detachment due to the tropical climate.

Transcutaneous creams produce similar effects as the oral form though metabolic changes related to the heart are less. Caution should be exercised to avoid inadvertent transfer to children and animals.

Subdermal estrogen implants are available in various sizes of 20, 50 and 100 mg estradiol each producing different durations of action. Tachyphylaxis is the biggest disadvantage. Testosterone implants are also available which help improve libido levels in postmenopausal women.

- Low dose vaginal estrogen therapy is useful for vaginal dryness, urinary problems such as incontinence and infection. Systemic absorption is minimal.[78,80,81]

ACTION OF ESTROGEN

The three major naturally occurring estrogens in women are estrone (E1), estradiol (E2), and estriol (E3). During the reproductive years, estradiol is the predominant estrogen. while estrone is predominant in menopause and estriol in pregnancy. Estradiol is the strongest estrogen with a potency of 80 times that of estriol.

The action of estrogen is mediated through receptors. The two distinct types of receptors, ERα and ERβ are similar but functionally different as they are expressed differently in the various parts of the body. ERα is predominant in the breast, uterus and vagina and is mainly involved in the reproductive events. ERβ is more general and is found in the ovary, brain, cardiovascular system and skin. When estrogen binds with these receptors, a conformational change occurs in the various end organs. Depending on the predominant receptor in the end organ, differing responses are then obtained.[82]

PRESCRIBING HORMONE THERAPY

Prior to starting HT, a detailed history along with a systemic review and a gynecological examination should be carried out. History should be directed to include potential indications and contraindications to HT along with a detailed family history of cardiovascular disease, migraines, VTE, cancers and osteoporosis. Blood pressure values, her height and weight measurements and BMI should be tabulated. A Pap smear (where relevant), a pelvic ultrasound and mammography is ideal as baseline investigations and again at regular intervals. Bone mineral density tests is encouraged for women with a high-risk of fracture.

Ideally, a risk/benefit assessment should be carried based on her existing health, medical and family history. The absolute risks/benefits based on the 50–59 year age group of the WHI study may be used as a guiding tool.[83]

Benefit or No Effect

- **Coronary heart disease:** 0.9 and 3.8 fewer cases per 1,000 women per five years for combined HT (estrogen + progestogen) users and estrogen only users, respectively
- **Mortality:** 5.3 and 5 fewer deaths per 1,000 women per five years for combined HT users and estrogen only users, respectively
- **Fracture:** 4.9 and 5.9 fewer cases per 1,000 women per five years for combined HT users and estrogen only users, respectively
- **Breast cancer:** 1.5 fewer cases per 1,000 women per five years for estrogen only users
- **Type 2 diabetes:** 11 fewer cases per 1,000 women per five years for all HT users
- **Colorectal cancer:** 1.2 fewer cases per 1,000 women per five years of use for combined HT users only.

Risk

- **Stroke:** 1.0 and 1.2 additional cases per 1,000 women per five years for combined HT users and estrogen only users, respectively
- **Venous thromboembolism:** 5 and 2 additional cases per 1,000 women per five years for combined HT users and estrogen only users, respectively
- **Breast cancer:** 6.8 additional cases per 1,000 women per five years for combined HT users
- **Cholecystitis:** 9.6 and 14.2 additional cases per 1000 women per five years for combined HT users and estrogen only users (data from HT users of all ages).

Contraindication to HT Use

- Known or suspected pregnancy or breast cancer
- Presence of estrogen dependent neoplasia
- Undiagnosed abnormal genital bleeding
- Active thromboembolic disorders.

Side Effects of Hormone Therapy

Breast tenderness and bloating are common when HT is initiated while headaches and nausea are uncommon. These initial side effects can be minimized by altering the doses and type of estrogen and progestogen. An increase in pigmentation may occur but allergic reactions are rare.

Women are often concerned that taking HT would exacerbate the weight gain that occurs in midlife. However, a meta-analysis of 28 trials found no evidence of increase in weight or body mass index with either estrogen only use or estrogen/progestogen use.[84]

Monitoring Treatment

Regular (yearly) blood profiles for lipids help monitor HT's effect on cholesterol levels and emphasizes the need for diet, exercise and possibly the use statins. Liver functions may be simultaneously assessed.

Combined HT may increase mammographic density. To reduce diagnostic difficulties, discontinuation of HT 2–4 weeks before the scheduled mammogram can be considered. A breast ultrasound can be added as an additional diagnostic tool. Women on HT should have regular mammograms 1–2 yearly.[17]

Women on combined HT often bleed during the first 3–6 months of treatment. If bleeding is prolonged beyond this, or is heavy and prolonged, a transvaginal ultrasound along with endometrial sampling is advised. A diagnostic hysteroscopy may become warranted. Once endometrial safety is confirmed, reduction of the estrogen/progestogen dose resolves this issue.

Bone mineral density measurements, preferably with dual-energy X-ray absorptiometry (DEXA) may be useful for long-term monitoring of treatment response. The minimal interval between DEXA measurements to show significant improvement is 18 months. Short-term responses can be assessed with bone turnovers.[17]

HORMONE THERAPY AND CANCERS

Breast Cancer

Though, cardiovascular disease is the leading cause of death in women, breast cancer appears to be more a health concern. Risk factors for breast cancer should also be considered in evaluating one's risk in developing breast cancer (Table 34.3).

Breastfeeding for more than 18 months and being physically active reduces the risk of breast cancer.

Mammographic density is known to decrease with age as the ratio of fatty tissue to glandular and fibrous tissue increase. Estrogen increases breast cell proliferation, breast pain and mammographic density which is then thought to delay the diagnosis of breast cancer.

The present data of HT on breast cancer is based on the HT regime used.[85]

Table 34.3: Risk factors for breast cancer.

Modifiable risks	Nonmodifiable risks
• Nulliparity • Having children after 30 years of age • Use of oral contraceptives for more than 15 years • Current use of medroxyprogesterone acetate contraceptive • Long-term use of combined HT (>5 years) • Drinking 2-5 glasses of alcohol daily • Being overweight (>25 kg/m^2)	• Breast cancer in first degree relative before the age of 50 years • Having the *BRCA 1* or *BRCA 2* gene • Being Caucasian • Having dense breast tissue • Having certain breast conditions such as fibrosis, mild hyperplasia, adenosis, ductal ectasia, phylloides • Early menarche • Late menopause • Exposure to diethylstilbestrol

In Combined HT Users

- There are 8 additional breast cancers per 10,000 women when HT is taken for 5 years and more.[50]
- Observational studies have suggested a higher risk in continuous combined users rather than in sequential therapy.[86]
- Evolving evidence suggests that the increased risk is due to pre-existing cancers that are too small to be diagnosed by imaging studies or clinical examination prior to HT onset.[78]
- Long-term follow-up found that the risk of new diagnosis of breast cancer dissipated within 3 years of cessation of combined HT[87]
- Women starting combined HT soon after menopause for more than 5 years showed a higher risk of breast cancer. The WHI trial showed a HR of 2.75, the French E3N also reported a greater risk of breast cancer in women who initiated HT within 3 years of menopause when compared to those with a long gap time.[88,89]

In Estrogen only Users

- There was no increased risk of breast cancer after an average 7.1 years of use
- The decrease in risk was noted in all age groups[52]
- There was a reduction in ductal carcinoma (HR 0.71; 95% CI 0.52-0.99)[90]
- Women who did develop invasive breast cancer, fewer breast cancer presented with localized disease and the tumors were larger and more likely to be node positive compared to those in the placebo group[90]
- There was a continued decreased risk after stopping estrogen (HR 0.77; 95% CI 0.62-0.95).[91]
- When estrogen was continued beyond 15 years, breast cancer incidence increased with an RR of 1.56 for more than 15 years of use.[92]

The hypothesis for the decreased risk in estrogen only users is the apoptotic effect that estrogen has on breast cancer cells in a low estrogen environment. However, the longer the breast cancer cells are estrogen deprived, the more probable the physiological estrogen will have a tumoricidal effect.[89]

Hormone therapy is not recommended for breast cancer survivors. Though, observational studies show no increased risk of recurrence of breast cancer, an RCT of HT use in women with breast cancer history (with bothersome vasomotor symptoms) was terminated after only 2 years of follow up, when significantly more new breast cancer events were diagnosed.[93,94] Targeted non-hormonal treatment such as antidepressants are now available for vasomotor symptoms.

Endometrial Hyperplasia and Cancer

Women with an intact uterus considering HT need both estrogen and progestogen. The addition of a progestogen is to negate the increased risk of endometrial cancer. Progestogen when given either in a sequential regime (10-12 days per month) or continuously, equally suppresses the risk of both endometrial hyperplasia and cancer.

Treatment with unopposed estrogen in postmenopausal women would provoke the following changes:

- Increase the risk of endometrial hyperplasia by 20-50% in one year[95]
- Cause a "duration related" increase in endometrial cancer by 17% per year of estrogen therapy to an odds ratio of greater than 8 after 10 years. This increased risk can persist 5 years or more after cessation of therapy[96]
- Increase the risk of both localized and widespread disease[97]
- Cause tumors which are less aggressive and with a better survival rate[98]
- Cause a "dose related" increase in endometrial cancer. Lower doses (esterified estrogens 0.3 mg) for two years did not increase the incidence of endometrial cancer compared to placebo but when given for 8 years, there was an eight-fold increase of endometrial cancer. Doses of 0.625 mg and 1.25 mg of esterified estrogens increased endometrial cancer risk by 28 and 53%, respectively[98]
- Equivalent doses of transdermal and oral estrogen have similar effects on the endometrium. Ultra low doses of transdermal estrogen results in low rates of endometrial proliferation and endometrial hyperplasia[99]
- A minimum of 10-12 days of progestogens (in cyclical regimes) must be given for adequate protection.[96,100]

OVARIAN CANCER

Recent data has emerged associating ovarian cancer with HT. The relative risk of ovarian cancer in current HT users (<5 years) is 1.43 (95% CI 1.31-1.56) while the risk for all HT users (current and past) is 1.37 (95% CI 1.29-1.46). The risk is similar for estrogen only users and combined HT users. The two most significant types of ovarian cancer were the serous variety (RR 1.53, 95% CI 1.40–1.66) and endometroid variety (RR 1.42, 95% CI 1.2–1.67).[101]

In the WHI combined HT study, a non-significant increased risk of ovarian cancer was seen with no differences in the tumor grade, stage or histology.[50] In estrogen only users, prolonged use (>10 years) found a small but significant increase in ovarian cancer.[102] However in a small study of women with *BRCA* 1 or *BRCA* 2 mutations, HT did not appear to increase the ovarian cancer risk (RR 0.93, 95% CI 0.56–1.56).[103]

The link between HT and ovarian cancer is still considered causal. There would be one extra case of ovarian cancer per 1,000 users and if the prognosis is typical, about one extra, ovarian cancer death per 1,700 users. Women who are at an increased risk of ovarian cancer should be counselled accordingly.

COLORECTAL CANCER

Observational studies have shown a reduced risk of colorectal cancer with oral HT use. There is no data on nonoral HT with risk of colorectal cancer.

In the WHI trial, the estrogen only users showed no effect on colorectal cancers with a suggestion of an increased risk in the older age group (70–79).[104]

The combined HT arm showed a reduced risk (RR 0.56; 95% CI 0.38–0.81)[50] which was predominantly for local disease. Where spread had occurred, there was more node involvement and a more advanced stage of diagnosis amongst the HT users.[105]

The reduced risk of colorectal cancers persisted for 4 years after cessation of therapy.[106]

LUNG CANCER

Lung cancer is a leading cause of mortality in women. Smoking (active or passive) plays a significant role. Though, large observational studies have reported a protective effect of HT on lung cancer risk, the results of the WHI study were differing.

The estrogen only arm of the WHI study did not show an increase in the risk of lung cancers (non-small cell variety). However, there was a non-significant trend towards an increase in risk in the combined HT arm. The age specific trend of the WHI study showed no increased risk in the 50–59 year age group with an increased risk of 1.8 extra cases of lung cancer per 1,000 women in the 60–69 year group.

The risk of death was also higher in the HT users especially if they smoked.[107,108]

Counseling regarding cessation of smoking is essential, especially if they are older women with present or past use of HT.

Hormone Therapy, Cognitive Aging and Dementia

Available data do not show evidence that HT increases or decreases the rate of cognitive decline or dementia risk.

Estrogen when initiated immediately after surgical menopause may show improvement in cognition.[109] Observational studies have shown a reduced risk of developing Alzheimer's disease (AD) with initiation of HT in the younger woman, suggesting an early window during which HT might reduce AD risk.[110]

In the older postmenopausal women, HT has been shown not to improve memory and that combined HT may be more harmful.[111] There was increased risk in dementia in the WHI Memory Study of women aged 65–79 years, especially in the combined HT group.[112]

The WHI Study of Cognitive Aging, an ancillary of the WHI and WHI Memory Study continued to show a worsening verbal memory but a positive trend towards figural memory in the combined HT users.[113]

HORMONE THERAPY AND DIABETES

Hormone therapy significantly reduces the incidence of type 2 diabetes mellitus. The postmenopausal estrogen and progestin intervention trial, revealed a lowered fasting glucose level but an elevated 2 hour post challenge test in HT users.[114]

In the WHI study, there were 15 lesser cases of type 2 diabetes mellitus in the combined HT arm compared to 14 lesser cases in the estrogen only arm.[115] Changes in the fasting glucose and insulin during the first year suggested a decrease in insulin resistance in the hormone group.

However, there is still inadequate evidence to recommend HT for the sole or primary indication of the prevention of type 2 diabetes mellitus in the perimenopausal or postmenopausal woman.

HORMONE THERAPY AND GALLBLADDER DISEASE

Both the WHI study and HERS trial showed a significantly increased risk of biliary tract disease and gallbladder surgery in postmenopausal women on oral HT.

After four years, the women on HT in the HERS were marginally higher at risk for biliary tract surgery when compared to the placebo group.[116] The WHI study showed an attributable risk of 9.6 and 14.2 additional cases per 1,000 women per five years for cholecystitis in their combined HT users or estrogen only users respectively.[117] Women receiving estrogen only were more likely to experience cholecystitis and undergo cholecystectomy.[30]

OTHER EFFECTS OF HORMONE REPLACEMENT THERAPY

1. **Recurrent urinary tract infections:** Vaginal estrogen reduces the frequency of recurrent urinary tract infections in postmenopausal women, while oral estrogen therapy has no role. Vaginal estrogen therapy is recommended for women who have three of more urinary tract infections per year. Localized estrogen would normalize the vaginal flora and increase the prevalence of lactobacilli and decrease *E. coli* vaginal colonization.[118,119]
2. **Urinary incontinence:** Both the WHI and HERS studies have shown worsening urinary incontinence in their oral HT users.[120]
3. **Falls:** Estrogen may improve balance and reduce tendency to fall, which in turn reduces the risk of fracture.[121]
4. **Osteoarthritis:** Postmenopausal women receiving long-term estrogen therapy (>5 years) had a 40% lower risk of hip osteoarthritis along with lower rates of subsequent arthroplasty.[122,123]
5. **Teeth:** Estrogen preserves teeth with the relative risk of edentia being 0.6 in postmenopausal HT users along with a lesser risk of osteoporosis of jaw.[124]
6. **Bronchospasm:** In the Nurses' Health study, the RR of new onset asthma was significantly greater in HT users compared to placebo. Other studies have shown conflicting data. Estrogen is not contraindicated for women with obstructive lung disease but worsening bronchospasm is a possibility.[125,126]
7. **Systemic lupus erythematosus:** Postmenopausal estrogen may increase the risk of mild to moderate flares. There is a 2.5 times risk of developing SLE for current estrogen users and a non-significant risk of 1.8 for past estrogen users.[127]
8. **Eyes:** The risk of cataract formation is decreased by 60% with long-term estrogen use (>10 years). Subcapsular and nuclear opacities were also decreased by 70–80% in estrogen users. HT has also been shown to reduce intraocular pressure and lower the risk of open angle glaucoma.[128–130]

The risk of dry eye syndrome was noted to be higher in postmenopausal HT users in some observational studies.[131]

Age-related macular degeneration, a leading cause of blindness in the elderly is also reduced by 48% in HT users when compared to the non-users.[132]

DURATION OF USE

The two main factors that have questioned the duration of use of HT is the increased risk of breast cancer and the effect of HT on coronary heart disease.

Combined HT users showed a higher risk of breast cancer and breast cancer mortality with 4–5 years of use in the WHI study, while the estrogen only users did not show any increased risk.[50,51] However long-term use of estrogen only HT (15–20 years) can be expected to increase breast cancer risk.[92]

Younger postmenopausal women do not have an increased cardiovascular, stroke and VTE risk with both estrogen and combined HT preparations. An initial increased risk was noted in the older woman. Observational studies have suggested a pattern of lower risk of heart disease when HT is used for 5 years and more.[133] The WHI estrogen only arm showed a significantly lower risk of CHD and MI in the 50–59 year age group.

General recommendations advice HT use is safe in the younger menopausal woman (within 10 years of menopause). There is presently no time limit for the duration of HT use. Every woman on HT should be regularly followed up and should have a risk/benefit assessment carried out yearly.

Premature Menopause/Primary Ovarian Insufficiency

Premature menopause (menopause before 40) or primary ovarian insufficiency (POI) is associated with:

- Lower risk of breast cancer
- Earlier onset estrogen related bone loss
- Possible increased risk of coronary heart disease (CHD). Observational studies show an increased risk of CHD with early menopause. However, the Framingham data reveal that women with CHD risk tend to menopause early.[134,135]

Normal data on hormone therapy effects cannot be used for women who menopause early, as physiological dosing of HT in these women convey minimal risks.

Women who have premature menopause or POI should be actively encouraged to take HT due to its positive effects on bone along with general protection for age-related issues. The use of HT is encouraged until the normal age of menopause.[78]

Bioidentical Hormone Therapy

These are custom made formulations that are compounded for an individual, based on the healthcare provider's prescription. These formulations may contain several hormones in combination (such as estradiol, estrone and estriol) and may be administered in the form of tablets, creams and sprays. The dosing of progesterone is difficult to assess because the levels in serum, saliva and tissue are markedly different.[136]

Some of these compounds are not government approved and the product information is not usually given with the preparation. Due to its non standardized regimes and delivery systems, studies are difficult to be carried out.

Until this data is available, the effect of bioidentical hormone therapy (BHT) should not be considered similar to conventional HT on the postmenopausal woman.

BHT is not recommended by international menopause societies.[78]

Tibolone

Tibolone is a synthetic steroid with weak estrogenic, progestogenic and androgenic properties. It can only be given for women with established menopause (no periods for one year) for relief of vasomotor symptoms and increase in bone mineral density. Due to its testosterone properties, libido is improved and it seems to have a better effect on the vaginal epithelium than the oral estrogen.

The Long-term Intervention on Fracture with Tibolone (LIFT) trial, which was designed to study the risk of tibolone on vertebral fractures was stopped early due to the increased risk of stroke.[137]

The data on breast is conflicting. Though, tibolone does not increase breast density, the Million Women Study reported an increased risk of breast cancer in current users of tibolone (RR 1.45, 95% CI 1.25–1.68) while in the LIFT trial, a decreased risk was seen.[138]

The Livial Intervention following Breast cancer, Efficacy, Recurrence and Tolerability Endpoints (LIBERATE) trial showed an increased risk of breast cancer in women with a previous history of breast cancer.[139]

Tibolone does not cause endometrial stimulation and has a better bleeding profile than combined HT users. Though, the Million Women Study showed an increase in endometrial hyperplasia with tibolone, the Tibolone Histology of the Endometrium and Breast Endpoints Study (THEBES) did not confirm this.[140]

RECOMMENDATIONS

The woman in menopausal transition goes though physical, mental, emotional and health changes. Primary prevention is important and should be emphasized. Key lifestyle changes in diet and exercise, maintaining ideal body weight, being proactive about regular health checkups, carrying our regular mammograms and targeted investigations as deemed necessary (such as DEXA screening) help ease the changes into the postmenopausal era.

HT should be encouraged for the younger postmenopausal woman with moderate to severe vasomotor symptoms. A risk-benefit assessment should be carried out prior to its commencement and at regular intervals thereafter.

Non-hormonal treatment for vasomotor symptoms are available, while vaginal estrogen creams which have minimal systemic absorption is available for vaginal atrophy. HT helps improve BMD and treat osteoporosis but should not be considered as the first line therapy for the osteoporotic woman. The risk of HT on cancers should be carefully evaluated against the background risk of the woman.

The Global consensus statement on menopausal hormone therapy (MHT) has put together present recommendations for HT use.

It states that in women less than 60 years of age or within 10 years of menopause, MHT:[141]

- Is the most effective treatment for vasomotor symptoms associated with the menopause
- Is effective for the prevention of osteoporotic fractures in "at risk" women
- May decrease coronary heart disease and all cause mortality in estrogen only users
- In combined HT users, there is a similar trend for mortality with no increase or decrease in the risk of coronary heart disease
- Local low dose estrogen therapy is preferred for women with vaginal dryness or dyspareunia
- Increases the risk of VTE and ischemic strokes however, the risk is rare below the age of 60
- May increase the risk of breast cancer in combined HT users and this risk is duration related. The risk decreases after treatment is stopped
- In the form of estrogen is sufficient for women who have had a hysterectomy
- Should be a decision based on the expectations, quality of life and health priorities as well as personal risk factors such as age, time since menopause and the risk for VTE, stroke, CHD and breast cancer
- Dose and duration of MHT should be consistent with treatment goals and safety issues and should be individualized
- Should be encouraged in women with premature ovarian insufficiency until the average age of menopause
- In the form of custom compounded bioidentical hormone therapy is not recommended
- Is not advice for breast cancer survivors with vasomotor symptoms.

REFERENCES

1. Burger HG, Cahir N, Robertson DM, et al. Serum inhibins A and B fall differentially as FSH rises in perimenopausal women. Clin Endocrinol (Oxf). 1998; 48:105.
2. Harlow SD, Gass M, Hall JE, et al. Executive summary of the stages of reproductive aging workshop +10: addressing the unfinished agenda of staging reproductive aging. Fertil Steril. 2012; 97(4):843-51.
3. McKinlay SM. The normal menopause transition: an overview. Maturitas. 1996;23:137.
4. Ismael NN. A study of menopause in Malaysia. Maturitas. 1994;19:205-09.
5. Premitha D, Nadkarni P, Nathan ST, et al. Malaysian women with regards to menopause and hormone replacement therapy. Abstract. 9th Malaysian Congress of Obstetrics and Gynaecology. 1999;29.
6. Fleming LE, Levis S, LeBlanc WG, et al. Earlier age at menopause, work and tobacco smoke exposure. Menopause. 2008;15:1103.
7. de Bruin JP, Bovenhuis H, van Noord PA, et al. The role of genetic factors in age at natural menopause. Hum Reprod. 2001;16:2014.
8. Henderson KD, Bernstein L, Henderson B, et al. Predictors of the timing of natural menopause in the multiethnic cohort study. Am J Epidemiol. 2008;167;1287.
9. Torgeson DJ, Avenall A, Russell IT, Reid DM. Factors associated with onset of menopause in women aged 45-9. Maturitas. 1994;19:83-92.
10. Faddy MJ, Gosden RG, Gougeon A. Accelerated disappearance of ovarian follicles in midlife: implications for forecasting menopause. Human Reprod. 1992;7:1342-6.
11. Richardson SJ, Senikas V, Nelson JF. Follicular depletion during the menopausal transition: evidence for accelerated loss and ultimate exhaustion. J Clin Endocrinol Metab. 1987;65:1231.
12. Vasomotor Symptoms. Society of Obstetrician and Gynaecologists of Canada (SOGC) Clinical Practice Guidelines. JOGC. 2014;36:S31-34.
13. Grisso JA, Freeman EW, Maurin E, Garcia-Espana B, Berlin JA. Racial differences in menopause information and the experience of hot flashes. J Gen Int Med. 1999;14(2):98-103.
14. Damodaran P, Subramaniam R, Omar SZ, Nadkarni P, Paramsothy M. Profile of a menopause clinic in an urban population in Malaysia. Sing Med Journal. 2000;41(9):431-5.
15. Kronenberg F. Hot flashes: epidemiology and physiology. Ann N Y Acad Sci. 1990;592:52-86.
16. Utian WH. Psychosocial and socioeconomic burden of vasomotor symptoms in menopause: a comprehensive review. Health Qual Life Outcomes. 2005;3:47.
17. Birkhauser MH, Panay N, Archer DF, et al. Updated practical recommendations for hormone replacement therapy in peri and post menopause. Climacteric. 2008;11:108-23.
18. MacLennan AH, Broadbent JL, Lester S, Moore V. Oral estrogen and combined estrogen/progestin therapy versus placebo for hot flushes. Cochrane Database Syst Rev. 2004;(4):CD002978.
19. Prior JC, Nielsen JD, Hitchcock CL, et al. Medroxyprogesterone and conjugated estrogen are equivalent for hot flushes: a 1 year randomized double-blind trial following premenopausal ovariectomy. Clin Sc (Lond). 2007;112:517-25.
20. Loprinzi CL, Sloan J, Stearns V, et al. Newer antidepressants and gabapentin for hot flashes: an individual patient pooled analysis. J Clin Oncol. 2009;27:2831.
21. Rada G, Capurro D, Pantoja T, et al. Non hormonal interventions for hot flushes in women with history of breast cancer. Cochrane Database Syst Rev. 2010;CD004923.
22. Reddy SY, Warner H, Guttuso T Jr, et al. Gabapentin, estrogen and placebo for treating hot flushes: a randomized controlled trial. Obstet Gynecol. 2006;108:41.
23. Santen RJ, Loprinzi CL, Casper RF. Menopausal hot flashes. 2015 www.uptodate.com Wolters Kluwer Health.
24. Freeman EW, Sammel MD, Lin H, Nelson DB. Associations of hormones and menopausal status with depressed mood in women with no history of depression. Arch Gen Psychiatry. 2006;63:375.
25. Soares CN, Frey BN. Is there a role for estrogen in treating depression during menopause? J Psychiatry Neurosci. 2010;35:E6-7.
26. Casper RF. Clinical manifestations and diagnosis of menopause. 2014 www.uptodate.com Wolters Kluwer Health.
27. Hajji SN. Pelvic relaxation and procedentia. In: Hajji SN, Evkans WJ (Eds). Clinical Reproductive Gynecology. Norwalk, Conn: Appleton and Lange; 1993;112-17.
28. Bachmann G, Santen RJ. Treatment of vaginal atrophy. 2014. www.uptodate.com Wolters Kluwer Health.
29. Suckling J, Lethaby A, Kennedy R. Local estrogen for vaginal atrophy in post-menopausal women. Cochrane Database Syst Rev. 2006;:CD001500.
30. Santen RJ, Allred DC, Ardoin SP, et al. Postmenopausal hormone therapy: an Endocrine Society Scientific Statement. J Clin Endocrinol Metab. 2010; 95:s1.
31. Cardozo L, Bachmann G, McClish D, et al. Meta-analysis of estrogen therapy in the management of urogenital atrophy in postmenopausal women: second report of the Hormones and Urogenital Therapy Committee. Obstet Gynecol. 1998;92:722.
32. Barnabei VM, Cochrane BB, Aragaki AK, et al. Menopausal symptoms and treatment related effects of estrogen and progestin in the Women's Health Initiative. Obstet Gynecol. 2005;105:1063.
33. Bachmann GA, Komi JO, Ospemifene Study Group. Ospemifene effectively treats vulvovaginal atrophy in postmenopausal women: results from a pivotal phase 3 study. Menopause. 2010;17:480.
34. Portman DJ, Bachmann GA, Simon JA, Ospemifene Study Group Ospemifene, a novel selective estrogen receptor modulator for treating dyspareunia with postmenopausal vulvar and vaginal atrophy. Menopause. 2013;20:623.
35. Brincat MP, Collagen GR. The significance in skin, bone and carotid arteries. In: Lobo RA (Ed). Treatment of the postmenopausal woman. Basic and Clinical aspects. 2nd edn. Philadelphia: Lippincott Williams and Wilkins; 1999;203-12.
36. Maheus R, Naud F, Rioux M, et al. A randomized, double-blind, placebo-controlled study on the effect of conjugated estrogens on skin thickness. Am J Obstet Gynecol. 1994;170:642.

37. Wolff EF, Narayan D, Taylor HS. Long term effects of hormone therapy on skin rigidity and wrinkles. Fertil Steril. 2005;84:285.
38. Phillips TJ, Symons J, Menon S, HT Study Group. Does hormone therapy improve age-related skin changes in post-menopausal women? A randomized, double-blind, double-dummy, placebo-controlled multicenter study assessing the effects of norethindrone acetate and ethinyl estradiol in the improvements of mild to moderate age related skin changes in the post-menopausal women. J Am Acad Dermatol. 2008;59:397.
39. Griffiths CE. The role of retinoids in the prevention and repair of aged and photoaged skin. Clin Exp Dermatol. 2001;26:613.
40. D'Agostino RB Sr, Vasan RS, Pencina MJ, et al. General cardiovascular risk profile for use in primary care: the Framingham Heart Study. Circulation. 2008;117(6):743-53.
41. Goff DC, Lloyd-Jones DM, Benett G, et al. 2013 ACC/AHA Guideline on the assessment of cardiovascular risk. J Am Coll Cardiol. 2014;63:2935-59.
42. Walsh BW, Schiff I, Rosner B, et al. Effects of post-menopausal estrogen replacement on the concentrations and metabolism of plasma. N Engl J Med. 1991;325:1196.
43. Binder EF, Williams DB, Schechtman KB, et al. Effects of hormone replacement therapy on serum lipids in elderly women: a randomized controlled trial. Ann Intern Med. 2001;134:754.
44. Rosano GM, Vitale C, Fini M. Hormone replacement therapy and cardioprotection: what is good and what is bad for the cardiovascular system? Ann N Y Acad Sci. 2006;1092: 341.
45. Brosnan JF, Sheppard BL, Norris LA. Haemostatic activation in post-menopausal women taking low dose hormone therapy: less effect with transdermal administration? Thromb Haemost. 2007;97:558.
46. Sumino H, Ichikawa S, Kasama S, et al. Different effects of oral conjugated estrogen and transdermal estradiol on arterial stiffness and vascular inflammatory markers in postmenopausal women. Atherosclerosis. 2006;189:436.
47. Reuben DB, Pala SL, Hu P, et al. Progestins affect mechanism of estrogen induced C reactive protein stimulation. Am J Med. 2006;119:167.e1.
48. Hurley S, Grady D, Bush T for the Heart and Estrogen/Progestin Replacement study (HERS Research Group). Randomised trial for the estrogen plus progestin for secondary prevention of coronary heart disease in post-menopausal women. JAMA. 1998;280;605-13.
49. Grady D, Herrington D, Bittner V for the HERS Research Group. Cardiovascular disease outcomes during the 6.8 years of hormone therapy: Heart and estrogen replacement study follow-up (HERS II). JAMA. 2002;288:49-57.
50. Rossouw JE, Anderson GL, Prentice RI, et al. Risks and benefits of estrogen plus progestin in healthy postmenopausal women: principal results from the Women's Health Initiative randomized controlled trial. JAMA. 2002;288:321.
51. Anderson GL, Limacher M, Assaf AR, et al. Effects of conjugated equine estrogen in postmenopausal women with hysterectomy; The Women's Health Initiative randomized controlled trial. JAMA. 2004;297:1465.
52. Rossouw JE, Prentice RL, Manson JE, et al. Postmenopausal hormone therapy and risk of cardiovascular disease by age and years since menopause. JAMA. 2007;297:1465.
53. Manson JE, Allison MA, Rossouw JE, et al. Estrogen therapy and coronary artery calcification. N Eng J Med. 2007;356;2591.
54. Schierbeck LL, Rejnmark L, Tofteng CL et al. Effect of hormone replacement therapy on cardiovascular events in recently postmenopausal women: randomized trial. BMJ. 2012;345:e6409.
55. Harman SM, Brinton EA, Cedars M, et al. KEEPS: The Kronos Early Estrogen Prevention Study. Climacteric. 2005;8(1):3012.
56. Harman SM, Black DM, Naftolin F, et al. Arterial imaging outcomes and cardiovascular risk factors in recently menopausal women: a randomized trial. Ann Intern Med. 2014;161:249
57. Cardiovascular disease. Society of Obstetrician and Gynaecologists of Canada (SOGC) Clinical Practice Guidelines. JOGC. 2014;36:S16-22.
58. de Villiers TJ, Pines A, Panay N, et al. Updated 2013 International Menopause Society recommendations on menopausal hormone therapy and preventive strategies for midlife health. Climacteric, 2013; 16:316 -37.
59. Simon JA, Hsia J, Cauley JA, et al. Postmenopausal hormone therapy and risk of stroke: the heart and estrogen-progestin replacement study (HERS). Circulation. 2001;103:638.
60. Viscoli CM, Brass LM, Kernan WN, et al. A clinical trial of estrogen replacement therapy after ischemic stroke. N Eng J Med. 2001;345:1243.
61. Martin KA, Rosenson RS. Menopausal hormone therapy and cardiovascular risk. Sept 2014. www.uptodate.com. Wolters Kluwer Health.
62. de Villiers TJ, Gass MLS, Haines CJ, et al. Global consensus statement on menopausal hormone therapy. Climacteric. 2013;16:203-4.
63. Hologic Inc. Normative data base. Waltham, Mass; 1995.
64. Lee JK, Khir ASM. The incidence of hip fracture in Malaysians above 50 years of age: variation in different ethnic groups. J Rheum Volume 10, Number 4, December 2007, pp. 300-305(6)
65. Clinical Practice Guidelines on Management of Osteoporosis. Ministry of Health, Malaysia. Malaysian Osteoporosis Society. Academy of Medicine, 2012.
66. Physician's Guide to Prevention and Treatment of Osteoporosis: National Osteoporosis Foundation, 1999.
67. Rosen HN. Calcium and Vitamin D supplementation in osteoporosis. Feb 2015. www.uptodate.com. Wolters Kluwer.
68. Autier P, Gandini S. Vitamin D supplementation and total mortality: a meta-analysis of randomized controlled trials. Arch Intern Med. 2007;167:1730-7.
69. Bischoff-Ferrari HA, Dawson-Hughes B, Willett WC, et al. Effect of vitamin D on falls: a meta-analysis. JAMA. 2004;291:1999-2006.
70. Lees B, Stevenson JC. The prevention of osteoporosis using sequential low dose hormone replacement therapy with estradiol 17 beta and dydrogesterone. Osteoporosis Int. 2001;12:251-8.
71. Heiss G, Wallace R, Anderson GL, et al. WHI Investigators. Health risks and benefits 3 years after stopping randomized treatment with estrogen and progestin. JAMA. 2008;299:1036-45.
72. Delmas PD, Ensrud KE, Adachi JD, et al. Efficacy of raloxifene in vertebral fracture risk reduction in postmenopausal women

with osteoporosis. Four year results from a randomized clinical trial. J Clin Endocrinol Metab. 2002;87(8):3609-17.

73. Cauley JA, Norton L, Lippman ME, et al. Continued breast cancer reduction in postmenopausal women treated with raloxifene: 4 year results from the MORE trial. Breast Cancer Res Treat. 2001;65:125-34.

74. Response to the Women's Health Initiative study Results by the American College of Obstetrician and Gynaecologists. Statement from the ACOG. August 2002.

75. Report for the NAMS Advisory Panel on post-menopausal hormone therapy. Statement from the North American Menopause Society. October 2002.

76. Hollihn Uwe K. Hormone replacement therapy. In: Schering AG(Ed). Hormone replacement therapy and the menopause. 1997;84-116.

77. Lobo RA. The role of progestins in hormone replacement therapy. AJOG. 1992;166:1997-2004.

78. The 2012 Hormone Therapy Position Statement of the North American Menopause Society. Menopause. 2012;19(3):257-71.

79. Jaakola S, Lyytinen H, Pukkala E, Ylikorkala O. Endometrial cancer in postmenopausal women using estradiol progestin therapy. Obstet Gynecol. 2009;114:1197.

80. Steunkel CA, Gass M. Results from 2010 NAMS survey on secondary transfer of transdermal estrogen preparations. Abstract P-85.menopause 011;18:1371

81. Lokkegaard E, Andreasen AH, Jacobsen RK, et al. Hormone therapy and risk of myocardial infarction; a national register study. Eur Heart J. 2008;29:2660-8.

82. Scughrus PJ, Lane MV, Scrimo PJ. Comparative distribution of estrogen receptor a (ERa) and b(ERb) mRNA in rat pituitary, gonad and reproductive tracts. Steroids. 1998;63:498-504.

83. Martin KA, Barbieri RL. Menopausal hormone therapy: benefits and risks. Feb 2015. www.uptodate.com. Wolters Kluwer Health.

84. Norman RJ, Flight IH, Rees MC. Oestrogen and progestogen hormone replacement therapy for perimenopausal and postmenopausal women: weight and body fat distribution. Cochrane Database Syt Rev. 2000;CD001018.

85. Stefanick ML, Anderson GL, Margolis KL; WHI Investigators. Effects of conjugated equine estrogens on breast cancer and mammography screening in postmenopausal women with hysterectomy. JAMA. 2006;295:1647-57.

86. Fournier A, Mesrine S, Boutron-Ruault MC, Clavel-Chapelon F. Estrogen-progestogen menopausal hormone therapy and breast cancer: does delay from menopause onset to treatment initiation influence risks? J Clin Oncol. 2009;27:5138-43.

87. Chlebowski RT, Anderson GL, Gass M, et al. Estrogen plus progestin and breast cancer incidence and mortality in postmenopausal women. JAMA. 2010;304:1684-92.

88. Anderson GL, Chlebowski RT, Rossouw JE, et al. Prior hormone therapy and breast cancer risk in the Women's Health Initiative randomized trial of estrogen plus progestin. Maturitas. 2006;55:103-15.

89. Jordan VC, Ford LG. Paradoxical clinical effect of estrogen on breast cancer risk: a 'new' biology of estrogen induced apoptosis. Cancer Prev Res (Phila). 2011;4:633-7.

90. Stefanick ML, Anderson GL, Margolis KL, et al. for the WHI investigators. Effect of conjugated equine estrogens on breast cancer and mammography screening in post-menopausal women with hysterectomy. JAMA. 2006; 295:1647-57.

91. LaCroix AZ, Chlebowski RT, Manson JE, et al. for the WHI investigators. Health outcomes after stopping conjugated equine estrogens among postmenopausal women with a prior hysterectomy: a randomized controlled trial. JAMA. 2011;1305-14.

92. Colditz GA, Rosner B. Cumulative risk of breast cancer to age 70 years according to risk factor status: data from the Nurses' Health Study. Am J Epidemiol. 2000;152:950-64.

93. Col NF, Kim JA, Chlebowski RT. Menopausal hormone therapy after breast cancer: a meta-analysis and critical appraisal of the evidence. Breast Cancer Res. 2005;7:R535-40.

94. Holmberg L, Iversen OE, Rudenstam CM, et al. for the HABITS Study Group. Increased risk of recurrence after hormone replacement therapy in breast cancer survivors. J Natl Cancer Inst. 2008 ; 100:475-82.

95. Woodruff JD, Pickar JH. Incidence of endometrial hyperplasia in postmenopausal women taking conjugated estrogens (Premarin) with medroxyprogesterone acetate or conjugated estrogens alone. The Menopause Study Group. Am J Obstet Gynecol. 1994;170:1213.

96. Weiderpass E, Adami HO, Baron JA, et al. Risk of endometrial cancer following estrogen replacement with and without progestins. J Natl Cancer Inst. 1999;91:1131.

97. Shapiro S, Kelly JP, Rosenberg L, et al. Risk of localized and widespread endometrial cancer in relation to recent and discontinued use of conjugated estrogens. N Eng J Med. 1985;313:969.

98. Chu J, Schweid AI, Weiss NS. Survival among women with endometrial cancer: a comparison of estrogen users and non-users. Am J Obstet gynecol. 1982;143:569.

99. Schiff I, Sela HK, Cramer D, et al. Endometrial hyperplasia in women on cyclic or continuous estrogen regimens. Fertil Steril. 1982;37:79.

100. Furness S, Roberts H, Marjoribanks J, Lethaby A. Hormone Therapy in postmenopausal women and risk of endometrial hyperplasia. Cochrane Database Syst Rev. 2012;8:CD000402.

101. Collaborative group on Epidemiological Studies of Ovarian Cancer. Menopausal hormone use and ovarian cancer risk: individual participant meta-analysis of 52 epidemiological studies. Lancet. 2015;9980:1835-42.

102. Garg PP, Kerlikowske K, Subak L, Grady D. Hormone replacement therapy and the risk of epithelial ovarian carcinoma: a meta-analysis. Obstet Gynecol. 1998;92:472.

103. Kotsopoulos J, Lubinski J, Neuhausen SL, et al. Hormone replacement therapy and the risk of ovarian cancer in BRCA1 and BRCA2 mutation carriers. Gynecol Oncol. 2006;100:83.

104. Ritenbaugh C, Standford J, Wu L, et al. Conjugated equine estrogens and colorectal cancers incidence and survival: the Women's Health Initiative randomized controlled trial. Cancer Epidemiol Biomarkers Prev. 2008;17:2609-18.

105. Freedman ND, Lacey JV, Hollenack AP, et al. The association of menstrual and reproductive factors with upper gastrointestinal tract cancers in the NIH-AARP cohort. Cancer. 2010;116:1572-81.

106. Delillis HK, Duan L, Sullivan-Halley J, et al. Menopausal hormone therapy and risk of invasive colon cancer; the California Teachers Study. Am J Epidemiol. 2010;171:415-25.
107. Chlebowski RT, Schwartz AG, Wakelee H, et al. for the Women's Health Initiative Investigators. Oestrogen plus progestin and lung cancer in postmenopausal women (Women's Health Initiative trial): a post-hoc analysis of a randomized trial. Lancet. 2009;374:1243-51.
108. Chlebowski R, Anderson G, Manson J, et al. Lung cancer among postmenopausal women treated with estrogen alone in the Women's Health Initiative randomized trial. J Natl Cancer Inst. 2010;102:1413-21.
109. Phillips SM, Sherwin BB. Effects of estrogen on memory functions in surgically menopaused women. Psychoneuroendocrinology. 1992;17:485-95.
110. Yaffe K, Sawaya G, Lieberburg I, Grady D. Estrogen therapy in postmenopausal women: effects on cognitive function and dementia. JAMA. 1998;279:688-95.
111. Resnick SM, Maki PM, Rapp S, et al. Effects of combination estrogen plus progestin hormone treatment on cognition and affect. J Clin Endocrinol Metab. 2006; 91:1802-10.
112. Shumaker S, Legault C, Rapp S, et al. Estrogen plus progestin and the incidence of dementia and mild cognitive impairment in postmenopausal women: the Women's Health Initiative Memory Study: a randomized controlled trial. JAMA. 2003; 289:2651-62.
113. Resnick SM, Espeland MA, An Y, et al. Effects of conjugated equine estrogens on cognition and affect in postmenopausal women with prior hysterectomy. J Clin Endocrinol Metab. 2009;4152-61.
114. Espeland MA, Hogan PE, Fineberg SE, et al. Effects of postmenopausal hormone therapy on glucose and insulin concentrations. Diabetes Care. 1998;21:1589-95.
115. Bonds DE, Lasser N, Qi L, et al. The effect of conjugated equine estrogen on diabetes incidence: the Women's Health Initiative randomized trial. Diabetologia. 2006;49:459-68.
116. Simon JA, Hunninghake DB, Agarwal SK, et al. Effect of estrogen plus progestin on risk for biliary tract surgery in postmenopausal women with coronary heart disease. The Heart and Estrogen/progestin replacement Study. Ann Intern Med. 2001;135:493.
117. Cirillo DJ, Wallace RB, Rodabough RJ, et al. Effect of estrogen therapy on gallbladder disease. JAMA.2005;293:330.
118. Brown JS, Vittinghoff E, Kanaya AM, et al. Urinary tract infections in postmenopausal women: effect of hormone therapy and risk factors. Obstet Gynecol. 2001;98:1045-52.
119. Stamm WE. Estrogens and urinary tract infections. J Infect Dis. 2007;195:623.
120. Waetjen LE, Brown JS, Vittinghoff E, et al. The effect of ultralow: dose transdermal estradiol on urinary incontinence in postmenopausal women. Obstet Gynecol. 2005;106:946.
121. Hammar ML, Lindgren R, Berg GE, et al. Effect of hormonal replacement therapy on the postural balance among postmenopausal women. Obstet Gynecol. 1996;88:955.
122. Nevitt MC, Cummings SR, Lane NE, et al. Association of estrogen replacement therapy with the risk of osteoarthritis of the hip in elderly white women. Study of Osteoporotic Fractures Research Group. Arch Intern Med. 1996;156:2073.
123. Cirillo DJ, Wallace RB, Wu L, Yood RA. Effect of hormone therapy on risk of hip and knee joint replacement in the Women's Health Initiative. Arthritis Rheum. 2006;54:3194.
124. Paganini-Hill A. The benefits of estrogen replacement therapy on oral health. The Leisure World Cohort. Arch Int Med. 1995;155:2325.
125. Troisi R, Speizer FE, Willett WC, et al. Menopause, postmenopausal estrogen preparations and the risk of adult onset asthma. A prospective cohort study. Am J Respir Crit Care Med. 1995;152:1183.
126. Hepburn MJ, Dooley DP, Morris MJ. The effects of estrogen replacement therapy on airway function in postmenopausal, asthmatic women. Arch Intern Med. 2001;161:2717.
127. Sanchez-Guerrero J, Liang MH, Karlson W, et al. Postmenopausal estrogen therapy and the risk of developing systemic lupus erythematosus. Ann Intern Med. 1995;122:430.
128. Worzala K, Hiller R, Sperduto RD, et al. Postmenopausal estrogen use, type of menopause and lens opacities. Arch Intern Med. 2001;161:1448.
129. Affinito P, Di Spiezo Sardo A, Di Carlo C, et al. Effects of hormone replacement therapy on ocular function in postmenopause. Menopause. 2003;10:482.
130. Newman-Casey PA, Talwar N, Nan B, et al. The potential association between postmenopausal hormone use and primary open angle glaucoma. JAMA Opthalmol. 2014;132:298.
131. Schaumberg DA, Buring JE, Sullivan DA, Dana MR. Hormone replacement therapy and dry eye syndrome. JAMA. 2001;286:2114.
132. Haan MN, Klein R, Klein BE, et al. Hormone therapy and age-related macular degeneration: the Women's Health Initiative Sight Exam Study. Arch Opthalmol. 2006;124(7):988-92.
133. Prentice RL, Manson JE, Langer RD, et al. Benefits and risk of postmenopausal hormone therapy when it is initiated soon after menopause. J Epidemiol. 2009;170:12-23.
134. Parker WH, Broder MS, Chang E, et al. Ovarian conservation at the time of hysterectomy and long term health outcomes in the Nurses' Health Study. Obstet Gynecol. 2009;113:1027-37.
135. Koh HS, van Asselt KM, van der Schouw YT, et al. Heart disease risk determines menopausal age rather than the reverse. Am Coll Cardiol. 2006;47:1976-83.
136. Bhavnani BR, Stanczyk FZ. Misconception and concerns about bioidentical hormones used for custom-compounded hormone therapy. J Clin Endocrinol Metab. 2012; 97(3):756-9. Epub 2011.
137. Cummings SR, Ettinger B, Delmas PD, et al. The effects of tibolone in older postmenopausal women. N Engl J Med. 2008; 359:697.
138. Beral V, Million Women Study Collaborators. Breast cancer and hormone-replacement therapy in the Million Women Study. Lancet. 2003; 362:419.
139. Kenemans P, Bundred NJ, Foidart M, et al. Safety and efficacy of tibolone in breast cancer patients with vasomotor symptoms: a double- blinded, randomized, non inferitory trial. Lancet Oncol. 2009;10:1315.
140. Archer DF, Hendrix S, Gallagher JC, et al. Endometrial effects of tibolone. J Clin Endocrinol Metab. 2007;92:911.
141. de Villiers TJ, Gass ML, Haines CJ, et al. Global consensus statement on menopausal hormone therapy. Climacteric. 2013; 16(2):203-4.

SECTION 3
Gynecologic Oncology

35. Gynecological Cancer Screening
36. Preinvasive and Invasive Cancer of the Cervix
37. Ovarian Cancer
38. Uterine Malignancy
39. Vulvar Cancer
40. Gestational Trophoblastic Neoplasia
41. Radiotherapy and Systemic Anticancer Therapy in Gynecological Malignancy
42. Palliative Care

CHAPTER 35

Gynecological Cancer Screening

V Sivanesaratnam

Overview

- The aim of screening is to detect the disease before symptoms occur, i.e. at the pre-invasive or more curable stage, when timely treatment can avert disability and mortality.
- The uterine cervix is the most frequent site in the genital tract affected by cancer. Cervical cancer is easily detected in the preinvasive or cervical intraepithelial neoplasia (CIN) phase by cervical cytology; cervical cancer is thus perhaps the only cancer that is preventable.
- The Papanicolaou (Pap) smear test fulfills the most important criteria of a useful screening test: good sensitivity and specificity, low cost, and little risk or discomfort to the patient.
- Newer terms low- and high-grade squamous intraepithelial lesion (SIL) have emerged.
- Low-grade precursor lesions usually regress, and in a compliant low-risk population, this can be managed by repeat cytology.
- Colposcopy would be the next step as it would help assess the site, extent and severity of the lesion, enabling "targeted" biopsies.
- The availability of vaccines against the 'high risk' human papilloma virus (HPV 16 and 18) is an important milestone in the prevention of cervical cancer.
- Ovarian cancer is a leading cause of death. The paucity of early symptoms and the intrapelvic location of the ovaries which limits their accessibility to physical examination makes this an elusive disease. This results in the majority presenting in an advanced stage.
- There are no proven screening tests for ovarian cancer. A high index of suspicion is essential for early diagnosis.
- The risk factors for endometrial cancer are obesity, use of estrogen after menopause, history of anovulation and nulliparity, breast cancer and tamoxifen therapy. Routine screening of women for endometrial cancer is not of any proven benefit. No screening test has been evaluated for its impact on endometrial cancer mortality, even amongst "high-risk" women.

INTRODUCTION

The genital tract is one of the most common situations of primary malignant disease in women. Such malignancies continue to be a major cause of mortality amongst women worldwide. The *aim of screening* is to detect the disease before symptoms occur, i.e. at the preinvasive or more curable stage, when timely treatment can avert disability and mortality. The screening test is not intended to be diagnostic, but rather to differentiate the population likely or not likely to have the disease; the former will subsequently require further tests to confirm the diagnosis. A suitable screening test should have high specificity, sensitivity and positive predictive value and should not be costly.

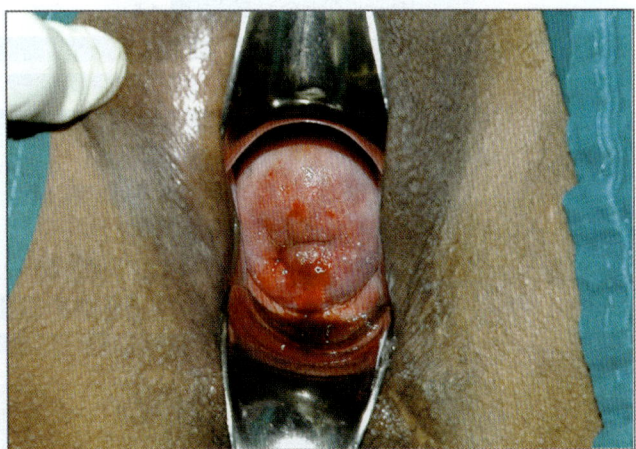

Fig. 35.1: Unhealthy cervix.

The three most prevalent gynecological cancers in the Asia-Oceania region are cervical, ovarian and endometrial cancers. Methods of screening these cancers will now be discussed.

CERVICAL CANCER

The uterine cervix is the most frequent site in the genital tract affected by cancer. It is important to note that all preinvasive and very early invasive lesions of the cervix are completely asymptomatic. Figure 35.1 shows picture of an unhealthy cervix. Cervical cancer is easily detected in the preinvasive or cervical intraepithelial neoplasia (CIN) phase by cervical cytology; *"cervical cancer is, thus, perhaps the only cancer that is preventable".* Yet in many parts of the developing and underdeveloped world cervical cancer is diagnosed in a late stage and as a consequence results in a high mortality. About 50% of all women in the industrialized countries would have had at least one Pap smear test during a 5-year period, compared to only 5% in developing countries.[1] Thus, in the industrialized world cervical cancer is uncommon, ranking 10th after more common cancers, such as breast, lungs, colon, etc.[1] Data from several Scandinavian studies showed that organized screening programs resulted in sharp reductions in incidence and mortality from cervical cancer; an 80% reduction in mortality was observed in Iceland, whilst a reduction in mortality of 50 and 34% occurred in Finland and Sweden. Similar reductions have been observed in the US and Canada.[2]

In contrast, cervical cancer continues to be a leading cause of mortality and morbidity in developing countries. In Malaysia, it is the third most common cancer in females (after breast cancer and colorectal cancer). The peak incidence is 60–69 years; the disease is more common amongst Chinese compared to Malays and Indians[3] (Fig. 35.2).

Papanicolaou Smear

The Papanicolaou (Pap) smear fulfills the most important criteria of a useful screening test: good sensitivity and specificity, low cost, and little risk or discomfort to the patient. Furthermore, effective modes of therapy are available when abnormal cells are detected.

Taking a Cervical Smear

Invasive cervical cancer begins in the transformation zone, the area at or just outside the squamocolumnar junction, which was originally lined by columnar epithelium, and which by the process of metaplasia becomes covered by squamous epithelium. It is this area that is at risk of carcinogenic attack and which may show abnormal changes. As these changes may occur in just small foci of the transformation zone, sweeping the sampling device a full 360° to cover the whole transformation zone is essential for proper sampling. It is obvious that the cervix must be well-visualized first, as occasionally obvious carcinoma may give "negative" smears because blood, necrotic material and leukocytes may obscure the often poorly preserved malignant cells.

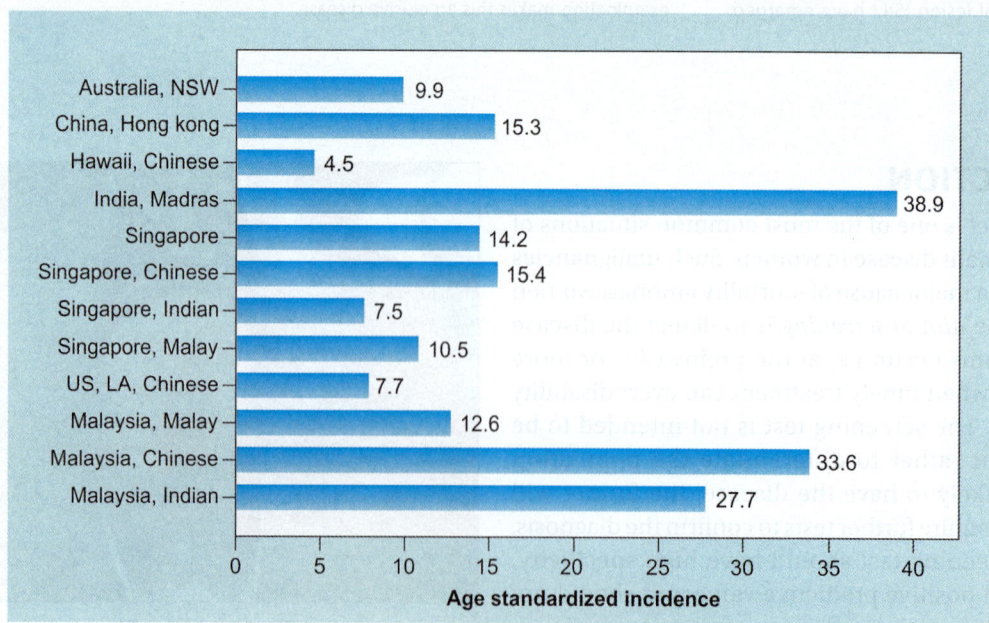

Fig. 35.2: Cervical cancer age—standardized incidence per 100,000 population.
Source: First Report of the National Cancer Registry—Malaysia, 2002

The use of traditional lubricants to aid speculum examination is best avoided as these may induce artifact and interfere with the interpretation of the smear. If necessary water can be used as a lubricant.

Whilst various techniques have been used for obtaining a cervical smear, we have found the use of a wooden spatula to scrape the ectocervix and moist cotton tip application to obtain an endocervical sample, will adequately sample the whole transformation zone. Such combined endocervical and ectocervical samples halves the false negative rate. Slides should be immediately fixed to avoid drying artifact resulting in loss of staining specificity and morphological detail.

Significance of Endocervical Cells in Smear

The importance of the presence of endocervical cells in cervical smears has been stressed; the use of the cytobrush does significantly increase the yield of endocervical cells. It is often said that the presence of endocervical cells in a cervical smear implies that the squamocolumnar junction has been adequately sampled. It appears that the pursuit of endocervical cells as an indication of an adequate smear has been overemphasized. In 10% of premenopausal and 50% of postmenopausal women, endocervical cells may not be obtained even on repeat smears. There is no doubt that complete sampling of the transformation zone where CIN begins is essential to reduce the number of false negative smears; thus, the importance of visualization of the cervix and taking an adequate ectocervical smear should not be overlooked. In postmenopausal women, an additional smear with a cytobrush will be of help as the transformation zone usually recedes into the cervical canal.

False-negative Smears

This may arise from:
- A sampling error by the clinician
- A screening error by the cytotechnician who has failed to recognize the abnormal cells
- An error in interpretation.

Clinician sampling error accounts for two-thirds of false negative smears, primarily due to failure to obtain an adequate smear from the transformation zone. Screening errors of 17–58.5% have been reported.

Liquid-based Cytology

This test (Thinprep) aims to reduce the incidence of false-negative results by optimizing the cell collection and preparation by removing mucus, protein and red blood cells from the preparation; this allows for cells to be uniformly distributed, improves fixation and preserves cellular architecture. This is new technology requiring technicians and cytopathologists to be retrained. Other disadvantages include difficulty in assessing glandular abnormalities.

Automated Cytological Screening

As most Pap smears do not contain atypical cells, a semi-automated system, such as PAPNET might help minimize the tedious aspects of the cytotechnician's tasks. The use of PAPNET may facilitate identification of high grade squamous intraepithelial lesions missed during standard cytological screening. Whilst this method of screening is more accurate than the Pap smear, this is very expensive and may not be cost-effective in developing countries.

The Bethesda System (TBS)

Recently, the terms low- and high-grade squamous intraepithelial lesion (SIL) have emerged from the TBS system of reporting cervical/vaginal smears.[4] Under this system are defined:

- Atypical squamous cells of undetermined significance (ASCUS)
- Inclusion of changes associated with human papilloma virus (HPV) (i.e. koilocytosis) with CIN 1 as low-grade squamous intraepithelial (LSIL) lesion
- Use of only two terms, LSIL and high-grade squamous intraepithelial lesion (HSIL) to encompass the spectrum of squamous cell carcinoma precursors, in lieu of the degrees of dysplasia/CIS and the three grades of CIN.

Low-grade precursor lesions usually regress, and in a compliant low-risk population, this can be managed by repeat cytology. However, whatever method of classification is used for reporting cervical smears, clinicians must take note that this does not confirm the diagnosis. Any form of atypia seen on the smear is significant and needs further evaluation.

Adenocarcinoma

Screening programs probably have little effect on detection of adenocarcinomas. At least 40% of adenocarcinoma or adenosquamous carcinoma were not detected on cervical cytology in an Australian study.[6] In a case-control study in Japan,[7] the risk of adenocarcinoma of the cervix was reduced by only 55% by cervical cytology compared to 86% reduction in the risk of squamous cell carcinoma.

Nevertheless, it is important to note that an increasing number of adenocarcinoma are now being seen, particularly in young women. An incidence of 26.9% of invasive adenocarcinoma has been reported by Sivanesaratnam et al.[8]

Who are the Women "at risk"?

There is no single ideal screening program at present. A balance of good medicine and practical/financial aspects needs to be considered. The population "at risk" needs to be screened. These include:

- Early age of coitus
- Experience with multiple sexual partners
- "High-risk" males and their multiple exposures.

The above factors would help promote the development and spread of sexually transmitted diseases (STDs).

Human Papilloma Virus (HPV)

Epidemiological studies indicate that cervical cancer and its precursor are caused principally, if not exclusively, by HPV infection.[9] Of more than 90 subtypes of HPV so far detected, about 20 infect the cervix. The *"high-risk" HPV types* are 16, 18, 31, 33, 35, 39, 45, 51, 52, 56 and 58 and the *"low-risk" types* are 6, 11, 42, 43 and 44. Reid et al.[10] demonstrated that almost all patients who had HPV type 6 and 11 had CIN 1 or 2 lesions, whilst 90% of patients with CIN 3 and invasive lesions were infected with HPV 16, 18 or 31.

Human papillomavirus infection is much more common in the younger than older patients. Recent evidence[9] suggests that in many women HPV infection is transient and is cleared within the first 12–24 months. Thus, whilst the presence of HPV infection in the young is an indication of sexual activity rather than a cervical cancer risk, in older women persistence of HPV is an indication of increased cervical cancer risk. A combination of *Pap smear* and *HPV DNA screening* can help detect 95% of patients with high-grade lesions, 100% with invasive cancers and 70% with low-grade lesions.[5, 11] This method is being considered as a primary screening method in some countries.

In the University of Malaya Medical Center, Kuala Lumpur, HPV16 was present in 56.4% of squamous cell carcinoma and in 35.5% of adeno-/adenosquamous carcinoma of the cervix; HPV18 was seen in 5.5% squamous cell carcinoma and in 17.6% adeno-/adenosquamous carcinoma.

HPV Vaccines

Vaccines have been developed against the two common viruses—HPV16 and HPV18; this is an important milestone in the prevention of cervical cancer. Currently, there are two vaccines available:

- Gardasil (HPV 6,11,16,18)
- Cervarix (HPV 16,18).

Many countries have commenced vaccination programmes, vaccinating young adolescent girls. Hopefully with the wide use of these vaccines against HPV, cervical cancer incidence will be reduced and ultimately eliminated.

Other "risk factors" include:

- Smoking—nicotine and cotinine were noted to be concentrated in the cervical mucus in patients with CIN 3; this may represent a mechanism for the association of cervical neoplasia and smoking.[12]
- Oral contraceptives—a firm statement on its role in causation of cervical cancer cannot yet be made.

Clearly, the multifactorial etiology of cervical carcinoma must be accommodated in screening programs.

What should the Pap Smear Screening Interval be?

As squamous cell carcinoma of the cervix is related to sexual activity, screening should commence at onset of sexual activity. There is no agreement as to how frequently it should be done. The Canadian Task force, noting that dysplasia may predate CIN 3 by a decade or so, suggested that in "low risk" women smears at 3-yearly interval may be adequate. The American Cancer Society and the American College of Obstetricians and Gynecologists similarly permit less frequent screening in a "low risk" woman after she has had 3 annual satisfactory cytological smears.

A large retrospective study on invasive cervical carcinoma by Morrell et al.[13] found at least 2 negative smears in 20% of cases in the 3 years prior to diagnosis of cancer. Similarly, an Alaskan study[14] noted 52% of native women who developed invasive cervical cancer had a normal Pap smear 3 years prior to diagnosis. Although sampling error is a possibility, these developments suggest a rapidly developing carcinoma. This means that clinicians must deal with two groups of patients: one with rapidly growing CIN lesions and the other with slow growing ones. Annual screening would thus appear appropriate.

When should Screening Stop?

This is still under debate. For women who have had regular negative smears, 60 years has been suggested as a safe cut-off point. Ashley[14] pointed out the existence of two different forms of cervical cancer:

- Those with a recognizable preinvasive stage occurring in young women
- A less common type occurring in older women which develops without a detectable precancerous phase.

16.6% of women with early invasive carcinoma of the cervix undergoing radical hysterectomy were noted by us to be between 50 and 69 years.[8] Furthermore, the peak incidence of cervical carcinoma in Malaysia is between 60 and 69 years.[3] Age should, therefore, be no barrier for cervical screening, particularly when the woman has had no previous Pap smear.

The Pap smear test is not a helpful screening test for cervical cancer in the following groups of women:
- Women <21 years of age
- Women who have had a total hysterectomy for a benign lesion of the uterus
- Women >65 years of age who have had a Pap test showing no abnormal cells. These women are unlikely to have an abnormal Pap test in future.

The Abnormal Smear—What is the Next Step?

The cervical smear detects that an abnormal area exists and provides an estimate of its severity. Colposcopy would be the next step as it would help assess the site, extent and severity of the lesion, enabling "targeted" biopsies without resort to cone biopsy or more radical measures. Flowchart 35.1 outlines the plan of management.

When no lesion is visible and the whole transformation zone has been visualized, a false positive smear has to be considered. The time and expense involved in performing colposcopic evaluation makes colposcopy less effective than cytology for routine cervical cancer screening. It is, however, useful for following up women with an abnormal smear in pregnancy to help monitor the progression, if any, of the lesion; absence of appearance of invasion will allow a conservative approach leaving the definite treatment to be considered after delivery.

Other Methods of Screening for Cervical Cancer

- *Cervicography:* This colpophotographic screening technique, which photographs the cervix after application of acetic acid, has a very high false positive rate and is costly compared with Pap smear; it is, thus, inappropriate as a primary screening tool
- *'Down staging' for cancer of the cervix:* Lack of laboratory facilities or resources for cytological screening is largely responsible for the late stage at diagnosis of cervical cancer in developing countries. An active attempt should be instituted to detect the cancer at an early stage when it is curable. This approach of "clinical downstaging" by visualization of the cervix with a speculum and recognizing cervical abnormalities would require training of nurses and other paramedics. However, a recent evaluation found unaided visual inspection not very promising either as a preselection procedure for cytology or as a low-technology measure for cervical cancer screening.[15]

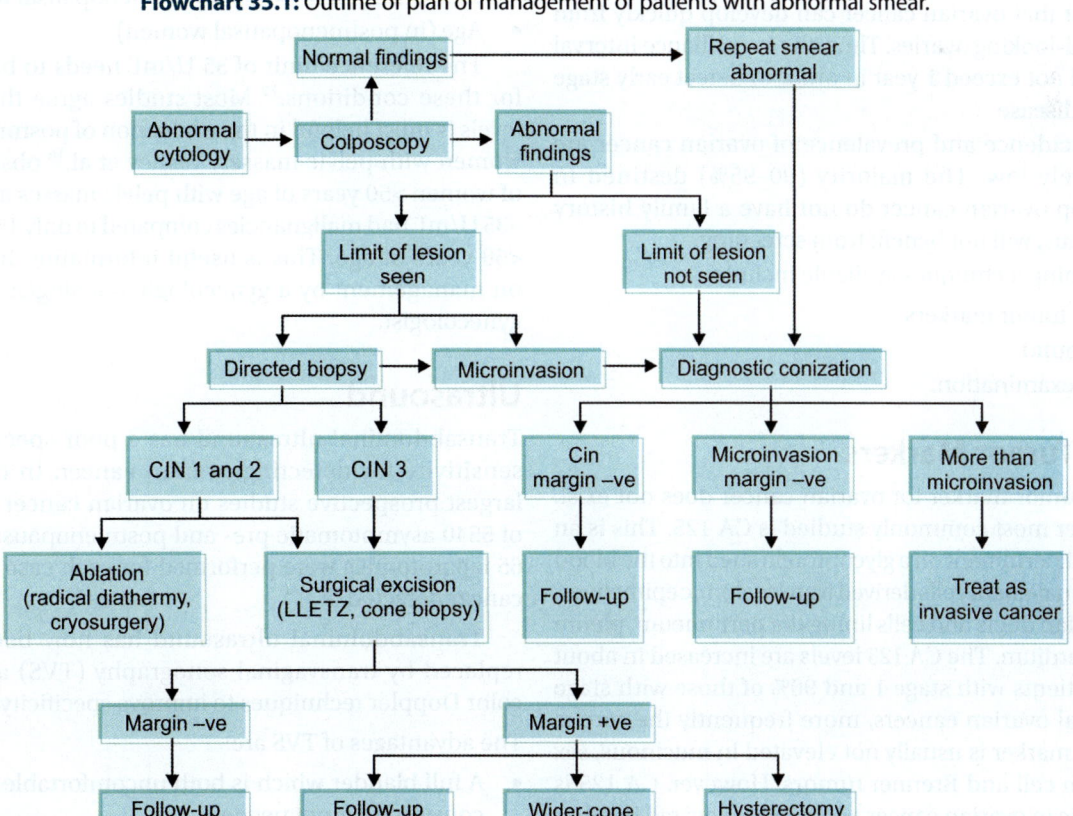

Flowchart 35.1: Outline of plan of management of patients with abnormal smear.

(LLETZ: Large loop excision of the transformation zone)

OVARIAN CANCER

Ovarian cancer is a leading cause of death amongst women both in the West and in the Asia-Oceania region, and other parts of the world. In spite of advances in surgical staging and debulking surgery and the use of modern chemotherapeutic regimes, the overall survival for ovarian cancer is only 41.6%.[16] The paucity of early symptoms and the intrapelvic location of the ovaries which limits their accessibility to physical examination makes this an elusive disease. This results in the majority presenting in an advanced stage. A major reduction in mortality will not occur until patients can be identified with early stage disease; the 5-year survival in stage 1 epithelial ovarian cancer is 80–90%.[16] A reliable screening test is, therefore, essential.

Attempts to screen the disease have often resulted in frustration; this is accounted for by several factors:

- The anatomic location of the ovaries is not amenable to any direct inspection
- Unlike cervical cancer, ovarian cancer lacks any defined precursor lesion
- Little is understood of the natural history, and time interval for progression from early to advanced disease is not known. Several reports in the literature of advanced ovarian cancer developing within months of a negative laparoscopy and peritoneal cytology, would suggest that ovarian cancer can develop quickly from normal-looking ovaries. Thus, the surveillance interval should not exceed 1 year in order to detect early stage of the disease
- The incidence and prevalence of ovarian cancer are relatively low. The majority (90–95%) destined to develop ovarian cancer do not have a family history and, thus, will not benefit from screening.

The screening techniques available include:
- Serum tumor markers
- Ultrasound
- Pelvic examination.

Serum Tumor Markers

An ideal tumor marker for ovarian cancer does not exist. The marker most commonly studied is CA 125. This is an antigenic determinant on a glycoprotein shed into the blood stream by malignant cells derived from coelomic epithelium, i.e. Müllerian ducts and cells lining the peritoneum, pleura and pericardium. The CA 125 levels are increased in about 50% of patients with stage 1 and 90% of those with stage 2 epithelial ovarian cancers, more frequently the serous type. This marker is usually not elevated in mucinous, sex cord, germ cell and Brenner tumors. However, CA 125 is not specific to ovarian cancer as it can be elevated in other malignancies and nongynecological tumors as well as in benign disorders (Table 35.1).

The serum CA 125 levels may be influenced by various factors:
- It fluctuates during the menstrual cycle
- Menopausal status
- Previous hysterectomy (in premenopausal women)
- Age (in postmenopausal women).

The reference limit of 35 U/mL needs to be adjusted for these conditions.[17] Most studies agree that CA 125 levels is most helpful in the evaluation of postmenopausal women with pelvic masses. Vasilev et al.[18] observed 80% of women >50 years of age with pelvic masses and CA 125 >35 U/mL had malignancies compared to only 15% in those <50 years of age. This is useful information in deciding on management by a gynecologic oncologist or general gynecologist.

Table 35.1: Conditions associated with elevated CA 125 levels.

Malignancies	Nonmalignant conditions
Gynecological	*Gynecological*
• Epithelial ovarian carcinoma	• Uterine leiomyomata
• Endometrial carcinoma	• Pelvic inflammatory disease
	• Early pregnancy
	• Benign ovarian cysts
	• Endometriosis
	• Ovarian hyperstimulation
Nongynecological	*Nongynecological*
• Carcinoma of pancreas	• Acute pancreatitis
• Breast carcinoma	• Cirrhosis
	• Pericarditis
	• Colitis
	• Peritonitis
	• Abdominal tuberculosis

Ultrasound

Transabdominal ultrasound has a poor specificity and sensitivity for detecting ovarian cancer. In one of the largest prospective studies on ovarian cancer screening of 5540 asymptomatic pre- and postmenopausal women, 65 laparotomies were performed for each case of ovarian cancer detected.[19]

Transabdominal ultrasound has now been largely replaced by transvaginal sonography (TVS) along with color Doppler techniques to improve specificity.

The advantages of TVS are:
- A full bladder which is both uncomfortable and time-consuming is not needed

- Obese patients can be easily scanned
- The transducer probe is close to pelvic organs resulting in better images.

There can be difficulties associated with differentiating benign from malignant ovarian cysts on ultrasonography. De Priest et al.[20] proposed a "morphology index"—based on tumor volume, cyst wall structure and structure of septa—that may increase the specificity of TVS as a screening tool. Van Nagell[21] recently reported on 57,214 patients who had annual TVS and 180 patients were subjected to surgical intervention. Of the 17 cases of ovarian cancer detected, 11 were in stage 1, 3 in stage 2, and 3 in stage 3. In this study, the use of TVS was associated with a sensitivity of 81%, specificity of 98.97%, positive predictive value of 9.4% and negative predictive value of 99.97%. Annual TVS screening appeared to achieve the primary objective of earlier detection of disease.

The risk of malignancy in a unilocular ovarian cyst <10 cm in diameter is essentially nonexistent, whilst that in complex ovarian tumors is significant requiring their early removal.

The presence of neovascularization in malignant ovarian tumors has prompted the use of Doppler ultrasound as a screening tool. Malignant tumors on color Doppler have a low resistance index (RI) and low pulsatility index (PI) than benign tumors. However, low impedance flows are normal in the luteal phase and in inflammatory process and some benign lesions and these should be kept in mind. Further, some carcinomas have high impedance flow. A recent European randomized study for ovarian cancer screening found that color Doppler did not reduce the false positive rate.

Whilst ultrasound has no hazards, the disadvantages to take note of are time, costly equipment and trained personnel needed to carry out the examination. The available data suggests that on its own ultrasonography does not exhibit adequate specificity for screening the general population.

Pelvic Examination

Routine pelvic examination for the early detection of ovarian cancer is disappointing and is of limited value in screening asymptomatic women. Despite the limitations, it is reasonable to examine the ovaries at any opportunity during cervical screening, antenatal booking, postnatal visits or family planning clinics. Physicians must have a high degree of suspicion especially on women with vague pelvic symptoms and perform a pelvic examination as part of routine gynecological examination. 10% of postmenopausal women with palpable ovaries have an ovarian neoplasm; palpable ovaries more than one year before menarche and in postmenopausal period are abnormal.

Multimodal Strategy

A critical factor for ovarian cancer screening is achieving a predictive value that is sufficiently high because of the rarity of the disease and the need for invasive procedures to evaluate a positive test. A positive predictive value of less than 10% is unacceptable in clinical practice. The low predictive values obtained with either CA_{125} or ultrasound do not justify their individual use for population screening, particularly when data documenting a decrease in mortality because of screening is lacking.

Jacob et al.[22] concluded after a large randomized trial that there was no significant difference in mortality rate between asymptomatic postmenopausal women subjected to annual CA 125 followed by TVS (if CA 125 was > 30 U/mL for 3 years) and controls and stated there was no justification in this type of multimodal ovarian cancer screening of the general population.

What then is the Current Status of Ovarian Cancer Screening?

Screening techniques may be appropriate in patients with a documented significant family history of ovarian cancer; these, however, comprise <1% of all ovarian cancers. The current screening modalities to identify highly curable early stage ovarian cancer in asymptomatic women have been rather disappointing. The high false positive tests can result in unnecessary investigations including surgical intervention in otherwise healthy women resulting in unnecessary morbidity and adverse psychological effects. No conclusion can be drawn as to the efficacy of any screening method at the moment; we have to await the results of several on-going large scale prospective randomized studies using multimodal strategy. At the current moment, in view of the low prevalence of the disease in the general population and the lack of scientific evidence that deaths from ovarian cancer are decreased by screening, routine screening for ovarian cancer cannot be recommended. It is, however, prudent to examine the adnexae when performing gynecological examination for other reasons; in fact, all women should have an annual rectovaginal examination as part of medical care.

Attention should also be directed at prevention of ovarian cancer instead. All women should be encouraged to engage in risk reducing lifestyle—breastfeeding, oral contraceptives and tubal ligation. Increased contraceptive usage in the UK had resulted in a parallel decrease in ovarian cancer incidence.[22]

ENDOMETRIAL CANCER

In Malaysia, this constitutes 3.4% of all female cancers. Mortality from this disease is low largely because of the early development of symptoms; it primarily manifests as postmenopausal or abnormal uterine bleeding which triggers an evaluation with an endometrial sampling. Majority of cases are thus, diagnosed when the disease is confined to the uterus.

Risk factors associated with the development of endometrial carcinoma include:

- Obesity
- Use of estrogen after menopause
- History of anovulation and nulliparity
- Breast cancer and tamoxifen therapy
- Hereditary non-polyposis colorectal cancer (Lynch type II syndrome).

Routine screening of women for endometrial cancer is not of any proven benefit. No screening test has been evaluated for its impact on endometrial cancer mortality, even amongst "high-risk" women.

Cytology

The Pap smear test is too insensitive for detection of early endometrial cancer; occasionally this may pick up exfoliated endometrial cells. The presence of such cells in a Pap smear of a postmenopausal woman, not on exogenous hormones, is abnormal and requires further assessments. Endometrial cytology has not been evaluated in women who do not have symptoms of endometrial cancer.

Endometrial Biopsy

Pipelle endometrial sampling is a convenient office procedure; whilst the overall accuracy is high, the efficacy of the technique in asymptomatic women has not been evaluated.

Ultrasonography (TVS)

Whilst this has been used to evaluate women with abnormal vaginal bleeding, its efficacy in screening for endometrial cancer in asymptomatic women is unknown.

Thus, much remains to be done in developing a safe, sensitive and specific screening test for endometrial cancer.

CONCLUSION

The goal of screening programs is to make a diagnosis before invasive cancer develops. The only gynecological malignancy where cytological screening has proven its value is in cervical cancer, but as yet, there is no reliable, cost-effective screening tests available for ovarian and endometrial cancers. An annual Pap smear test will not only allow for early detection of malignancies of the cervix, but will also give an opportunity to physicians to screen for breast lumps by palpation, for ovarian malignancies and pelvic abnormalities by bimanual and rectovaginal examinations, and for vulval neoplasm by careful inspection.

REFERENCES

1. Richart R. Screening—the next century. Cancer. 1995;76: 1919-27.
2. Benedet JL, Anderson MB, Matistic JP. A comprehensive program for cervical cancer detection and management. Am J Obstet Gynecol. 1992;166:1254-9.
3. Lim GCC, Yahaya H, Lim TO. The first report of the National Cancer Registry—Cancer incidence in Malaysia. 2002.
4. Kurman RJ, Soloman DJ. The Bethesda system for reporting cervical/vaginal cytological diagnosis. Definitions, criteria and explanatory notes terminology and specimen adequacy. New York: Springer Verlag; 1993.
5. Anderson GH, Boyes DA, Bendect JH, et al. Organization and results of cervical cytology screening program in British Columbia, 1955-85. MBJ. 1988;296:975-78.
6. Mitchell H, Medley G, Drake M. Quality control measures for cervical cytology laboratories. Acta Cytol. 1988;32:288-92.
7. Makino H, Sato S, Yajima A, Fukao A. Case-control study of the effectiveness of mass screening in reducing invasive cervical cancer. Nippon Sanka Fujunka Gakkai Zasshi. 1991;43:1226-32.
8. Sivanesaratnam V, Sen DK, Jayalakshmi, Ong G. Radical hysterectomy and pelvic lymphadenectomy for early invasive cancer of the cervix—14 years experience. Int J Gynecologic Cancer. 1993;231-6.
9. Schiffman MH. Recent progress in defining the epidemiology of human papilloma virus infection and cervical neoplasia. J Nat Cancer Inst. 1992;84:394-98.
10. Reid R, Greenberg M, Jenson, et al. Sexually transmitted papillomaviral infection. The anatomic distribution and pathological grade of neoplastic lesions associated with different viral types. Am J Obstet Gynecol. 1987;156: 212-22.
11. Meijer CJLM, Snijders PJF, Van der Brule AJC, et al. Can cytologic screening be improved by HPV screening? In: J Monsenego, AB Miller (Eds). Papillomavirus in Human Pathology. Paris: Ares-Serono Symposia Publications; pp493-498.
12. Hellberg D, Nilson S, Haley MJ, et al. Smoking and cervical intra-epthelial neoplasia: nicotine and cotinine in serum and mucus in smokers and nonsmokers. Am J Obstet Gynecol. 1988;158:910.
13. Morell ND, Taylor JR, Synder RN, et al. False-negative cytology rates in patients in whom invasive cervical cancer subsequently developed. Obstet Gynecol. 1982;60:41-4.
14. Davidson M, Schnitzer PG, Bulkow LR, et al. The prevalence of cervical infection with human papilloma-viruses and cervical dysplasia in Alaska native women. J Infact Dis. 1994;169:792-800.

15. Wesley R, Sankaranarayanan R, Mathew B, et al. Evaluation of visual inspection as a screening test for cervical cancer. Br J Cancer. 1997;75:436-40.
16. Pecorelli S, Odicino F, Maisonneve P, et al. Carcinoma of the ovary. J Epidemiol and Biostatics. 1998;3:75-102.
17. Grover S, Guinn M, Weidman P, Koh H. Factors influencing serum CA 125 levels in normal woman. Obstet Gynecol. 1992; 79:511.
18. Vasilev SA, Schlaerth J, Campeau J, Morrow CP. Serum CA 125 levels in preoperative evaluation of pelvic masses. Obstet Gynecol. 1998;71:751-56.
19. Campbell S, Bhan V, Royston P, et al. Transabdominal ultrasound screening for early ovarian cancer. BMJ. 1989;299: 1363-7.
20. De Priest PD, Shenson D, Fried A, et al. 24th Annual Meeting of the Society Gynecologic Oncologists. Abstract No 21. 1993.
21. Van Nagell JR, De Priest PD, Reedy MB, et al. The efficacy of transvaginal sonographic screening in asymptomatic women at risk for ovarian cancer. Gynecol Oncol. 2000;77: 350-6.
22. Dos Santos Silva I, Swerdlow AJ. Recent trends in incidence of and mortality from breast, ovarian and endometrial cancer in England and Wales and their relation to changing fertility and oral contraceptive use. Br J Cancer. 1995;75:485.
23. Cheah PL, Looi LM, Sivanesaratnam V. Human papilloma virus in cervical cancer in Malaysia. J Obstet Gynecol Res. 2011;37:489-96.

CHAPTER 36

Preinvasive and Invasive Cancer of the Cervix

V Sivanesaratnam

Overview

- The majority of CIN lesions are of squamous origin. As the proliferation of these abnormal cells rises to the surface, the grade of the lesion increases like CIN I, II, and III.
- The etiology is multifactorial—the human papilloma virus (HPV) appears to have a crucial role.
- The availability of vaccines against HPV is an important milestone in the prevention of CIN and invasive carcinoma of the cervix
- The management of CIN can be broadly divided into—ablative techniques and excisional techniques.
- Routine hysterectomy in the primary treatment of CIN is not justified.
- Squamous cell carcinoma accounts for 75% of all invasive lesions.
- Radical hysterectomy and pelvic lymphadenectomy as well as radical radiotherapy (external pelvic radiation + brachytherapy) are equally effective forms of therapy for Stage IB and early IIA.
- Radical hysterectomy and pelvic node dissection (Wertheim's radical hysterectomy) involves removal of the uterus, upper-third of the vagina, parametria and paracolpos and a thorough pelvic lymphadenectomy (common iliac, external iliac, obturator, internal iliac, gluteal, and pre-sacral nodes).
- In selected young patients with squamous cell carcinoma of the cervix (exocervical lesions <2cm, negative nodes) 'fertility sparing' radical trachelectomy and pelvic lymphadenectomy is possible. However, the primary aim of curing the cancer should not be compromised.
- Most patients with stage IIB lesions and beyond will be treated with pelvic radiation (external beam and brachytherapy).

INTRODUCTION

The female genital tract is one of the most common sites for primary malignant disease and the cervix uteri is the most common site affected by cancer. As shown in Figure 36.1, more than 75% of invasive cancer of cervix occurs in developing countries.

In Malaysia,[1] it is the third most common cause of death from cancer amongst women after breast cancer and colorectal cancer (Fig. 36.2) and constitutes 12.0% of the total female cancers. In the West, the incidence has decreased markedly as a result of effective screening programs; in many parts of Asia-Oceania, on the other

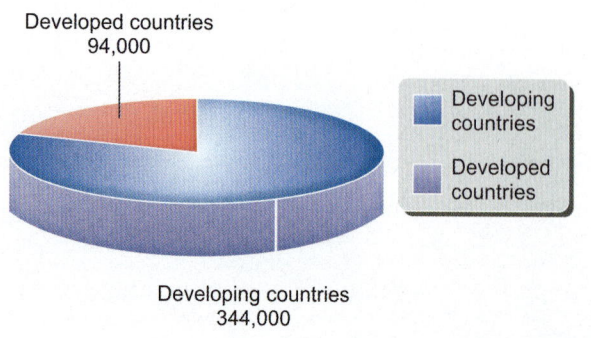
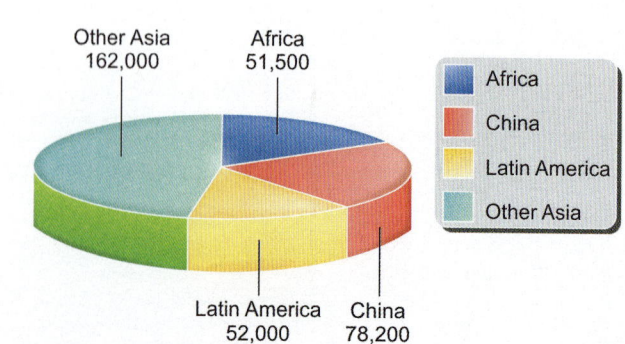

Fig. 36.1: Estimated number of new cervical cancer cases per year, 1985.
Source: Parkin' et al. 1993

CHAPTER 36 Preinvasive and Invasive Cancer of the Cervix

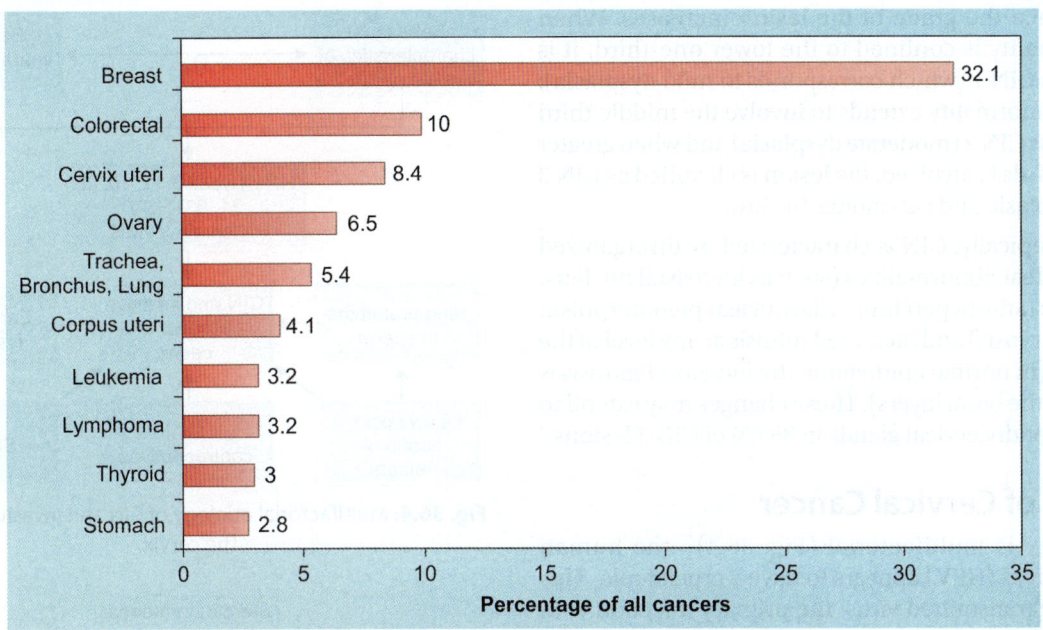

Fig. 36.2: Ten most frequent cancers in females in Malaysia.
Source: NCR Report 2007, Ministry of Health, Malaysia. 2011

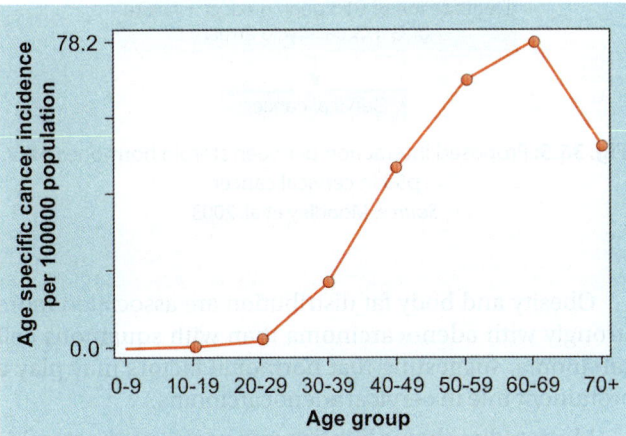

Fig. 36.3: Carcinoma cervix: Age specific cancer incidence per 100,000 population, Peninsular Malaysia 2002.
Source: The first report of the National Cancer Registry, Cancer Incidence in Malaysia, 2002

hand, invasive cervical cancer is relatively high with most of the patients presenting in an advanced stage.

The reasons for the late presentation are:
- Fear of cancer
- Cultural taboos
- Ignorance
- Lack of appropriate facilities for early detection.

This is despite the fact that cervical cancer is the only preventable cancer. In Malaysia, the incidence of cervical cancer peaks at 60 to 69 years of age (Fig. 36.3). With changing trends, this cancer is being seen in younger patients in many parts of the world, including the Asia-Oceania region.

PREINVASIVE LESIONS OF THE CERVIX

These by themselves are completely asymptomatic; only routine screening will help to detect these lesions (Details of screening for cervical cancer are discussed in the Chapter on "Gynecologic Cancer Screening").

Concept of Cervical Intraepithelial Neoplasia

An active process of squamous metaplasia occurs within the transformation zone of the cervix in adolescence during periods of endocrine change; although this is a normal physiological process, under the influence of a carcinogenic agent cellular alterations resulting in an atypical transformation zone may occur.

The concept of cervical intraepithelial neoplasia (or CIN) was introduced by Richart[2] to represent a spectrum of intraepithelial abnormalities which were previously called dysplasia and carcinoma-in situ. The two latter terms imply that carcinoma-in situ is more serious than dysplasia; one might, therefore, assume they represent two different entities resulting in over-treatment of the former and under-treatment of the latter. This is obviously unsatisfactory. The CIN terminology helps to emphasize the concept of a single disease process.

Pathology

The majority of CIN lesions are of squamous origin. The presence of abnormal immature basal cells above the lowermost layer in the epithelium indicates a dysplastic process. As the proliferation of these abnormal cells rises to the surface the grade of the lesion increases. When the abnormality is confined to the lower one-third, it is classified as CIN 1 (which corresponds to mild dysplasia); when the abnormality extends to involve the middle third it is known as CIN 2 (moderate dysplasia) and when greater than two-thirds is involved, the lesion is classified as CIN 3 (severe dysplasia and carcinoma-in situ).

Microscopically, CIN is characterized by disorganized growth, nuclear abnormalities (such as increased nucleus: cytoplasmic ratio, hyperchromasia, nuclear pleomorphism and anisokaryosis) and increased mitosis at any level of the epithelium (in normal epithelium, the increased mitosis is confined to the basal layers). These changes may extend to involve the endocervical glands in 88.6% of CIN 3 lesions.[3]

Etiology of Cervical Cancer

The etiology is multifactorial (Fig. 36.4)—the human papilloma virus (HPV) appears to have a crucial role. This is a sexually transmitted virus; the primary infection with the virus occurs mostly in young adults. The chance of an HPV infection during life is estimated at 80–85%; thus, the prevalence of the infection is high and a large proportion of women and men would be infected by the age of 30 years.[4] The mucosal types of HPV which have strong affinity for the epithelium of the transformation zone are of two types:

- High-risk HPV (hrHPV)
- Low-risk HPV

hrHPV or oncogenic viruses cause 95% of cervical cancer. 80% of hrHPV infections are transient and asymptomatic with mean duration of 6–14 months and with no epithelial abnormalities. Only 20% cause morphological changes in epithelium of the cervix (CIN); only few without intervention will progress to cervical cancer. The only risk factor for progression of a premalignant lesion is persistence of hrHPV infection resulting in development and maintenance of CIN 3 lesions.[5] These hrHPV types include types 6, 11, 16, 18, 31, 33. A Bangkok study reported HPV 16 in 5% normal cervical cytology, 46% in CIN and 61% in cervical cancer. In a Malaysian study, HPV-DNA was detected in 95.7% of cervical carcinoma (HPV 16 in 73.9% and HPV 18 in 65.2% of cancer).[6]

More recently,[7] we reported the presence of HPV16 in 56.4% of squamous cell carcinoma and 35.3% in adeno-/adenosquamous carcinoma of the cervix; HPV18 was seen in 5.5% of squamous cell carcinoma and 17.6% adeno-/adenosquamous cell carcinoma of the cervix. An important milestone in the prevention of cervical cancer is the availability now of vaccines against the 'high risk' HPV16 and 18 viruses.

The number of sexual partners is the most important risk factor for acquisition of hrHPV infection. Age at first coitus and smoking are not independent risk factors for progressive disease.

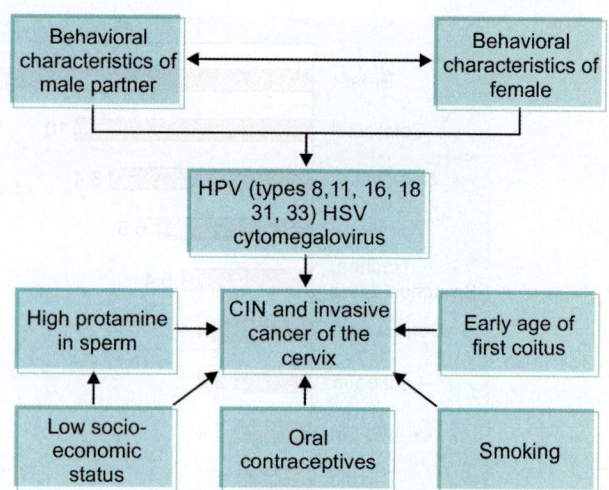

Fig. 36.4: Multifactorial etiology of CIN and invasive cancer of the cervix.

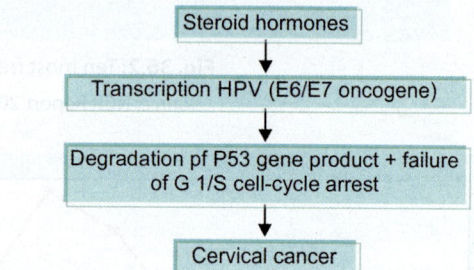

Fig. 36.5: Proposed interaction between steroid hormones, HPV, p53 in cervical cancer.
Source: Moodley et al. 2003

Obesity and body fat distribution are associated more strongly with adenocarcinoma than with squamous cell carcinoma, suggesting that hormonal factors may play a prominent role in cervical adenocarcinoma.

Most studies show a link between *contraceptive* steroids and cervical cancer and presence of hormone receptors in cervical tissue; the duration of steroid usage is the variable most closely linked to development of cervical neoplasia. The WHO collaborative study[8] (1985) reports relative risk of 1.3 to 1.8 for users of 5 or more years of pill usage. Figure 36.5 illustrates the possible interaction between steroid hormones, HPV, and p53 in cervical cancer.

Natural History of Cervical Carcinoma

The current understanding of the natural history of the disease is illustrated in Figures 36.6 and 36.7. CIN 3 precedes invasive carcinoma of the cervix in most cases. If CIN 3 is untreated, 25% may regress, but majority will develop invasive carcinoma—30% at 10 years, 70% at 12 years and 80% at 30 years. However, it is important to bear in mind that this transit time need not always be slow.

CHAPTER 36: Preinvasive and Invasive Cancer of the Cervix

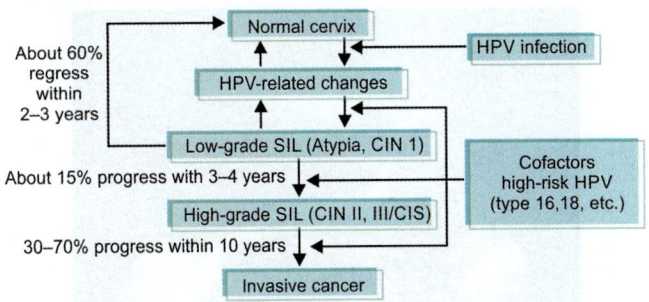

Fig. 36.6: Natural history of cervical cancer.
(CIN: cervical intraepithelial neoplasia; SIL: squamous intraepithelial lesion; CIS: carcinoma in situ)

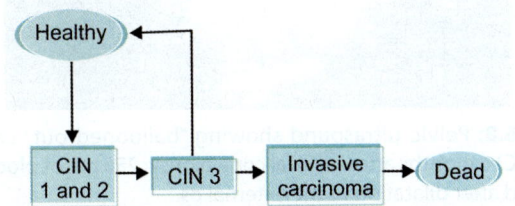

Fig. 36.7: Natural history of cervical cancer and its precursor stages as a compartmental model.

Management of CIN

An outline of the plan of management of an abnormal smear is given in the Chapter on "Gynecological Cancer Screening".

The management can be broadly divided into:
- Ablative techniques
- Excisional techniques.

Most patients with CIN lesions can be treated by local ablative techniques; however, certain criteria have to be met:
- The lesion must be seen in its entirety at colposcopy
- Colposcopic assessment must be consistent with a CIN lesion; any suggestion of preclinical invasion contraindicates local destructive therapy; a cone biopsy is required
- There must be no suspicion on colposcopy of abnormal endocervical cells
- Close follow-up examination (cytology and colposcopy) is essential particularly in the first year after treatment.

The *ablative techniques* available include:
- Radical electrocoagulation diathermy
- Cryosurgery
- CO_2 laser ablation.

Prior to the procedure, the atypical area is defined by colposcopy and the Schiller iodine staining test. Iodine is not taken up by the glycogen-deficient epithelium which contains CIN lesions. Any local destructive procedure must encompass all the iodine negative (Schiller positive) areas.

Radical Electrocoagulation Diathermy

The procedure usually require general anesthesia and is an extremely effective way of treating all forms of CIN. The author routinely excises the abnormal area(s) initially to provide tissue for further evaluation. The cervix is then dilated to Hegar 9 dilator; this provides adequate exposure of the endocervical canal and discourages postoperative cervical stenosis. The epithelium in the crypts and distal canal is then coagulated by numerous insertions (15 to 20) of the needle electrode to a depth of one cm in the long axis of the cervix, each insertion lasting for at least 1–2 seconds. The ball electrode is then systematically used to fulgurate the epithelial surface until the mucus stops bubbling. A heavy vaginal discharge may persist for about 2 weeks, but other complications are minimal. Up to 98% are cured by this procedure.

Cryosurgery

This can be performed in an outpatient setting without anesthesia. Because of its anatomical configuration and easy accessibility, the cervix is an ideal organ for cryosurgery. A gun-type appliance with interchangeable probe tips of variable shape designed to approximate with the surface area of the atypical epithelium delivers the cryogen (liquid nitrogen, nitrous oxide or carbon dioxide) directly onto the cervix.

Once the probe tip is in place, the refrigerant is circulated until the edge of the iceball extends at least 3–5 mm onto the normal cervix. The tip is defrosted and the cervix examined by colposcopy to ensure that all atypical areas are treated. With carbon dioxide a freeze-thaw-freeze technique is recommended.

A watery discharge may last 10–14 days after the procedure.

The primary success rate in treating CIN 3 with cryosurgery is about 95%. The concern is that large lesions with glandular involvement may not be cured by this treatment.

CO_2 Laser Ablation

In the 1980s, this was a popular method in the West to treat CIN; the method is performed in the outpatient setting, usually with no anesthesia and if necessary a paracervical block. High cure rates of 95% were reported. However, the high cost of laser equipment and advanced training required are major drawbacks; cryosurgery and radical diathermy coagulation, at a fraction of the cost, give equally good results.

The *excisional methods* available are:
- Large loop excision of the transformation zone (LLETZ)
- Cold-knife conization

- Laser-excisional conization
- Hysterectomy.

Large Loop Excision of the Transformation Zone (LLETZ)

Recently this has become a cost-effective alternative to traditional approaches to therapy of CIN lesions. This can be performed in an outpatient setting using a paracervical block analgesia. Using a diathermy loop connected to a low-voltage output, the whole transformation zone including 10 mm or more of the endocervical canal can be excised; diathermy fulguration of the exposed stroma can help hemostasis.

The resulting thermocoagulation artefact at the margins may interfere with histopathological evaluation. Colposcopic directed biopsies may miss the most significant lesion, especially if taken by the 'average' colposcopist. One of the obvious advantages of LLETZ is in providing more tissue for histological evaluation resulting in increased recognition of those at risk of glandular involvement and early invasive lesions so that appropriate additional therapy can be carried out and management improved; it would have a place in patients for whom local destructive therapy is contraindicated. In a transient population where a high proportion of patients may be lost to follow-up, LLETZ appears reasonable.

Excisional Conization

This is a combined diagnostic/therapeutic approach. The tissue removed must include the whole transformation zone, including free upper endocervical and lower ectocervical margins. Colposcopy and Schiller's test will help determine how large or small the zone should be. *There is no place today for conization not preceded by colposcopy and colposcopically directed biopsies.*

The main *indications* for cone biopsy after colposcopic assessment are:

- Inability to visualize the whole transformation zone (upper limit extends into the cervical canal)
- Colposcopic suspicion of occult invasion, even if target biopsies show only CIN 3
- Cytology suspicious of adenocarcinoma in situ
- Lesions where cervical cytology indicates a greater possibility of invasive disease than is indicated by colposcopy or the directed biopsy
- Repeated abnormal cytology suggesting neoplasia in the absence of colposcopic abnormality
- Microinvasion on punch biopsy.

Cold-knife Conization

In this technique, the circumferential ectocervical incision is made several millimeters beyond the outer limit of the

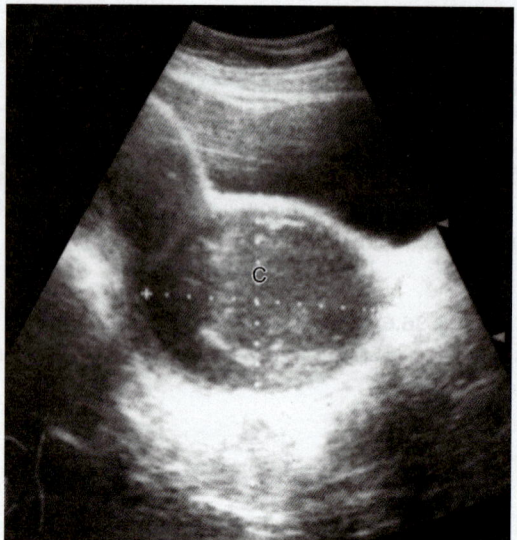

Fig. 36.8: Pelvic ultrasound showing "ballooned-out" cervical canal (C) 6 months after cervical cone biopsy; 250 mL of blood was drained after dilatation of the external os.

transformation zone and the cone is then fashioned as dictated by the colposcopic findings. The cone bed is then inspected and bleeding points are diathermized; deep lateral sutures at 3 and 9 o'clock position will help occlude the descending branches of the uterine artery.

The overall complication rate is 23–25%; this includes hemorrhage, pelvic infection and cervical stenosis. Very rarely, a hematocervix/hemotometra may result from severe stenosis of the external os (Fig. 36.8).

Whilst it is important to ensure adequate surgical margins, it is also important not to remove more than is necessary of the endocervical canal to achieve a complete excision of the lesion. This is because of three reasons:

- Control of hemorrhage is easier if a small length of endocervical canal is removed
- A slightly reduced length of endocervical canal will not compromise fertility
- Maintenance of internal os is important.

The result of a properly planned therapeutic conization are excellent; long-term follow-up is obligatory. The dilemma arises when the cone biopsy margins are involved by CIN; 50–80% of such patients have been reported to have residual disease at hysterectomy.[9] The author routinely curettes the endocervix and lower part of endometrial cavity immediately after cone biopsy. When 'cone tip' is positive, the findings in the curettage specimens are used to decide whether to follow-up the patient, repeat the cone biopsy or perform a hysterectomy.

Laser Excisional Conization

This requires skill and experience with use of CO_2 laser and excellent clinical judgement. When compared to cold-knife conization, the intraoperative and immediate postoperative bleeding are reduced. The high cost of the equipment, its maintenance and hazards to the surgeon are disadvantages. LLETZ cone is a simple and cheaper alternative that is now being performed in many clinical units.

Hysterectomy

Routine hysterectomy in the primary treatment of CIN is not justified. The *indications* for the procedure are mainly relative:

- Pre-existing gynecological problems: Uterine myoma, uterovaginal prolapse, dysfunctional uterine bleeding. Invasive cancer must be adequately excluded prior to hysterectomy
- Resection margins of cone biopsy show evidence of CIN; the alternatives have been discussed earlier
- The lesion extends to vaginal fornix.

Follow-up is essential in all cases.

ADENOCARCINOMA IN SITU

This is a difficult lesion to diagnose occurring often in association with squamous CIN or at the edge of an invasive adenocarcinoma. The diagnosis is based on the presence of cellular atypia, abnormal mitoses, stratification, papillary projections and outpouchings; the normal architectural pattern of the endocervical crypts is preserved and often only the superficial crypts are involved. Stromal reaction, such as inflammatory infiltrate or edema, are absent, and the adjacent glands should be normal. A punch biopsy alone is insufficient for diagnosis; a cone biopsy, which may be therapeutic, is essential to establish the diagnosis and exclude the possibility of an invasive adenocarcinoma. Like CIN, adenocarcinoma in situ (AIS) may be present for several years before invasive carcinoma develops.

INVASIVE CARCINOMA OF THE CERVIX

The most common *symptoms* are:

- Abnormal vaginal bleeding
- Vaginal discharge.

Abnormal bleeding occurs in 80–90% of patients; this may be postcoital bleeding, intermenstrual spotting, irregular vaginal bleeding, and postmenopausal bleeding. Some patients may present with only a vaginal discharge—serous or mucoid; some patients may have a foul smelling discharge. Pelvic pain and leg edema are usually seen in advanced disease. A minority of patients are completely asymptomatic.

On vaginal speculum examination, the cervix may appear normal in early (microinvasive) cervical cancer, and if the lesion is endocervical. Visible disease takes *two main forms—exophytic* (Fig. 36.9) or *ulcerative*, which

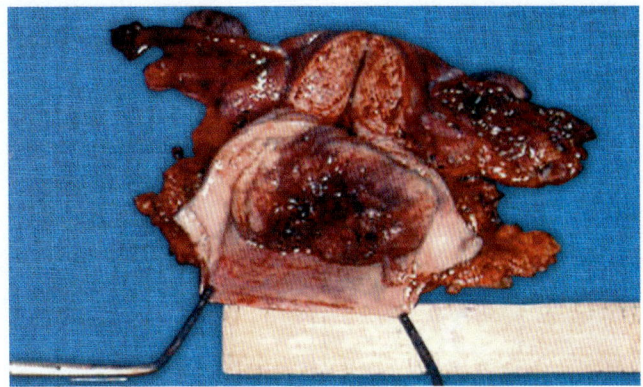

Fig. 36.9: Radical hysterectomy specimen showing a large exophytic growth in cervix *(Stage 1B2 disease).*

often bleeds easily on contact. The tumor may completely replace the cervix which may be distorted. The lesion may extend down the vagina and/or extend laterally into the parametrium; parametrial involvement may result in obstructive uropathy. In order to determine the extent of the disease, a rectovaginal examination is essential; this would help determine the degree of cervical expansion and extent of parametrial and uterosacral ligament involvement.

Clinical Staging

This is based on the official staging classification by International Federation of Gynecology and Obstetrics which is based on physical examination and noninvasive tests (Table 36.1 and Fig. 36.10). These tests include biopsies, cystoscopy, sigmoidoscopy, chest radiographs and intravenous urography. Where facilities are available, a CT scan of the chest, abdomen and pelvis will give useful information not detected by above tests and may influence management.

Pathology

Squamous cell carcinoma accounts for 75% of all invasive lesions; there are *2* types—the much more common and better differentiated large cell carcinoma (nonkeratinizing and keratinizing types) and the much rarer small cell carcinoma, which is a poorly differentiated lesion.

About 25% of invasive cervical cancers are adenocarcinoma or adenosquamous carcinomas. The rest involves rarer types, such as transitional cell, lymphomas and sarcomas, and melanoma and together these account for fewer than 1% of cases.

Management

Stage 1A (Microinvasive Carcinoma)

There is still controversy over the management of microinvasive cervical cancer. The risk of lymph node metastases depends on the depth of invasion (negligible

SECTION 3 Gynecologic Oncology

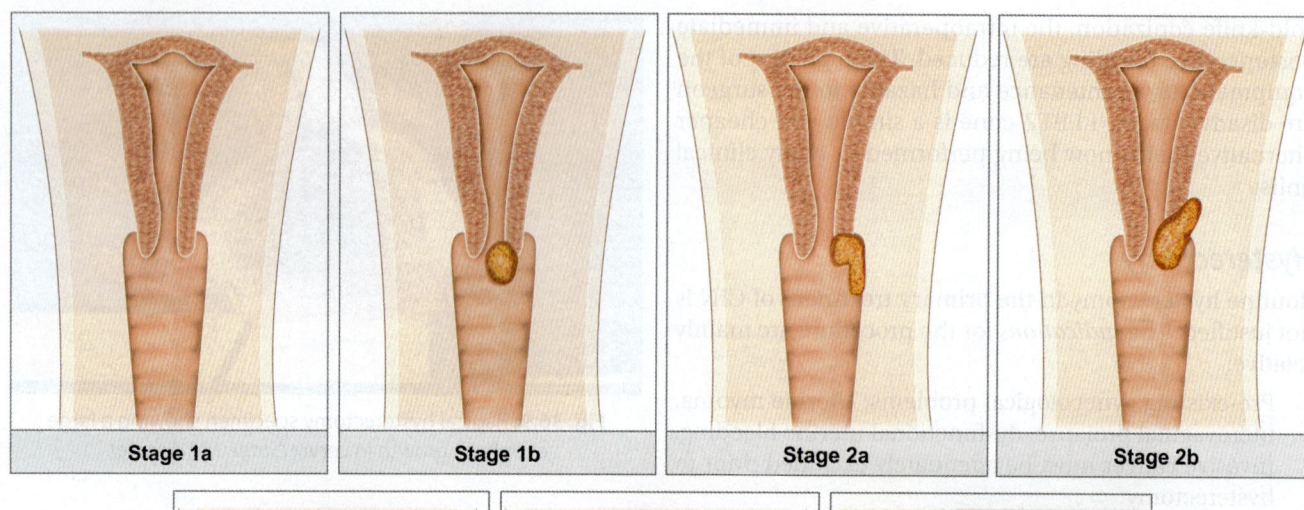

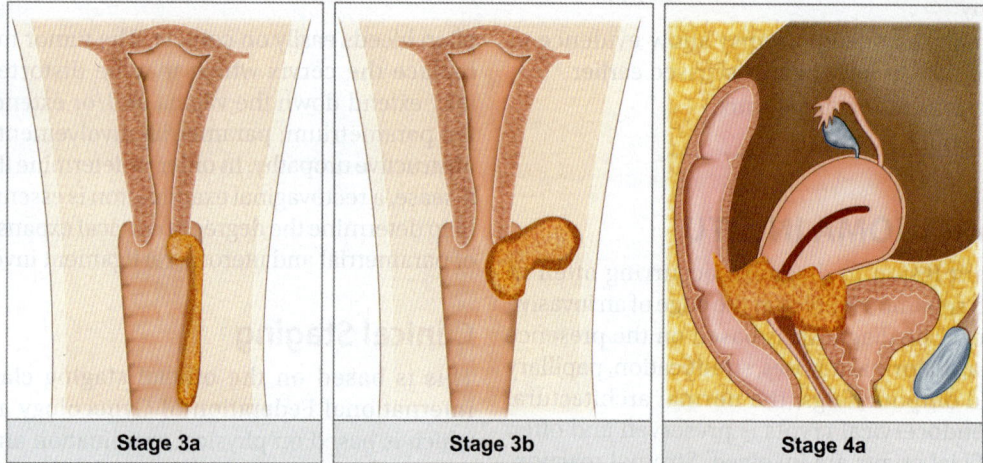

Fig. 36.10: Clinical staging of cervical carcinoma (diagrammatic representation).

Table 36.1: The International Federation of Gynecology and Obstetrics Staging for Cervical Carcinoma (2009).

Stage 1	**The carcinoma is strictly confined to the cervix (extension to the corpus is disregarded)**
1A	Invasive carcinoma diagnosed only by microscopy (Preclinical carcinoma)
1A1	Measured stromal invasion of not >3 mm in-depth and horizontal extension of not >7 mm
1A2	Measured stromal invasion of >3 mm but not >5 mm in-depth and horizontal extension of not >7 mm (The diagnosis of stage 1A1 and 1A2 should preferably be made on cone biopsy which includes the entire lesion. Vascular space involvement should not alter the staging but may influence mode of therapy)
1B	Preclinical lesions greater than stage 1A2 and clinically visible lesions confined to the cervix
1B1	Clinically visible lesions not >4 cm
1B2	Clinically visible lesions >4 cm
Stage 2	**The carcinoma extends beyond the cervix, but not to the lateral pelvic wall or to the lower third of the vagina**
2A1	Involvement of the upper two-third of vagina without parametrial involvement; <4 cm in greatest dimension
2A2	>4 cm in greatest diameter
2B	With parametrial involvement
Stage 3	**The carcinoma extends to the lateral pelvic wall and/or the tumor involves the lower third of vagina. All the cases of hydronephrosis or a nonfunctioning kidney are included**
3A	No extension to pelvic wall
3B	Extension to pelvic wall (as detected by no cancer-free space between the tumor and the pelvic wall on rectovaginal examination) and/or hydronephrosis or nonfunctioning kidney
Stage 4	**The carcinoma has extended beyond the pelvis or has clinically involved the mucosa of bladder or rectum (Bullous edema does not permit the case to be allotted as stage 4)**
4A	Spread of growth to bladder or rectum
4B	Spread to distant organs

if <1 mm, 1% if invasion is 1–3 mm, and 4% if it is 3–5 mm). Hence, if the invasion is <3 mm, hysterectomy can be avoided—a cone biopsy would suffice. For lesions >3 mm and in those with lymphovascular permeation an extrafascial hysterectomy and pelvic lymphadenectomy would appear advisable.

Stage 1B and Early 2A

Radical hysterectomy and pelvic lymphadenectomy as well as radical radiotherapy (external pelvic radiation + brachytherapy) are equally effective forms of therapy. The advantages of radical hysterectomy are, it would allow for:
- Preservation of ovarian function
- Preservation of coital function.

Both these important aspects will be compromised if radiotherapy is given. The incidence of ovarian metastases in stage 1B squamous cell carcinoma is 0–1% allowing for conservation of normal looking ovaries in young women; the conserved ovaries are best transposed (paracecal on the right and paracolic on the left) thus, to protect the ovaries pelvic radiation should be needed subsequently. The incidence of ovarian metastases in adenocarcinoma of the cervix is higher (4.3%); in such cases it would not be wise to conserve the ovaries.[10]

Radical hysterectomy and pelvic node dissection (Wertheim's radical hysterectomy) involves removal of the uterus, upper-third of the vagina, parametria and paracolpos and a thorough pelvic lymphadenectomy (common iliac, external iliac, obturator, internal iliac, gluteal, and presacral nodes) (Fig. 36.11). In older women, a bilateral salpingo-oophorectomy is done.

Complications of radical hysterectomy include:
- Urinary problems
    - Urinary tract infection
    - Bladder atony
    - Urinary fistula (vesicovaginal, ureterovaginal).
- Bowel problems
    - Atony of rectum, constipation.
- Lymphedema (Fig. 36.12) (in about 1% of cases).

The most serious of these complications is *urinary fistula*; fortunately this occurs in only 2–3% of patients. The above complications can be minimized with improved surgical technique and appropriate postoperative care; early ambulation and chest physiotherapy are important adjuncts in the prophylaxis against postoperative *thromboembolism*.

Adjuvant Treatment

The following features seen on histopathological evaluation will adversely affect survival:
- Lymph node metastasis
- Full thickness stromal invasion
- Lymphovascular tumor permeation
- Microscopic parametrial metastases.

In order to improve overall survival in these patients, adjuvant treatment is necessary. Adjuvant pelvic irradiation in these instances might decrease the incidence of local pelvic recurrences, but the development of distant metastases is not prevented, resulting in no improvement in overall survival. The addition of whole pelvic irradiation

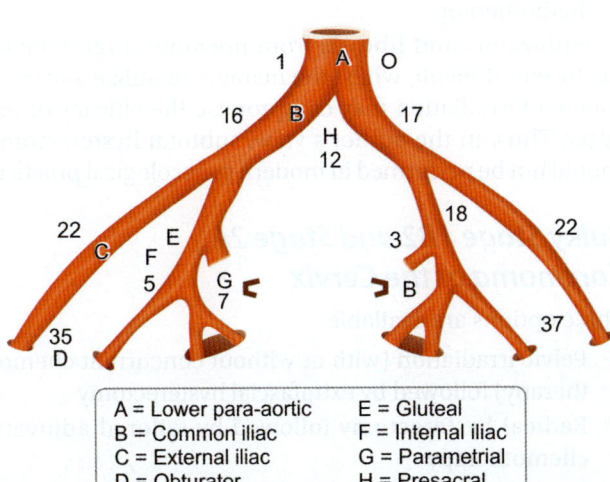

Fig. 36.11: Distribution of positive pelvic nodes in 66 patients with stage 1B and early stage 2A carcinoma of the cervix (overall incidence 16.6%).

A = Lower para-aortic
B = Common iliac
C = External iliac
D = Obturator
E = Gluteal
F = Internal iliac
G = Parametrial
H = Presacral

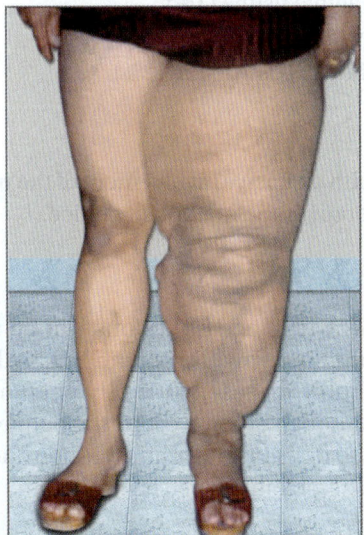

Fig. 36.12: Severe lymphedema. The patient had Wertheim radical hysterectomy and pelvic lymphadenectomy. She developed pelvic recurrence 3 years later and was treated by pelvic irradiation. She remains otherwise well 20 years later.

to radical surgery also carries a high risk of morbidity and mortality.

Patients with above poor prognostic features can be regarded as having systemic disease requiring systemic measures; in these instances it is fair to assume the presence of micrometastases not only within the pelvis but also at extrapelvic sites. Using adjuvant chemotherapy, we reported 10-year survivals of 86.1% in patients with risk factors; survival in those with squamous cell carcinoma was better if mitomycin C + 5-fluorouracil (5FU) was used and for adenocarcinoma and adenosquamous carcinoma, better survivals were obtained with cisplatinum, vinblastine and bleomycin (PVB regime). Patients without risk factors have survivals of 98%.[11]

Primary radiation therapy for early stage cervical carcinoma is based primarily on the extent and distribution of the disease; treatment is directed to upper vagina, cervix and parametria, as well as lymph nodes on pelvic wall. Treatment usually begins with external radiation in an attempt to shrink the central tumor; this will help improve the application of subsequent intracavitary cesium therapy.

The complications of radiation therapy can be divided into:

- Acute complications (occurring during or immediately after therapy)
  - Perforation of the uterus
  - Sigmoiditis (8%)
  - Hemorrhagic cystitis (3%).
- Chronic complications (occurring as late as 12–18 months)
  - Vaginal stenosis (70%)
  - Rectovaginal fistula (1%)
  - Vesicovaginal fistula (1%)
  - Small bowel obstruction (2%).

Stage IIa

In patients with extensive involvement of the upper vagina, radiation therapy is the method of choice.

Stage IIb

Most patients with stage IIb lesions will be treated with pelvic radiation (external beam and brachytherapy). For those with bulky disease, currently chemoradiation is advocated, although in some centers neoadjuvant chemotherapy is used to shrink the primary lesion and is followed by radical hysterectomy or pelvic irradiation.

Stage IIIa and IIIb

These patients are treated by pelvic irradiation (external beam brachytherapy). In the presence of bulky disease chemoradiation is used.

Stage IVa

Pelvic irradiation is used in most instances. Pelvic exenteration is rarely performed, usually when a rectovaginal or vesicovaginal fistula is present.

Stage IVb

Pelvic radiation may be used for palliation of bleeding from vagina, bladder or rectum. As distant metastases are present, chemotherapy is often employed; this is only palliative.

The *5-year survivals* for *radiotherapy* are 86.6% for stage 1, 69.9% for stage II, 42.5% for stage III and 12.3% for stage IV.[12]

More recently, concurrent *chemoradiation* has been used with improved survivals.

Special Situations

Invasive cervical carcinoma found incidentally after simple hysterectomy.

With minimal invasive disease no further treatment is needed. For more severe lesions there are two options:

- Immediate postoperative radiotherapy
- Radical excision of the upper vagina and pelvic lymphadenectomy.

Positive surgical margins and when residual disease is left behind at radical hysterectomy.

Here, pelvic irradiation is the method of choice.

Cervical Stump Carcinoma

There are two options:

- Radical cervicectomy with bilateral lymphadenectomy
- Radiotherapy.

Adhesions and fibrosis from previous surgery make the former difficult, whilst the inability to utilize a uterine source of irradiation may compromise the efficacy of the latter. Thus, in the author's view, subtotal hysterectomy should not be performed in modern gynecological practice.

Bulky Stage 1B2 and Stage 2A Carcinoma of the Cervix

Three options are available:

- Pelvic irradiation (with or without concurrent chemotherapy) followed by extrafascial hysterectomy
- Radical hysterectomy followed by tailored adjuvant chemotherapy
- Neoadjuvant chemotherapy followed by radical hysterectomy and pelvic lymphadenectomy.

Currently, there has been great interest in the third option. A randomized trial will help decide which is the best option.

CHAPTER 36 Preinvasive and Invasive Cancer of the Cervix

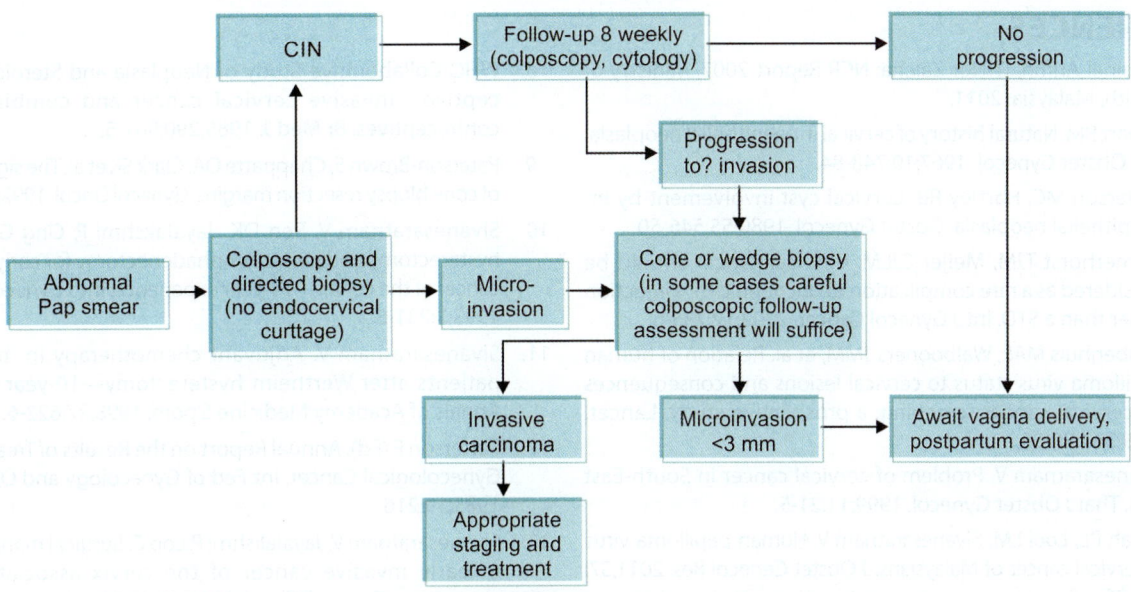

Fig. 36.13: Scheme of evaluation of an abnormal smear in pregnancy.

Fertility Sparing Surgery

Radical hysterectomy remains the mainstay of treatment for stage 1B and early 2A cervical carcinoma. Recently, there has been a great interest in performing conservative (fertility-sparing) surgery in young women with small 1B1 lesions. A laparoscopic/retroperitoneal lymphadenectomy is performed; if frozen section of the nodes show no metastases, a radical trachelectomy, vaginoisthmic anastomosis with a prophylactic cerclage around the isthmus is carried out. The essentials for cure and preservation of fertility are 1 cm upper tumor free margin and 1 cm residual cervical canal. The *contraindications* for the procedure are:

- Presence of L/V permeation
- +ve nodes
- Tumors >2 cm
- Upper endocervical involvement.

Cervical Cancer in Pregnancy

This is rare, occurring 1 in 4077 deliveries. About 55% of patients with cervical cancer in pregnancy are asymptomatic. Pregnancy presents an ideal time for cervical screening. The management of an abnormal smear in pregnancy is shown in Figure 36.13. The treatment options available are:

- Radiotherapy
- Radical hysterectomy and pelvic lymphadenectomy.

For stage 1B and early 2A lesions diagnosed before 24 weeks of pregnancy, the pregnancy is disregarded and definitive therapy instituted. Radical hysterectomy and pelvic lymphadenectomy is our preferred choice. The dilemma arises when patients present between 24 and 28 weeks gestation; treatment may be delayed until the fetus has a better chance of survival. When sufficient maturity has been achieved (32–43 weeks) a classical cesarean section is performed, the placenta is left in situ. The uterine incision is closed and the radical hysterectomy and pelvic lymphadenectomy is then performed.

For more advanced disease (stage IIB, III and IV) radiotherapy is the treatment of choice. In early pregnancy, external beam radiation results in an abortion; after the uterus is empty, brachytherapy completes therapy. Treatment may be delayed in those in the latter part of second or third trimester to achieve fetal viability; the fetus is then delivered by classical cesarean section before radiotherapy.

We observed a 5-year survival of 92.8% in our antenatally diagnosed patients, which is similar to the non-pregnant patient; only 25% of those diagnosed and treated in the puerperium survived. Hence, early diagnosis and therapy during pregnancy is important, rather than in the puerperium.[13]

Follow-up

All patients will need long-term follow-up assessments, for reassurance, psychosexual counseling symptomatic relief and early detection of recurrence.

REFERENCES

1. O Zainal Ariffin, IT Nor Zaleha: NCR Report 2007, Ministry of Health, Malaysia. 2011.
2. Richart RM. Natural history of cervical intraepithelial neoplasia. Clin Obstet Gynecol. 1967;10:748-84.
3. Anderson MC, Hartley RB. Cervical cyst involvement by intraepithelial neoplasia. Obstet Gynecol. 1980;55:546-50.
4. Helmerhorst TJM, Meijer CJLM. Cervical cancer should be considered as a rare complication of oncogenic HPV injection rather than a STD. Int J Gynecol Cancer. 2002;12:235-6.
5. Nabbenhuis MAE, Walbooners JMM, et al. Relation of human papilloma virus status to cervical lesions and consequences for cervical-cancer screening; a prospective study. Lancet. 1999;354:20-25.
6. Sivanesaratnam V. Problem of cervical cancer in South-East Asia. Thai J Obstet Gynecol. 1999;11:21-5.
7. Cheah PL, Looi LM, Sivanesaratnam V. Human papilloma virus in cervical cancer of Malaysians. J Obstet Genecol Res. 2011;37:489-96.
8. WHO Collaborative Study of Neoplasia and Steroid Contraceptives: Invasive cervical cancer and combined oral contraceptives. Br Med J. 1985;290:961-5.
9. Paterson-Brown S, Chappatte OA, Clark SK et al. The significance of cone biopsy resection margins. Gynecol Oncol. 1992;46:182-5.
10. Sivanesaratnam V, Sen DK, Jayalakshmi P, Ong G. Radical hysterectomy and pelvic lymphadenectomy for early invasive cancer of the cervix—14-year experience. Int J Gynecol Cancer. 1993;3:231-8.
11. Sivanesaratnam V. Adjuvant chemotherapy in "high risk" patients after Wertheim hysterectomy—10-year survival. Annals of Academy Medicine S'pore. 1998;27:622-6.
12. Patterson F (Ed). Annual Report on the Results of Treatment in Gynecological Cancer. Int Fed of Gynecology and Obstetrics. 1985;19:216.
13. Sivanesaratnam V, Jayalakshmi P, Loo C. Surgical management of early invasive cancer of the cervix associated with pregnancy. Gynecol Oncol. 1993;48:68-75.

CHAPTER 37

Ovarian Cancer

V Sivanesaratnam, Lim Boon Kiong

Overview
- Epithelial ovarian cancer comprise 80–85% of all ovarian tumors. The overall survival is only 41.6%. The elusive nature of the disease results in 70% of the cases to be in the advanced stage at presentation.
- Surgery is the main modality of treatment, however, advanced or aggressive the disease.
- Chemotherapy has an important role—adjuvant treatment after primary surgery or as neoadjuvant in chemo-debulking of tumors assessed to be inoperable to facilitate subsequent optimal debulking.
- In selected young patients surgery can be tailored to preserve fertility.

INTRODUCTION

Ovarian cancer is the fourth common cancer among Malaysian women and is a leading cause of death from gynecological cancer. Epithelial ovarian cancer comprise 80–85% of all ovarian tumors. The exact etiology is unknown; increasing parity, use of oral contraceptive pills and breastfeeding appear to have a protective effect, whilst low parity/subfertility, use of fertility drugs and genetic factors increase the risk.

The overall survival is only 41.6%. The elusive nature of the disease results in 70% of the cases to be in the advanced stage at presentation. A thorough clinical examination and the aid of imaging techniques—ultrasound, CT scan—will help determine the extent of the disease preoperatively and the subsequent planning of treatment.

Surgery is the main modality of treatment, however, advanced or aggressive the disease. The extent of surgery should be individualized. This would be influenced by age, reproductive status, histological type of tumor, stage of the disease and general medical status.

A second-look laparotomy has little place in the routine management. In patients with persistent or recurrent disease, secondary salvage surgery may be performed in suitable patients. Minimally invasive surgery (laparoscopic surgery) for ovarian masses can do harm if patient selection is not carefully done.

Fertility sparing surgery is possible in patients with germ cell tumors; it is also a viable option for selected patients with stage 1 epithelial ovarian carcinoma after a comprehensive surgical staging.

Chemotherapy has an important role—adjuvant treatment after primary surgery and as neoadjuvant in chemo-debulking of tumors assessed to be inoperable to facilitate subsequent optimal debulking.

Survival rate is much better when the cases are managed by gynecologic oncologists.

Ovarian carcinoma is the leading cause of death from gynecological cancer in the US. In Malaysia, ovarian carcinoma is the fourth most common cancer among women in Peninsular Malaysia in the year 2002 (after cancers of the breast, cervix uteri and colon) and constituted 5% of total female cancers.[1] It is a leading cause of death from gynecological cancer because it is difficult to detect before it disseminates; approximately 70% of cases present in advanced stage.

EPIDEMIOLOGY

Malignant neoplasms of the ovaries occur at all ages, including infancy and childhood. Malignant germ cell tumors are most commonly seen in females younger than 20 years, whereas epithelial cancers of the ovary are primarily seen in women older than 50 years. The probability of developing ovarian cancer before the age of 75 is 0.4–1.7%. The incidence of epithelial ovarian cancer in women between the age of 40 and 44 is 15 to 16 per 100,000. Epithelial ovarian cancer is infrequent in women below the age of 40, after which the rate increases; in Malaysia the age specific incidence peaks at 60–69 years at 27.0 per 100,000 population.[1] The disease appears to be more common amongst the Chinese (9.9 per 100,000 population) compared to the Malays (8.1 per 100,000 population) and Indians (7.4 per 100,000 population).[1] The lifetime risk of developing ovarian cancer was 1:100 for Chinese, 1:125 for Indians and 1:125 for Malays. It was the third commonest cancer diagnosed in Malay women (after cancers of breast and cervix uteri).

ANATOMY

The ovaries are a pair of solid oval-shaped organs measuring 2–4 cm in diameter; they are situated in the "ovarian fossa" on either side of the pelvis between the bifurcation of the common iliac vessels and medial to bony pelvis. Hence, these are not palpable per abdomen because of this deep location in the pelvis; neither are they easily palpable on pelvic examination, unless they are enlarged. They are connected by a peritoneal fold to the broad ligament, by the infundibulopelvic ligament to the lateral wall of the pelvis and by the ovarian ligament to the cornu of the uterus which continues anteriorly as the round ligament.

Mode of Spread

Ovarian cancer spreads mainly by two routes:
- Transperitoneal
- Via lymphatics.

The visceral and parietal peritoneum, and the omentum are common sites for metastases; subdiaphragmatic and liver surface involvement are also common.

The lymphatic drainage occurs mainly by the ovarian lymphatics to the para-aortic nodes; via accessory external iliac lymphatic channels this may drain into the external iliac, common iliac, hypogastric and lateral sacral nodes and occasionally via the round ligaments into the inguinal nodes.

ETIOLOGICAL FACTORS

The exact etiology of ovarian cancer is unknown but it has been known to have a close association with several factors.

- *Parity:* The risk of developing ovarian cancer reduces with parity. The relative risk for a nulliparous woman is 1.5 while a woman with parity of more than three has a relative risk of 0.73.[2] An associated factor that also reduces the risk is a history of breastfeeding, although no consistent relationship has been established between breastfeeding duration and decreased risk

- *Oral contraceptive pill (OCP):* Taking OCP has been associated with the reduction in the risk of developing ovarian cancer. The relative risk of women taking OCP for more than 36 months is 0.4. It has been estimated that oral contraceptives may have prevented over 1,700 cases of ovarian cancer per year in the US.[3] The risk of ovarian cancer is also increased in women with breast cancer and vice versa[2]

- *Years of ovulation:* The risk of ovarian cancer increases with number of years of ovulation. Therefore, women with low parity/subfertility, early menarche and late menopause have higher risk of developing ovarian cancer

- *Hormonal:* Risk of developing ovarian cancer is said to be increased in patients taking fertility drugs, e.g. clomiphene citrate of more than one year duration. The use of clomiphene for more than 12 ovulatory cycles is associated with a 2- to 4- fold elevated risk. Most of the tumors in this group of patients are borderline malignancy.[4]

- *Genetic factors:* Women with genetic risk for ovarian cancer can be divided into two groups:
  - Familial ovarian cancer
  - Hereditary ovarian cancer.

  Hereditary ovarian cancer syndrome is defined as women with at least 2 first-degree relatives with ovarian cancer. Approximately 5% of ovarian cancer has a hereditary basis.[5]

  The lifetime risk for ovarian cancer in the normal population is approximately 1.6%. With one relative affected, the lifetime risk rises to 5%. Lifetime cumulative risk of developing ovarian cancer increases to 7% in patient with at least 2 relatives suffering from ovarian cancer.[5] Approximately 3% of these women have hereditary ovarian cancer syndrome which carry a lifetime risk of 25–50% in developing ovarian cancer. At least 2 genes have been identified to be involved in the development of ovarian cancer, i.e. BRCA1 (location 17q21) and BRCA2 (13q12). BRCA1 is a tumor-suppressor gene that acts as a negative regulator of tumor growth. Mutation of this gene causes dysfunction leading to development of cancer.

  There are two types of hereditary ovarian cancer syndrome that has been identified:[6]

  Hereditary breast-ovarian cancer syndrome (HBOC) (85–90%). The vast majority is due to mutation of BRCA1 gene with a small proportion due to mutation of BRCA2 gene.

  Hereditary nonpolyposis colorectal syndrome (HNPCC). This is also an autosomal dominant condition and previously known as Lynch syndrome II. Ovarian cancer occurs in 5–10% of HNPCC. It also increases predisposition to endometrial and stomach cancer.

In breast-ovarian cancer syndrome, women with either the mother or a sister suffering from breast and/or ovarian cancer has a 50% risk of developing ovarian cancer in her lifetime. Therefore, women less than 35 years of age with a history of hereditary ovarian cancer syndrome should be monitored with a pelvic examination, ultrasound scan and CA 125 every 6 months. For those above 35 years of age and have completed their family, they should be encouraged to consider prophylactic removal of the ovaries.

Other hereditary factors that has been linked to the occurrence of ovarian cancer are mutation of p53 gene, abnormalities of dominant oncogenes, e.g. c-myc, H-ras and Ki-ras.[7]

- *Environmental factors:* A diet high in meat and animal fat, characteristic of industrialized nations, has been reported in some studies to be associated with an increased risk of ovarian cancer.[2] Some studies disputed the above findings.[8] There have been conflicting reports regarding the association of the use of talcum powder and development of ovarian cancer[9,10]
- *Others:* White race and residence in North America and Northern Europe are also at higher risk of developing ovarian cancer.[11] A meta-analysis of 21 studies has shown that there is a small increase (not statistically significant) in overall risk of ovarian cancer in women taking HRT (RR 1.15; CI 1.05–1.27).[12]

The protective effect of factors 1, 2 and 3 which produce periods of *ovulatory rest* support the *incessant ovulation* hypothesis for the etiology of ovarian cancer. According to this hypothesis, ovarian cancer develops from an aberrant repair process of the surface epithelium, which is ruptured and repaired during each ovulatory cycle.[13] The other hypothesis of primary etiology of ovarian cancer is excessive gonadotropin secretion leading to excessive stimulation of ovary.

SCREENING FOR OVARIAN CANCER

Ovarian cancer is curable when detected at an early stage, but most cases are diagnosed after spread from the ovary has taken place. The typically late diagnosis of ovarian cancer is due to the paucity of symptoms in the early stage as well as the deep location of the ovaries in the pelvis. Screening for ovarian cancer is one way to detect the occurrence of ovarian cancer at the premalignant or early stage. This will be discussed in the Chapter 35 "Gynecological Cancer Screening".

PREVENTION OF OVARIAN CANCER

As ovarian cancer cannot be detected early, attention should be directed to its prevention.

- *Oral contraceptive pills:* Most of what is known about role of oral contraceptive pills in prevention of ovarian cancer is based on epithelial tumor which comprise 80–85% of all ovarian cancers
- OCP usage reduces the risk of familial and hereditary ovarian cancer. The exact mechanism of risk reduction by OCPs remains to be defined. Decreased ovulation may be its main mechanism but progestational components of OCPs may also exert independent protective effects, including inducing apoptosis on epithelial cells[14]
- Synthetic *retinoid* (fenretinide) may also protect women from ovarian cancer[15]
- *Tubal ligation* (RR 0.33) and *hysterectomy* (RR 0.67) may have some protective effect to the occurrence of ovarian cancer.[16] This could be explained by prevention of passage of carcinogens (e.g. talc) via vagina to the ovaries
- Prophylactic oophorectomy, generally reduced the risk of ovarian cancer in women. However, this may not be protective to all women especially those with hereditary ovarian cancer syndrome. Follow-up studies have shown that approximately 10% of women in this category developed disseminated intra-abdominal carcinomatosis despite prophylactic oophorectomy.[17] Prophylactic oophorectomy may not be justifiable for women below 50 years without the risk of ovarian cancer.

CLASSIFICATION OF OVARIAN NEOPLASMS

Neoplasm of the ovary can arise from:
- Surface epithelium/serosa
- Ovarian stroma
- Secondary deposit/metastatic.

Surface epithelium: During embryonic life, the coelomic cavity forms and is lined by a mesothelial lining of mesodermal origin, parts of which become specialized to form the serosal epithelium covering the gonadal ridge. By process of invagination, this same mesothelial lining gives rise to Müllerian duct. Müllerian duct is the origin of fallopian tubes, uterus and vaginal wall. Therefore, it is not surprising that epithelial ovarian carcinoma may show histological features resembling those from these genital organs. Epithelial ovarian tumor which comprise 80–85% of all ovarian tumors can be classified into the following types (Box 37.1).

Ovarian stroma: The second group of ovarian tumors arise from specialized cells in the ovarian stroma. These have been classified into three categories, i.e. germ cell tumors, sex-cord stromal tumors and those of nonspecific mesenchymal origin (Box 37.2).

Box 37.1: Classification of epithelial ovarian tumors (80–85%).

- Serous tumor (resembles fallopian tube)
- Mucinous tumor (resembles endocervix)
- Endometrioid tumors
- Clear cell tumors (resembles endometrial glands during pregnancy rich in glycogen)
- Transitional-cells or Brenner tumors
- Mixed epithelial tumors
- Undifferentiated carcinoma

Box 37.2: Classifications of germ-cell, sex-cord stromal and non specific mesenchymal tumors.

Germ-cell tumors (10–15%)
- Dysgerminoma
- Yolk-sac tumor (Endodermal sinus tumor)
- Embryonal carcinoma
- Polyembryoma
- Choriocarcinoma
- Immature teratomas
- Mixed germ-cell tumor

Sex-cord stromal tumors (3–5%)
- Granulosa—stromal cell tumors
  - Granulosa cell tumor
  - Thecoma
  - Sclerosing stromal tumor
- Sertoli-stromal cell tumors
  - Sertoli-cell tumor
  - Leydig-cell tumor
  - Sertoli-Leydig cell tumor
- Gynandroblastoma
- Steroid-cell tumors
- Unclassified

Nonspecific mesenchymal tumors (<1%)
- Fibroma, hemangioma leiomyoma, lipoma
- Lymphoma
- Sarcoma

DIAGNOSIS

Symptoms and Signs

- Asymptomatic: Unfortunately ovarian cancer in its early stages does not produce any symptoms or signs that would alert the clinician to this diagnosis. This explains why approximately two-thirds of all ovarian cancers are already in stage 3 or 4 at diagnosis (Figs. 37.1 to 37.3)
- Gastrointestinal symptoms: Most frequent symptoms are those associated with gastrointestinal upset including bloating, abdominal distention and abdominal discomfort
- Abdominal mass
  - Respiratory symptoms due to abdominal distention, pleural effusion or metastases
  - Abnormal uterine bleeding due to hormone producing ovarian cancer, such as granulosa cell tumors

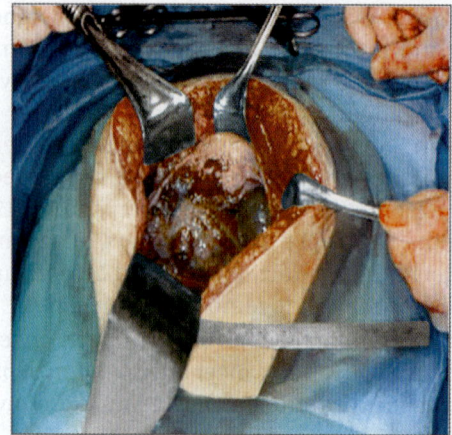

Fig. 37.1: Notice the right ovarian tumor (immature teratoma) that has extended anteriorly to the right broad ligament; it had infiltrated part of the bladder and was densely adherent to the rectum posteriorly. The patient was 28 years of age.

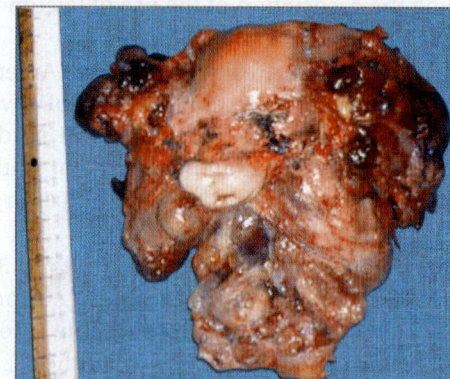

Fig. 37.2: The tumor (immature teratoma) has been removed en bloc with the uterus via a retroperitoneal approach; notice that it has eroded through the capsule.

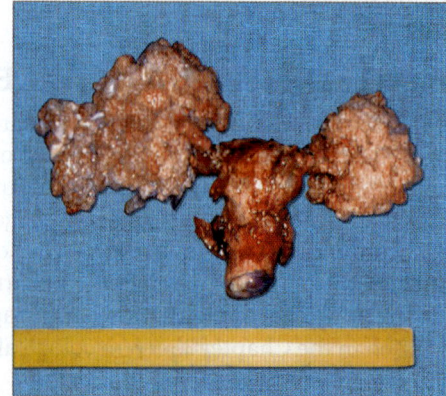

Fig. 37.3: Bilateral papillary serous cystadenocarcinoma of the ovary in a 38-year old patient. Notice the capsule has been completely eroded. There are deposits on the back of the uterus. The patient had ascites, "omental cake" and intraperitoneal deposits.

- Constitutional symptoms, such as loss of appetite, loss of weight, lethargy, etc. are an indication of progressing and advancing disease
- Acute symptoms are rare; this results from pain due to torsion, rupture, infection or intracystic hemorrhage.

EXAMINATION
General Examination
Pallor, loss of weight, palpable left supraclavicular lymph nodes and cachexia are late manifestations.

Specific Examination
Pleural effusion and reduced air entry may indicate lung involvement.

Abdominal distention may be due to ascites (shifting dullness in mild ascites, fluid thrill in gross ascites) or pelvic/abdominal mass. There may also be a palpable abdominal mass (omental cake) (Fig. 37.4) or organomegaly.

Pelvic examination may reveal the presence of an adnexal mass and if the tumor has spread to the bladder and rectum or other surrounding structures, the mass will become fixed/immobile (Figs. 37.1 to 37.3). In these instances, patients may also present with bowel and urinary symptoms. In addition to a vaginal examination, rectal or rectovaginal examination is useful in the evaluation of these masses.

PREOPERATIVE EVALUATION
Biochemical
Patients could be anemic, hypoproteinemic and suffering from electrolyte deficiencies in advanced stage of ovarian cancer; these need assessment prior to surgery. The tumor markers may be raised. Different type of ovarian cancers produced different tumor markers. As 80% of ovarian cancers are epithelial in origin, CA125 is a common tumor marker to be raised and this should be a routine investigation in a patient with suspected ovarian neoplasm.

Tumor marker is useful in aiding diagnosis but more importantly, it is very useful in assessment of the response to therapy. It can also be used for early detection of recurrence. Overall, approximately 85% of patients with epithelial ovarian cancer have a CA125 level of >35 iu/mL. However, elevated CA125 is found only in 50% of patient with stage 1 disease. In advanced stage, >90% will have elevation of CA125.[18-20] CA125 is less often elevated in mucinous, than serous tumors.[21] Other tumor markers are carcinoembryonic antigen(CEA), alpha-fetoprotein (AFP), human chorionic gonadotropin (hCG), inhibin, estrogen and androgen. The CEA level may be elevated in mucinous and Brenner tumor. The AFP level is elevated in endodermal sinus tumor (100%), immature teratoma (62%) and dysgerminoma (12%). The hCG level is invariably elevated in choriocarcinoma. Inhibin and estrogen levels may be elevated in granulosa cell tumor, whilst androgen levels are raised in Sertoli-Leydig cell tumors.

Imaging
Ultrasound is a very useful tool in aiding the diagnosis of ovarian tumors. The ultrasound features of ovarian malignancy are bilaterality, presence of solid areas, papillary projections, ascites, hydronephrosis or liver secondaries. CT scan may be able to identify lymphadenopathy, and detect peritoneal tumor deposits and is useful in the assessment of operability and extent of surgery anticipated preoperatively. CT scan, however, may not be able to detect lesions smaller than 1 cm size.

Endoscopy
In those with occult blood in stools or significant intestinal symptoms, colonoscopy needs to be done to exclude a primary colonic cancer with ovarian metastases. Similarly, an upper gastrointestinal endoscopy is important if there are significant gastric symptoms.

Breast Examination
Breast cancer may also metastasize to the ovaries. It is, therefore, important to examine the breasts in all cases; if there are suspicious palpable breast masses bilateral mammograms should be obtained.

STAGES OF OVARIAN CANCER
This is based on the **FIGO staging of ovarian cancer (2014)**:

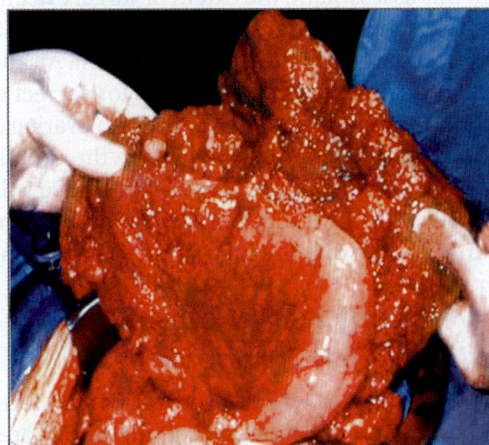

Fig. 37.4: "Omental cake" in a patient with advanced ovarian cancer. Notice the tumor deposits in the omentum and mesocolon.

Stage 1: *Tumor limited to the ovaries*

    1A Tumor limited to one ovary; capsule intact, no tumor on ovarian surface; negative peritoneal washings.

    1B Tumor involves both ovaries; otherwise like 1A.

    1C Tumor limited to one or both ovaries
- 1C1 There is surgical spill
- 1C2 Capsule rupture before surgery or tumor on ovarian surface
- 1C3 Malignant cells in ascites or peritoneal washings

Stage 2: *Tumor involves one or both ovaries with pelvic extension (below the pelvic brim) or primary peritoneal carcinoma*

    2A Extension and/or implants on uterus and/or Fallopian tube(s).

    2B Extension to other pelvic intraperitoneal tissues.

Stage 3: *Tumor involves one or both ovaries with cytologically or histologically confirmed spread to the peritoneum outside the pelvis and/or metastases to the retroperitoneal lymph node.*

    3A Positive retroperitoneal lymph nodes and/or microscopic metastasis beyond pelvis
- 3A1 Positive retroperitoneal nodes only

        3A1(i) Metastases $\leq$ 10 mm

        3A1(ii) Metastases > 10 mm

        3A2 Microscopic, extrapelvic (above the brim) peritoneal involvement +/- positive peritoneal lymph nodes.

    3B Macroscopic, extrapelvic, peritoneal metastasis 2 cm or less +/- positive retroperitoneal nodes. Includes extension to capsule of liver and spleen

    3C Macroscopic, extrapelvic, peritoneal metastasis >2 cm +/- positive retroperitoneal lymph node. Includes extension to capsule of liver and pelvis

Stage 4: A Pleural effusion with positive cytology

    B *Hepatic and/or splenic parenchymal metastases, metastases to extra-abdominal organs* (including inguinal lymph nodes and lymph nodes outside of the abdominal cavity).

Other points to note regarding staging are:
- Histological type including grading should be designated at staging
- Primary site (ovary, Fallopian tube or peritoneum) should be designated where possible
- Tumors that may otherwise qualify for stage 1 but involved with dense adhesions justify upgrading to Stage 2 if tumor cells are histologically proven to be present in the adhesions.

TREATMENT OF OVARIAN CARCINOMA

Surgery is the main modality of treatment of ovarian carcinoma, however, advanced or aggressive the tumor is. The extent of surgery is individually tailored, taking into consideration the patient's wishes. As the surgery may include resection of bowel and bowel anastomosis, the preoperative preparation of both small and large bowel is important.

Several factors will influence the extent of surgery in ovarian carcinoma. These are:
- Age and reproductive status
- Histological type of tumor
- Stage of disease
- General medical status.

Staging Laparotomy

The components of a comprehensive surgical staging are:[22]
- A thorough and systematic exploration of the whole peritoneal cavity—this should include examinations of the undersurface of the diaphragm, liver, spleen, stomach and intestines, para-aortic nodes and pelvic structures
- Cytological/histological sampling of paracolic gutters, subdiaphragmatic and pelvic peritoneal surfaces
- Omentectomy
- Para-aortic and pelvic node sampling.

This will help decide whether the disease:
- Is confined to one or both ovaries
- Has spread locally with metastases confined to pelvis
- Is more advanced with intra-abdominal metastases
- Is primary or secondary ovarian carcinoma.

From this assessment, the extent of surgery needed can be individually tailored. A Pfannenstiel incision (Fig. 37.5) is not adequate to allow this detailed assessment. An adequate upper abdominal exposure is essential for correct staging and optimal tumor excision in patients with ovarian cancer. A vertical incision extending well above the umbilicus is essential. The use of a laparoscopic light source will allow easy visualization of the upper surface of the liver and undersurface of the diaphragm—sites for early metastases.

Surgery for Early Well-encapsulated Epithelial Ovarian Carcinoma

In the young patient where preservation of fertility is desired, a unilateral or bilateral salpingo-oophorectomy (if there are bilateral tumors present) is performed; ideally these are sent for "frozen section". About a third of these

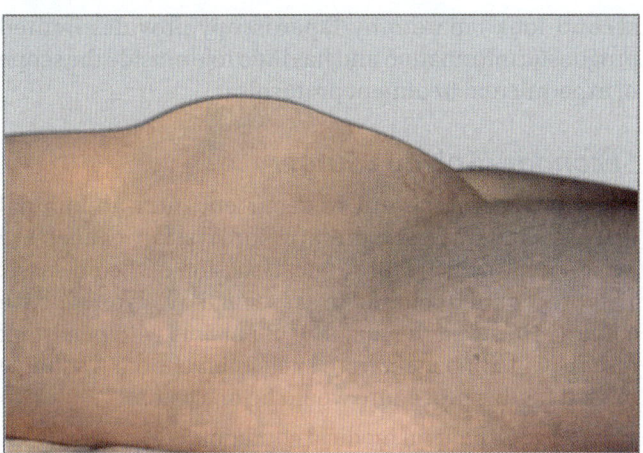

Fig. 37.5: The patient has a large suprapubic mass. She was referred after laparotomy via a Pfannenstiel incision showed the tumor to be fixed. This is not an appropriate incision for ovarian cancer surgery. The tumor is illustrated in Figures 37.1 and 37.2.

"apparent stage 1 cases" will be understaged if only a unilateral salpingo-oophorectomy is carried out.[23] If the tumor is grade 1 or 2 and the tumor is limited to one or both ovaries without capsular invasion and the peritoneal fluid cytology is negative for malignant cells, *(low-risk* cases) the above surgery would suffice; the uterus may be conserved, provided endometrial tumor is excluded. Adjuvant chemotherapy is not necessary.

In the presence of a poorly differentiated carcinoma (grade 3), clear cell carcinoma or positive peritoneal cytology *(high-risk* cases) conservative surgery is best avoided and a total hysterectomy, omentectomy with or without pelvic/para-aortic node dissection is performed. Adjuvant chemotherapy in these cases improves survival.

Deliberate puncture and aspiration must be avoided because this is dangerous and can result in iatrogenic tumor spread; malignant ovarian cysts must be removed intact.

In the management of *ovarian germ cell tumors,* the availability of effective chemotherapeutic regimes, such as PEB (cisplatinum, etoposide, bleomycin) and VAC (vincristine, actinomycin D and cyclophosphamide) has made conservative surgery possible even in advanced staged disease in young women.

Surgery for Ovarian Carcinoma with Local Extension (Figs. 37.1 and 37.2)

Maximal clearance is only possible via a primary extraperitoneal approach; a total hysterectomy, omentectomy pelvic/para-aortic lymphadenectomy is performed. This needs competence. Adjuvant chemotherapy improves survival.

Surgery for Ovarian Carcinoma with Disseminated Intraperitoneal Disease

The aim is cytoreductive surgery to achieve no macroscopic residual disease or to residual lesions <1 cm. To achieve this, the surgery should not increase operative mortality. The initial surgical approach influences survival and, therefore, it should be correctly done. Optimal debulking requires judgement and experience in addition to aggressive skills. Thus, advanced ovarian cancers are best not handled surgically by those not familiar with the radical approach to achieve optimal results.

The *benefits* of optimal cytoreduction are:

- Improves patient comfort
- Improves functional and nutritional status
- Improves oxygenation and blood flow resulting in delivery of cytotoxic drugs to residual tumor
- Small volume tumor needs fewer cycles of chemotherapy
- Decreases chance of chemo-resistance.

The median survival is significantly related to the residual tumor size at conclusion of surgery; the FIGO Annual Report 1998 reported 5 years survival of 56.5% when no microscopic residual disease was achieved, 32.5% when the residual disease was less than 2 cm and 13.1% when this was >2 cm. The best results are achieved when these cases are managed by gynecologic oncologists.

Place of Chemotherapy

Chemotherapy plays a very important *adjuvant* role in the treatment for ovarian cancer.[24] Except for a small group of patients with stage 1A, well and moderately differentiated tumors, the rest will require chemotherapy in the postoperative period (adjuvant chemotherapy). The overall 5-year survival in the small group of patients (stage 1A) is greater than 90%, and these patients can be spared the toxicity of chemotherapy.[25]

Surgery alone is rarely, if ever, curative for patients with advanced ovarian cancer. The choice of adjuvant chemotherapy depends on the histological type of cancer, i.e. epithelial or germ cell tumor. The platinum compound remains the most active agent in the treatment of epithelial ovarian cancer. It is also the cornerstone of combination drug regimens. Carboplatin is a second generation platinum compound. It is less nephrotoxic, less neurotoxic and less emetogenic than cisplatinum.[26] It can be administered in an out-patient basis. It's dose limiting toxicity is myelosuppression, especially thrombocytopenia.

Single agent carboplatin and combination regimes like paclitaxel and carboplatin along with cisplatinum, adriamycin (doxorubicin) and cyclophosphamide (PAC) are widely used regimes in the treatment of epithelial ovarian cancer.[27,28] In a recent randomized trial carried out by the International Collaborative Ovarian Neoplasm (ICON) group, all the 3 regimes were found to be equally effective.[29]

For germ cell tumors, cisplatinum, etoposide and bleomycin (PEB) is the most effective combination.

In selected patients who are poor operative risks with massive, pleural and peritoneal effusions or those who have been assessed preoperatively to have extensive, fixed pelvic tumors where optimal debulking is unlikely to be achieved, *neoadjuvant chemotherapy* has a role to achieve chemo-debulking and allow optimal surgery to be performed subsequently.

Massive Ovarian Cyst

These tumors are best removed intact. The malignancy rate has been reported to be 27%;[23] thus, siphonage prior to removal is to be avoided because of the risk of spillage of malignant cells. The tumor illustrated in Figure 37.6 was removed intact and weighed 41 kg; it was a mucinous cystadenocarcinoma.

"Second Look" Surgery

The role of 'second look' operations remain controversial. In the 1970s, this was used to assess patients after adjuvant chemotherapy for complete response both surgically and pathologically. A high complication rate of 63% has been reported previously.[30] A review of the literature shows that 4–53% of patients who had histologically negative second-look procedures subsequently succumbed;[25,26,29,31,32] thus,

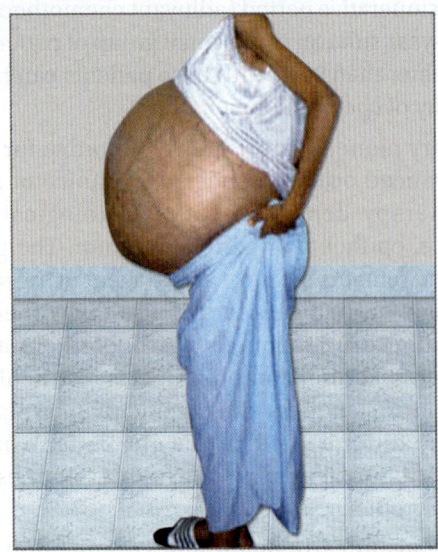

Fig. 37.6: Massive ovarian cyst in a 60-year-old lady, it weighed 41 kg and was a mucinous cystadenocarcinoma.

second-look laparotomy/laparoscopy provides limited prognostic information and has little role outside the scope of experimental treatment protocols.

Secondary Salvage Surgery

Patients with persistent or recurrent intra-abdominal disease after primary therapy for ovarian cancer are occasionally suitable for surgical excision of their disease. This procedure is referred to as "secondary" cytoreductive surgery. However, the majority of patients with persistent disease will not benefit from such intervention. A suitable patient for this procedure would be one who:

- Is in good general medical condition
- Has no ascites
- Has not had cisplatinum combination therapy
- Has had a reasonably long interval (>9–12 months) since primary surgery.

Optimal debulking should be the aim; only then are patients likely to respond to second-line chemotherapy.

Fertility Preservation in Young Patients with Ovarian Cancer

Approximately 7–8% of patients with stage 1 epithelial ovarian cancer are under 35 years of age.[33] Correct intraoperative histopathological diagnosis ('frozen section') will help prevent over- or under-treatment of these patients. Conservative surgery has been recommended for both malignant (Stage 1 or 2, non-clear cell) and borderline tumors in these young women. Subsequent successful pregnancy outcomes have been reported.[34] With the advent of highly innovative developments in assisted conception, it has become possible for women without ovaries to reproduce.[35,36]

Malignant germ cell tumors are extremely sensitive to chemotherapy with cure rates of 95% for early stage disease and 75% for advanced disease.[37,38] Fertility sparing surgery is possible even in those with advanced disease. Excellent pregnancy outcomes have been reported in patients with malignant germ cell tumors who have had conservative surgery with chemotherapy.[34,38,39]

It must be borne in mind that such conservative surgery is appropriate only in selected young women for the purpose of preserving reproductive function. It is generally not recommended when the patient is in the peri- or postmenopausal age.

CONCLUSION

Ovarian cancer continues to have an overall poor prognosis compared to other genital cancers; this is primarily due to the advanced stage at presentation.

Several advances have transformed the surgical approach to ovarian cancer management in the past two decades. For the vast majority of patients considered inoperable in the past, a wide range of surgical procedures are available today; these require experience, fine judgment and aggressiveness on the part of the surgeon. Although surgical cytoreduction is the main modality of therapy today, the importance of adjuvant chemotherapy should not be overlooked. Only a combination of these two modalities will help improve survival in these cases. Individualized management should be the objective to obtain cure in some and palliation in others with advanced disease.

REFERENCES

1. The First Report of the National Cancer Registry. Cancer incidence in Malaysia. 2002;148-50.
2. Green MH, Clark JW, Blayney DW. The epidemiology of ovarian cancer. Semin Oncol. 1984;11(3):209.
3. Cramer DW, Hutchison GB, Welch WR. Factors affecting the Association of Oral Contraceptives and Ovarian Cancer. N Engl J Med. 1982;307:1047.
4. Rossing MA, Daling JR, Weiss NS, et al. Ovarian tumor in a cohort of infertile women. N Engl J Med. 1994;331:771.
5. Lynch HT, Bewtra C, Lynch JF. Familial ovarian cancer clinical nuances. Am J Med. 1983;81:1073.
6. Schildkraut JM, Thompson WD. Familial ovarian cancer: A population-based case control study. Am J Epidemiology. 1988;128:456.
7. Auersperg N, Edelson MI, Mok SC, Johnson SW, Hamilton TC. The biology of ovarian cancer. Semin Oncol. 1998;25(3):281.
8. Slattery ML, et al. Nutrient intake and ovarian cancer. Am J Epidemiol. 1989;130.:497.
9. Longo DL, Young RC. Cosmetic talc and ovarian cancer. Lancet 1979;2:349.
10. Piver MS, Baker TR, Jishi MF, et al. Familial ovarian cancer. A report of 658 families from the Gilda Radner Familial Ovarian Cancer Registry 1981-1991. Cancer. 1993;1:582.
11. Daly M, Obrams GI. Epidemiology and risk assessment for ovarian cancer. Semin Onco. 1998;25:255.
12. Garg PP, Kerlikowske K, Subak L, et al. Hormone replacement therapy and the risk of epithelial ovarian cancer: A meta-analysis. Obstet Gynecol. 1998;92:472.
13. Fathalla MF. Incessant ovulation—factor in ovarian neoplasia. Lancet. 1971;2:163.
14. Rodriguez G. Biologic effect of progestins on the ovarian epithelium: Cancer prevention through apoptosis? 1999 (in press).
15. Janerich DT. Can fenretinide protect women against ovarian cancer? J Natl Cancer Inst. 1995; 87:146.
16. Hankinson SE, Hunter DJ, Colditz GA, et al. Tubal ligation, hysterectomy, and risk of ovarian cancer. A Prospective study. JAMA. 1993;270:2813.
17. Tobacman JK, Tucker MA, Kase R, Greene MH, Costa J, Fraumeni JF. Intra-abdominal carcinomatosis after pro-phylactic oophorectomy in ovarian-cancer-prone families. Lancet. 1982;2:795.
18. Bast RC, Klug TL, St John, et al. A radioimmunoassay using a monoclonal antibody to monitor the course of epithelial ovarian cancer. N Eng J Med. 1983;309:883.
19. Canney PA, Moore M, Wilkinson PM, James RD. Ovarian cancer antigen CA125: A prospective clinical assessment of its role as a tumor marker. Br J Cancer. 1984;50:765.
20. Jacobs I, Bast RC. The CA 125 tumor-associated antigen: A review of the literature. Hum Reprod. 1989;4:1.
21. Vergote IB, Bormer OP, Abeler VM. Evaluation of serum CA125 levels in the monitoring of ovarian cancer. Am J Obstet Gynecol. 1987;157:88.
22. Young RC, Decker DG, Wharton JT. Staging laparotomy in early ovarian cancer. JAMA. 1983; 250:3072.
23. Dottors DJ, Katz VL, Curvie J. Massive ovarian cyst. A comprehensive surgical approach. Obst Gynecol Surv. 1988;43:191.
24. Young RC, Walton LA, Ellenberg SS. Adjuvant therapy in stage I and II epithelial ovarian cancer. Results of two prospective randomized trials. N Engl J Med. 1990;322:1021.
25. Greco F, Julin CG, Richardson R, et al. Advanced ovarian cancer: Brief intensive combination chemotherapy and second look operations. Obstet Gynecol. 1981;58:199.
26. Jones S, Khoo IS, Whitaker S. Evaluation of ovarian cancer by second look laparotomy after treatment. Anst NZJ Surgery. 1981;51:30.
27. Canetta R, Bragman K, Smaldone L. Carboplatin: Current status and future prospects. Cancer Treat Rev. 1988;15:17.
28. The International Collaborative Ovarian Neoplasm Group. Paclitaxel plus carboplatin versus standard chemotherapy with either single agent carboplatin or cyclophosphamide, doxorubicin and cisplatin in women with ovarian cancer: The ICON 3 randomized trial. The Lancet. 2002;360:505.
29. Luseley DM, Chan KK, Fielding JWL, et al. Second-look laparotomy in the management of epithelial ovarian carcinoma: An evaluation of fifty cases. Obstet Gynecol. 1984;64:421.
30. Chambers S, Chambers JT, Kohorn ET. Evaluation of the role of second-look surgery in ovarian cancer. Obstet Gynecol. 1988;72:404.
31. Ho G, Beller U, Speyer JL, Columbo N, et al. A reassessment of the role of second-look laparotomy in advanced ovarian cancer. J of Oncol. 1988;5:1316.
32. Copeland IJ, Gershenson DM. Ovarian cancer recurrences in patient with no marcoscopic tumor at second-look laparotomy. Obstet Gynecol. 1988;68:873.
33. Novot D, Williams M, Brodman M, et al. The concept of uterine preservation with ovarian malignancies. Obstet Gynecol. 1991; 78:566-8.

34. Maltaris T, Boechim D, Dittrical R, et al. Reproduction beyond cancer: A message of hope for women. Gynec Oncol. 2006;103:1109-21.
35. Novot D, Laufer N, Kopolovic T, et al. Artificially-induced endometrial cycles and establishment of pregnancies in the absence of ovaries. N Eng J Med. 1986; 314:806-811.
36. Rosenwake Z. Donor eggs. Their application in modern reproductive technologies. Fertil Steril. 1987;47:885-90.
37. Tangir J, Zalterman D, Ma W, et al. Reproductive function after conservative surgery and chemotherapy for malignant germ cell tumors of the ovary. Obstet Gynecol. 2003;101:251-7.
38. Sivanesaratnam V, Sen DK, Peh SC. Cure of stage IV endodermal sinus tumor of the ovary with pulsed cyclophosphamide. Gynecol Oncol.1986;133-5.
39. Sivanesaratnam V. Third S.S. Ratnam Memorial Lecture 2007. Ovarian Cancer : Is there hope for women? J Obstet Gynecol Res. 2009;3:393-404.

CHAPTER 38

Uterine Malignancy

Christina Portelli, Tim Duncan

Overview

- Uterine malignancy is the fourth most common female cancer after breast, lung and bowel cancer in the UK and is the sixth most common worldwide. Uterine cancer incidence is the highest in North America and lowest in South-Central Asia. This may be partly reflected by varying data quality worldwide but more likely reflects the contrasting rates of obesity.
- The variation between countries may reflect different prevalence of risk factors, genetics and diagnostic methods.
- Endometrial cancer is the most common gynecological cancer in the UK principally affecting postmenopausal women.
- About 75% of cases are diagnosed in postmenopausal women.
- The peak incidence is 64–74 years with a subsequent reduction in incidence in those over 80 years old.
- The most common presenting symptom is abnormal or postmenopausal bleeding. This can be an early sign, often with the cancer being confined to the uterus. 8–10% of women presenting with postmenopausal bleeding have endometrial cancer.
- Diagnostic investigations may include an office based or hysteroscopic endometrial biopsy and transvaginal ultrasonography.
- Staging investigations may include a chest X-ray, MRI or CT.
- Staging is based on the surgico-pathological findings.
- The surgical management includes total hysterectomy and bilateral salpingo-oopherectomy, which increasingly is being performed via the laparoscopic route. Pelvic and para-aortic lymphadenectomy may be performed according local protocols. There is huge regional variation in practice relating to lymphadenectomy.
- Adjuvant therapy may be required according to the stage, grade and presence of lymphovascular invasion of the tumor. Adjuvant therapy has traditionally been in the form of external beam radiotherapy combined with the vaginal brachytherapy, although the rates are falling.
- Radiotherapy and hormonal treatment can be an option for those medically unfit for surgery and in the palliative setting to control symptoms of vaginal bleeding secondary to locally advanced disease.
- Salvage radiotherapy can be used successfully for localized pelvic recurrences.
- Systemic chemotherapy is increasing being used in high-risk cases, although data confirming a survival advantage have yet to be reported. Chemotherapy can also be used for women with disseminated primary disease and for recurrence.
- There might be a role for hormonal treatment in the form of progestogens in women diagnosed with recurrent tumors and also in selected cases as a fertility preserving treatment.
- The overall five-year survival is over 70%.

INTRODUCTION

Malignant disease of the uterus most commonly arises in the endometrium. In western countries, it is now the most common gynecological cancer. Postmenopausal bleeding is the most common complaint in women diagnosed with endometrial cancer. However, endometrial cancer can present in premenopausal women and presenting with new onset menorrhagia or intermenstrual bleeding. Such women may have a delay in diagnosis as they are often initially managed as a menstrual disorder. There is a strong etiological association with unopposed estrogen and uterine cancer. This should be considered in symptomatic younger women with polycystic ovarian syndrome (PCOS) and obesity and appropriate investigations organized. In general endometrial cancer presents at an early stage and hence carries a good prognosis. The cornerstone of treatment is a hysterectomy and removal of the ovaries. Surgery is often via the laparoscopic route, which carries huge advantages in this typically obese population. Radiotherapy and increasing chemotherapy is utilized in advanced and high-risk cases. Endometrial hyperplasia is a precursor to endometrial cancer and shares many of the same risk factors.

EPIDEMIOLOGY AND RISK FACTORS

5,300 cases of endometrial cancer are diagnosed each year in UK with approximately 1,650 deaths. The incidence varies between countries and different patient groups. The incidence has been found to be seven times higher in Caucasian North Americans compared to their Chinese counterparts. The median age of the endometrial cancer is 61 years with 75% occurring in the postmenopausal years. However, 3–8% are under the age of 45 when diagnosed.

HISTOPATHOLOGY

Endometrial Hyperplasia

Hyperplasia of the endometrium is characterized by an increased glandular component. The gland and stroma ratio is often increased. The International Society of Gynaecological Pathologist and World Health Organization (WHO) have a proposed classification system based on the architectural and cytological features (Table 38.1). The simplified system is being increasingly adopted and hinges on the presence or absence of cytological atypia, which is the key feature in relation to risk of malignant transformation. If nuclear and cytological abnormalities exist then it is classified as atypical hyperplasia.

In the absence of cellular atypia hyperplasia has low-risk of malignancy potential (1–4% risk), although treatment with progestogens is usually recommended, especially if the patient is symptomatic. In the presence of cellular atypia the risk of concurrent, or progression to, endometrial cancer can be as high as 45%, these patients are treated in line with those with low grade endometrial cancer.

Uterine cancer commonly arise in glandular cells and are termed endometrial cancers (epithelial neoplasms), the remainder are at least in part derived from the connective tissue, namely stroma and muscle (non-epithelial or mixed nonepithelial neoplasms).

Epithelial Tumors

There are two main types of endometrial cancer:

Type 1: Estrogen related endometroid adenocarcinoma this is the more common type (75%). Overall 5 year survival is around 85%. These are associated with endometrial hyperplasia.

Type 2: Non-estrogen related (papillary serous, clear-cell and adenosquamous carcinoma). Recently, a precursor lesion for papillary serous carcinoma, termed endometrial intraepithelial carcinoma, has been described. These subtypes tend to behave more aggressively with earlier metastasis and consequently more advanced disease. A much poorer prognosis is observed with 5 year survival being around 50%.

Endometriod adenocarcinomas are graded based on the varying degree of nuclear atypic, mitotic activity and stratification appearance of the tumor. There are three grades well, moderate and poorly differentiated which corresponds to grade I-III respectively. All type 2 endometrial cancers are deemed to be grade III. Grade III tumors are the most aggressive and likely to recur. The grade of the cancer is a crucial feature in determining the extent of surgical staging required and type of adjuvant postoperative treatment offered.

Nonepithelial Tumors

Endometrial Stromal and Undifferentiated Sarcoma

Endometrial stromal neoplasms, a subset of uterine mesenchymal neoplasms account for less than 10% of uterine sarcomas and approximately 1% of all uterine malignant neoplasms. Endometrial stromal neoplasms are classified into three categories (WHO):

- Endometrial stromal nodule (ESN)
- Endometrial stromal sarcoma (ESS)
- Undifferentiated endometrial sarcoma (UES).

Simple hysterectomy is curative for ESN however, ESS and UES are neoplasms with malignant and metastatic potential. Historically, they were characterized as either low or high-grade ESS. However, high-grade endometrial stromal tumors are now referred to as undifferentiated endometrial sarcomas (UES) or high-grade undifferentiated uterine sarcomas (HGUS), reflecting their composition of anaplastic cells with little or no evidence of endometrial stromal differentiation. Stage 2 and more advanced ESS

Table 38.1: Classification system based on architectural and cytological features.

Pattern	Cytological atypia	WHO	Simplified WHO
Rounded glands with regular outlines	None	Simple hyperplasia	Endometrial hyperplasia
Closely packed glands with irregular outlines	None	Complex hyperplasia	Endometrial hyperplasia
Rounded glands with regular outlines	Focal	Simple hyperplasia with atypia	Atypical endometrial hyperplasia
Closely packed glands with irregular outlines	Multifocal or diffuse	Complex hyperplasia with atypia*	Atypical endometrial hyperplasia

*This pattern has about 25% risk of progressing to carcinoma

tumors are treated with adjuvant endocrine regimes (e.g. medroxyprogesterone). Radiotherapy may be administered to reduce the risk of locoregional disease recurrence. As UES are high grade tumors, they have a high-risk of recurrence regardless of the stage. All patients with UES diagnosis are offered adjuvant chemotherapy, although due the varity if the disease data on the most effective regimes is limited.

Observation alone for early stage is a reasonable treatment option. Due to the lack of high quality data participation in clinical trials should be encouraged.

LEIOMYOSARCOMA

Histologically, leiomyosarcomas typically have prominent cellular atypia, abundant mitoses (≥10 per 10 high power fields), and areas of coagulative necrosis. As these smooth muscle neoplasms arise in the stroma, they are more difficult to classify as benign (without metastatic potential) or malignant (with metastatic potential). Cellular atypia, mitosis, and "coagulative necrosis" are known as the Stanford criteria. In the largest retrospective study, which resulted in the development of these criteria, the presence of two of the three features indicated a risk of metastatic spread of >10% (Table 38.2). However, opinions vary as to the exact level of mitotic activity required for diagnosis of sarcoma. Other common features, which may be used in borderline cases, are hypercellularity features and an infiltrative border.

Leiomyosarcomas are typically large (>10 cm) yellow or tan solitary masses. They have a soft fleshy cut surface with hemorrhagic and necrotic areas. The mass may bulge into the uterine cavity, but the epicenter is in the myometrium.

Leiomyosarcomas and leiomyomas are independent entities. Leiomyosarcomas are rare, while they may coexist with benign leiomyomas (fibroids), they exhibit distinctive cytogenetic abnormalities. Fibroids do not appear to be a precursor to leiomyosarcomas. Both neoplasms may express estrogen and progesterone receptors.

The majority of leiomyosarcomas present in postmenopausal women, with classical symptoms being pain, bleeding and a rapidly increasing pelvic mass. Such features in a postmenopausal woman with "fibroids" should raise suspicion. There are no reliable diagnostic tests as endometrial biopsies are often normal due to the tumor arising deep to the uterine lining. In addition magnetic resonance imaging (MRI), computed tomography (CT) and ultrasound have very poor predictive values, although the presence of necrosis within a fibroid, which can be seen on MRI, should be considered as suspicious. Following a prominent legal case in the US, the difficulty in differentiating benign leiomyoma from their malignant counterpart, has led to a rapid reduction in uterine morcellation during laparoscopic surgery for fibroids.

Mixed endometrial stromal and smooth muscle tumor are also referred to as stromomyomas, and are defined as having at least 30% each of endometrial stromal and smooth muscle components. There is very little data on this type of tumor.

Mixed Epithelial-Nonepithelial Tumors

Uterine adenosarcoma is a rare mixed epithelial-nonepithelial neoplasm. This accounts for 5–9% of all uterine sarcomas. On histological analysis, adenosarcomas have a benign epithelial component mixed with a malignant

Table 38.2: Classification of problematic uterine smooth muscle tumors based on pathologic features.

Group	Mitotic index (per 10 HPF)	Atypia	Coagulatve tumor cell necrosis	Designation	Metastatic or recurrent disease
I	≥5 to <20	None or mild	None	Leiomyoma with increased MI	1/89
II A	<10	Diffuse, moderate or severe	None	Atypical leiomyoma with low-risk percent or recurrence	2/46
II B	≥10	Diffuse, moderate or severe	None	Leiomyosarcoma	4/10
III	≤20	Diffuse, moderate to severe	Present	Leiomyosarcoma	19/33
IV A	<10	None to mild	Present	Smooth muscle tumors of low malignant potential, limited experience	1/4
IV B	≥10	None to mild	Present	Leiomyosarcoma	3/4
V	≥1 to ≤20	Multifocal, moderate to severe	None	Atypical leiomyoma, limited experience	0/5

(MI: mitotic index; HPF: high power fields)
Source: Bell SW et al. Am J Surg Pathol. 1994; 18:535.

stromal (i.e. sarcomatous) element. Uterine adenosarcoma present as solid, typically edematous, polypoid mass usually arising from the fundus. They are typically considered as low grade neoplasms with a low malignant potential with a good prognosis. The majority of adenosarcomas are diagnosed at stage I with an overall survival of over 80%. Most commonly adenosarcomas arise in the endometrium, but they may also present in the myometrium, cervix, or extrauterine Müllerian tissues.

PATTERNS OF SPREAD

Disease dissemination occurs through the myometrium and into the lymphovascular space. Lymphatic spread can occur to the pelvic and para-aortic lymph nodes and occasionally the inguinal and supraclavicular nodes. The cervix, ovaries and fallopian tubes can be involved though lymphatic and direct invasion. There may also be an associated estrogen secreting primary ovarian tumor, e.g. granulosa cell tumor

Endometrial cancer may also spread transperitoneally through the myometrium, breaching the uterine surface or via the fallopian tubes. This can lead to a carcinomatosis picture with diffuse peritoneal involvement similar to that seen in advanced ovarian cancer. This pattern of spread is more commonly seen with papillary serous cancers.

Hematogenous spread leading most commonly to liver and lungs metastases can also be seen.

RISK FACTORS

- Obesity
- Polycystic ovarian disease
- Nulliparity
- Unopposed estrogen hormonal replacement therapy
- Personal or family history of breast, bowel, uterine cancer (e.g. Lynch syndrome)
- Some selective estrogen selector modulators (Tamoxifen)
- Estrogen secreting ovarian tumors, e.g. thecoma, granulosa cell tumor
- Diabetes
- Hypertension
- Endometrial hyperplasia (premalignant condition)
- Late menopause.

Endometrial cancer is uncommon in premenopausal women and genetic factors account for only 1% of newly diagnosed cases. Lynch syndrome or hereditary nonpolyposis colorectal cancer syndrome (HNPCC) is associated with a relative risk of 1.5 for the development of endometrial cancer before the menopause. Women with Lynch syndrome have a 27–71% risk of developing endometrial cancer. These women have a germline

Box 38.1: Amsterdam II Criteria.

Each of the following is required
- Three or more relatives with colorectal, endometrial, small intestine, ureter, or renal pelvis cancer
- Two or more successive generations affected
- One or more relatives diagnosed before age 50
- One patient should be a first-degree relative of the other two
- Exclusion of familial adenomatous polyposis in cases of colorectal cancer
- Pathological verification of tumors

mutation in one mismatch repair allele. The second allele is inactivated through mutation, loss of heterozygosity, or epigenetic silencing by promoter hypermethylation. Inactivation of both alleles causing dysfunction in DNA repair mechanisms which produces increased DNA mutations and alteration of microsatellite regions in the tumor compared to normal tissue. Microsatellite instability is found in 90% of tumor tissue from patients with Lynch syndrome. *MSH2* and *MLH1* account for 90% of the identified mutuations, however, other mutations in *PMS1*, *MSH6*, and *MLH3* have also been described. The median age of diagnosis in women with Lynch syndrome is 46–54 years. Most are of endometroid subtype, although non-endometrioid tumors have also been reported, with the majority diagnosed at an early-stage. Women with Lynch syndrome are at risk for other cancers. The Amsterdam Criteria have been developed to identify families at risk for Lynch syndrome (Box 38.1). The Society of Gynecologic Oncologists published committee guidelines for genetic testing of individuals at risk for Lynch syndrome (Box 38.2).

Protective factors against endometrial cancer:
- Combined contraceptive pill
- Progestogens
- Early menopause
- Multiparity.

CLINICAL FEATURES

The most common presenting symptom is postmenopausal bleeding (PMB), although 90% of women with this symptom will not have cancer. Atrophic vaginitis is the most common cause of PMB. However, as this is so commonly seen in postmenopausal women full investigation to exclude other cuases is still required, i.e. this is a diagnosis of exclusion. 10% of women presenting with postmenopausal bleeding have endometrial cancer. Abnormal vaginal discharge may precede vaginal bleeding.

As well as abnormal bleeding women with sarcomas can present with increasing abdominal girth, pelvic pain and abnormal vaginal discharge.

CHAPTER 38 Uterine Malignancy

Box 38.2: Society of Gynecologic Oncologists Statement Guidelines on Risk Assessment for Lynch Syndrome.

Genetic evaluation strongly recommended if risk of Lynch syndrome is 20–25%
- Pedigree meeting Amsterdam Criteria
- Patients with synchronous or metachronous colorectal and endometrial or ovarian cancers before age 50 years
- Patients with first- or second-degree relative with germline mutation in an MMR gene

Genetic assessment may be "helpful" if risk of Lynch syndrome is 5–10%
- Patients with endometrial or colorectal cancer before age 50 years
- Patients with endometrial and/or ovarian cancer and another Lynch-associated malignancy before age 50 years
- Patients with endometrial or colorectal cancer and a first-degree relative with a Lynch syndrome–associated malignancy before age 50 year
- Patients with endometrial or colorectal cancer at any age with 2 or more first- or second-degree relatives of any age with a Lynch syndrome–associated malignancy
- Patients with first- or second-degree relative who meets above criteria

Premenopausal women presenting with irregular and intermenstrual bleeding may also uncommonly have endometrial cancer. This should be suspected in particularly in women with the previously described risk factors, in particular obesity. Abnormal cervical cytology due to presence of endometrial malignant cells is a represents a more unusual presentation of endometrial cancer.

A rapid increase in size of the fibroid is a worrying feature, particularly in postmenopausal women and warrants further investigations as malignant transformation may be occurring. Advanced disease may present with pelvic pain, hematuria, abdominal distension or pulmonary symptoms.

DIAGNOSIS AND INVESTIGATIONS

An endometrial biopsy sample is required for diagnosis and this can often be achieved in the outpatient setting using an endometrial sampler (e.g. Pipelle©). This is tolerated reasonably well by most by women, with an accuracy of 90%.

A transvaginal ultrasound measurement of the endometrial thickness (ET) in postmenopausal women helps to stratify the risk of endometrial cancer. The thicker the endometrium the greater the risk. If the ET is less than 4 mm endometrial cancer is very unlikely, with the risk being reduced from 10% to less than 1%. Most centers will therefore not perform a biopsy if the ET is less than 4 mm. Considering the negative predictive value is not 100%, patients with recurrent PMB should have a biopsy performed regardless of the ET.

Hysteroscopy and biopsy is an alternative to sampling and maybe be carried out in the outpatient setting. This has the advantage of being able to visualize the uterine cavity with directed biopsies of suspicious areas and resection of any polyps identified. Hysteroscopy and curettage under anesthesia may be performed if the outpatient setting is unsatisfactory or unsuitable.

The role of MRI is still debatable in staging, however it can provide valuable information on extrauterine disease, depth of myometrial invasion, cervical involvement and the presence of lymphatic spread. In combination with tumor grade, the depth of myometrial invasion determined by pelvic MRI, can aid in determining the risk of lymphatic involvement and hence whether a lymphadenectomy is indicated. It is also invaluable in planning radiotherapy as it allows accurate assessment of tumor volumes. CT imaging may evaluate the presence of distant metastases and this is more commonly utilized where the risk of distant spread is greater, such as type 2 endometrial cancer and sarcomas. The role of PET CT is yet to be established.

REVISED FIGO STAGING 2009

Endometrial cancer staging is based on the surgical and pathological findings.

Carcinoma of the Endometrium

IA	Tumor confined to the uterus, no or <½ myometrial invasion
IB	Tumor confined to the uterus, >½ myometrial invasion
II	Cervical stromal invasion, but not beyond uterus
IIIA	Tumor invades serosa or adnexa
IIIB	Vaginal and/or parametrial involvement
IIIC1	Pelvic node involvement
IIIC2	Para-aortic involvement
IVA	Tumor invasion bladder and/or bowel mucosa
IVB	Distant metastases including abdominal metastases and/or inguinal lymph nodes.

Uterine sarcomas (Leiomyosarcoma, endometrial stromal sarcoma, and adenosarcoma)

IA	Tumor limited to uterus <5 cm
IB	Tumor limited to uterus >5 cm
IIA	Tumor extends to the pelvis, adnexal involvement

IIB	Tumor extends to extrauterine pelvic tissue
IIIA	Tumor invades abdominal tissues, one site
IIIB	More than one site
IIIC	Metastasis to pelvic and/or para-aortic lymph nodes
IVA	Tumor invades bladder and/or rectum
IVB	Distant metastasis.

PROGNOSTIC FACTORS

An appreciation of prognostic factors will aid patient counseling and determine the need for adjuvant therapy. Patients can be stratified into the following groups according to surgical and final pathological analysis of the uterus, lymph nodes and omentum (Box 38.3).

Low-risk Group

These are cancers with grade I differentiation, no myometial invasion or intraperitonenal spread of the disease. The risk of pelvic lymph node disease is less than 1%.

Intermediate Risk Group

The Gynecologic Oncology Group stratifies this group of women who have disease within the myometrium or occult cervical stromal invasion. This group is further divided with an intermediate high-risk group consisting of cancers with invasion into the outer third of the myometrium, grade 2 or 3 tumors, or evidence of lymphovascular space invasion. This group of patients often receives adjuvant therapy.

Women with myometrial invasion, high-grade tumor and/or intraperitoneal disease can have a risk of nodal disease of up to 60%.

High-risk Group

These patients have evidence of lymph node involvement, serous uterine cancer or clear cell carcinoma at any stage. These are considered at high-risk of recurrence and often receive adjuvant therapy.

MANAGEMENT

In presumed early stage disease surgical management consists of hysterectomy, bilateral salpingo-oopherectomy and evaluation of the peritoneal cavity. The inspection of the abdomen includes assessment of the peritoneal surfaces, liver surface and omentum. This can be carried out through open or laparoscopic surgery. There are numerous randomized controlled trials (RCT), e.g. LACE trial, advocating the use of laparoscopic surgery due to the reduction in complications and improvement in quality of life scores. The RCTs comparing traditional

Box 38.3: Prognostic factors.

- Lymph node involvement
- Lymphovascular space invasion
- Histological subtype
- Peritoneal cytology*
- Steroid receptor
- Stage of the disease
- Tumor differentiation
- Ploidy status
- Tumor size
- Age
- Performance status

* No longer part of FIGO staging

open hysterectomy with a laparoscopic approach all give consistent conclusions. Firstly, the perioperative risks are reduced with a laparoscopic approach in particular the reduction in venous thromboembolic disease, wound infections and the need for blood transfusions. Secondly, the patients length of stay, pain scores and numerous quality of life measures are superior with laparoscopic surgery. Importantly, there is no difference in progression free and overall survival. Many consider a laparoscopic approach to be the gold standard.

Patients presenting with more advanced disease, with evidence of disease outside of the uterus may be a candidate for more extensive surgery. In patients with cervical involvement some advocate a radical hysterectomy that involves removal of the uterus, cervix, parametria and upper vagina. An alternative is to administer radiotherapy following a more standard hysterectomy. There is no convincing data to suggest which approach is most effective. In women where the is macroscopic disease in lymph nodes or other sites within the peritoneum, a debulking approach to surgery similar to that performed for ovarian cancer can be considered. A number of studies suggest there may be a survival advantage to complete macroscopic resection of disease followed by adjuvant therapy. Clearly the more extensive surgery must be balanced against a patient's wishes and performance status.

The role of pelvic and para-aortic lymphadenectomy is controversial. The indications vary between institutions but tend to be restricted to the high-risk subtypes. There is limited evidence of a therapeutic role for lymphadenectomy with macroscopically normal nodes. Most clinicians performing lymphadenectomy use nodal status to triage the use of adjuvant therapies. The a study in treatment of endometrial cancer (ASTEC) study has not supported the use of lymphadenectomy to improve outcome. Those undergoing lymphadenectomy were associated with more complications such as lower limb lymphedema (5–10%) and vascular injury (0.5–1.0%). The risk of lymphedema was greatest in those patients receiving adjuvant radiotherapy following nodal surgery. The trial has been criticized due to poor lymph node counts observed and a disregard for the nodal status in determining the need for adjuvant treatment. This issue forms the basis of many current and forthcoming endometrial cancer trials. Other clinical trials are focusing on the potential application of sentinel lymph node techniques to endometrial cancer.

Radiotherapy for endometrial cancer is given as external beam therapy (EBRT) and vaginal brachytherapy (VB). Radiotherapy has traditionally formed the basis of adjuvant therapy in endometrial cancer. EBRT side effects are common, although they are improving with newer more accurate radiotherapy systems such as image modulated radiotherapy treatment (IMRT). Radiotherapy side effects include long-lasting adverse effects to vagina, bowel and urinary tract including fibrosis, stricture, fistula formation, and second malignancies.

Some international RCTs, most notably the PORTEC trials, have led to a significant change in practice. A number of RCTs have demonstrated that whilst radiotherapy reduces the incidence of local recurrence it fails to improve overall survival. This is due to the high radiotherapy salvage rate that can be achieved in radiation naïve patients with pelvic recurrence. In addition, radiotherapy fails to reduce the risk distant relapse. The PORTEC 2 trial also demonstrated that VB was as effective as EBRT at controlling local relapse with a fraction of the toxicities. Hence, the use of adjuvant radiotherapy in early stage endometrial cancer, with exception of VB, is used much less commonly.

Palliative radiotherapy can be used for symptomatic vaginal bleeding control and those medically unfit for surgery.

The use of chemotherapy is increasing common in patients with extrauterine disease and type 2 cancers. The evidence is still developing, with large trials, e.g. PORTEC 3, still waiting to report. However, chemotherapy is already creeping into standard practice in conjunction with radiotherapy or in isolation.

Fertility Sparing Treatment

Up to 5% of endometrial carcinomas are diagnosed in premenopausal, nulliparous women. In such cases there is an evolving role for fertility preserving treatment using progestogens. Management is based on the tumor grade, cell type, hormone receptor status and depth of myometrial invasion. Fertility sparing treatment options are not recommended for high-risk patients, e.g. grade 3 and type 2 carcinomas, high-risk because of the poor response rate and high-risk of distant disease.

Fortunately young women are more likely to have low-grade endometroid carcinomas type that convey a more favorable prognosis. Such tumors are more likely to express progesterone receptors and thus, are more likely to respond to progesterone therapy. Oral medroxyprogesterone and megestrol acetate are used for such hormonal treatment options. Less data is available for the IUS but this is showing some promising initial response rates of up to 75%. Surveillance with repeated 3 monthly endometrial sampling is recommended to assess response and surgery recommended if there is disease progression or persistence.

Follow-up

The most common site of recurrence is the vaginal vault with an overall risk of 15–20%. This is reduced by adjuvant radiotherapy in the form of brachytherapy.

There is no evidence to support a survival advantage from routine follow-up for women treated for endometrial cancer. However, these women are more likely to need physiological support and management of post-treatment toxicities. All patients should have access to specialist nurse and palliative team specialists if required. There is no evidence that routine radiological imaging offers any benefit. The additional aim of follow-up is to detect any recurrent disease and initiate treatment as early as possible, although the evidence that early detection and treatment of recurrence confers any prognostic benefit is lacking.

CONCLUSION

Most uterine cancers arise in the endometrium. The incidence is rising rapidly, which is thought to be directly linked to the epidemic of obesity in the developed world. Prognosis depends upon the stage, grade and subtype of the cancer (Table 38.3). The treatment is based on total hysterectomy and bilateral salpingo-oophorectomy, which is increasingly performed via the laparoscopic route. Lymphadenectomy is utilized to varying degrees. Considering that PMB is the most common and very obvious symptom, the majority of patients present at an early stage. This leads to a favorable prognosis for the majority. There is a reducing role for adjuvant radiotherapy and an increasing role for chemotherapy. Uterine sarcomas have a poor prognosis but are fortunately rare.

Table 38.3: FIGO staging and overall 5 year survival.

Stage	5 year survival
IA	88%
IB	75%
II	69%
IIIA	58%
IIIB	50%
IIIC	47%
IVA	17%
IVB	15%

BIBLIOGRAPHY

1. Abeloff's Clinical Oncology, Fifth Edition Niederhuber, John E., MD John F. Boggess and Joshua E. Kilgore 88, 1575-1591.e4.
2. Bell SW, Kempson RL, Hendrickson MR. Problematic uterine smooth muscle neoplasms. A clinicopathologic study of 213 cases. Am J Surg Pathol. 1994;18(6):535-58.
3. Department of Pathology, Stanford University Medical Center, CA 94305. [1994, 18(6):535-558]
4. FIGO staging for endometrial and uterine cancer- The International Federation of Gynecology and Obstetrics (FIGO).
5. Gynaecological Oncology for the MRCOG and Beyond Second edition Edited by Nigel Acheson and David Luesley RCOG.
6. Pecorelli S. Revised FIGO staging for carcinoma of the vulva, cervix, and endometrium. Int J Gynaecol Obstet. 2009; 105: 103-4. cancerresearch.org.uk
7. Society of Gynecologic Oncologists Education Committee statement on risk assessment for inherited gynecologic cancer predispositions. Gynecol Oncol. 2007;107(2):159–62. Lancaster JM, et al. National Cancer Data Base as published in the AJCC Staging Manual in 2010.

CHAPTER 39

Vulvar Cancer

V Sivanesaratnam

Overview

- Malignancies in the vulva are uncommon and comprise 3–4% of genital tract malignancies.
- The most common symptom is long standing vulva pruritus and a recognizable lesion which is usually raised, fleshy, ulcerated or warty in appearance.
- The management of early vulvar lesions should be individualized with emphasis on carrying out the most conservative procedure that will achieve cure for the patient.
- For advanced disease a multidisciplinary team approach is needed in the surgical management of such patients for optimal results.

INTRODUCTION

Malignancies in the vulva are uncommon and comprise 3–4% of genital tract malignancies. Internationally, the incidence of vulva cancer varies, the highest rates being seen in Portuguese South America and in Portugal; the lowest rates are seen in Asian countries.[1] Asian women who have migrated to Australia continue to be at significantly lower risk for this malignancy.[2] The true incidence in Malaysia is not known. The University of Malaya Medical Center is a major referral center for gynecological malignancies. Of the 3,125 gynecological malignancies managed during a 12-year period, vulva malignancies comprised 2.8% (Table 39.1); thus, this malignancy is rare in Malaysia.

Table 39.1: Gynecological malignancies managed at the University of Malaya Medical Center, KL 1991-2002.

Malignancy	Number	%
Carcinoma cervix	1,466	47.0
Carcinoma of ovary	960	30.7
GTD	284	9.1
Carcinoma endometrium	269	8.6
Carcinoma vulva	88	2.8
Carcinoma of vagina	16	0.5
Others	42	1.3
Total	3,125	100.00

It is essentially a disease of the elderly with a mean age of 56 years in Malaysian women. Over the past two decades a subset of women younger than 50 years with squamous cell carcinoma has emerged.[3]

About 90% of the malignancies seen are squamous cell carcinomas; melanomas, adenocarcinoma, basal cell carcinoma and sarcomas are far less commonly seen.

ETIOLOGY

Most vulva cancers occur in postmenopausal women; more recently there is a trend towards a younger age at presentation. No specific etiological factor has been identified for vulva cancer. Recent studies suggest two different etiological types of vulva cancer:

- *One occurring in younger women:* This is related to human papilloma virus (HPV) and smoking, and commonly associated with vulval intraepithelial neoplasia (VIN)
- *The other occurring in older women:* This is the more common type and is unrelated to smoking or human papilloma virus infection, and concurrent VIN is uncommon.

Other diseases associated with vulva cancer include lymphogranuloma venereum and granuloma inguinale. A positive serology for syphilis is present in 5% of vulva cancers; these patients tend to have more poorly differentiated tumors. Vulva cancer has also been associated with immunosuppression and a history of cervical neoplasia.

SQUAMOUS CELL CARCINOMA

This accounts for 90% of vulva cancers.

Clinical Presentation

The most common symptom is long standing vulva pruritus and a recognizable lesion which is usually raised, fleshy, ulcerated or warty in appearance (Figs. 39.1 and 39.2).

Other symptoms include vulva pain, bleeding, dysuria and discharge. In many parts of Asia-Oceania at the time of diagnosis, squamous cell carcinoma of the vulva is often large and exophytic and fungating (Figs. 39.2 and 39.3) because of delay in treatment. Such late presentations are often due to:

- Fear of cancer
- Cultural taboos
- Ignorance
- Lack of appropriate facilities.

Many seek traditional treatment first, thus delaying definitive therapy. In contrast to the exophytic type, some tumors may grow as endophytic masses with ulceration.

Most of the lesions occur in the labia majora, favoring the medial aspect (see Fig. 39.1); primary involvement of the labia minora is seen in less than 30% of patients. Primary clitoral (Figs. 39.4A and B) and periurethral sites are less common.

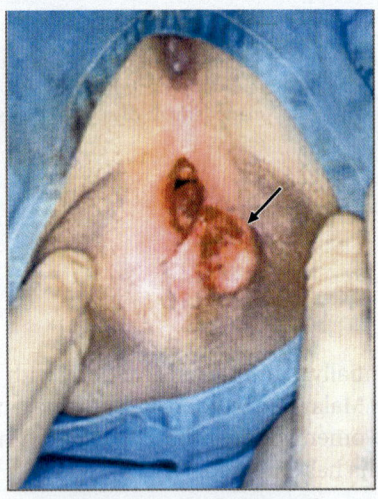

Fig. 39.1: The 2 cm lesion arises in the left labium majus; note the typical irregular surface and superficial ulceration of a squamous cell carcinoma.

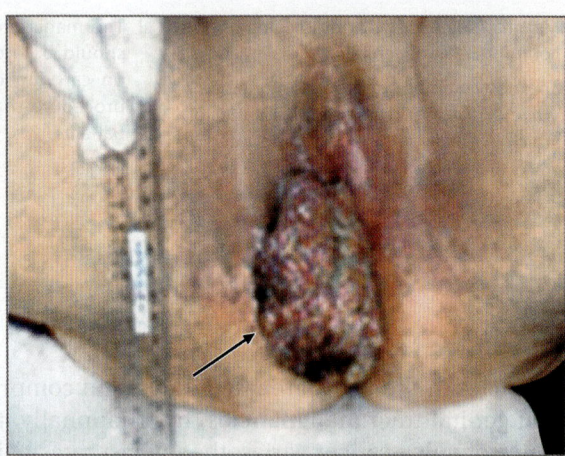

Fig. 39.2: This patient ignored her symptoms for more than 1 year in spite of an obvious tumor in the lower vulva. Such late presentations are not unusual amongst Asian patients.

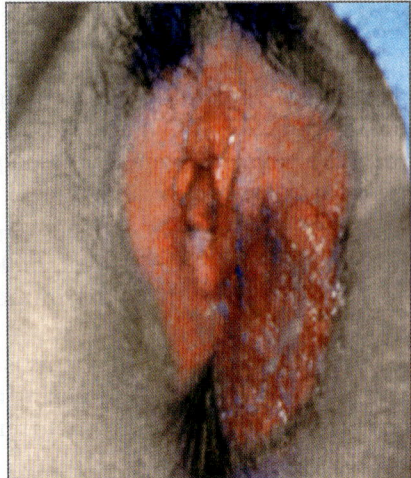

Fig. 39.3: Squamous cell carcinoma of vulva involving both labia majora, anus and medial aspect of upper thigh.

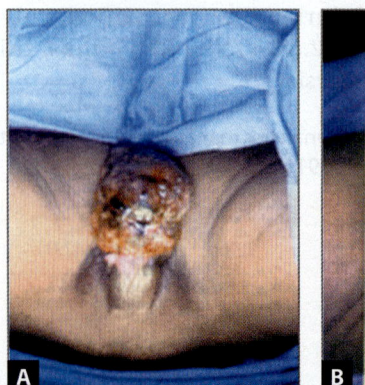 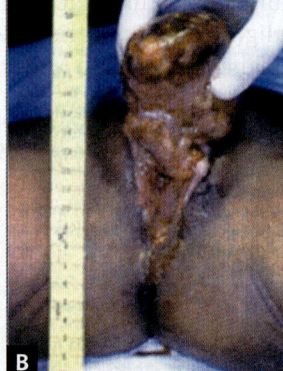

Figs. 39.4A and B: A large clitoral squamous cell carcinoma. This is relatively uncommon.

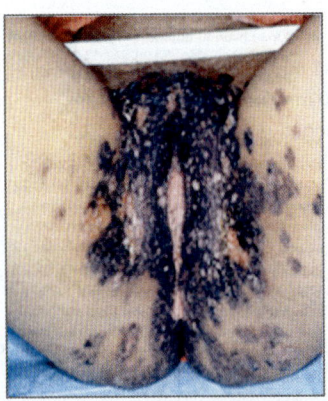

Fig. 39.5: Extensive squamous cell carcinoma of vulva. Note the multifocal lesions extending to the medial aspects of both thighs and buttocks. Such an occurrence is extremely rare.

In approximately 5% of cases the lesions are multifocal (Fig. 39.5).

The *clinical examination* should include a thorough examination of the vulva, vestibule, introitus, perineum and anus. Because neoplasms of the lower female genital tract are often multicentric, the vagina and cervix should be evaluated; a complete pelvic examination including cervical cytology is essential. The groins should be carefully palpated for lymph node involvement.

DIAGNOSIS

This requires a wedge biopsy which can be carried out as an office procedure under local anesthesia; this should include surrounding normal skin and underlying connective tissue. For small lesions, an excisional biopsy is preferred.

In those with a large primary tumor, a computed tomography (CT) is useful to determine extent of spread of disease. Where there is involvement of the vestibule a cystoscopic evaluation is useful to determine extent of urethral and bladder involvement. If the anus is involved a proctosigmoidoscopy is useful.

PATTERN OF SPREAD

There are three modalities of spread:
- Direct extension to adjacent organs such as urethra, vagina and anus (*see* Fig. 39.3)
- Lymphatic embolization to regional lymph nodes
- Hematogenous spread to distant sites (lungs, liver, bone).

The predominant method of spread is by lymphatic embolization. As demonstrated by Perry-Jones,[4] the lymphatics of the vulva course superiorly to the area of the mons pubis and then turn to drain in the ipsilateral superficial inguinal nodes located between the Camper's fascia and fascia lata; lymphatics from here perforate through the cribriform fascia to the deep inguinal (femoral) nodes. The latter number 1 to 4; the Cloquet node (Rosenmuller), which is the most cephalad of the femoral nodes, is absent in 50% of cases. These nodes are situated medial to the femoral vein within the fossa ovalis, there are no nodes distal to the lower margin of the fossa ovalis. Thus, there is no need to remove the fascia lata lateral to the femoral vessels; this reduces risk of injury to the femoral nerve. From the inguinofemoral nodes the lymphatics drain into the pelvic nodes, and in particular the external iliac nodes. The lymphatics from *laterally situated lesions* drain to the ipsilateral nodes; the vulva lymphatic channels do not cross labiocrural folds on to the medial aspects of the thigh, and drainage to the contralateral groin is rare.

Lymphatics from *the clitoris and anterior aspect of vulva and perineum* drain to both groins. Direct lymphatic pathways from the clitoris and Bartholin's glands to the pelvic nodes have also been observed. This pattern of spread is illustrated in Figure 39.6.

An Australian study using bipedal lymphangiograms[5] demonstrated no nodes medial to the pubic tubercle and no nodes in outer 15–20% of a line drawn from the anterior aspect of the anterosuperior iliac spine to the pubic tubercle. Occasional lymphatics from the leg traverse this outer area to join axillary lymphatics; thus, limiting the lateral extent of groin incision will help reduce postoperative lymphedema.

Lymph Node Metastases

The incidence of groin lymph node metastasis is approximately 30%; this is related to the size of the tumor and stage of the disease. The incidence of pelvic lymph node involvement is approximately 5–6%, such patients usually have three or more positive inguinal nodes. The occurrence of pelvic node metastases without groin node metastasis is extremely rare.

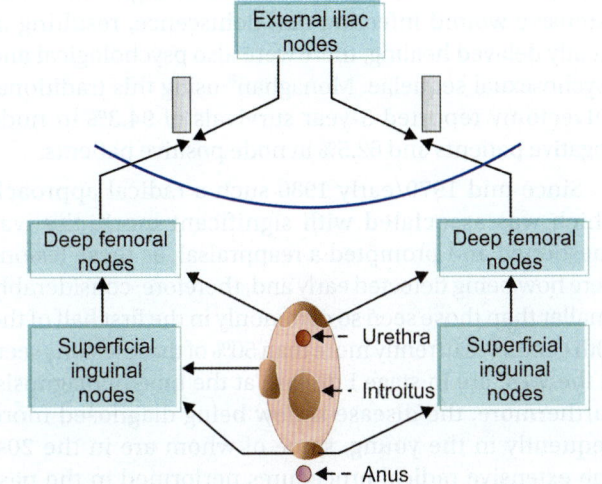

Fig. 39.6: Schematic representation of potential lymphatic spread from vulva cancer.
Source: Stanley Way

Box 39.1: 2009 FIGO staging for vulvar cancer.

- 1A Tumor confined to the vulva or perineum or both, 2 cm or < in size, stromal invasion 1 mm or <, no nodal involvement
- 1B Tumor confined to the vulva or perineum, >2 cm in size or with stromal invasion >1.0 mm, negative nodes
- 2   Tumor of any size with adjacent spread (1/3 lower urethra, 1/3 lower vagina, anus), negative nodes
- 3A Tumor of any size with positive inguino-femoral lymph nodes:
  - (i) 1 lymph node metastasis greater than or equal to 5 mm
  - (ii) 1–2 lymph node metastases of less than 5 mm
- 3B (i) 2 or more lymph node metastases greater than or equal to 5 mm
  - (ii) 3 or more lymph node metastases less than 5 mm
- 3C Positive nodes with extracapsular spread
- 4A (i) Tumor invades other regional structures (2/3 upper urethra, 2/3 upper vagina) bladder mucosa, rectal mucosa, or fixed to pelvic bone.
  - (ii) Fixed or ulcerated inguino-femoral nodes
- 4B Any distant metastases including pelvic lymph nodes

Hematogenous spread occurs late in the disease; the absence of lymphatic metastases in such patients is rarely seen.

Staging

This is now based on a surgical-pathological staging (Box 39.1).

MANAGEMENT

The surgical approach to vulvar cancer has continued to change over the past 4 to 5 decades. In 1912, Basset proposed *en bloc* resection of the vulvar tumor and inguinofemoral nodes; the lines of excision were inadequate resulting in poor survival. Tausig[6] and Way[7] advocated a more radical surgical excision which included the entire vulva and mons and extended laterally over and including the inguinal nodes and inferiorly extending to the urogenital diaphragm. This had been extremely successful from a curative point of view, with overall survival rates of 65%. However, the postoperative morbidity was extremely high; there was extensive wound infection and dehiscence, resulting in greatly delayed healing; there were also psychological and psychosexual sequelae. Monaghan[8] using this traditional vulvectomy reported 5-year survivals of 94.3% in node negative patients and 62.5% in node positive patients.

Since mid 1970/early 1980 such a radical approach which was associated with significant morbidity was questioned and prompted a reappraisal, as these lesions were now being detected early and, therefore, considerably smaller than those seen so commonly in the first half of the 20th century. Currently more than 50% of these lesions seen in the West are in stage I disease at the time of diagnosis. Furthermore, the disease is now being diagnosed more frequently in the young, some of whom are in the 20s. The extensive radical procedures performed in the past have helped define the patterns of local lymphatic spread, incidence of nodal metastases and pathological features of the primary tumor; these accumulated data have helped in predicting the risk of nodal metastases allowing for customization of extent of surgery based on:

- Lesion size
- Location
- Depth of invasion
- Clinical suspicion of lymph node metastasis.

For instance, for small T1 squamous cell carcinoma there are no positive nodes if the depth of invasion is <1 mm; the incidence of nodal metastases increases as the depth of invasion increases, 7.7% for depth of 1.1 to 2 mm to 34.2% for depth >5 mm.[9] The incidence of lymph node metastases according to clinical stage[9] are:

Stage I	10.7%
Stage II	26.2%
Stage III	64.2%
Stage IV	88.9%

Management of Early Vulvar Cancer

The management of early vulvar lesions should be individualized with emphasis on carrying out the most conservative procedure that will achieve cure for the patient.

Thus, for small lesions (<2 cm) that are laterally situated with <1 mm depth of invasion a wide radical excision (with 10 mm clear margins) would suffice; there is no need to perform a lymphadenectomy, thus sparing the patient the potential morbidity.

For laterally situated lesions with depth of invasion exceeding 1 mm or lesions >2 cm in size, a wide radical excision may be performed with an ipsilateral inguinofemoral lymphadenectomy; if a metastatic deposit is noted, the contralateral lymphadenectomy should also be performed (*see* Fig. 39.6). In the presence of an otherwise normal-looking vulva, such vulvar-sparing surgery is a safe surgical option regardless of the depth of invasion. Conserve the clitoris where possible.

For midline lesions (*see* Figs. 39.4 and 39.6) the resection should include bilateral inguinofemoral lymphadenectomy. Metastases to the femoral nodes can occur without involvement of the superficial inguinal nodes. Thus, if groin node dissection is indicated a thorough inguinofemoral lymphadenectomy is mandatory. It is also important to bear in mind that patients who develop recurrent disease in an undissected or incompletely dissected groin have a very high mortality (92%).

Incision

Recently there has been a shift to the *triple incision* technique (separate groin incision for lymphadenectomy) to reduce postoperative morbidity (Fig. 39.7). The advantages are:

- Primary closure is easily achieved
- Primary healing occurs in > 65% of cases
- Mean hospital stay is markedly reduced.

Whilst such a conservative approach is generally safe, *skin bridge metastases* has been reported; this results from two possible mechanisms:

- Transit metastatic emboli
- Retrograde permeation of lymphatics

Thus, separate groin incisions are probably not advisable when more than microscopic lymph node metastases are present.

Modified Twombley-Ulfelder Technique

As stated earlier, unlike in the West, a majority of our patients present with large bulky tumors. We have used the modified Twombley-Ulfelder technique which helps preserve sufficient skin to achieve primary skin closure (Figs. 39.8 to 39.11).

SPECIAL SITUATIONS

- *Lesion in close proximity to the urethra:* Here, the distal 1 cm of urethra can be resected; this does not compromise urethral continence.
- *Lesion close to or involving the clitoris:* Here, anterior vulvar irradiation is an option; it will sterilize the tumor without interfering with clitoral sensitivity.
- *Proximity of the lesions to the anus:* When the lesion is extensive and involves the anus as shown in Figure 39.12, a more radical procedure is necessary.

An alternative approach in the management of such lesions is *irradiation* to the vulva which would help preserve the vulval contour as well as the anus (Figs. 39.13 to 39.15).

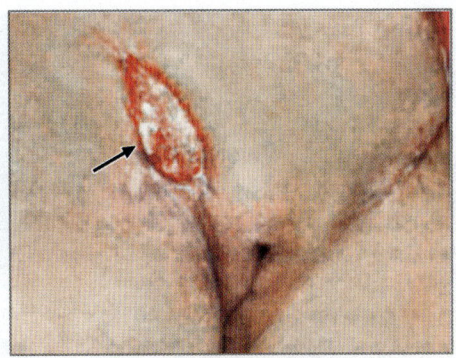

Fig. 39.7: Wide radical excision of 2 cm lesion over the perineum and bilateral groin node dissection had been done. Note the superficial breakdown of wound in right groin. The normal vulva appearance is preserved.

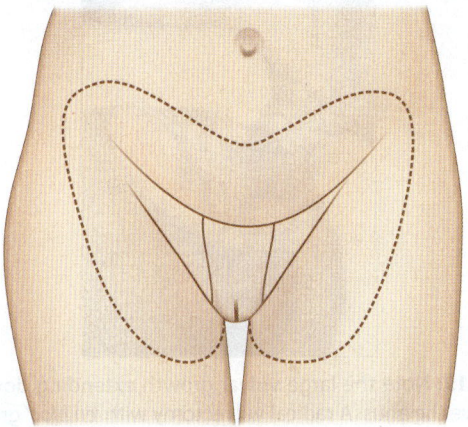

Fig. 39.8: Skin incision for radical vulvectomy. The dotted lines indicate the limits of the superficial groin dissection (*Adapted from Twombley GH, Cancer*).

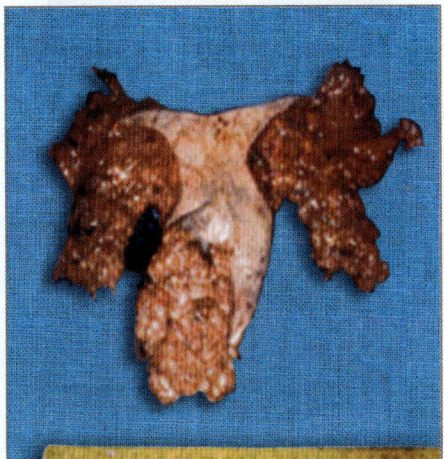

Fig. 39.9: Radical vulvectomy specimen (using the technique above) from patient shown in Figure 39.2.

406 SECTION 3 **Gynecologic Oncology**

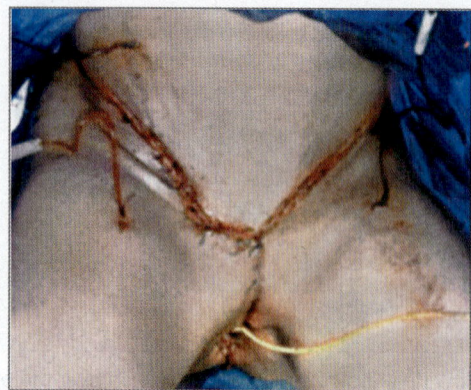

Fig. 39.10: Primary skin closure is easily obtained.

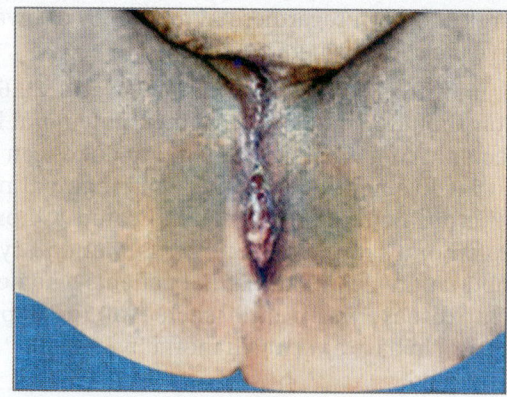

Fig. 39.11: Appearance of the operation site 6 months later. Satisfactory healing is obtained.

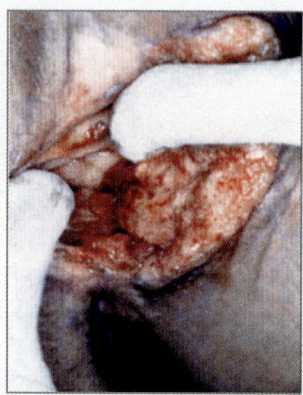

Fig. 39.12: Note the large vulvar growth extending downwards to involve the anus. A radical vulvectomy with 'en bloc' groin node dissection and posterior exenteration was done (see Figs. 39.13 and 39.14).

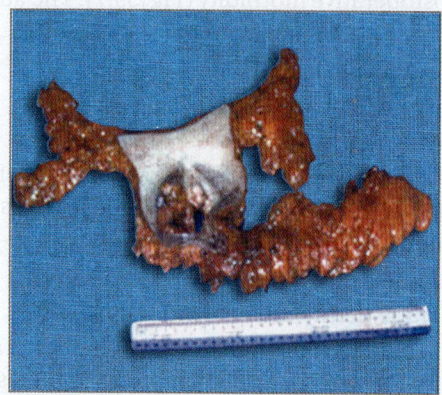

Fig. 39.13: Radical vulvectomy specimen 'en bloc' with groin nodes and rectum and anus.

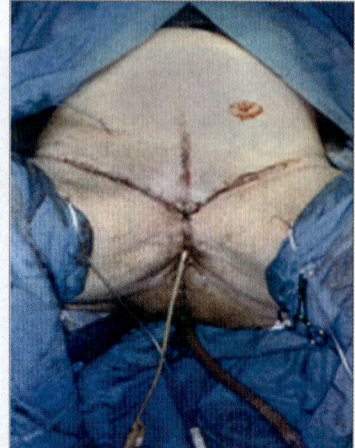

Fig. 39.14: Primary skin closure has been achieved with subsequent satisfactory healing. Note the colostomy in the left iliac fossa.

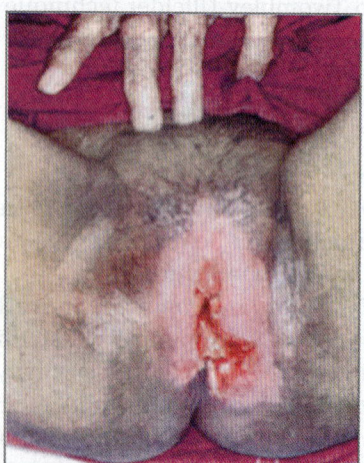

Fig. 39.15: Please refer to Figure 39.3. Surgical excision for the lesion which had extended to the medial aspect of the thigh would have required reconstructive surgery to close the large raw area. Note the satisfactory response after radiotherapy and preservation of vulvar appearance 6 months later.

- *Carcinoma of the vulva in pregnancy:* This is extremely rare. The first case of squamous cell carcinoma of the vulva in Malaysia and possibly the second in Asia was reported by us.[10] Treatment is individualized; radical excision with or without ipsilateral or bilateral inguinal lymphadenectomy is carried out as in the non-pregnant patient until 36 weeks, beyond which the definitive therapy is deferred into the puerperium. These tumors can be aggressive and grow rapidly during pregnancy as observed by us (Fig. 39.16).

LYMPHATIC MAPPING (FIG. 39.17)

Recently there has been a great interest in locating the sentinel node using intraoperative mapping with lymphoscintigraphy. Selective sentinel node biopsy in early vulvar cancer is done using this technique; if this was negative for metastases it would spare the patient lymphadenectomy with the associated morbidity. Whilst this is reliable in a majority of cases, occasional false-negative sentinel nodes have been reported.

OTHER VULVAR MALIGNANCIES

Malignant Melanoma of Vulva

This is rare in Malaysia; in the West this is the second most common type of vulvar cancer, occurring predominantly in postmenopausal white women and involving the labia minora or clitoris. Diagnosis is based on an excisional biopsy (for small lesions) for histological diagnosis. The overall prognosis is poor with 5 year survival of 30%; hence, the surgical approach now is towards vulvar conservation with radical excision of the primary tumor.

Verrucous Carcinoma

This is a variant of squamous cell carcinoma. This cauliflower tumor may be difficult to distinguish from condylomata acuminata or squamous papilloma. It is a locally aggressive tumor that pushes into, rather than invades, the underlying structures; metastasis to regional nodes is rare. Treatment is radical excision; radiation therapy is contraindicated as it may induce anaplastic transformation.

Basal Cell Carcinoma

This is locally invasive, non-metastatic tumor is rare; it is usually present as a 'rodent' ulcer and involves the labium majus. Treatment is wide local excision.

Bartholin's Gland Carcinoma

Primary carcinoma of *Bartholin's* gland accounts for 5% of all vulvar cancers. The histological types noted are adenocarcinomas, squamous cell carcinomas and rarely transitional cell carcinomas. Current therapy consists of hemi-vulvectomy, ipsilateral inguinofemoral lymphadenectomy; pelvic lymphadenectomy is performed for those with positive groin nodes.

Vulvar Sarcomas

These constitute 1 to 2% of vulvar cancers; leiomyosarcomas are the most common. Wide local excision is the recommended initial treatment. Recurrences are likely with lesions > 5 cm diameter with infiltrating margins.

Transitional Cell Carcinoma

This may be a primary tumor of the vulva, arising from the Bartholin's glands. Rarely, it may be an extension of a primary tumor in bladder or urethra on to the vulva (Figs. 39.18 to 39.20).

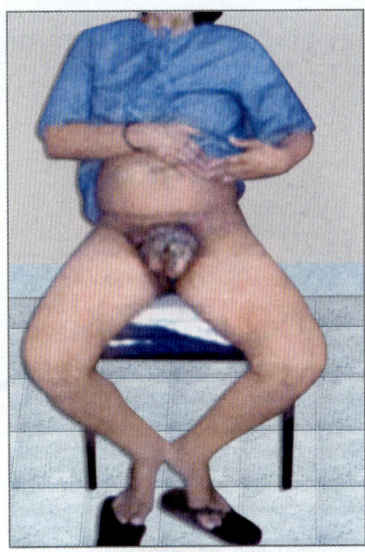

Fig. 39.16: Carcinoma of the vulva in pregnancy. The 28-year-old patient was referred soon after a term vaginal delivery. Notice the large exophytic growth and groin node enlargement. Radical vulvectomy and bilateral inguinofemoral lymphadenectomy was performed; there was metastases to 17 nodes. She succumbed 6 months later.

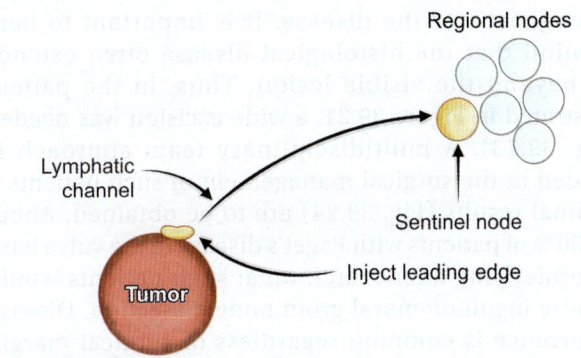

Fig. 39.17: Illustrating the principle of sentinel node localization.

SECTION 3 Gynecologic Oncology

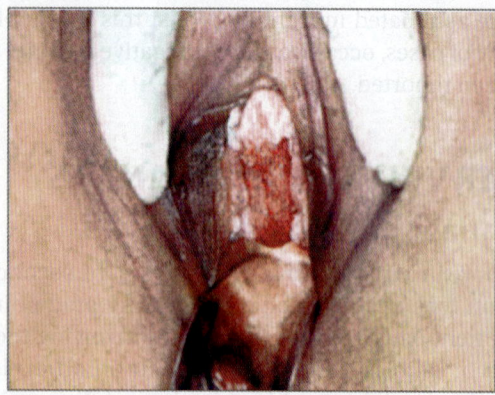

Fig. 39.18: Transitional cell carcinoma of bladder extending to involve the clitoris, vestibule and labia minora. An anterior exenteration, radical vulvectomy and bilateral inguinofemoral node dissection and ileal conduit were done (Fig. 39.19). The posterior vaginal wall was preserved and swung forward to create a vaginal lumen (Fig. 39.20).

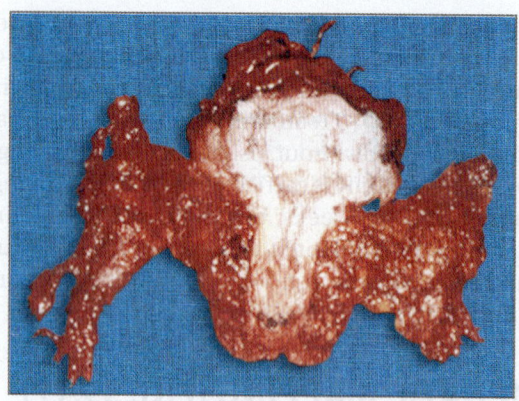

Fig. 39.19: Operative specimen (anterior exenteration and radical vulvectomy) of above showing transitional cell carcinoma of bladder extending down to the urethra.

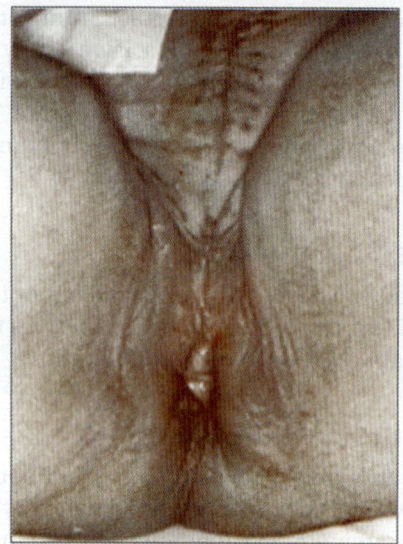

Fig. 39.20: The above patient 6 months after surgery. There is satisfactory healing with a functioning ileal conduit and satisfactory vaginal lumen.

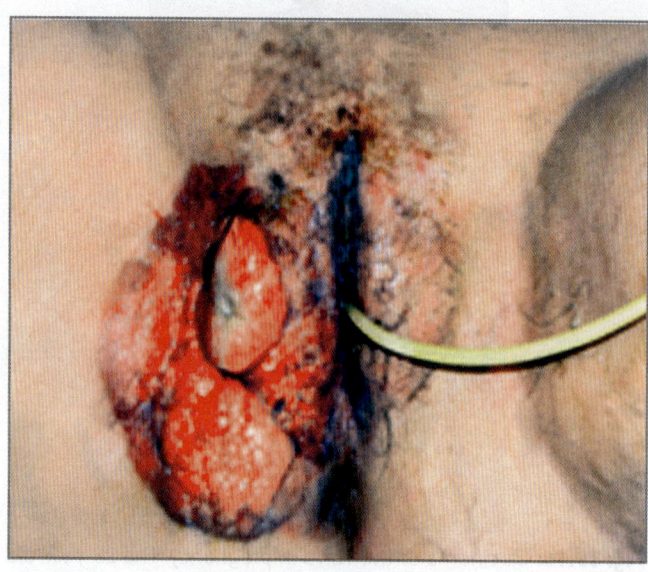

Fig. 39.21: Extramammary Paget's disease of the vulva. Note the typical extensive, reddish appearing lesions; the lesion extends into the medial aspect of the right thigh, the perineum, the mons and the left labia majora requiring extensive excision (Fig. 39.22).

Extramammary Paget's Disease of the Vulva

This is a rare neoplasm that usually occurs in postmenopausal women and comprises 1-2% of vulvar malignancies. Patients may present with vulvar pruritus, vulvar irritation, vulvar burning or a noticeable vulvar lesion. The lesions appear well defined, moist and reddish eczematoid lesions. The lesions can appear eroded or look like an ulcerated plaque, or in some cases appear raised and uneven (Fig. 39.21).

A biopsy of the lesion is needed to confirm the diagnosis; the typical intraepithelial *"Paget cells"* (Fig. 39.22) is diagnostic of the disease. It is important to bear in mind that the histological disease often extends far beyond the visible lesion. Thus, in the patient illustrated in Figure 39.21, a wide excision was needed (Fig. 39.23). A multidisciplinary team approach is needed in the surgical management of such patients if optimal results (Fig. 39.24) are to be obtained. About 20-30 % of patients with Paget's disease of the vulva have an underlying adenocarcinoma; such patients would require inguinofemoral groin node dissection. Disease recurrence is common regardless of surgical margin status. Long-term monitoring is advised and repeat surgical excision carried out if necessary.

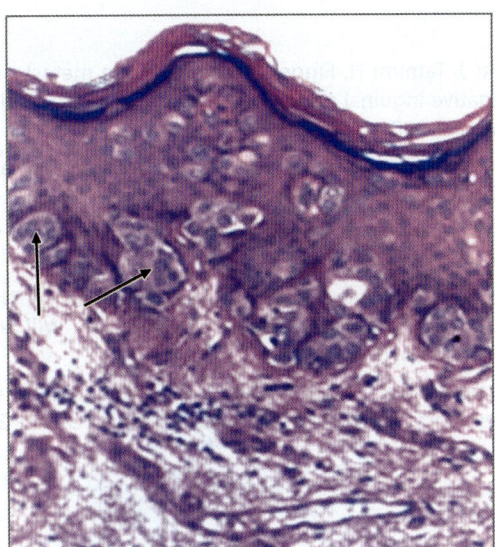

Fig. 39.22: Paget's disease of the vulva. The typical '*Paget cells*' on histological evaluation of the biopsy confirms the diagnosis; these changes often extend beyond the margin of the visible lesion.

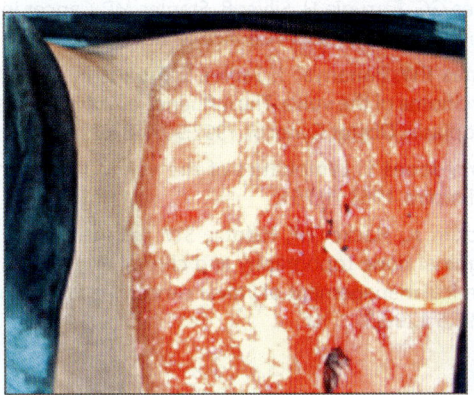

Fig. 39.23: Extramammary Paget's disease of the vulva. A wide excision beyond the margin if the visible lesion has been done. Reconstructive surgery is now needed (*see* Fig. 39.24).

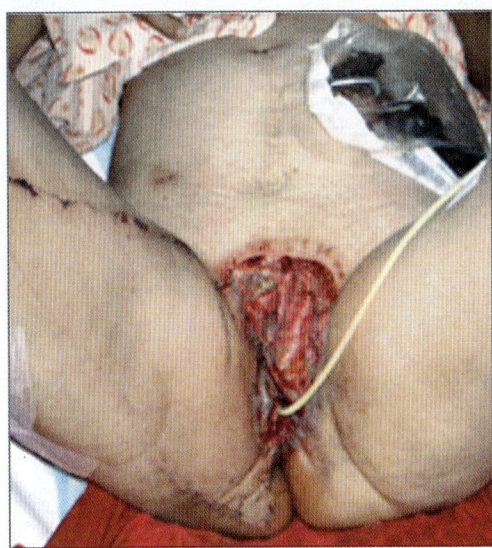

Fig. 39.24: The extensive raw area following wide excision of the vulval lesion (*see* Fig. 39.23) now requires reconstructive surgery. A musculocutaneous graft from the right thigh has been used to cover the raw area with split skin graft over the mons pubis. The temporary colostomy seen was closed subsequently. Notice the satisfactory healing and appearance of the vulva 4 weeks after surgery. As the histological evaluation of the operative specimen revealed an underlying adenocarcinoma, bilateral inguinofemoral groin node dissection was subsequently done; this revealed metastases to one lymph node on the right side.

SUMMARY

Recent advances in the surgical approach to vulvar malignancies suggest the following:

- More limited resection of primary lesion for unifocal tumors and, otherwise, normal vulva
- Omission of groin node dissection for T1 tumors and <1 mm stromal invasion
- Elimination of routine pelvic lymphadenectomy
- Use of separate groin incisions for inguinofemoral lymphadenectomy
- Omission of contralateral groin node dissection for lateral T1 lesions/negative ipsilateral nodes
- Use of postoperative radiation to groin recurrence in those with multiple positive groin nodes
- Care should be individualized.

REFERENCES

1. Parkin M, Muir CS, Wheelan SL, et al. Cancer incidence in five continents. Vol VI. Lyon International Agency for Research on Cancer, 1993.
2. Giles GG, Farrugia H, Silver B, Staples MP. Cancer in Victoria, Melbourne: Anticancer Council of Victoria, 1992.
3. Jones RW, Bananyai J, Sables S. Trends in squamous cell carcinoma of the vulva: The influence of vulvar intraepithelial neoplasia. Obstet Gynecol. 1997;90:448-52.
4. Parry-Jones E. Lymphatics of the vulva. J Obstet Gynecol Br Empire. 1963;70:751.
5. Nicklin JL, Hacker NF, Heintze SW. An anatomical study of inguinal node topography and clinical implications for the surgical management of vulvar cancer. Int J Gynecol Cancer. 1995;5:128-33.
6. Chu J, Tamimi H, Figge D. Femoral node metastases with negative inguinal nodes in early vulvar cancer. Am J Obstet Gynecol. 1981;140:337-39.
7. Taussig F. Carcinoma of the vulva: An analysis of 155 cases. Am J Obstet Gynecol. 1940;40:764.
8. Way S. Carcinoma of vulva. Am J Obstet Gynecol. 1960;79: 692.
9. Hacker NF. Vulvar cancer. In Berek JS and Hacker NF (Eds). Practical Gynecologic Oncology, 2nd edn. Williams and Wilkinson, Sydney; 1994.
10. Sivanesaratnam V, Pathmanathan R. Carcinoma of the vulva in pregnancy, a rare occurrence. Asia-Oceania J Obstet Gynecol. 1990;16:207-10.

CHAPTER 40

Gestational Trophoblastic Neoplasia

V Sivanesaratnam

Overview

- Gestational trophoblastic neoplasia (GTN) encompasses a spectrum of clinical and histological entities and comprise a group of neoplastic disorders arising from trophoblastic tissue of the placenta.
- Hydatidiform mole: *Vaginal bleeding* is the most common presenting symptom of Ist trimester of pregnancy, occurring in 97% of cases. *Excessive uterine enlargement* is seen in about 70% of patients.
- *Pre-eclampsia* is observed in about 25% of patients. The diagnosis of hydatidiform mole should be considered whenever pre-eclampsia develops before 20 weeks gestation. *Hyperemesis gravidarum* occurs in 25% of patients, particularly in those with excessive uterine enlargement and markedly elevated hCG levels.
- The diagnosis of a *complete mole* is nearly always made by the typical 'snow storm' appearance on ultrasonography.
- Once the diagnosis of hydatidiform mole is confirmed (by ultrasound) the uterine cavity must be emptied; *suction curettage* is the preferred method.
- The risk of choriocarcinoma developing is one thousand fold higher after mole evacuation. Hence, careful follow-up with beta hCG needs to be done. If patient has irregular bleeding later in life choriocarcinoma has to be ruled out by doing beta hCG levels.
- Chemotherapy is the treatment of choice for choriocarcinoma/ GTN.
- Gestational trophoblastic neoplasia is highly curable.

INTRODUCTION

Gestational trophoblastic disease encompasses a spectrum of clinical and histological entities and comprise a group of neoplastic disorders (Box 40.1) arising from trophoblastic tissue of the placenta.

The term 'gestational trophoblastic tumor' (GTT/GTN) has been applied collectively to the latter 3 conditions, all of which have various propensities for local invasion and metastasis, and lead to death if left untreated.

Hydatidiform mole and choriocarcinoma are common gynecological problems in Malaysia and other South-East Asian countries (Table 40.1). Due to the lack of a Tumor Register in many of these countries, the true incidence is unknown. Currently, worldwide a decreasing incidence of GTN has been noted; the contributory factors include: decreasing parity, improved socioeconomic status and increased use of early pregnancy ultrasound scans.

Box 40.1: Gestational trophoblastic disease (GTD).

- Hydatidiform mole (partial and complete)
- Invasive mole (chorioadenoma destruens)
- Gestational choriocarcinoma
- Placental site trophoblastic tumor (PSTT)
- Epithelial trophoblastic tumor (ETT)

Table 40.1: Incidence of hydatidiform mole in Asia.[1]

Center	Author	Year	Rate per 1000	Type of denominator
Singapore	Teoh et al	1971	1.2	Deliveries
Japan	Takeuchi	1982	1.96	Pregnancies
Indonesia	Farid Aziz	1984	12.9	Pregnancies
Malaysia	Sivanesaratnam	1991	2.8	Deliveries
Philippines	Panlilio	1987	7.0	Deliveries

HYDATIDIFORM MOLE

Hydatidiform mole is more prevalent in Indonesia and Philippines (Table 40.1). In Malaysia, the incidence was reported as 2.8 per 1000 deliveries; a significantly higher incidence among the Chinese was observed (5.52 per 1000 deliveries, $p < 0.001$)[2] (Table 40.2).

On the basis of gross morphology, histopathology and karyotype (Table 40.3) hydatidiform mole may be categorized into:

- Complete hydatidiform mole
- Partial hydatidiform mole.

A complete mole is a hydatidiform mole without an embryo or fetus. Macroscopically, it is characterized by clusters of "grape-like" vesicles of varying sizes (Fig. 40.1).

Table 40.3 shows the histological differences between complete and partial moles. These features are often subject to inter- and intra-observer variations.

Clinical Features

The classical clinical features include:
- Vaginal bleeding
- Anemia
- Excessive uterine enlargement
- Hyperemesis gravidarum
- Hyperthyroidism
- Toxemia of pregnancy
- Theca-luteal cysts.

Vaginal bleeding is the most common presenting symptom, occurring in 97% of cases. This occurs in the early second trimester of pregnancy and is often intermittent and prolonged. (In ectopic tubal pregnancy a similar pattern of bleeding occurs but in the early first trimester). Molar tissue may separate from the decidua and disrupt maternal vessels; this results in large volume of retained blood within the uterine cavity causing the excessive uterine enlargement seen in about 70% of patients and anemia in 50% of patients.

Pre-eclampsia is observed in about 25% of patients. The diagnosis of hydatidiform mole should be considered whenever pre-eclampsia develops before 20 weeks gestation. Hyperemesis gravidarum occurs in 25% of patients, particularly in those with excessive uterine enlargement and markedly elevated hCG levels.

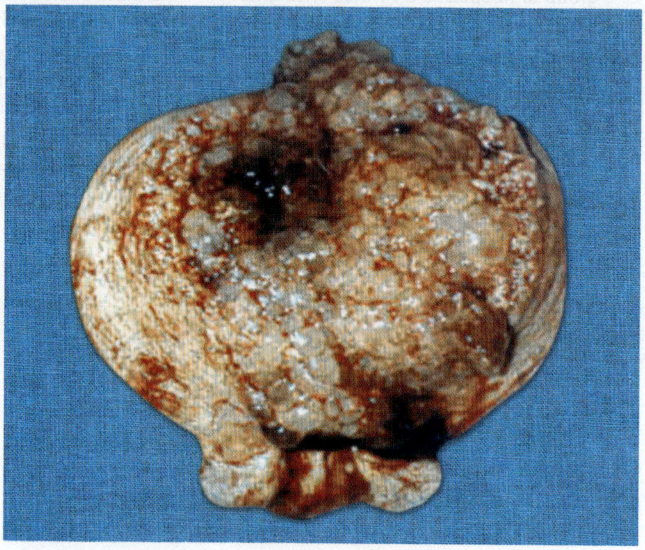

Table 40.2: Hydatidiform mole—racial incidence (University Hospital, Kuala Lumpur 1978-1987).

Race	No. with molar pregnancy	Total deliveries	Incidence per 1000 deliveries
Malay	91	34,344	2.66
Chinese	51	9,247	5.52*
Indian	12	13,497	0.89
Others	5	344	14.70
Total	159	57,430	2.78

* $p <0.001$

Fig. 40.1: Notice the clusters of "grape-like" vesicles within the uterine cavity. The patient had a hysterectomy performed (Today, hysterectomy is seldom performed for hydatidiform mole).

Table 40.3: Differences between complete and partial mole.

Features	Complete mole	Partial mole
Fetal or embryonic tissue	Absent	Present
Hydatidiform swelling and cavitation of villi	Diffuse	Focal
Circumferential trophoblastic proliferation with or without atypia	Diffuse	Focal
Scalloping of chorionic villi	Absent	Marked
Stromal trophoblastic inclusions	Absent	Marked
Fetal stromal vessels	Absent	Absent
Karyotype	46XX; 46XY (entirely paternal origin)	69XXY; 69XYY (triploid—extrahaploid set paternal origin)

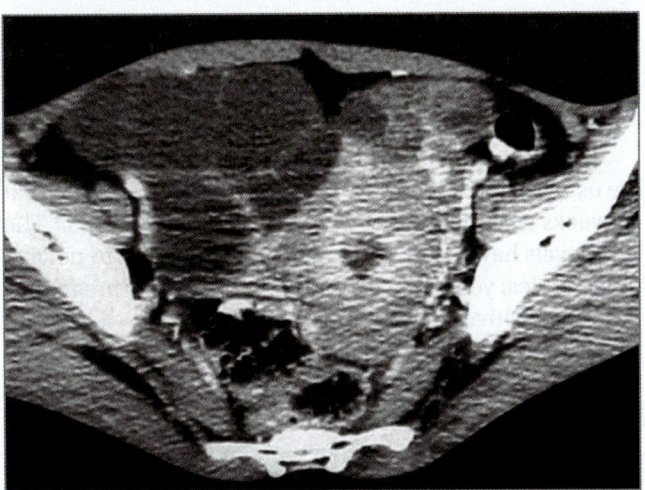

Fig. 40.2: Notice the typical large thin-walled multiloculated cysts. The patient had uterine evacuation for complete mole 1 week earlier.

Hyperthyroidism occurs in about 5% of patients; tachycardia, warm skin and tremor may be present. The diagnosis is confirmed by detection of elevated levels of free thyroxine (T_4) and triiodothyronine (T_3). These clinical and biochemical features rapidly revert to normal soon after uterine evacuation, confirming the features are transient.[3] The therapy, therefore, need not be prolonged.

Theca-luteal cysts (>6 cm) are present in about 50% of patients with complete mole. These are thin-walled multiloculated cysts that are often bilateral (Fig. 40.2).

Their formation is related to the high level of circulating hCG. Because the uterus is often excessively large, these cysts may not be easily palpable. Spontaneous regression occurs after molar evacuation within 8–10 weeks. Continued persistence of these cysts would indicate persistence of trophoblastic mole.

Diagnosis of Molar Pregnancy

The diagnosis of a complete mole is nearly always made by ultrasonography; the chorionic villi of complete hydatidiform moles proliferate diffusely with hydropic swelling and produce a characteristic vesicular sonographic pattern or "snow-storm" pattern. The increasing use of high resolution ultrasound has led to the earlier diagnosis of molar pregnancy when the patient is asymptomatic; in the first trimester the typical appearance of the complete mole has been reported as a complex, echogenic, intrauterine mass containing many small cystic spaces.

Management of Molar Pregnancy

Once the diagnosis of hydatidiform mole is confirmed (by ultrasound) the uterine cavity must be emptied; suction curettage is the preferred method. An oxytocin infusion (20 units in 500 mL saline) is commenced soon after induction to aid in the uterine evacuation and minimize the risk of uterine perforation. The aim in the management is to prevent malignant sequelae; thus, complete evacuation of the uterus is essential. In 25% of our cases, complete evacuation was not achieved at the first attempt.[2] A routine ultrasound examination one week later should be performed. If residual molar tissue is still present a second evacuation needs to be done; the uterus is now smaller and firmer and can be curetted without fear of perforation. The danger of repeated curettage is the development of Asherman's syndrome; fertility in these patients can be restored by lysis of intrauterine adhesions.[4]

Acute respiratory distress occurring in 27% of cases during or after evacuation of uteri larger than 16 weeks has been reported.[4] This is caused by a combination of factors—trophoblastic embolization, pre-eclampsia, anemia, fluid overload and hyperthyroidism.[5] With cardiovascular and respiratory support in intensive care, response is usual within 72 hours.

The occurrence of a hydatidiform mole and a coexistent fetus is rare, one in 22,000–100,000 pregnancies. In such a twin pregnancy, where there is one viable fetus and the other pregnancy is molar, there are no clear guidelines of management. The patient should be counselled regarding the increased risk of post-molar GTN/metastatic disease. In addition these patients are at increased risk of medical complications—hyperthyroidism, hemorrhage, and pregnancy induced hypertension. Soper et al.[6] suggested that if the fetal karyotype is normal, major fetal malformations excluded, and there is no evidence of metastatic disease, pregnancy can be allowed to continue if the mother wishes, unless complications force delivery. Whilst the probability of achieving a viable pregnancy is 40%, there are risks of complications such as pulmonary embolism and pre-eclampsia. No increased risk of developing GTN after such twin pregnancy has been reported.[7]

Follow-up

The patients should be seen weekly. At these visits a pelvic examination looking for vaginal nodules, and regression in size of uterus and theca-luteal cysts are noted and the serum hCG levels assessed. These weekly visits are continued till the hCG levels return to normal (<2 mIU/mL), after which the patient is seen 2 weekly for the next 3 months and monthly for the next 9 months.

Contraception after Molar Pregnancy

The potential for persistent trophoblastic proliferation after initial evacuation of a hydatidiform mole is well-recognized. The failure to note a progressive decline in the serum hCG after molar evacuation is generally indicative of trophoblastic malignancy.

In the UK, the use of combined oral contraceptives pill (OC) in such patients before hCG levels returned to normal resulted in a 2-fold increase of postmolar tumor requiring chemotherapy.[8] However, it can be used safely after the hCG levels have returned to normal;[9] we prefer to advise the use of barrier method of contraception till the hCG levels return to normal. It must, however, be noted that OCs do not postpone the occurrence of choriocarcinoma; thus, women on OC in the postmolar period run the same risk of developing choriocarcinoma as their counterparts not on OC. Close follow-up is, therefore, essential.

Partial Hydatidiform Mole (PHM) (Fig. 40.3)

As a result of lack of awareness and the lack of detailed routine histopathological evaluation of the placenta and products of conception evacuated at abortion, resulting in under-reporting, the true incidence of PHM is unknown. In our own institution we reported[10] that 30% of all molar pregnancies were, in fact, PHM. The histopathological differences from a complete mole are shown in Table 40.3.

Whilst the ultrasound features of a complete mole are reliable, the ultrasound diagnosis of a partial mole is more complex. The finding of cystic spaces in the placenta and a ratio of transverse to anteroposterior diameter of the gestation sac >1.5 is required for the reliable diagnosis of partial molar pregnancy.[11]

The clinical features characteristic of complete mole are usually absent in PHM. However, one of our patients at 19 weeks gestation had a 24 weeks' enlarged uterus.[1] The hCG levels have been said to be not higher than in normal pregnancies; yet in one of our cases the urinary pregnancy test was positive at a dilution of 1: 4096.

Until as recently as 1988, various authors have claimed that no choriocarcinoma has been associated with PHM.[12,13] This is in spite of the first documented case by us in early 1981[14] of malignant evolution with fatal outcome in a patient with PHM. The partial mole is, thus, part of a spectrum of GTN and not an entity by itself and is potentially malignant. It, therefore, requires close follow-up as for complete moles.

Invasive Mole

The diagnosis of an invasive mole cannot be made on evacuation of the uterus alone; the exact incidence is not known. At a time when hysterectomy was considered proper for molar pregnancy, Acosta-Sison[15] reported 18 histologically proven cases in a series of 210—an incidence of 8.6%.

Recent advances in treatment and the current practice of uterine conservation in a majority of cases of molar pregnancy mean that a pathological diagnosis of an invasive mole cannot be made; abdominal or transvaginal scans are not always helpful in detecting myometrial invasion. Deep myometrial invasion can result in uterine perforation and massive intraperitoneal hemorrhage. The gross appearance of hemorrhage and necrosis in the uterine wall can be confused with choriocarcinoma. Detailed histopathological evaluation showing persistence of villous structures confirm an invasive mole as was shown in one of our patients.[16]

Although invasive mole is generally less malignant than choriocarcinoma, 3.4% of documented cases of invasive mole have subsequently died from histologically varified choriocarcinoma.[17] Thus, chemotherapy should not be withheld in the presence of metastases, or failure of hCG regression and persistence of theca-luteal cysts as we have observed.[16]

Table 40.4: Gestational trophoblastic tumor/choriocarcinoma (University Hospital, 1981–1990)—Racial distribution).

Race	No. of cases	Total delivery	Incidence per 1000 deliveries
Malay	40	37,380	1.07
Chinese	44	9,581	4.58*
Indian	13	14,210	0.91
Others	1	510	1.96
Total	98	61,681	1.59

* p < 0.001

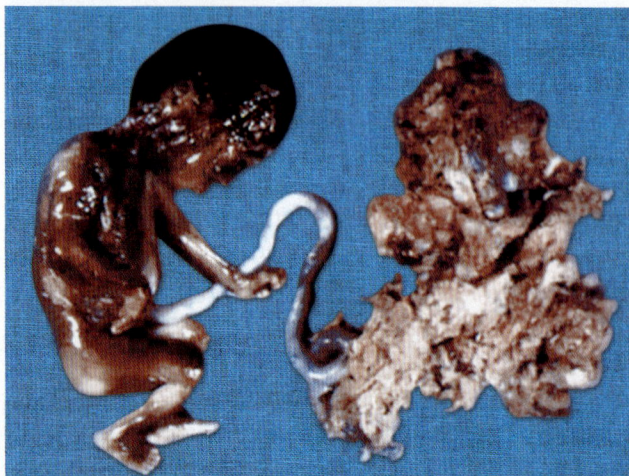

Fig. 40.3: Partial mole—note the macerated fetus and vesicles in the placenta.

PROPHYLAXIS AGAINST CHORIOCARCINOMA

Selective Preventive Chemotherapy

It is well-known that embolization of trophoblasts occurs during uterine contraction, stimulation by oxytocics and during evacuation of the uterus. The role of chemotherapy at the time of molar evacuation remains controversial.[18] However, we have shown that such prophylaxis is not justified as it does not significantly reduce the malignancy rate;[17] this study showed that the neoplasia takes longer to be detected.

The disadvantage of routine chemotherapy is that a large number of patients (80–90%) who are unlikely to develop persistent GTN, will be unnecessarily exposed to the toxic effects of these drugs. *Selective preventive chemotherapy* has been practiced by us for the past 25 years.[19] This is used in patients identified at risk of developing GTN/choriocarcinoma, i.e.

- Those with a very slow decline in hCG levels
- Those with an initial fall but subsequent rise in hCG levels
- Those in whom an initial fall is followed by a plateau.

These patients will receive the "low-risk" regime chemotherapy[20] (methotrexate 50 g IV on day 1, 3, 5, 7, 9 with oral folinic acid 12 mg 24–30 hours after each dose of methotrexate; course repeated after 7–10 days). The justifications for such an approach are:

- A long period of observation without treatment often results in many seeking non-effective traditional native treatment, so that we may see them only when the disease is already well-advanced
- The 'low-risk' chemotherapy regime above has minimal toxicity; the risk is definitely less than that of metastatic GTN
- The theoretical risk of development of tumor resistance is obviated by the administration of full course of chemotherapy in all instances until biochemical remission is achieved
- Normal reproductive function and normal offspring have been shown in long-term follow-up studies after chemotherapy.[21]

Follow-up of patients receiving 'selection preventive chemotherapy' for more than 10 years showed none developed choriocarcinoma, indicating the value of such therapy

Role of Prophylactic Hysterectomy

In 1966 Tow[22] advocated prophylactic hysterectomy in patients with molar pregnancy at 40 years or more, or in those para 3 or more, as the rate of subsequent malignancy in such patients was significantly increased 3½ times. Hence, it is not unusual to see this practice adopted in many developing countries of Asia.

The subsequent development of widespread metastasis to brain and lungs observed as late as 9 years[20] after hysterectomy and the need for close follow-up of patients with radioimmunoassay even after hysterectomy, means that 'prophylactic hysterectomy' is less justified today.

PLACENTAL SITE TROPHOBLASTIC TUMOR

Placental site trophoblastic tumor (PSTT) very rare tumor is now recognized as a variant of gestational trophoblastic neoplasia; most PSTT's follow non-molar pregnancy. It is composed of only one type of trophoblastic cell (cytotrophoblast); as syncytial cell which are the source of hCG are absent, the hCG production in PST is variable or absent. Curettage is needed to confirm the diagnosis. The clinical course is variable; the only case we have seen in the past 25 years presented with nephrotic syndrome.[20]

Hysterectomy is the primary treatment for PSTT; multi-agent chemotherapy play a major role in the clinical management of this tumor.[23,24] However, these tumor have a poor response to chemotherapy. High levels of expression of VEGF (vascular endothelial growth factor) has been reported in these tumors; inhibition of VEGF may be a novel approach in treatment of this condition.[25]

EPITHELIOID TROPHOBLASTIC TUMOR

Epithelioid trophoblastic tumor is a rare variant of PSTT. It appears to develop from neoplastic transformation of chorionic–type intermediate trophoblasts. Most present several years after a full-term delivery.[26] Mildly elevated hCG may be present. Extra-uterine sites of disease are rare. The primary treatment is hysterectomy.

CHORIOCARCINOMA

The risk of choriocarcinoma is 1000-fold higher after hydatidiform mole than after an abortion or normal pregnancy. Choriocarcinoma is, thus, more prevalent in the countries of South-East Asia. An incidence of gestational trophoblastic tumor/choriocarcinoma of 1.59 per 1000 deliveries was reported in our center.[1] As shown in Table 40.4, choriocarcinoma is also more commonly seen among the Chinese (4.59 per 1000 deliveries) compared to Malays and Indians.

The most common sites of disease are the uterus and lungs (Table 40.5).

In view of the various sites of disease, choriocarcinoma may present with:

- Genital tract manifestations
- Extragenital tract manifestations.

Table 40.5: Choriocarcinoma—sites of disease (n =98), (University Hospital Kuala Lumpur, 1981-1990).

Genital	Number	Extragenital	Number
Uterus	36	Lungs	78
Vagina	8	Brain	14
Paravaginal	8	Liver	11
Cervix (Fig. 40.9)	3	Porta hepatis	2
Fallopian tube	2	Kidney	1
Stomach	1		
Spleen	1		
Para-aortic nodes	1		

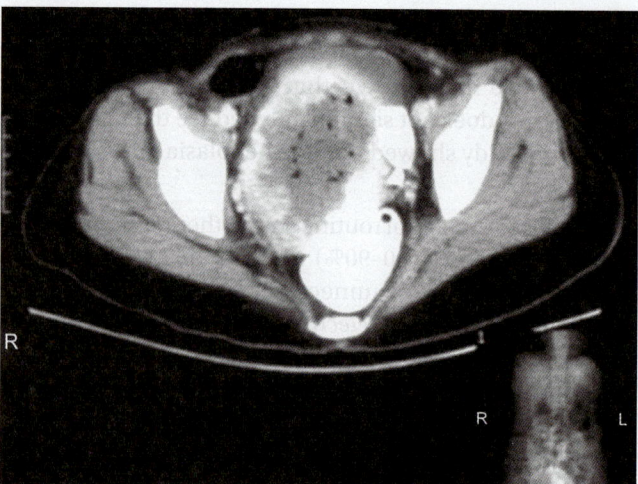

Fig. 40.4: CT scan of pelvis showing appearance of uterine choriocarcinoma.

Genital Tract Manifestations

The most common site is the uterus. There is enlargement of the uterus to a varying degree. The symptoms include:

Amenorrhea

The occurrence of amenorrhea after molar evacuation may indicate choriocarcinoma. An ultrasound assessment of the uterus would exclude an intrauterine pregnancy as the cause of the amenorrhea.

Vaginal Bleeding

This could be intermittent and prolonged. If such bleeding occurs after evacuation of a mole, abortion or normal delivery, possibility of uterine choriocarcinoma should be borne in mind (Fig. 40.4).

Intraperitoneal Hemorrhage

Choriocarcinoma is invasive; thus, the uterine wall can be perforated by tumor resulting in intraperitoneal hemorrhage. The presence of prior amenorrhea can make distinction from a ruptured ectopic pregnancy difficult; the diagnosis is often discovered only at surgery.

Vaginal Metastasis

The commonest location is at the introitus, suburethral in position (Fig. 40.5). The differential diagnosis of a bluish nodule at this location include endometriosis, and melanoma.

Extragenital Manifestations

The *lungs* are the commonest sites for extragenital metastasis. 'Canon-ball' lesion, either single or multiple, on chest radiograph or CT scan are typical (Fig. 40.6). Miliary lesions are also sometimes seen; if this is associated with

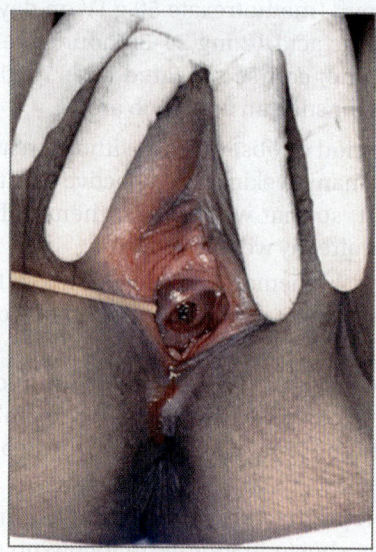

Fig. 40.5: Typical location of vaginal metastasis of choriocarcinoma (an endometriotic nodule or melanoma at this site will also have a similar appearance).

hemoptysis such patients may be mistaken to have miliary TB. If the lesion is pleural based, hemothorax could occur causing respiratory difficulty.

The *brain* is the next most common site for extragenital metastases (Fig. 40.7). Depending on the location the patient may have varied neurological symptoms and signs and may be mistakenly diagnosed as having a primary brain tumor, cerebrovascular accident or even psychosis.

Secondaries can also occur in the *liver*. If the liver involvement is extensive, or if lesions occur in the bile duct or portahepatis, jaundice may be the mode of presentation (Fig. 40.8).

CHAPTER 40 Gestational Trophoblastic Neoplasia

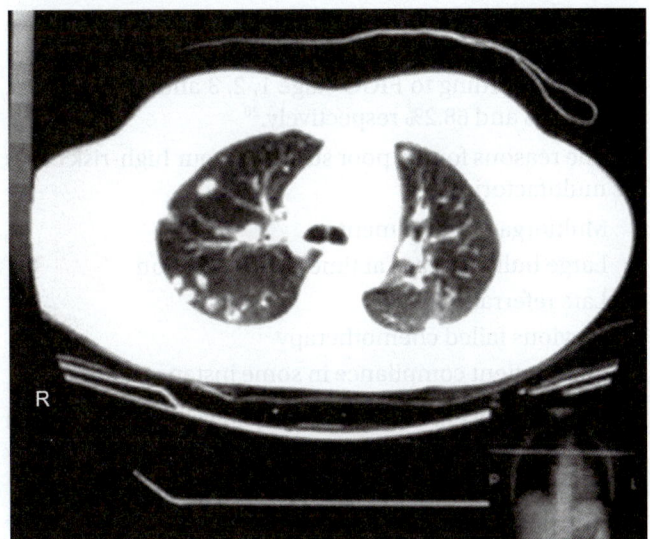

Fig. 40.6: CT scan of thorax showing typical rounded metastatic lesions in the lungs in a patient with choriocarcinoma.

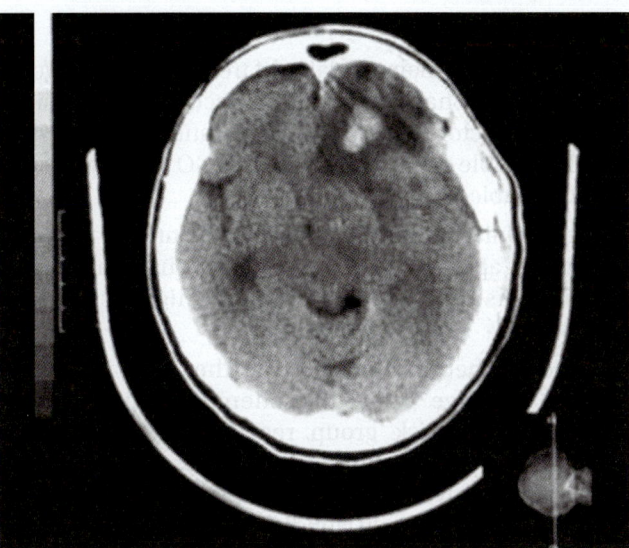

Fig. 40.7: Choriocarcinoma with brain metastases. Note the rather hyperdense lesion with surrounding edema in the right frontal lobe. She also had severe jaundice (see Fig. 40.8).

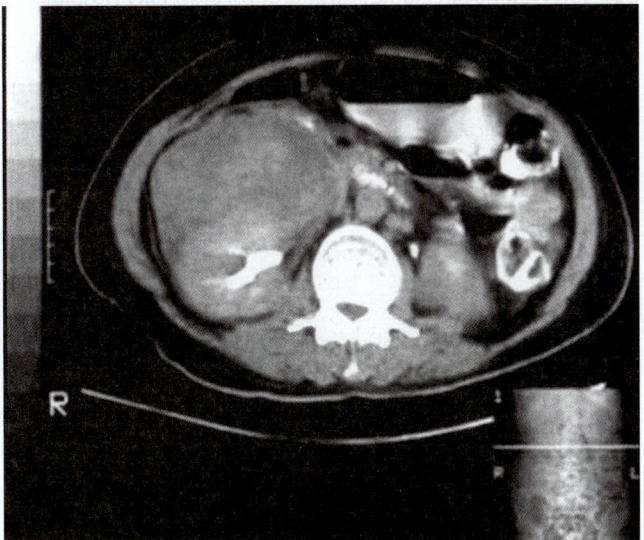

Fig. 40.8: Choriocarcinoma. Note the large tumor mass in the region of portahepatis. She was intensely jaundiced and had brain and lung metastases (see Figs. 40.6 and 40.7). She responded to chemotherapy.

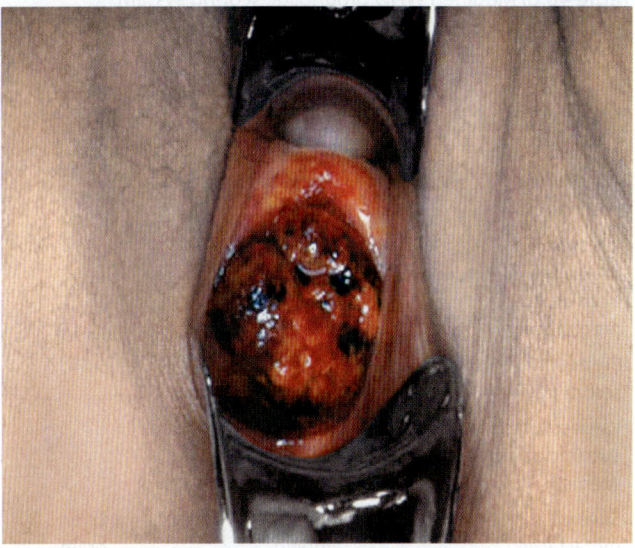

Fig. 40.9: Note the large hemorrhagic/blackish tumor in the cervix. The patient also had liver, lung and brain metastases (see Fig. 40.10 shows the appearance of the cervix after treatment).

Other sites for metastases include the upper *gastrointestinal tract* (presenting as hematemesis), lower gastrointestinal tract (presenting as malena), and *kidneys* (presenting as hematuria). Figure 40.9 shows large hemorrhagic/blackish tumor in the *cervix*. The patient also had liver, lung and brain metastases.

Choriocarcinoma is, thus, one of the great mimics of other diseases. A high index of suspicion is crucial for early diagnosis. Clinicians must, therefore, keep in mind the possibility of choriocarcinoma in all women in the reproductive age group. A test for hCG should be a reflex response to any such presentation.

Management of Choriocarcinoma

The strategies in therapy include:
- Chemotherapy
- Interventional surgery in localized resistant disease
- Radiotherapy.

Chemotherapy

This remains the main modality of treatment. The severity of the disease has been graded according to various prognostic factors. The WHO prognostic scoring system (1983)[27] (Table 40.6) and revised FIGO staging system (1992)[28] (Table 40.7) are shown next.

At the University of Malaya Medical Centre for purposes of assigning appropriate chemotherapy we have categorized our patients into low, medium and high risk groups (Box 40.2).[20]

As described earlier, those in the 'low-risk' group receive selective preventive chemotherapy. Patients in the 'medium-risk' group, receive methotrexate and actinomycin D with folinic acid. Those in the 'high-risk' group receive the modified CHAMOCA or EMA–PE regimes. For the severely jaundiced patient we have found cisplatinum/etoposide/bleomycin combination safe and effective. For details of these regimes please refer to our publication.[20] We reported survivals of 98% in patients in the 'medium-risk' group and 61.7% in 'high-risk' group. Survival according to FIGO stage 1, 2, 3 and 4 were 100%, 80%, 78.6% and 68.2% respectively.[20]

The reasons for the poor survival in our high-risk cases are multifactorial:
- Multiorgan involvement
- Large bulky disease at time of presentation
- Late referrals
- Previous failed chemotherapy
- Poor patient compliance in some instances.

We also observed significantly lower survival (50%) when the interval between the antecedent pregnancy (mole) and the development of GTN exceeded 24 months.[1]

Chemotherapy administered optimally is generally very effective therapy for choriocarcinoma, as shown by the remarkable response noted in Figures 40.9 and 40.10.

Table 40.6: Modified WHO prognostic scoring system.

Risk factors	Score			
	0	1	2	4
Age (year)	<40 years	=> 40 years	–	–
Antecedent pregnancy	Mole	Abortion	Term	–
Interval (months from index pregnancy)	<4	4–6	7–12	> 12
Pretreatment serum hCG IU/l	$<10^3$	10^3–10^4	10^4–10^5	$>10^5$
Largest tumor size (including uterus)	<3 cm	3–5 cm	=>5 cm	-
Sites of metastases	Lung	Spleen, kidney	GI tract	Liver, brain
No. of metastases	–	1–4	5–8	>8
Prior chemotherapy	–	–	Single drug	=>2 drugs

Source: FIGO[27,28] (2010)

Table 40.7: Revised FIGO anatomical staging system for GTN[27,28] (2009).

Stage	
1	Disease confined to the uterus
2	GTN extends outside uterus but is limited to the genital tract structures (adnexa, vagina, broad ligament)
3	GTN extends to the lungs, with or without known genital tract involvement
4	Disease at all other metastatic sites

Box 40.2: Choriocarcinoma—'risk' groups, University Hospital, Kuala Lumpur classification.[20]

Low-risk
- Persistent trophoblastic disease after molar evacuation (no radiological evidence of disease)

Medium-risk
- Lesions in the uterus (uterine size <8 weeks)
- Vaginal nodule
- <3 lung nodules (each <2 cm size)

High-risk
- >3 lung nodules
- Metastases to brain, liver or kidneys
- Uterine tumor (uterine size >8 weeks)
- Paravaginal masses
- Failed chemotherapy

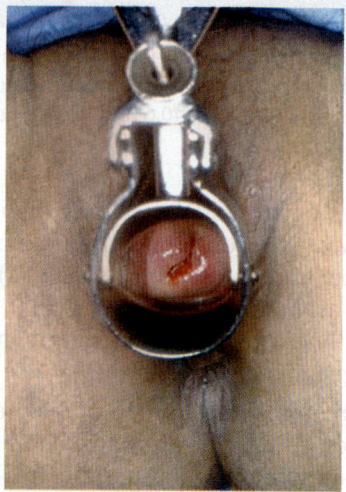

Fig. 40.10: Normal appearance of the cervix (*see* Fig. 40.9 which shows the cervix prior to treatment) after successful treatment with combination chemotherapy.

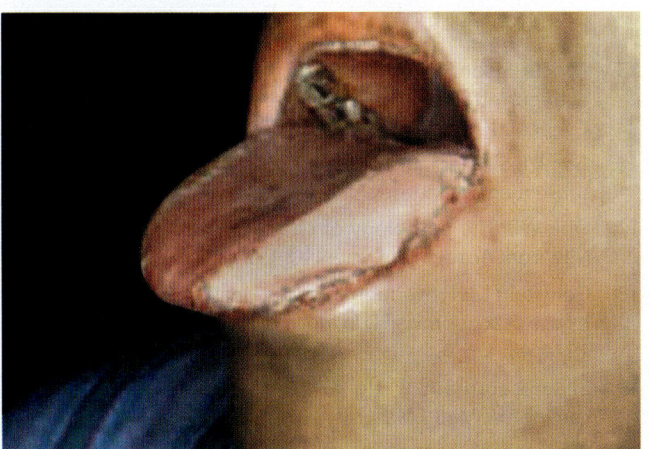

Fig. 40.11: Note the severe oral mucositis after high dose MTX. This could be prevented with appropriate doses of folinic acid.

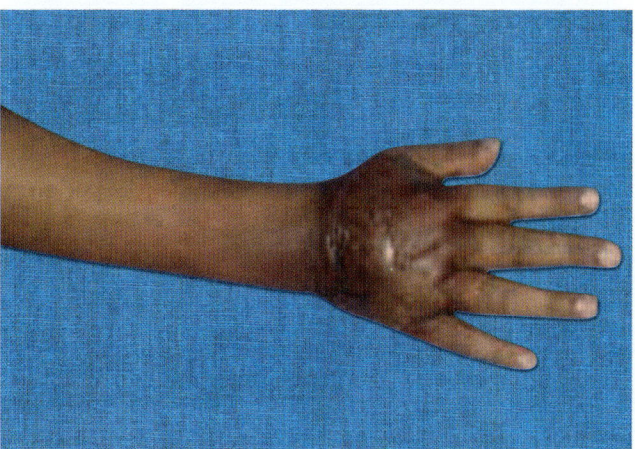

Fig. 40.12: Extravasation of drug causing skin necrosis. This is preventable.

Side Effects of Chemotherapy

Apart from nausea and vomiting, the severe side effects include *severe mucositis* (Fig. 40.11) and *extravasation of drugs* causing skin necrosis (Fig. 40.12). Patient compliance will be enhanced if these side effects are minimized.

Another uncommon side effect following chemotherapy is *'transient menopause'* characterized by amenorrhea, and elevated FSH and LH levels; with the use of cyclical oral contraceptives, return of normal ovulatory cycles is the norm.[1]

Cerebral Metastases

Patients with central nervous system metastases have one of the worst prognosis, with variable survival rates. The use of chemotherapy (with intrathecal MTX) as the main modality, with craniotomy and excision of metastasis or whole brain irradiation in a few, resulted in an overall survival rate of 84.6%.[1]

Role of Surgery

As chemotherapy is effective as primary treatment, surgery has only a limited role. Solitary nodules in the lungs not responding to chemotherapy can be excised at thoracotomy. Similarly, hysterectomy need not be performed routinely; it is only indicated for resistant disease or severe hemorrhage (Fig. 40.13). Continued per vaginal bleeding after biochemical remission has been obtained in a patient with uterine choriocarcinoma may be due to an *A-V malformation* in the uterine wall. A pelvic arteriogram will help confirm the diagnosis; with ipsilateral uterine artery embolization or ligation this bleeding stops. Successful pregnancy outcomes have been reported after such a fertility sparing procedure.[20]

Future Pregnancies

Women after molar evacuation should be advised not to conceive until their hCG levels have been normal for 6

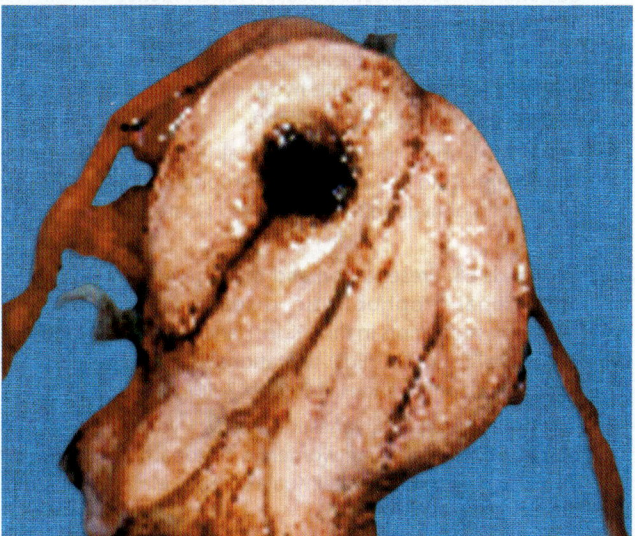

Fig. 40.13: Hysterectomy specimen for resistant choriocarcinoma. Note the blackish lesion in wall of uterus; the ovaries were conserved. Biochemical response was achieved soon after.

months. Those who have had chemotherapy are advised not to conceive for one year after completion of treatment.

Pregnancies can occur after treatment of gestational trophoblastic tumors; in one large study[21] 86% succeeded in having at least one live birth. Successful pregnancies are even possible in patients who have had choriocarcinoma with cerebral metastases.[1, 29, 30]

CONCLUSION

Gestational trophoblastic neoplasia is highly curable. Best results will not be achieved unless these cases are referred promptly to specialized centers where appropriate facilities are available to determine the correct diagnosis, the extent of the disease and where optimal care during chemotherapy is available.

REFERENCES

1. Sivanesaratnam V. Gestational trophoblastic disease in Malaysia and the Pacific Basin. Contemp Rev Obstet Gynecol. 1995;7:179-84.
2. Sivanesaratnam V. The President's Lecture: Gestational trophoblastic disease—the Malaysian experience. Proceedings of the 3rd Malaysian Congress of Obstetrics and Gynecology, Kuala Lumpur 1991.
3. Sivanesaratnam V. Transient hyperthyroidism complicating molar pregnancy. New Zealand J Med. 1978; 84:436-7.
4. Sivanesaratnam V. Asherman's syndrome successfully treated by the insertion of a multiload copper 250 device. J Obstet Gynecol. 1986;7:22-23.
5. Twiggs LB, Morrow DP, Schlaerth JB. Acute pulmonary complications of hydatidiform mole. Am J Obstet Gynecol. 1979;135:189-94.
6. Soper JT, Mutch DG, Schink JC. Diagnosis and treatment of gestational trophoblastic disease: ACOG Practice Bulletin No. 53. Gynaecologic Oncology. 2004;93:575-85.
7. Sabire NJ, Foskett M, Paradinas FJ, et al. Outcome of twin pregnancies with complete hydatidiform mole and healthy co-twin. Lancet. 2002;359:2165-66.
8. Stone M, Dent J, Kardona A, et al. Relationship of oral contraception to development of trophoblastic tumor after evacuation of hydatidiform mole. Br J Obstet Gynecol. 1976; 83:913-6.
9. Newlands ES. Presentation and management of persistent gestational trophoblastic disease and gestational trophoblastic tumors in the UK. In: Hancock BW, Newlands ES, Berkowitz RS, Cole IA. (Eds). Gestational Trophoblastic Disease London: Chapman and Hall 1997;143-56.
10. Cheah PL, Looi LM, Sivanesaratnam V. Hydatidiform molar pregnancy in Malaysian women, a histopathological study from the University Hospital, Kuala Lumpur. Malaysian Journal of Pathology. 1993;15:59-63.
11. Fine C, Bundy AL, Berkowitz R, et al. Sonographic diagnosis of patient hydatidiform mole. Obstet Gynecol. 1989;73: 414-8.
12. Szulman AE. Trophoblastic disease: clinical pathology of hydatidiform mole. Obstet Gyne Clinics of North America. 1988;15:443-56.
13. Bagshawe KD. Trophoblastic neoplasia—current results and therapeutic issues. In: Magreth 1 (Ed). New Directions in Cancer Treatment. London: Springer, 1988;514.
14. Looi LM, Sivanesaratnam V. Malignant evolution with fatal outcome in a patient with partial hydatidiform node. Aust NZJ Obstet Gynecol. 1981;21:51-52.
15. Acosta-Sison H. Indications for immediate hysterectomy with currettage in cases of hydatidiform mole. Am J Obstet Gynecol. 1961;81:715-7.
16. Goh JYL, Sivanesaratnam V, Peh SC. Perforating invasive mole with subsequent metastases. Sing J Obstet Gynecol. 1987;18:151-3.
17. Obir WB. The pathology of choriocarcinoma. Annals of the New York Academy of Sciences. 1971;172:299-426.
18. Goldstein DP. Prevention of gestational trophoblastic disease by use of actinomycin D in molar pregnancies. Obstet Gynecol. 1974; 43: 475-9.
19. Sivanesaratnam V, Ng KH. Prophylaxis against choriocarcinoma. Med J Malaysia. 1977; 3: 219-31.
20. Sivanesaratnam V. Management of gestational trophoblastic disease in developing countries. Best Practice & Research Clinical Obstetric and Gynecology. 2003;17:925-42.
21. Rustin GJ, Booth M, Dent J. et al. Pregnancy after cytotoxic chemotherapy for gestational trophoblastic tumors. Br Med J. 1984;288:183-206.
22. Tow WSH. The influence of the primary treatment of hydatidiform mole on its subsequent course. J Obstet Gynecol Br Cwlth. 1966; 77:544-52.
23. Newlands ES, Bower M, Fisher RA, Paradinas FJ. Management of placental site trophoblastic tumors. J Reprod Med. 1998;43:53-9.
24. Feltmate CM, Genest DR, Wise L, et al. Placental site trophoblastic tumor: 17-year experience at New England Trophoblastic Disease Centre. Gynecol Oncol. 2001;82:415-9.
25. Berkowitz RS, Goldstein DP. Current advances in management of gestational trophoblastic disease. Gynecol Oncol. 2014; 128:3-5.
26. Alison KH, Love JE, Garcia RL. Epitheloid trophoblastic tumor: review of a rare neoplasm of the chorionic type intermediate trophoblast. Arch Path Lab Med. 2006;130:1875-7.
27. Edge SB, Byrd DR, Compton CC, et al. Gestational trophoblastic tumors in AJCC Cancer Staging Manual. 7th Edn. New York, NY Springer. 210;439.
28. FIGO Committee on Gynaecologic Oncology. Current FIGO staging of cancer of the vagina, fallopian tube, ovary and gestational trophoblastic neoplasia, Int J of Gynecol and Obstet. 2009;105:3-4.
29. Sen DK, Sivanesaratnam V, Chuah CY, et al. Cerebral metastases from choriocarcinoma. Acta Obstet Gynecol Scand. 1987;66:425-8.
30. Sivanesaratnam V, Sen DK. Normal pregnancy after successful treatment of choriocarcinoma with cerebral metastases. J Reprod Med. 1988;33:402-3.

CHAPTER 41

Radiotherapy and Systemic Anticancer Therapy in Gynecological Malignancy

Robert Wade

Overview

- Successful treatment of gynecological cancer is multimodality and involves surgery, radiotherapy and systemic anticancer therapy.
- Radiotherapy is the treatment of patients with ionizing radiation. It can be delivered externally most commonly with a linear accelerator, or by the use of radioisotopes directly to the tumor (brachytherapy).
- Systemic anticancer therapy is used as a radio-sensitizer, adjuvantly to reduce the risk of reoccurrence and palliatively.
- Cervical cancer can be effectively treated with a combination of chemoradiotherapy and brachytherapy.
- Endometrial cancer of grade 3/ Stage 1b and above has traditionally been treated with surgery and adjuvant radiotherapy. The role of chemotherapy is under investigation in the adjuvant setting.
- Ovarian cancer treatment involves a combination of surgery and chemotherapy with survival improving with increased surgical effort and the addition of cycles of carboplatin paclitaxel chemotherapy.
- Vaginal cancer is radiosensitive and effectively treated with radiotherapy.
- Adjuvant radiotherapy has a role in treating node positive vulval cancer.

RADIOTHERAPY

Ionizing radiation can be used to treat systemic disease, particularly malignant disease. Radiotherapy can be electromagnetic (photons), particulate (electrons, protons, ions) or can be the consequence of radioactive decay (alpha, beta or gamma rays).

Radiotherapy can be delivered from outside the patient, i.e. shining radiotherapy beams through a patient to reach the relevant targets or directly into the target (brachytherapy) where radioactive isotopes are inserted directly into the tumor.

In clinical practice, photons are the most widely used form of radiotherapy. Their energy determines how they interact with matter and their penetrating power. Kilovoltage photons (the basis of diagnostic X-rays) and megavoltage photons (generated by linear accelerators) interact in different ways. MV photons have much more penetrating power and as the dose builds up several centimeters in matter allow skin sparing and have advantages in treating pelvic anatomy.

Radioactive isotopes deliver their radiation dose directly to the chosen target. Gamma rays are the most clinically useful in gynecological cancer. Their main advantage is the dose delivered falls off very quickly following the inverse square law. The energy of gamma rays varies according to the radioisotope. Iridium-192 has replaced caesium-137 as the radioisotope of choice for delivering gynecological brachytherapy. It produces high energy gamma rays [High dose rate (HDR) brachytherapy (12Gy/hr)] as opposed to cesium [Low dose rate (LDR) brachytherapy (0.5-1Gy/hr)].

The aim of radiotherapy is to cause lethal DNA damage in tumors. Radiotherapy induces double-stranded DNA breaks in DNA strands to make cancer cells nonviable. Similar damage also occurs in normal tissues. The aim of treatment is to exploit the differences between cancer cells and normal tissues to cause as much cancer cell lethality as possible but to minimize damage to normal tissues. The side effects of radiotherapy reflect normal tissue damage. Five different radiobiological factors determine tumor and normal tissue response to radiotherapy. Normal tissues and tumors have different inherent **radiosensitivity**.

Repair processes are different in cancer cells and normal cells, with repair being more effective in non-proliferating cells. **Repopulation** can occur quickly in rapidly dividing cells. **Reoxygenation:** Hypoxic cells are relatively radio resistant so correction of anemia increases oxygenation. Short radiation treatments may be less effective due to persistence of hypoxic cells. **Redistribution:** Cancer cells have different sensitivities to radiation in different phases of the cell cycle. Curative radiotherapy schedules over an extended time take advantage of these differences to maximize anticancer effect and allow normal tissue repair to occur during treatment.

The delivery of radiotherapy is constantly improving and becoming more targeted exploiting modern imaging modalities to the full. Computerized tomography and magnetic resonance imaging scans are used to plan radiotherapy treatments (usually the tumor, high-risk areas and draining lymph nodes). Traditional three-dimensional conformal techniques are being replaced by intensity modulated radiotherapy (IMRT) with image guidance. This allows more complicated volumes to be treated (rectangular volumes verses volumes and treatments which match the anatomy more closely). It has the advantage of reducing normal tissue damage. Target movement during a course of radiation treatment can be considerable. IMRT requires some form of imaging during treatment to ensure treatment accuracy. This forms the basis of image-guided radiotherapy (IGRT).

Side effects of radiotherapy reflect normal tissue damage and repair. The side effects can occur during a treatment course (early side effects) or some months to years later (late side effects). They vary depending on the site being treated.

The following are common early side effects in treating the pelvis.

Skin reactions are more common when it is desirable to bring the radiation dose close to the skin surface especially when treating vulval and vaginal cancer. Reactions vary from erythema to moist desquamation.

Pelvic radiotherapy can cause bowel damage. Bowel side effects are common with bowel radiotherapy. Anorexia and nausea are best treated with ondansetron. Diarrhea is usually managed with loperamide/codeine. More significant bowel damage requiring admission and IV fluids occurs very occasionally.

Bone marrow toxicity is uncommon as modern radiation treatments minimize the dose to the bone marrow. It can occur if systemic anticancer therapy is administered as a radiation sensitizer. This can be an issue with curative treatment for cervical cancer. In this situation, oxygenation is important and it is important to maintain hemoglobin levels at 120 g/dL or greater.

Late side effects associated with pelvic radiotherapy include the following:

- Lymphedema can occur and requires symptomatic treatment from a specialist lymphedema clinic
- The most common bowel side effect following radiotherapy is a change in bowel habit
- Rarely more significant bowel damage can occur
- Bleeding from the bowel due to telangiectasia and malabsorption states can occur but are not common. These need to be investigated and treated on their own merits
- Very significant side effects such as bowel stenosis and fistulae are very uncommon.

Similar late effects can affect the bladder and urinary system.

Vaginal dilators are advised to reduce the risk of vaginal stenosis.

Ovarian failure following curative pelvic radiotherapy is inevitable in patients of reproductive age where the ovaries remain in situ.

SYSTEMIC ANTICANCER CANCER THERAPY

Systemic anticancer therapy (SACT) covers a variety of different anti-cancer treatments including traditional chemotherapy, biological therapy, hormone therapy and immunotherapy.

Chemotherapy covers a widerange of compounds that act at various points in the cell cycle to induce cancer cell lethality. The side effects of chemotherapy reflect damage to normal cells.

Alkylating agents such as ifosfamide form covalent linkages with DNA.

Cisplatin and carboplatin cause cross links with DNA and other cellular components.

Gemcitabine is an example of an antimetabolite, resulting in premature DNA chain termination.

Paclitaxel is an example of an antimicrotubule agent.

Side effects of chemotherapy reflect the populations of cells with a rapid turn over as well as direct effects on organs.

Nausea and vomiting are common. This perhaps is not surprising as most of these agents are natural poisons. Combinations of powerful antiemetics are often required to make chemotherapy tolerable (5HT3 inhibitors, steroids, dopamine antagonists). Bone marrow effects are common and can be life-threatening. The most serious complication is neutropenic sepsis. The highest risk of this is at 7–14 days postchemotherapy and carries a small risk of mortality.

CHAPTER 41 Radiotherapy and Systemic Anticancer Therapy in Gynecological Malignancy

Prompt treatment with intravenous antibiotics is indicated in appropriate patients. Anemia and symptomatic thrombocytopenia are treated supportively with blood and platelet transfusions.

Skin toxicity and mucositis can occur. Nerve damage (peripheral neuropathy) is agent specific. Bowel toxicity (mainly diarrhea) can be an issue. Direct organ damage can also occur (e.g. kidney toxicity with cisplatin).

More targeted treatments have become available in the last few years. Bevacizumab is an inhibitor of the endothelial growth factor receptor (EGFR). It inhibits angiogenesis and has some efficacy in ovarian and cervical cancer.

Poly (ADP-ribose) polymerase (PARP) inhibitors may also have a role in the treatment of ovarian cancer. *BRCA 1* and *BRCA 2* genes give rise to errors in the homologous DNA repair pathway. If single strand DNA break repair is inhibited by poly (ADP-ribose) polymerase inhibitors (PARPs), this increases likelihood of cancer death.

Antiestrogens and progesterone's have a role in the palliative treatment of some gynecological malignancies.

ONCOLOGICAL TREATMENT OF SPECIFIC CANCERS

The general principles of oncological treatment depend on the inherent individual sensitivity of a tumor to the different treatment modalities, the stage (and whether the aim is cure or palliation) and on patient factors (willingness to undergo treatment and degree of comorbidities).

CERVICAL CANCER

Early stage cervical cancer is treated with surgery alone. Adjuvant radiotherapy is reserved for patients with features suggesting a high-risk of reoccurrence (close margins under 4 cm or lymph node involvement). Bulky stage 1 and stage 2b-4 cervical cancer is treated with a combination of chemoradiotherapy and brachytherapy. There has been a trend towards more complex radiotherapy and brachytherapy to improve local control and cure rates. Treatment involves radiotherapy to the cervix, endometrium, parametrium, draining pelvic and occasionally para-aortic lymph nodes. The aim is to give a dose of 45 Gy in 25 daily fractions. IMRT combined with IGRT can be utilized to spare bowel (Fig. 41.1). Endometrial movement can be considerable between fractions so some form of image guidance is required to ensure accurate treatment. Weekly cisplatin is used as a radiation sensitizer and improves outcomes by 10%. Oxygenation is maintained by keeping hemoglobin levels above 12.

Brachytherapy follows chemoradiotherapy. The patient undergoes a general anesthetic. Under anesthetic an

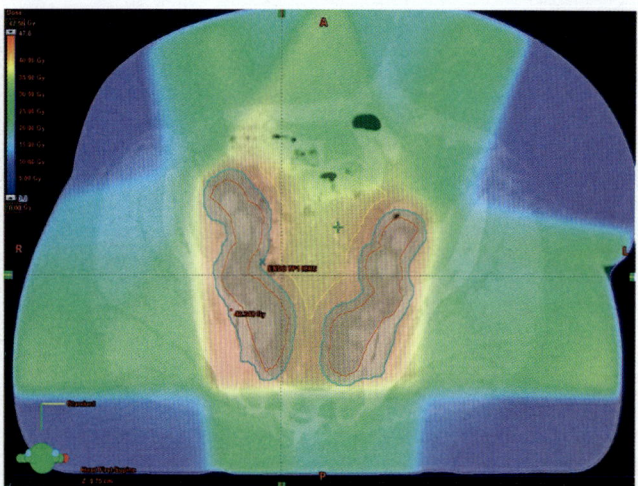

Fig. 41.1: Axial image of a CT IMRT plan. The blue contour represents the planning target volume and encompasses the lymph node drainage area delineated by a red line with a margin for interfractional movement and other variables. The red area represents the 45 Gy volume. Of note the center of the scan is cooler representing less dose being delivered to the abdominal cavity IMRI, intensity modulated radiation therapy.

intrauterine applicator is inserted. Some form of imaging to check position is undertaken and the treatment is prescribed. The old Manchester system where the dose was prescribed to point A (2 cm lateral and above the cervical os) is in the process of being superseded by the more conformal Vienna system. In this system, a series of volumes are delineated [High-risk clinical target volume (HRCTV), Intermediate risk-target volume (IRCTV), organs at risk (OAR)]. The dose is then prescribed to the volume. The applicator has an intrauterine tube that sits in the intrauterine cavity, a ring applicator that abuts the cervix and interstitial needles that are inserted into the parametrium. An MRI scan is performed with the applicator in situ to delineate the target volume. The treatment plan is modelled on a planning computer and optimized before treatment is delivered. This technique allows higher doses to be delivered to the cervical tumor with lower doses administered to the organs at risk (bladder, rectum, sigmoid, bowel). Iridium is the most common radioisotope used. It produces highly energetic gamma rays so radiation treatments are normally fractionated. The source is delivered to the patient by an afterloading system to ensure no radiation exposure to staff members. Four fractions are delivered prescribed to the HRCTV at least 6 hours apart with a view to delivering doses of 85 Gy or greater to the primary tumor (Fig. 41.2). Outcome is dependant on tumor size. Currently, there is interest in neoadjuvant chemotherapy prior to radiotherapy. The interlace trial is looking at whether the addition of carboplatin paclitaxel upfront improves long-term outcomes.

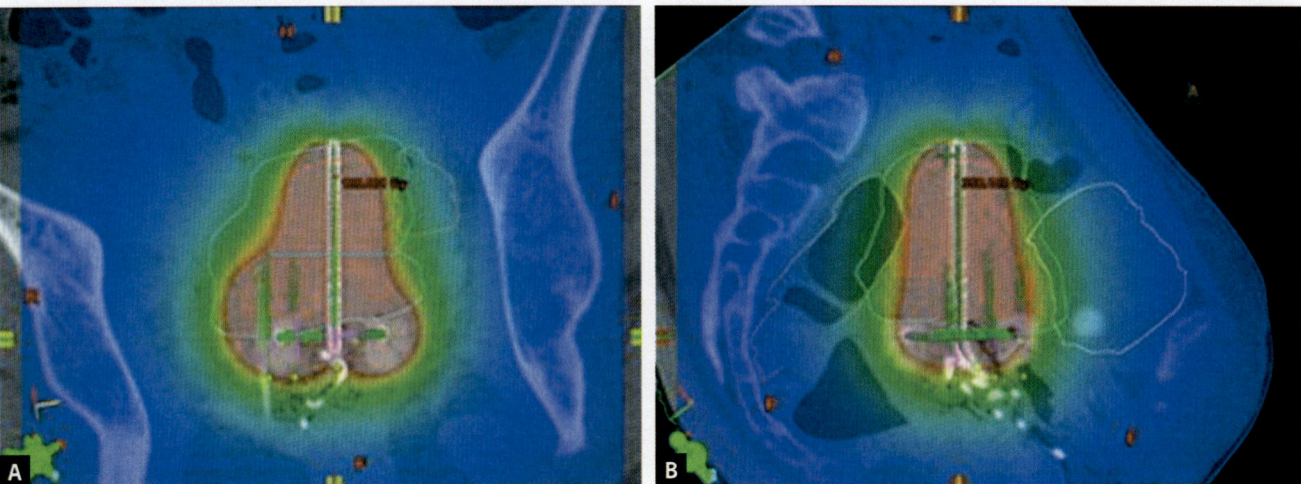

Figs. 41.2A and B: (A) Sagittal and (B) coronal views of a CT brachytherapy plan. The red contour represents the HRCTV. The blue contour represents the IRCTV. The intrauterine tube and ring applicator can be seen in the center of the image. Interstitial needles are used to improve coverage and allow sparing of the bladder and bowel.

(HRCTV: High-risk clinical target volume; IRCTV: intermediate-risk clinical target volume)

Chemotherapy is used in the palliative setting for cervical cancer. The prime aim here is symptom control. Carboplatin paclitaxel and cisplatin topotecan are both regimens that have activity in the palliative setting.

ENDOMETRIAL CANCER

Curative treatment for endometrial cancer is multimodality. Surgery is the treatment of choice for early stage disease. The role of radiotherapy has become less clear since the publication of the ASTEC trial. This demonstrated a local control benefit for radiotherapy but no corresponding survival benefit. Surgical practice has also changed with pelvic lymph node dissections being carried out for high-risk disease. Traditionally, adjuvant radiotherapy has been offered for G3 or 1b tumors and above. The aim is to deliver 45 Gy to the pelvic lymph nodes and tumor bed with brachytherapy using a vaginal cylinder to the vaginal vault. Brachytherapy doses vary but 11 Gy in 2 fractions is an example of an adjuvant fractionation. If, however, the pelvic lymph nodes have been removed and are negative then brachytherapy on its own is an acceptable local treatment. The role of chemotherapy is currently being investigated in clinical trials. PORTEC 3 looked at whether adjuvant chemotherapy adds a survival benefit for high-risk endometrial cancer. Carboplatin paclitaxel was the test chemotherapy in this trial. Results are awaited.

Chemotherapy has a role in the palliative treatment of endometrial cancer. Carboplatin paclitaxel has become the first choice regimen, with other single agents such as epirubicin also offering some activity. Hormonal therapy also has a palliative role. Progesterone's and antiestrogens can be used in estrogen sensitive tumors.

OVARIAN CANCER

Treatment for ovarian cancer is multimodality. Early stage serous ovarian cancers are treated with surgery. Patients with stage 1c tumors are offered single agent carboplatin. Stage 2 and greater tumors are treated with a combination of surgery and chemotherapy either upfront, at an interval or adjuvantly. The exact order of treatment depends on operability and likelihood of achieving optimal cytoreduction. The radicality of surgery is certainly increasing with evidence that where optimal cytoreduction is possible 5-year survival rates are better than optimal debulking. Carboplatin paclitaxel is the preferred chemotherapy with the aim of delivering six, three weekly cycles around surgery.

There has been interest in bevacizumab in the curative setting. Bevacizumab improves progression free survival and is currently being investigated further in clinical trials. The newly reopened ICON 8 trial is investigating the role of bevacizumab in the adjuvant setting as well as investigating the role of dose dense chemotherapy.

Traditionally, chemotherapy has been the sole treatment offered on relapse of ovarian cancer with the choice dependant on whether the cancer is deemed platinum sensitive or not (relapse after 6 months of previous treatment). There is also interest in secondary debulking. Palliative chemotherapy tends to be offered sequentially. Active treatments include weekly paclitaxel, carboplatin and liposomal doxorubicin, liposomal doxorubicin on its own, weekly topotecan and gemcitabine carboplatin.

PARP inhibitors are currently the subject of clinical trials.

CHAPTER 41 Radiotherapy and Systemic Anticancer Therapy in Gynecological Malignancy

VULVAL CANCER

Surgery is the treatment of choice for vulval cancer. The role of adjuvant nodal radiotherapy in high-risk disease is currently under investigation in the groins trial. Cisplatin is sometimes used as a radiation sensitizer. Radiotherapy with electrons is sometimes offered adjuvantly if surgical margins are close in areas where further resection may be difficult (i.e. around anus).

VAGINAL CANCER

Localized lower vaginal cancers are treated with some form of radiation therapy alone. The general principle is to give doses of 64 Gy 32 fractions to the primary tumor with lower adjuvant dose of radiation treatment to the draining nodes. There may be an advantage to concomitant cisplatin as a radiation sensitizer. Interstitial brachytherapy is an alternative.

TROPHOBLASTIC TUMORS

Management of these rare but highly curable tumors is very specialist and offered in very specialist centers. They are treated with chemotherapy.

CONCLUSION

Successful treatment of gynecological malignancy is multimodality. Advances in surgery, radiotherapy and in systemic treatment are improving survival rates but requires an increasingly more multidisciplinary approach.

BIBLIOGRAPHY

1. Barrett A, Dobbs J, Morris S, Roques T. Practical radiotherapy planning 4th edition. HodderArnold 4th edn. 2009.
2. DeVita VT, Lawrence TS, Rosen berg SA. DeVita, Hellman and Rosenberg. Cancer: Principles and Practice of Oncology. 8th edition. Lippincott Williams and Wilkins; 2008.
3. Potter R, et al. Recommendations from gynaecological (GYN) GEC ESTRO working group (II): concepts and terms in 3D image-based treatment planning in cervix cancer brachytherapy–3D volume parameters and aspects of 3D image-based anatomy, radiation physics, radiobiology. Radiother Oncol. 2006;78(1): 67-77.

CHAPTER 42

Palliative Care

Claire Stewart, Onnig Tamizian

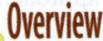
Overview

- Palliative care is not the same as terminal care; it encompasses the time period from when curative treatment is no longer possible through to end of life care and death. Clearly its duration is very variable, as is the patient's outlook and needs.
- The emphasis is to maintain the best quality of life achievable for the patient, and therefore meticulous attention should be paid to symptom control at all times.
- Optimum palliative care requires holistic assessment and multidisciplinary input to make best use of all available resources and expertise.

INTRODUCTION

Death and dying is seen in every area of medicine and the vast majority of healthcare professionals will care for dying patients at some point in their career. Palliative care relates specifically to the control of distressing symptoms and should not be viewed as synonymous to terminal care. At the 58th World Health Assembly in 2005, palliation was recognized as an essential component of cancer care; equally as important as measures, such as surgery, medical care and radiation/chemotherapeutic oncology; and the integration of palliative care into national cancer strategies was strongly recommended. For maximum benefit, patients should have contact with the palliative team for at least 3 months prior to death and, therefore, palliative referrals should be considered early in the disease course, especially if patients have difficult to control, severe or ongoing symptoms.

Palliative care aims to help the patient lead as normal a life as possible, with effective relief from pain and other distressing symptoms. Meticulous attention to symptom control is essential and a holistic assessment of each individual patient is paramount. Even if the underlying disease cannot be cured, patients may still enjoy a fruitful and rewarding life if they are comfortable. There should be frequent re-evaluation of symptoms and the effectiveness of treatments reviewed regularly to ensure well-being is maintained. In order to elicit specific, relevant details about the problems, fears and anxieties suffered by each individual patient, it is essential to develop excellent communication skills. Making a cancer diagnosis and breaking this news to the patient is one of the doctor's first responsibilities, and as such, the manner in which it is performed influences the course of the doctor-patient relationship. Patients need sensitive, clear and sometimes repeated explanations of the diagnosis and its implications, along with honest, balanced discussion regarding the potential effects of any treatments, both curative and palliative, on their general well-being and ability to continue with normal activities of daily living.

SYMPTOM MANAGEMENT

The principles involved in symptom management are based around a thorough evaluation and assessment of each problem. Patients with advanced gynecological cancer frequently report pain, weakness, anorexia, nausea, vomiting, constipation, dry mouth and psychological distress. Symptoms need to be appreciated in the context of the beliefs of the individual, their understanding of the situation, their coping mechanism and expectations. A full history should be taken of each individual symptom, as understanding the pathophysiology enables more appropriate management plans to be initiated. Combining treatment both for the underlying cause and the symptom is generally the best approach, as it prevents recurrence or worsening of the problem. It is essential to elicit the patient's key treatment priorities and for the physician and patient to negotiate achievable goals. Open discussions about the possible benefits and side effects of all treatments, including any changes in lifestyle that the patient may need to consider, are important. The actual benefit of any intervention should be assessed after implementation and ineffective therapies discontinued to minimize side effects.

Drug Administration in Palliative Care

In the majority of cases, the oral route is preferred first line as it is the least invasive and disruptive option, and gives the patient maximal control in the management of their symptoms. However, it is essential to have alternative routes available for urgent use or when oral routes fail. As their illness progresses, patients will become increasingly weak and may struggle to take oral medications, even in syrup or dispersible format. Furthermore, gastric stasis is common in many advanced cancers and, therefore, the absorption and bioavailability of medication will be compromised. In these cases, it is common to use the subcutaneous route for administering essential drugs (usually given into the upper arm), although intramuscular injections may rarely be needed if the patient has severe extensive peripheral edema. In patients who need regular doses of medication, it is preferred to use a continuous subcutaneous infusion (CSCI) as this avoids repeated injections but also provided a steady state dose for the patient, avoiding the peaks and troughs that may precipitate side effects or breakthrough symptoms. If these options are not acceptable or are unavailable, then some drugs are available in rectal preparations or as transdermal patches. Care should be taken when changing preparations as the drug dose may vary according to the route of administration. For example, when morphine is given via the subcutaneous, intramuscular or intravenous route, the dose is typically half that of the oral dose. When the patient is approaching the end of life, it is also wise to have essential 'anticipatory' drugs prescribed subcutaneously (SC) so that there is no delay if an expected symptom does arise. It is common to prescribe a strong opiate for pain, Midazolam 2.5 mg for agitation or distress, Haloperidol 1.5–2.5 mg for nausea or agitation/hallucinations; and Hyoscine butylbromide 20 mg for respiratory secretions or colicky pain. These can obviously be tailored according to local drug availability and individual patient need.

Pain Control

Pain is not just a physical experience—it has emotional, psychological, social and spiritual components. Pain will be perceived more intensely if the patient is frightened, anxious, angry, depressed, isolated or fatigued. It is essential that these holistic interactions are acknowledged and addressed since this may enable more rapid relief of pain with less use of medication, and hence fewer side effects. When setting treatment goals, ensuring a full night's sleep, undisturbed by pain, is a good initial aim. It is essential to engage the patient to understand what her key priorities are, so that treatments can be tailored to her, allowing her to maintain her social activities and lifestyle.

To treat pain appropriately and effectively, it is first necessary to determine the likely cause or mechanism of the pain. The basic principles of pain assessment need to be revisited, and detailed information about the site, radiation, onset, duration, nature, and relieving and exacerbating features need to be obtained. It is important to determine whether the pain is directly cancer related or secondary to another problem, such as constipation, severe ascites, gastroesophageal reflux, or infection. As part of the assessment it is important to ask what effect the pain is having on the patient's daily activities, what expectations or goals they have and what they think may be causing the pain. It is also essential to review which analgesics have been tried previously, how often they were taken and what consequences they had, both in terms of symptomatic relief and side effects. Investigations may assist in determining the cause of pain, but clearly a fine balance needs to be struck when dealing with a very ill patient. Investigations should only therefore be performed if they will significantly alter management and benefit the patient.

The importance of regular administration of analgesia in maintaining adequate pain relief cannot be sufficiently emphasized. Regular medication prevents the recurrence of pain, and analgesia should be given in appropriate doses at frequent intervals, as determined by the pharmacokinetics of the particular drug being used. Adverse effects may reduce the acceptability and tolerance of medication, so these should be anticipated and measures taken to prevent or ameliorate them.

Analgesic drugs can be broadly classified as nonopioid (simple), opioid and adjuvant. Each group has a different mechanism of action and may therefore be best suited to different types of pain. Drugs should be prescribed in a stepwise fashion, as guided by the World Health Organization (WHO) analgesic ladder:

Step 1: Start with nonopioid drugs ± adjuvant therapies

Step 2: Weak opioids (combined with non-opioids ± adjuvants), e.g. Codeine, Dihydrocodeine, Tramadol

Step 3: Strong opioids (combined with non-opioids ± adjuvants), e.g. Morphine, Diamorphine, Oxycodone, Fentanyl.

Simple (nonopioid) Analgesia

The WHO analgesic ladder suggests starting with regular doses of nonopioid drugs. These include paracetamol

(Acetaminophen) and Nonsteroidal anti-inflammatory drugs (NSAIDs), which include ibuprofen, naproxen, meloxicam and diclofenac. Prostaglandins are produced by malignant cells and macrophages, and act to stimulate or sensitize afferent peripheral nerve endings in pain fibers. NSAIDs work by reducing inflammation and prostaglandin synthesis, thereby reducing sensitization and pain. Paracetamol works centrally to reduce prostanoid production, but unlike NSAIDs, has no peripheral anti-inflammatory effect. Peripheral sensitization occurs with both nerve injury and tissue inflammation, therefore NSAIDs will be effective for most cancer-related pain, and should be given alongside opioids unless there is a significant contraindication. Long-term NSAID use may be limited by side effects which include GI ulceration, renal impairment, bronchospasm and a slight increase in the risk of myocardial infarction. It is advisable to use the lowest effective dose and to consider concomitant gastroprotection with a proton-pump inhibitor, such as Omeprazole. Both Paracetamol and NSAIDs have additional antipyretic properties and may be useful in relieving nonspecific cancer-related fever.

Opioid Analgesia

Opioids are thought to act both peripherally and centrally through inhibition of nociceptive transmission at spinal cord, brainstem and possibly at peripheral nerve level. There are four opioid receptor subtypes distributed throughout the body and each opioid has a slightly different receptor combination affinity. Opioids are not effective for pain related to muscular cramp/spasm, and only partially effective for neuropathic pain. Constipation is very common in patients taking opioids, so they should always be prescribed in combination with regular laxatives. Other recognized side effects include gastric stasis, nausea, sedation, urinary retention, confusion, agitation, hallucinations, myoclonus and pruritus. Some effects will ease after a few days, however, others may be persistent and require treatment; or even discontinuation of the opioid. In these cases, an alternative opioid can be tried, and oxycodone is often better tolerated than morphine.

When patients are commenced on strong opioids, it is advisable to begin with a regular, four hourly dose of an immediate release oral preparation, such as Oramorph or Sevredol. If the patient has been on weaker opiates previously, a reasonable starting dose would be 10 mg orally (every 4 hours), however a smaller dose is advisable in those with renal failure, hepatic impairment, the elderly, the very frail or those who are opiate naïve. For patients whose pain is not controlled with four hourly dosing, additional 'as required' (PRN) doses of a further 5–10 mg should be given, although care should be taken to monitor for side effects, such as drowsiness and toxicity. This regime should be continued for at least 48 hours, ensuring adequate pain relief is achieved. Once the pain is controlled, it is then possible to calculate the total daily opiate requirements and convert to a long-acting, modified release preparation, such as MST Continus or Zomorph. There should always be a fast, short-acting opioid available for breakthrough pain, and this should be prescribed on a PRN basis. However, the dose should be recalculated as one sixth of the total daily dose, not left at the default of 5–10 mg as initially used. See the worked example below for more details:

> Patient commenced on immediate release oral morphine, 10 mg four hourly and as required:
> Six regular doses given in 24 hour period = 60 mg
> Four additional 'as required' (PRN) doses needed = 40 mg
> Total 24-hour opiate requirement = (60 mg + 40 mg) = 100 mg
> Morphine changed to modified release/long acting oral preparation = 50 mg twice daily
> New PRN dose = (100 mg/6) = approximately 15 mg (may give range of 15-20 mg)
> → *Note:* immediate release oral morphine is still used for PRN doses

It is also helpful to have PRN medication available via alternative routes (usually subcutaneous or intramuscular) in case rapid relief is needed for severe breakthrough pain, or the patient is unable to take the oral option. The dose should be adjusted accordingly—parenteral morphine should be half the oral dose (so 7.5–10 mg in the above example), and if using Diamorphine, the dose is one third of the oral morphine dose (so 5–7.5 mg in the above example). When converting to a longer acting preparation, it may also be appropriate to change the route of administration, particularly if the condition of patient is deteriorating rapidly or struggling to tolerate oral medications. Options include continuous subcutaneous infusions (CSCI) or transdermal patches (only buprenorphine or fentanyl currently available in patch format). However, great care should be taken when using dose conversion tables and it may be wise to seek advice from a specialist pharmacist. Of particular note, fentanyl is 80–100 times more potent than Morphine and doses are in micrograms, not milligrams.

Neuropathic Pain

Pain originating from damage to the nervous system may be difficult to manage with conventional analgesia. Neuropathic pain in the context of gynecological malignancy may arise from sacral plexus infiltration in cervical or ovarian cancer, radiculopathy secondary to spinal cord compression or as a side effect from platinum-based cytotoxic chemotherapy or radiotherapy. A number of adjuvant drugs, which are not conventional analgesics, can be helpful in managing neuropathic pain, especially when combined with nonopioids. Neuropathic pain is thought to stem from neuronal hyperexcitability and spontaneous activity at the site of injury, combined with neurochemical changes in the central nervous system (CNS). Common adjuvant analgesic drugs therefore include antidepressants and antiepileptics. It is thought that by increasing serotonin (± noradrenaline/norepinephrine) levels in the central nervous system, antidepressants enhance the central inhibition of nociception. Within this group, Tricyclic antidepressants, such as amitriptyline, are the most effective and should be used first line, followed by Venlafaxine, then SSRIs like citalopram and paroxetine. If they are ineffective, then an antiepileptic drug should be tried instead. Antiepileptic drugs work through different mechanisms, including peripheral sodium channel blockade, calcium channel blockade and alterations in the glutamate and GABA systems. Gabapentin and pregabalin are increasingly being used with good effect, and can be safely combined with antidepressants if needed. Sodium valproate given at bed time is another reasonable option, but as with all antiepileptics, must be started at low dose and titrated up slowly. Improvements in sleep are often seen quickly with these drugs but it is important to warn patients that significant improvements in pain may not be evident for 1–2 weeks.

Corticosteroids, such as dexamethasone are also very helpful for treating pain and weakness secondary to nerve or spinal cord compression, and should be considered first line if neuropathic pain is associated with limb weakness. They have an anti-inflammatory effect and reduce the overall tumor mass through the reduction of peritumor edema. Typical doses of 4–8 mg once daily are used for nerve root compression, whilst suspected spinal cord compression requires higher doses and should prompt urgent specialist referral. Many patients have increased alertness and energy with steroids so it is preferable to administer the dose in the morning (or split between morning and early afternoon in higher doses) to prevent insomnia. Transient hyperglycemia is a common effect of steroids, as is increased appetite, and therefore diabetics should be monitored more closely during the treatment course. Rarely, there can be personality changes, disinhibition and psychosis with high dose steroids so it is also important to be vigilant for these symptoms.

Bone Pain

Although distant bony metastases are uncommon in gynecological malignancies, some tumors may directly invade into the surrounding pelvic bones causing severe pain. Bone pain can be difficult to treat and is not always relieved by opioids. However, it does respond particularly well to NSAIDs and radiotherapy, either in a single high dose fraction or in series of low dose fractions. In some cases of pathological fracture (or imminent fracture), surgery may be considered, although this is less common in advanced, progressive disease. Bisphosphonates are also increasingly being used for the treatment of bone pain, although the evidence for this comes from studies in patients with breast cancer and myeloma who have a relatively good prognosis.

Other Adjuvant Analgesics

Smooth muscle relaxants (anti-spasmodic) can be used to relieve colic and visceral distension pain. Within this group, Hyoscine butylbromide or Glycoperronium are generally preferred as they do not cross the blood brain barrier and are therefore not sedative. Morphine is ineffective at relieving muscular cramp and 'trigger point' pain; and nondrug treatments, such as massage, local heat and relaxation therapy should always be considered first line. If these are ineffective then skeletal muscle relaxants, such as baclofen, diazepam and tizanidine can be used. Topical lidocaine patches are typically used for post-herpetic neuralgia but can be used for localized superficial pain which is difficult to manage. Ketamine is an NMDA-receptor channel blocker which is occasionally used for severe neuropathic pain unresponsive to conventional treatment. However, it has several undesirable side effects and it is strictly limited to specialist use.

Invasive Techniques for Pain Control

These include nerve blocks, epidural/intrathecal administration of drugs, and neurodestructive procedures but all require the involvement of a specialist pain management team.

Alternative Therapies

Transcutaneous electrical nerve stimulation (TENS), local heat therapy (e.g. heat packs), acupuncture, aromatherapy, massage and hypnotherapy may be beneficial. Cognitive behavioral therapy and other psychological therapies may help patients adjust to living with chronic pain, and giving patients focused attention and time to talk can be therapeutic in itself. Immobilization of the painful area using a cervical collar, sling or surgical corset may be of help for some patient, and in some cases orthopedic surgery to pin or fuse an area may be a viable option.

Nausea and Vomiting (Table 42.1)

Nausea and vomiting has a major impact on quality of life, and alongside pain, is one of the most distressing symptoms for patients. It is helpful to ascertain whether the patient is suffering primarily from nausea, vomiting or if both symptoms are equally troubling. As with pain, it is beneficial to determine the likely causes in the individual, then tailor treatment accordingly. Nausea and vomiting may be secondary to biochemical disturbances (hypercalcemia, uremia), malignant GI involvement (tumor infiltration, obstruction, gastric stasis), raised intracranial pressure, chemotherapy, other drug effects; or may be of unclear/multifactorial origin. A multifaceted approach to management is therefore needed, simultaneously treating any underlying or preventable cause, while also providing symptom relief. Routes of

Table 42.1: Causes of nausea and vomiting, suitable medications and mechanism of action.

Cause of nausea and/or vomiting	Mechanism of action	Specific drugs and dosage
Gastric stasis Bowel dysmotility (functional)	Prokinetic	Metoclopramide 10 mg qds, higher doses suitable in CSCI Domperidone 10–20 mg tds
Gastritis	Prokinetic plus antacid	As above plus Ranitidine 150 mg bd or Omeprazole 20 mg od
Chemical/drug-induced Hypercalcemia Renal failure	Chemoreceptor trigger zone (Central)	Haloperidol 1–2.5 mg orally qds or 2.5 mg SC, or 2.5–10 mg in CSCI Prochlorperazine 3–6 mg buccal, 12.5 mg bd SC Ondansetron 4 mg qds (rarely used in palliative care) Metoclopramide also has a central effect
Mechanical bowel obstruction Raised intracranial pressure Motion sickness	Vomiting center (Central)	Cyclizine 50 mg tds, or 150 mg in CSCI Levomepromazine 6–12 mg orally or 6.25–12.5 mg SC, higher doses in CSCI Hyoscine butylbromide 20 mg qds, up to 120 mg in CSCI
Bowel spasm/colic Excess GI secretions	Vomiting center and antisecretory	Hyoscine butylbromide 20 mg qds, up to 120 mg in CSCI Octreotide 100 mcg SC, up to 250–500 mcg in CSCI
Unclear or multifactorial	Broadspectrum	Levomepromazine 6–12 mg orall or 6.25–12.5 mg SC, higher doses in CSCI

administration also need to be carefully considered as many patients with nausea have coexisting gastric stasis, resulting in poor absorption and bioavailability of oral medication.

Cyclizine, Haloperidol and Metoclopramide are most commonly prescribed in palliative care. However, antiemetics should not be prescribed at random, but according to their mechanism of action:

More than one agent with differing mechanisms of action may be required for effective symptom control. Centrally acting drugs are usually effective in treating biochemical and drug induced nausea, whilst prokinetics are particularly appropriate for cases of gastric stasis (providing there is no mechanical obstruction). Cyclizine has an antihistamine and anticholinergic effect and is a useful broad spectrum agent, whilst movement associated nausea also benefits from anticholinergic agents such as Hyoscine hydrobromide or butylbromide. The antiserotonergic agents, Ondansetron and Granisetron, are of particular value in chemotherapy associated emesis and their effects may be enhanced by coadministration of corticosteroids such as Dexamethasone. Anxiety or emotional distress will often exacerbate nausea so this must be addressed alongside conventional treatments.

Constipation (Table 42.2)

Constipation is a common cause of discomfort and distress in patients with gynecological malignancies. Although it is usually multifactorial, it is highly associated with the use of opioid analgesia; and is therefore predictable, and to some extent, preventable. All patients taking weak or strong opioids should be prescribed regular laxatives, and as the opioid dose increases, so too should the laxatives. Tricyclic antidepressants, often prescribed alongside opioids, are also associated with constipation so it is important to be proactive in preventing problems in these patients. Simple lifestyle measures should be used in tandem with pharmacological interventions, including maintaining mobility, encouraging adequate hydration (especially fruit juices) and adding bran/fiber to the diet. Local pain will inhibit bowel activity so ensure any anal fissures, hemorrhoids or perianal wounds are treated effectively. It is also important to ensure that the patient is comfortable and has adequate privacy when trying to open her bowels.

When assessing constipation, it is useful to ascertain what the normal bowel habit was prior to their illness. It is also important to ask specifically what the patient is experiencing, as this will help guide treatment—is it infrequent bowel motions? Hard stools that are difficult or painful to pass? Rectal pain and fullness; or perhaps just a feeling of general discomfort and bloating? Once this has been established, rational choices and combinations of laxatives can be commenced based on the different mechanisms of action of each drug:

Co-danthrusate and Co-danthramer were often used first line in palliative care as they combine stimulant and softening properties. However, Dantron is known to be carcinogenic in rodent studies, therefore is now only recommended for patients who are terminally ill. It is also contraindicated in patients with persistent anal leakage or incontinence due to the high risk of a Dantron skin burn. Consequently, Docusate sodium is becoming more popular as it too possess both softening and mild stimulant properties; however, the overall choice of laxative should be tailored to the individual. Suppositories or enemas may be particularly useful for patients with spinal cord

Table 42.2: Medication for constipation and mechanism of action.

Mechanism of action	Specific examples
Osmotic laxatives (Softeners)	• Lactulose syrup • Macrogols, e.g. Laxido, movicol • Magnesium hydroxide, e.g. Milk of magnesia • Magnesium sulfate, e.g. Epsom salts
Stimulant laxatives	• Senna • Bisacodyl • Dantron, e.g. Co-danthramer • Sodium picosulfate
Bulk-forming (Fiber)	• Isphaghula Husk, e.g. Fybogel, Regulan • Methylcellulose • Sterculia
Surface-wetting agents	• Docusate (also mild stimulant) • Poloxamer
Lubricants	• Liquid paraffin • Arachis oil • Mineral oils

compression, autonomic neuropathy or those who are having difficulty taking oral medications. If standard laxative treatment is ineffective, it is helpful to consider underlying causes, such as dehydration, hypercalcemia or partial obstruction. Methylnaltrexone is an opioid antagonist which may be used in terminally ill patients with opioid-induced constipation unresponsive to normal measures. However, it is expensive and needs to be given as a subcutaneous injection; and is contraindicated in known or suspected bowel obstruction.

Fecal Impaction

In cases of fecal impaction, rectal treatments (suppositories or enemas) are particularly beneficial and should be tailored according to the examination findings. If the rectum is full of hard stool, then a softening and lubricating agent should be used first line; if soft stool is present in the rectum, then a stimulant agent should be used primarily. Glycerol suppositories are softeners but may also stimulate local peristaltic action and are a good first line option for most patients. Arachis oil enemas (peanut/groundnut oil) are particularly effective for lubricating and softening hard impacted stool, but must be avoided in those with peanut allergies. Stimulant agents, such as Bisacodyl suppositories are useful for those patients who have not responded to Glycerol or who have severe impaction. To be effective, the Bisacodyl suppository needs to be in contact with the bowel mucosa so if this is not possible, a Docusate or phosphate enema may be more appropriate. If rectal measures are not acceptable to the patient, high dose oral macrogols (osmotic laxatives) can be used but this should be discussed with specialists. Rarely, manual evacuation of the impacted feces may be needed but this should also be discussed with specialists. In all cases, regular oral laxatives must be continued to prevent recurrence of the impaction.

Diarrhea

When diarrhea occurs in patients with advanced cancer, it is essential to exclude fecal impaction with overflow. A rectal examination is mandatory and a plain abdominal X-ray may be useful in looking for extensive constipation (or evidence of pseudomembranous colitis) depending on the clinical context. Other common causes of diarrhea in advanced cancer include tumor infiltration of the bowel wall, the effect of treatment, such as radiotherapy (radiation colitis) or antibiotic treatment, excessive laxative use and infection including *Clostridium difficile*. Patients should be encouraged to maintain adequate hydration, and once impaction has been excluded, laxatives should be temporarily stopped. Stool samples should be sent for microscopy and culture, especially if the patient has recently received antibiotics. For persistent noninfective diarrhea, regular Loperamide or Codeine (if not already taking opiates) can be used, whilst oral Metronidazole or oral Vancomycin will be required for *C. difficile* diarrhea.

Intestinal Obstruction

This is a recognized problem in patients with advanced ovarian cancer; they commonly have multiple sites of obstruction secondary to disseminated intra-abdominal disease. At each level the obstruction may be functional (due to bowel dysmotility) or mechanical; partial or complete; and transient or persistent. Management may be conservative or surgical depending on the degree and site of obstruction, the overall clinical situation and the patient wishes. Patients will typically complain of abdominal pain with persistent nausea and vomiting. Mechanical obstruction is associated with colicky pain, and abdominal distension is more likely with distal obstruction. There will be abnormal bowel habit but this may range from absolute constipation with absence of flatus, to liquid diarrhea secondary to impaction and overflow. In functional obstruction, bowel sounds may be absent whilst some mechanical obstructions cause hyperactive bowel sounds with borborygmi. Conservative treatment aims to reduce these symptoms, not the underlying obstruction; and it is preferable to try pharmacological management before considering a nasogastric tube. Patients should be made nil by mouth and given supplementary intravenous fluids to prevent dehydration, although regular mouth care is also needed to deal with the sensation of thirst. If patients are approaching the end of life, a more pragmatic approach is to allow small amounts of their favorite food and drinks, as tolerated. Prokinetic agents (including Metoclopramide and Domperidone) and laxatives should be stopped; and all essential medications changed to non-oral routes.

Regular antiemetics should be commenced (e.g. Cyclizine or Haloperidol, preferably as a CSCI) alongside appropriate analgesia, and Hyoscine hydrobromide or butylbromide should be added if there is colicky pain. In cases of persistent large volume vomiting, or in those who have not responded to these measures, it may be necessary to add Octreotide (or another somatostatin analogue) to reduce bowel secretions. If patients are passing flatus and have no colicky pain, prokinetics can be restarted but must be discontinued immediately if symptoms worsen.

Partial obstruction is particularly common in gynecological malignancy, and many patients have recurrent episodes which initially resolve after a few days of bowel rest. These patients can be advised to follow a light, low residue (low fiber) diet and Metoclopramide can be used, providing it does not cause colicky pain. However, as the obstruction progresses, the frequency and duration of these episode will increase until the obstruction becomes complete and irreversible. Surgical intervention may be appropriate to relieve mechanical obstruction and provide symptom alleviation, but can be associated with significant postoperative morbidity and mortality. It is best reserved for cases where a single site obstruction is suspected, and in patients with localized intra-abdominal disease with otherwise good nutritional and physical status. Self-expanding metal stents can be used for left-sided colorectal obstruction but they are also associated with complications including bleeding, perforation and incomplete stent expansion.

Anorexia

Anorexia is very common in advanced malignancy, and may be associated with significant weight loss and cachexia. In many cultures, eating is seen as a social activity and there may be considerable feelings of guilt or rejection if patients are not able to engage in family meals. Reassurance should be given, and it should be explained to patients and their families that in advanced disease, the body is often unable to process large amounts of food comfortably. Patients should be encouraged to eat small amounts of enjoyable food when wanted, and should not feel burdened or restricted by 'standard' meal times. A short trial of oral steroids may boost appetite and can be considered if appropriate. Dietary supplements can be prescribed and patients should, be encouraged to eat and drink full fat versions of foods, such as milk, ice cream and cheese. Antacid medications, such as Ranitidine or Omeprazole may also help reduce the discomfort of indigestion or acid reflux often associated with anorexia.

Dry Mouth/Oropharynx

A dry mouth is caused by reduced salivary gland action and occurs in over 80% of patients with advanced cancer. It can be exacerbated by many drugs, including opioids, antihistamines and antidepressants, and patients should be made aware of this. Saliva has many essential functions so a persistently dry mouth can cause significant discomfort and predispose patients to oral infections and dental decay. Speech may be difficult and dentures can become loose or uncomfortable causing significant embarrassment and frustration. Saliva is also essential for chewing and swallowing comfortably, and reduced oral lubrication negatively impacts on taste sensation leading to reduced appetite and reduced oral intake. Adequate hydration, regular mouth care and attention to oral hygiene is essential, as is the prompt diagnosis and treatment of glossitis, ulcers or oral *Candida* infection. Patients should be encouraged to drink small amounts regularly, and other useful treatment measures include chewing gum or sucking ice, acid sweets (like lemon drops) or pastilles. The proteolytic enzymes present in pineapple are particularly useful for those with a heavily coated tongue, and help improve comfort in many cases. For those with persistent oral dryness, artificial saliva preparations may provide relief although their benefit is short lasting and regular applications are needed. In moribund patients, the mouth should be moistened every 30 minutes with a small amount of water to preserve comfort.

Breathlessness

Breathlessness is one of the most common symptoms in advanced cancer, and is not limited to patients with intrathoracic malignancy. It may be defined as an unpleasant or uncomfortable awareness of the need to breathe, or a sensation of difficulty in achieving a 'proper' breath. It is often very frightening for the patient, and this needs to be acknowledged. A systematic approach using pharmacological and nonpharmacological treatment is important, and reversible causes should be treated; including infection, pulmonary edema, pleural effusions, pulmonary emboli and severe ascites. If suitable, the patient should be encouraged to remain physically active with an exercise program tailored to their abilities, and breathing retraining may be possible alongside education about the causes of breathlessness. Simple measures are often helpful and include making the patient sit upright, encouraging them to relax their shoulders downwards, loosening clothes, cooling measures and increasing air movement around the face (through the use of a fan or open window). During acute exacerbations, it is essential that someone stays with the patient, reassuring them and providing explanation. If the patient is hypoxic, oxygen replacement may be helpful, although some patients find the mask claustrophobic. If there is thick or purulent sputum which is difficult to expectorate, then inhaled saline (nebulized) may be helpful, and if appropriate, antibiotics may be considered. Bronchodilators, such as Salbutamol or Ipratropium can also be beneficial, especially if there is evidence of wheeze.

For longer term management, or in cases unresponsive to simple measures, low dose opioids may be considered (if opiate naïve, start at 2.5 mg oral morphine as required, and titrate up slowly). Oral or subcutaneous low dose benzodiazepines can also be helpful, especially if patients are particularly tense or anxious (Diazepam 1–2 mg bd orally, or Midazolam 2.5 mg SC as needed).

Ascites

Ascites is the accumulation of fluid in the peritoneal cavity and is commonly seen with advanced ovarian, endometrial and cervical cancer. Although not overtly painful, the accumulation of fluid does cause discomfort and may be associated with dyspnea, indigestion, nausea, vomiting and poor mobility. In severe cases, there may even be compression or obstruction of the ureters. Treatment of the underlying cause, such as palliative chemotherapy or radiotherapy, may help but usually these alternatives have already been exhausted. The simplest and most commonly used treatment is regular paracentesis, or the insertion of an ascitic drain to remove the excess fluid. This gives good symptomatic relief for the vast majority of patients. If there has been extensive surgery with a risk of adhesions or if the fluid is loculated, an ultrasound-guided procedure is recommended. Care should be taken to avoid large fluid shifts, particularly in elderly or frail patients, as the sudden depletion in intravascular volume may precipitate renal failure, severe hyponatremia and cardiovascular collapse. Slow drainage over several days should therefore be aimed for, with monitoring of patient observations and comfort. Spironolactone (a potassium sparing diuretic) may slow down the reaccumulation of ascites and is worth considering in certain cases, however, the renal function should be monitored to minimize the risk of hyperkalemia. Although the albumin level in patients with severe ascites is usually low, intravenous albumin replacement is not routinely indicated as the underlying pathophysiology is not reversible and there is no evidence that albumin replacement improves outcomes.

Obstructive Uropathy

The ureter is particularly susceptible to obstruction in gynecological malignancies due to its anatomical course through the pelvis and close proximity to the uterus. However, ureteric obstruction may pose a management dilemma depending on the overall clinical context. Percutaneous nephrostomy can easily be performed to decompress the kidney, preserving its function and prolonging the patient's life. However, obstructive uropathy may also be a terminal event, enabling the patient to gradually drift into unconsciousness and death. It is therefore important to determine whether relieving the obstruction and prolonging the patient's life is indeed in her best interests. For example, if obstructive renal failure is the presenting symptom in an otherwise asymptomatic patient with cervical cancer (denoting stage 3b disease), then a nephrostomy and palliative radiotherapy may be of value in giving her time to come to terms with the diagnosis and sort out her affairs. Conversely, if a patient develops obstructive uropathy secondary to progressive, recurrent disease, having previously exhausted all other treatment options, then an urgent nephrostomy may not be an appropriate intervention at that time. Honest, open discussion and informed consent is crucial in both of these examples but in reality, it may be very difficult when the patient is acutely unwell with an urgent need for treatment. It may therefore be wise to pre-empt this scenario and discuss the patient's wishes in advance. It is also essential to remember that doses of many drugs, including morphine, will need to be reduced to prevent accumulation and toxicity in patients with renal impairment. In patients with severe or ongoing renal impairment, Fentanyl is preferable to Morphine, although expert advice should be sought regarding dose titration and route of administration.

Hypercalcemia

Hypercalcemia is not particularly common in gynecological cancers but may be associated with clear cell and small cell ovarian carcinomas, or secondary to bony metastases. It can cause of a variety of nonspecific symptoms including lethargy, weakness, confusion, drowsiness, psychiatric disturbances, nausea, vomiting and constipation. The treatment of choice for those with severe or symptomatic hypercalcemia (typically levels >3.0 mmol/L) is aggressive intravenous rehydration with sodium chloride 0.9% followed by intravenous bisphosphonates. Pamidronate is most commonly used and is well tolerated, although repeated doses may be necessary. More expensive third generation bisphosphonates, such as Zolendronate are more potent so need to be given less frequently, and may be appropriate in some cases. Thiazide diuretics should be stopped but Furosemide can be given if there is significant underlying heart failure. Any Vitamin D/calcium compounds should also be discontinued. Definitive treatment involves removing the underlying cause, which is usually not an option in advanced disease. In persistent or refractory hypercalcemia, parenteral Calcitonin may be used, however it is unlikely to be effective if bisphosphonates have already failed. Furthermore, resistant hypercalcemia is a poor prognostic sign, indicating a short-life expectancy, so in these cases aggressive treatment may not be in the patients' best interests.

Fistulae

Enterocutaneous or enterovaginal fistulae may occur with advanced malignancy resulting in severe ulceration and irritation of the skin surrounding the fistula. Surgical diversion is the treatment best option, although this may not always be possible or appropriate. Conservative measures aim to reduce the production of the proteolytic enteral secretions using Somatostatin or Octreotide, and protect surrounding skin through the use of stoma bags and barrier creams, such as 1% silver sulphadiazine. With rectovaginal fistulae, the preferred treatment is an end colostomy or a loop colostomy but if neither are possible, barrier creams and attention to hygiene are essential. Fistulae are often associated with large amounts of necrotic tumor and even if surgical diversion has been possible, large amount of foul smelling discharge may persist. Regular douching with Betadine or Saline combined with oral and/or topical Metronidazole may help reduce the smell of anaerobic organisms. Patients may require pre-emptive pain relief prior to this and should be given appropriate psychological support at all times.

Fungating and Malodorous Wounds

Fungating or malodorous wounds occur when malignant tissue erodes through epithelial layers (including the skin) and the wound is unable to heal. In gynecological malignancies, the wounds are often deep and inaccessible, and can be very difficult to manage. They typically affect areas associated with sexual functioning or excretion and this may cause shame, disgust and fear amongst patients. It is therefore important to remember the psychosocial impact on the patient and her family. The basic management of these wounds includes regular thorough irrigation and desloughing. The dressings should be changed several times daily and expert advice sought regarding the dressing type used. Short-acting opiates may be needed to allow irrigation and dressing changes since it is often excruciatingly painful for the patient. Any infection should be treated promptly and as with fistulae, even in the absence of overt infection, topical or oral Metronidazole may be used to reduce the offensive odor associated with anaerobic colonization of the wound. Depending on the situation, local radiotherapy may be considered with the aim of slowing disease progression and reducing bleeding or exudate formation. However, radiation necrosis may worsen the problem so this should be carefully considered in conjunction with specialists.

Lymphoedema

This is the accumulation of lymphatic fluid in the subcutaneous tissues and is seen in up to 40% of patients undergoing radical hysterectomy and radiotherapy for cervical cancer. It most commonly affects the limbs and is usually a result of compression or damage to the lymphatic system through surgery, radiotherapy, postoperative infection or direct tumor involvement. In the initial stages, the swelling is soft and pitting, and often painless. However, with time, there is progressive protein deposition and chronic inflammation leading to interstitial fibrosis of the subcutaneous tissues. Subsequently, the swelling becomes tense and less pitting, and is associated with hyperkeratosis and lymphorrhea. At this stage, patients will often complain of severe discomfort and a sensation of tightness or heaviness along with reduced mobility. The impact of lymphoedema on body image, sexual relationships and social functioning should not be forgotten, so physical treatments should be complemented by appropriate psychological support.

In advanced cancer, lymphoedema cannot be cured and early treatment is essential to maintain limb comfort and function; and minimize deterioration. Preventative advice is paramount and daily skin care is required to improve and maintain the skin integrity, thereby reducing the risk of infection. The importance of regular light exercise and limb movement should be stressed, and women encouraged to elevate the affected limb when at rest. Swelling may be reduced by external compression bandaging, massage, manual lymphatic drainage or the use of intermittent positive pressure boots for 1–2 hours a day, although obviously the appropriateness of this depends on the overall clinical context. In the rapidly deteriorating patient, low compression garments alone may be the most realistic option for providing comfort. If there is coexisting fluid retention secondary to cardiac or venous insufficiency, diuretics can be considered but may make little difference.

Terminal Care

Continued involvement of the medical team is essential in the care of the dying patient, and time should be taken to identify the key wishes of the patient and their family. It is important that patients do not feel abandoned and that there is ongoing re-evaluation of problems as they arise. It is essential to continue supporting the family at this emotionally distressing time and explanations should be given around what to expect as the patient becomes weaker. Patients are likely to become increasingly drowsy with reduced oral intake, and may spend large parts of the day sleeping. It is helpful to address expectations around eating and drinking, explaining that artificial hydration and nutrition is not necessarily helpful to the dying patient and may in fact increase patient discomfort. The breathing may become labored, and excess respiratory secretions (death rattle) are often very distressing for the family, although less so for the patient themselves. Secretions can be reduced with anticholinergics, such as subcutaneous Hyoscine, however, they must be administered promptly and regularly if they are to work effectively. Agitation and confusion are common, and may have a variety of causes including hypoxia, hypotension or biochemical abnormalities. If the patient is distressed then sedation is appropriate via the subcutaneous or rectal route with Haloperidol or Benzodiazepines. If these are unsuccessful, Levomepromazine is a useful alternative which has both antiemetic and anxiolytic/sedative effects. It is important to remember agitation may be secondary to urinary retention, so it may be helpful to consider an indwelling catheter in patients approaching the end of life. Intractable breathlessness may be managed by low dose opioids and benzodiazepines, which can be given orally, rectally or parenterally depending on availability and appropriateness. Mouth care and appropriate repositioning need to be performed frequently, and all focus should move towards ensuring patient's comfort, so only interventions which improve symptoms should be continued. Nonessential treatments should be discontinued and the route of administration of relevant drugs changed as the patient becomes less able to tolerate oral medications. It is common for patients to be commenced on a portable syringe driver with a CSCI as this improves the steady state dosing of medications, limiting the likelihood of breakthrough pain. Additional doses of medication should still be given as needed, particularly prior to interventions that are necessary but may cause pain, such as dressing changes. Continued reassurance should be given, and the patient and family encouraged to report new or worsening symptoms promptly so that treatment can be modified as needed.

SUMMARY

Palliative care needs are common in patients with advanced gynecological cancer. Common problems include pain, nausea and vomiting, constipation, dry mouth, renal impairment and psychological suffering. Palliative care should not be reserved only for dying patients as distressing symptoms may be present at any stage of the disease process. Symptoms should be assessed and managed promptly to provide the best quality of life possible for patients. Relevant anticipatory drugs should be prescribed to avoid delays in administration. Pain is still the most feared symptom for many patients and it is essential that analgesia is given regularly; the dose and frequency should be tailored to the particular drug being used. Skilled clear communication is essential and holistic assessment is the key to identifying the most important and relevant problems for each individual patient.

Index

Page numbers followed by b refer to box, f refer to figure, fc refer to flowchart, and t refer to table

A

Abdomen, part of 119
Abdominal entry, site of 275f
Abdominal hysterectomy, types of 261
Abdominal pain
    causes of 64t
    types of 64t
Abdomino-pelvic
    examination 325
    masses 21b
    ultrasound 325
Abortion 105, 106t, 126, 133
    complications of 105
    related morbidities 105
    septic 121
    unsafe 105
Abscess 21
    tubo-ovarian 117, 245, 245f
Acanthosis nigricans 324
Acetaminophen 428
Aciclovir 134, 135
Acid-burn 21
Acid-fast bacilli 287
Acne 57, 58, 322
    microcomedonal 46
Acquired immunodeficiency
        syndrome 126, 144
Actinomycin D 389
Acute pelvic inflammatory disease,
        pathology of 118
Adenocarcinoma 365, 377, 401
    endometriod 394
    in situ 377
Adenoma 38
    pituitary 315
Adenomyoma 115, 235f, 236f
Adenomyosis 84, 85, 109, 114, 115, 236
    focal 239
    treatment of 116
Adenosarcoma 397
Adenosine deaminase 288
Adnexa 26, 234f, 261
Adnexal mass 287f
    transvaginal scan of 247f

Adnexal torsion 273
Adrenal hyperplasia
    congenital 46, 47, 54, 308, 313, 332,
        333, 335, 336
    lipoid 329
Adrenarche
    isolated premature 46
    precocious 59
    premature 46
Adrenocorticotropic hormone 61, 62
    testing 62
Adriamycin 389
Agenesis 8
Alcohol 23
Alkaline
    hematin technique 84
    pH 35
Allergic dermatitis 151
Allergic vulvitis 34
    treatment 34
Allergy 22, 70
Alopecia 58
    androgenic 313
Alprazolam 63
Alzheimer's disease 354
Ambiguous genitalia, etiology of 32
Ambo-sexual hair 323
Amenorrhea 56, 93, 94, 99, 104, 318, 416
    causes of 56
    diagnosis 56
    evaluation 56
    hypo-oestrogenic 312
    hypothalamic 97, 312
    management goals 58
    post-pill 98
    primary 94
        causes 94
    severe hypothalamic 49
    treatment of 99
American Association of Gynecologic
        Laparoscopists 273
American Fertility Society Classification
        of Endometriosis, modified 112f
American Society for Colposcopy and
        Cervical Pathology 71t

Amoxicillin 128, 138, 220
Ampicillin 122, 220
Anaerobes 121
Anal disease 70
Anal intercourse 129
Anal neuralgias 281
Anal sphincter 207f
    external 207f
Analgesia 427
    nonopioid 427
    opioid 428
    simple 427
Analgesic 111
    adjuvant 429
    drugs 427
Anastrozole 113
Ancillary instruments 301
Androgen 62, 189
    insensitivity 51, 333
        complete 32
        syndrome 50, 57, 96
    maternal 333
    producing
        adrenal tumors 69
        tissue, destruction of 317
    receptivity, peripheral 31
    receptor antagonists 326
    secreting
        adrenal 313
        suppression of 326
    stimulate hair follicles 323
Androstenedione 31, 58, 185
Anechoic cyst 40
Anemia 55b, 107, 268
    aplastic 53
    mild 55
    severe 89
        bleeding 55
Angiokeratoma 152
Ano-genital infection,
uncomplicated 130
Anorectal diseases 280
Anorectal disorders 281
Anorexia 52, 432
    nervosa 49, 308, 323

Anorgasmia 103
Anovaginal fistula 213f
Anovulation 58t, 59, 319
   chronic 318, 322
   diagnosis of 316fc
   management of 316fc
   normogonadotropic 313, 315
Anovulatory cycles 59
Anteflexion 290
Antepartum 145
Anterior vaginal wall 193, 198, 199, 200, 211f
   defects, repair of 202
   descent of 200
   prolapse 198
Anti-adhesion agents 114
Antiandrogens 326
Antibiotic 296
   oral 131
Antibody detection 127
Anticancer therapy, systemic 421, 422
Antidepressants 217, 430
Antidopaminergics 217
Antiepileptic drugs 60, 168
Antifibrinolytic agent 89
Antifungals
   agents, oral 132
   endoanal application of 281
   properties 326
Antigen detection 127
Antihypertensive 217
   therapy 336
Anti-Müllerian hormone 43, 60, 61, 329, 344
Antiprogesterones 156
Antiretroviral treatment 179
Antiviral 134, 135
   drugs, oral 134
   therapy, suppressive 134
   treatment 135
Anus 402
Anxiety 62, 188
Aphthous ulcers 151
   oral 280
Aplasia 7, 8
Apomorphine 189
Appendicitis 66, 120
Arcuate uterus 8, 234, 235f
Arcus tendineus levator ani 197
Aromatase inhibitor 68, 113, 316
Arrhenoblastoma 159
Arteriovenous malformation 238f, 240
Artery forceps points towards ureter 267f
Arthritis 127
   gonococcal 123
   sexually acquired reactive 123
Ascites 287f, 433
Ascitic fluid
   analysis of 288
   tapping of 288
Asherman's syndrome 22, 56, 98, 99, 236, 240, 277, 413

Ashknazic Jewish and Eskimo
   population 332
Aspiration 389
Assisted reproductive technology 114, 321
Asymptomatic gallstones, management
   of 280
Asymptomatic mobile retroversion 292
Asynchrony 94
Atresia 7
Autoimmune disease 313
Automated cytological screening 365
Autonomic nervous system 206, 207
Axillary hair development 309
Ayer's spatula 224, 224f
   uses 224
Azithromycin 122, 128, 130, 138, 141
Azole group antifungals 132

B

Babcock's forceps 228, 228f
Backache 129
   low 130
Bacteria, gram-negative facultative 121
Baden-Walker halfway system 194f
Baldy-Webster operation 293
Ballooned-out cervical canal 376f
Barbiturates 168
Barrier methods 165
Bartholin's abscesses 130
Bartholin's cysts 21, 151
Bartholin's gland 6, 407
   carcinoma 407
Bartholinitis 129
Basal body temperature 164, 339
   method 164
Basal cell
   abnormal immature 373
   carcinoma 401, 407
   papilloma 152
Basal serum hormone levels,
   evaluation of 61
Basson model of female sexuality 182f
Beads-on-a-string sign 245
Behavioral therapy 211
Behcet's disease 151
Belly button surgery 273
Benign ovarian cyst, laparoscopic
   appearance of 161f
Benzathine penicillin 138
Benzodiazepines 435
Beta adrenergics 80
Betamethasone 326
Bevacizumab 424
Bicornis bicollis 234
Bicornuate uterus 7, 8, 8f, 10, 11, 65,
   71, 234, 235f
Bilateral inguinofemoral node
   dissection 408f

Biliary tract
   disease 280
   risk of 354
Billings method 164
Bioidentical hormone therapy 355
Biopsy 140, 287
Bisphosphonates 433
Bladder 199, 206, 207f, 214f
   buttressing stitches 270, 271f
   catheterization, prolonged 214
   dome of 283f
   injuries 282
   muscle 207
   neurogenic 208
   syndrome 68
   transitional cell carcinoma of 408f
Blastocyst stage 341
Blastopores 131
Bleeding 55b
   intermenstrual 20, 393
   mild 55
   postmenopausal 20, 396
Bleomycin 380, 389
Blind uterine horn 65
Bloating, abdominal 62
Blood
   and blood products, transfusion of 145
   cyclical discharge of 13
   donors 146
   karyotyping, peripheral 95
   tests 50
Bloomer's shelf 26
B-mode trasvaginal scan 238f
Body mass index 23, 103, 347
Body odor 46
Bone
   density 170
   development of 310
   marrow effects 422
   mineral density 352
   pain 429
Bonney's and Marshall tests 209
Bowel
   disease, inflammatory 274, 279, 280, 308
   dysmotility 430, 431
   injuries 268, 283
   problems 379
   toxicity 423
Brachytherapy 421, 423
   external beam 380
   gynecological 421
   interstitial 425
Brain 416
   metastases 417f
Brainstem 428
Breast 396
   abscess, lactational 220
   budding 43
   cancer 219, 219t, 352, 353t

  during pregnancy, treatment of 220
  inflammatory 220
  pregnancy associated 219
 carcinoma 23
 development 43, 309
  premature 61
 diseases 216, 217
  common 216, 218
 drain, lymphatic of 216
 endpoints study 356
 engorgement 326
 examination 45, 387
 functioning of 216
 lesions 217t
 lump 217, 218
 milk 145
 ovarian cancer syndrome 385
  hereditary 384
 pain 216
 problems 220
 related symptoms 216
 tenderness 62
Breastfeeding 145
Breathlessness 432
Brenner's tumor 158, 247, 368, 387
Broad ligament 264f, 267
 medial leaf of 267f
Bromocriptine 217, 315
 side effects of 315
Bromoergocryptine 98
Bronchospasm 355
Bulky inhomogenous cervix 242f
Butylbromide 432

C

Cabergoline 315
Cachexia 20
Café-au-lait spots 37
Calcium
 antagonists 80
 channel blockade 429
Calendar method 164
Cancer 191, 352, 353
 colorectal 354
 vulval 425
Candida
 albicans 70, 131
 glabrata 131
 infection 432
 krusei 131
 parapsilosis 131
 tropicalis 131
Candidiasis
 investigation 34
 predisposing factors 34
 treatment 34
Cannula 300f
Canon-ball lesion 416

Carbamazepine 168
Carbohydrate metabolism 167
Carbon dioxide 301
 insufflation 276f
 laser ablation 375
Carboplatin 389
 regimes 389
Carcinoembryonic antigen 69
Carcinoma
 adenosquamous 374, 377, 394
 cervix 242f, 373f, 401
 endometrium 401
 in situ 373, 375
 microinvasive 377
 verrucous 407
Carcinomatosis, intra-abdominal 385
Cardinal ligament 198
 complex 266f
Cardiorespiratory disease, severe 274
Cardiovascular disease 343, 347, 352
 history of 351
 severe 298
 treatment 347
Cardiovascular disorders 22
Cardiovascular system 167
Cefotaxime 122
Cefotetan 122
Cefoxitin 122
Ceftizoxime 122
Ceftriaxone 122, 138, 141
Celiac disease 56
Cell
 hyperplasia 319
 non-proliferating 422
Cellular atypia, prominent 395
Central nervous system 37, 49, 419
 disorders 37
 symptoms 145
 tumors 37
Cerebral metastases 419
Cerebrospinal fluid 145
Cerebrovascular events 348
Cervarix 366
Cervical
 canal 166
 cancer 241, 364, 364f, 367, 374, 374f, 381, 423
  etiology of 374
  invasive 377
  natural history of 375f
  treatment of 261
 cap 166
 carcinoma 374
  clinical staging of 378f
 cone biopsy 376f
 cytology 70, 71t
 dilators 223
 disease, malignant 27
 erosion 152
 fibroids 154, 241

 intraepithelial neoplasia 126, 364, 373, 375
  concept of 373
 leiomyoma 237f, 242f
 mucus method 164
 obstruction 79
 polyps 152, 153f
 precancer 141
 rim 294
 smear 26f, 364
 stenosis 81
 stump carcinoma 380
 tear 105
Cervicitis 129
Cervicography 367
Cervicopexy, abdominal 272
Cervix 14, 87, 200, 261, 266f, 285, 286, 290
 absent 51
 after treatment, appearance of 417f
 benign lesions of 152
 cancer of 367
 carcinoma of 23, 380
 congenital elongation of 200
 diseases of 241
 epithelium of 374
 examination of 30
 invasive
  cancer of 372, 374f
  carcinoma of 377
 normal appearance of 418f
 preinvasive lesions of 373
 supravaginal portion of 198
 tuberculosis of 286
 unhealthy 363f
 uteri 372
 visualization of 25
Cesarean section 135
Chancre 135
Chancroid 139
 clinical features 139
 general advice 139
 investigations 139
 organism 139
 regimens to treat 139
 treatment 139
Chemical vaginitis 105
Chemotherapy 383, 417, 418, 419, 422, 424, 429
 neoadjuvant 390
 place of 389
 selective preventive 414, 415
 side effects of 419
Childbirth 107, 190, 212
Childhood cancer survivors 72
 chemotherapy 72
 radiation 72
Chlamydia 121-123, 129, 189
 clinical features 127
 deoxyribonucleic acid of 127
 infection 127

serology 140
trachomatis 35, 66, 67, 117, 118, 121, 127, 139
  diagnosis of 127
Chlamydial infection 126, 127
  clinical features 127
  investigations 127
  organism 127
  pathology 127
  route of spread 127
  treatment 128
Chocolate cyst 110, 111f
Cholecalciferol 349
Cholecystitis 352
Cholesterol 147
Choriocarcinoma 69, 248, 387, 411, 414, 414t, 415, 416t, 417, 417f, 418b
  gestational 411
  management of 417
  prophylaxis against 414
  resistant 419f
Chromotubation 299f
Chronic pelvic inflammatory disease 22, 123
  pathology of 118
Chronic pelvic pain 66-68
  causes of 66
Ciprofloxacin 130
Circadian rhythm, establishment of 308
Cisplatinum 389
Clamping cornual structures 270f
Clear cell 394
  tumor 158, 247
Climacteric symptoms 21
Clindamycin 122, 128
Clitorodectomy 103
Cloacal membrane 5f
Clomiphene citrate 315, 316, 321, 340
Clostridium difficile 431
Clotrimazole 132
Coagulation disorders 94
Cognitive-behavioral therapy 68
Cogwheel sign 245
Coital function, preservation of 379
Coitus
  interruptus 164
  triggers 126
Cold-knife conization 376
Colitis 279
  ulcerative 279
Color flow mapping 241f, 248
Colorectal syndrome, hereditary nonpolyposis 384
Colpectomy 203
Colpocleisis 203, 272
Colpoperineorrhaphy, posterior 269, 271
Colpopexy 203
Colporrhaphy
  anterior 202, 268, 270
  posterior 202
Colposcopy 190

Combined antiretroviral therapy 147
Complex adnexal mass 247f
  transvaginal scan of 245f
Condom 165
  female 166
  male 165
Condyloma
  accuminatum 281
  acuminata 35, 141, 152
Condylomata lata 136, 152
Confirmatory test 145
Congestion, hemorrhage of 160f
Conjunctivitis 127
Constipation 430
Contraception 162, 179
  after molar pregnancy 413
  efficacy of 162
  postabortal 171
Contraceptive
  agents, classification of 163
  failure 163
  implants 170
  non-oral estrogen-progestin 113
  precautions 337
  steroids 374
Contralateral superior vesical pedicle 283f
Core needle biopsy 218
Cornual structure 263f
Corpus luteal cyst 157
Corpus luteum 233f, 243
  cyst 243, 244f
Cortical tumors, adrenal 159
Corticosteroids 281, 324, 429
Cosmetic genital surgery, female 73
Co-trimoxazole 141
C-reactive protein 121
Crede's method 294
Creighton Model Fertility Care System 164
Crohn's disease 56, 151, 279
Cryosurgery 375
Cryptomenorrhea 9, 332
Cryptorchidism 335, 336
Cu T 380 A, insertion technique 173f
Cul-de-sac 200, 233, 241f, 245
Cusco's speculum 24, 25, 26f
  insertion of 25f
Cusco's vaginal speculum 221, 221f
  advantages 222
  disadvantage 222
  uses 222
Cushing's disease 56, 58, 62
Cushing's syndrome 49, 58, 60, 325
Cyclophosphamide 389
Cyclosporine 323
Cyproterone acetate 38, 61, 326
Cysts 40
  benign 157
  endometriotic 239
  functional 242, 243
  inclusion 152

mesonephric 151
multilocular endometriotic 245f
multiloculated 247f, 413f
papillary serous 158f
paraovarian 245
paratubal 245
pathological 157
peritoneal inclusion 245
physiological 157
small 244f
tubo-ovarian 119
Cystadenocarcinoma
  mucinous 390f
  serous 246
Cystadenoma
  endometrioid 158
  mucinous 158
  serous 158, 246f
Cystic teratomas, mature 247
Cystitis 129
  interstitial 68
Cystocele 201, 268
  repair 271f
Cystoscopy 210
Cytological atypia, absence of 394
Cytology 370
Cytotrophoblast 415

D

Danazol 65, 90, 217, 324
Danish Osteoporosis Prevention Study 348
Dantron 430
Deep vein thrombosis 268, 281
  risk of 351
Dehydration 268
Dehydroepiandrosterone 31, 54, 61
  sulfate 44, 185
Dementia 343, 354
Dense adhesions, laparoscopic appearance of 299f
Deoxycorticosterone 333
Deoxyribonucleic acid 134
  detection of 127
  screening 366
Depo-provera 56
Depot medroxyprogesterone 179
Depression 21, 62, 188
Dermatoses 151
Dermoid 158
  cyst 248f
  tumor 247f
Desire disorders 183
Desmopressin acetate 55
Dexamethasone 326
Dextrose water 91
Diabetes 23, 179, 188, 209, 354
  gestational 104
  mellitus 22, 131, 268, 308, 321
    non-insulin dependent 103, 321

Index

Diaper dermatitis 33
   candidiasis 33
   management 33
Diaphragm 165f
Diarrhea 423, 431
Diazepam 433
Diazoxide 323
Diclofenac 428
Dienogest 113
Dietary plus supplements 349
Dihydroepiandrostenedione 186
Dihydrotestosterone, metabolite 324
Dimethyl biguanide 321
Distorsions, architectural 217
Distress, psychological 426
Dominant follicle 233f
Domperidone 431
Donovania granulomatis 140
Dopamine 315
Doxorubicin 389
Doxycycline 122, 128, 138, 141
Doyen's retractor 227, 227f
Drug therapy 211
Dry mouth 432
Dry perianal skin 281
Ducrey's bacillus 139
Duct ectasia 217, 219
Dymenorrhea 93
Dysfunctional uterine bleeding 54, 54t
Dysgenesis 8
Dysgenetic male
pseudohermaphroditism 331
Dysgerminoma 69, 247, 331
Dyslipidemias 188
Dysmenorrhea 63, 67, 77, 79, 110, 113
   classification 78
   degree of 77
   early menarche 77
   etiology of 78
   examination 79
   heavy menstrual flow 77
   incidence 77
   management of 79, 79fc, 82fc
   membranous 78, 81
   primary 63, 64, 78
   risk factors for 77
   secondary 63, 65, 78, 81
   severity of 79t
   treatment of 67t
   types of 77, 78
Dyspareunia 67, 110, 113, 129, 130, 204, 291, 334
   presence of 22
Dysplasia 373
   mild 71
   moderate 71
   severe 71
Dysuria 280

E

Eating disorders 71
   menstruation 72
   prognosis 71
   sexuality 72
Econazole 132
Ectropion 152
Egg factor, investigation of 339
Ejaculatory ducts 329
Electric vacuum aspirator 224
Electronic pneumo-apparatus 300
Embryo 4f
   caudal half of 3f
Embryonal cell 156
   carcinoma 69
Embryonic period fetus 5
Emergency contraception 171
   mechanism of action 171
   methods 171
Emergency obstetric care 107
Endocervical
   cells, significance of 365
   crypts 377
   discharge 127
Endocrine 324
   causes 93, 94
   disorder, common 318
   gland disorders 56
   theory 78
Endocrinology 345
Endodermal sinus tumor 69, 387
Endometrial
   ablation 90
   aspirate 287
   biopsy 340, 370, 397
      curette 225, 225f
   cancer 59, 104, 369, 384, 396, 398, 399, 424
      types of 394
   carcinoma 350
   cavity 232f, 235f, 238f
   cycle 15
   events 17
   fluid 240
   growth 16f
   hyperplasia 104, 238f, 240, 353, 393, 394
   outline, irregular 238f
   pathology 94
   polyp 84, 238f, 239f, 240
   sampling 87
   stromal 394
      neoplasms 394
      sarcoma 397
   tissue 90
   tumor 240
Endometrioma 26, 110, 111f
Endometriosis 53, 65, 67, 81, 109, 111, 111b, 114, 152, 188, 245, 267, 291, 293, 298
   etiology of 109
   implantation 23
   prevalence of 109
   severe 299f
   staging of 111t
   symptoms of 100t
   therapy for 111b
   treatment of 65, 298
Endometritis 117, 238f, 240
Endometrium 94, 285, 356
   abnormal protrusion of 85
   benign tumors 236
   carcinoma of 23, 397
   diseases of 236
   hyperplasia of 394
   malignant tumor 236
   secretory 16
   thickened 238f
   transcervical resection of 90
   triple layered 231f
   tuberculosis of 286
Endopelvic fascia 206
Endosalpingitis 118
Endoscopic surgical methods 155
Endoscopy 273
Energy gamma rays 421
Enlarged uterus 414
   sagittal magnetic resonance image of 115f
   transvaginal sonogram of 115f
Enteritis, infective 279
Enterocele 201
   repair 202
Enzyme linked immunosorbent assay 127, 145
Epilepsy 72
Episiotomy scissor 227, 227f
Epithelial ovarian tumors, classification of 386b
Epithelial tumors
   benign 158
   common 157
Epithelium
   celomic 3
   squamous 128
   surface 385
Equine estrogen
   conjugated 88, 350
   oral 55
Erectile dysfunction 189
Ergocalciferol 349
Erythema 220
Erythromycin 128, 138, 141
   sterarte 128
Escherichia coli 34, 118
Estradiol 61, 69, 316, 355
   valerate 350
Estrogen 62, 104, 350
   action of 351
   conjugated 11
   intravenous conjugated 55
   only hormone therapy 350

progestogen combination 156
replacement
    study 348
    therapy 186
synthesis 28
therapy 88
types of 352
Estrogenization, lack of 29
Estrone 104, 355
Ethamsylate 89
Etoposide 389
Excessive androgen production,
    causes of 32
Excision 103
Exosalpingitis 118
Extended Manchester operation 269
External cephalic version 149
External genitalia 5, 6f
    development of 6
    examination of 45
    female 331
    feminization of 6f
    inspection of 24
    male 329
Eyes 355

F

Facial tissue, perirectal 271
Fallopian tube 14, 118, 233, 269, 285
    development of 5
    exterior of 118
    interior of 118
    investigation of 340
    normal 233
Falope ring 176, 177f
Famciclovir 134
Family planning clinics 369
Fascia, pubocervical 201f
Fatigue 62
Febrile illness 145
Fecal fistulae 213, 215
Fecal impaction 431
Fecal incontinence 206, 212
    treatment of 212
Fecal seepage 212
Female genital tract 125, 372
    defense mechanism of 125, 125b
    development of 3
    embryology of 3
    uterus 125
    vagina 125
    vaginal flora 125
    vulva 125
Female genitalia, normal 331
Female pelvis, normal 232, 232f
Female sterilization 175
    health benefits of 178
Feminizing functional
    mesenchymomas 158

Fentanyl 433
Ferriman and Gallwey scoring system 325f
Fertility
    control 104
    function 30
    preservation 390
    problems 274
    rate, adolescent 101
    sparing
        surgery 381, 383
        treatment 399
Fertilizable oocyte 93
Fertilization 4, 13
Fetal
    anomalies 126
    blood sampling 135
    hydrops 136
    pituitary luteinizing hormone 329
    ultrasound, routine 149
Fetus, sexual differentiation of 328
Fever
    low grade 129, 280
    postoperative 267
Fiber 431
Fibroadenoma 218
Fibrocystic
    disease 218
    disorder 218
Fibroid 84, 85, 154, 298, 299f, 395
    degenerated 121
    microscopic appearance of 154f
    multiple 22, 153f
    submucous 154, 154f
Fibromas 247
Fibrosis, cystic 51, 56, 338
FIGO staging 399t
Filshie clip 177f
Fimbriectomy 176
Finasteride inhibits 327
Fine needle aspiration cytology 218
Finger nails 132
Fistula 433
    enterocutaneous 433
    enterovaginal 433
    formation 213
    ureterovaginal 209, 213, 213f, 215
Fitz-Hugh-Curtis syndrome 23, 120, 123, 127
Fluconazole 132
Fluctuant lump 220
Fluid
    outlining normal endometrial
cavity 241f
    retention 44
    small amount of 236f
Fluorouracil 380
Fluoxetin 63
Flutamide 326, 327
Foley's bulb in situ 241f
Foley's catheter 225, 225f
Folinic acid 419f

Follicle
    different types of 14f
    growth of 14f, 15f
    multiple enlarged 244f
    preantral 14
    primordial 13
    stages of 14f
    stimulating hormone 14, 28, 47, 49,
        51, 54, 61, 165, 185, 313, 316, 338,
        343, 350
    serum 338
Follicular cyst 68, 157, 243
Follicular phase 14
    dominance 15
    mechanism of ovulation 15
    ovulation 15
    recruitment 15
    selection 15
Folliculogenesis 232, 233f
    dynamics of 15f
Forceps 228, 228f
Fossa of Waldeyer 232
Fothergill's operation 268, 269
Fothergill's repair 203
Fracture 352
Frank's dilation 9
Frank's technique 52
Frei's test 140
Full-blown syndrome 60
Fundal dimpling 235f
Fungus, gram-positive 131

G

Gabapentin 429
Galactocele 220
Galactorrhea 98
Gallbladder disease 354
Gardasil 366
Gardnerella vaginalis 118
Garland sign 244, 244f
Gartner's cyst 152
Gastric stasis 429, 430
Gastritis 430
Gastroesophageal reflux 427
Gastrointestinal system 110
Gastrointestinal tract 417
Gemcitabine carboplatin 424
Generation next vaginal prolapse 202
Genetic sex 328
Genital abnormalities, external 331
Genital dysplasia, olfactory 96
Genital fistulae 213
    classification 213
    etiology 213
    types of 213f
Genital herpes 134
    primary episode of 134
Genital hiatus 196f
Genital mucosa 28

Genital mutilation
   dies of 102
   female 102, 103*b*
Genital neoplasm 38
Genital organ prolapse, classification of 194*t*
Genital prolapse 20
   with cystocele 201*f*
Genital ridge 329
Genital sex 329
Genital tract 150, 262, 363
   anatomic abnormality of 52
   lower 27, 129
   manifestations 416
   tuberculosis of 94, 98
   upper 129
   uterus didelphys 7
Genital tuberculosis 97, 98, 285, 286
   clinical manifestation of 286*t*
   female 285
   pathology 285
Genital ulcerative diseases 133
Genital ulcers 141*f*
Genital warts 126, 141
   clinical features 141
   organism 141
   specific treatment 141
   treatment 141
Genitalia, abnormalities of 49
Genitourinary tract 5, 21
Gentamicin 122
Germ cell 368
   classifications of 386*b*
   migrate 3
   number of 5
   primordial 3
   tumors 157, 243, 247, 386
      malignant 390
Gestational trophoblastic
   disease 411, 411*b*
   disorders 248
   neoplasia 411, 419
   tumor 411, 414*t*
Gestrinone 90, 113
Gilliam's ventrosuspension 293
Gland, pituitary 43
Glandular epithelium 127
Global reproductive health strategy 102
Global sex survey 102
Glucocorticoid 39
   excess of 323
   replacement 336
   therapy 326
Glucose 147
   tolerance test 320
Glycerine 201
Glycogen deficient epithelium 375
Gonadal differentiation, disorders
   of 329, 330
Gonadal dysgenesis 48, 331, 335
   partial 331
   syndromes of 329, 331

Gonadal failure, early 48
Gonadal primordia 329
Gonadal sex 329
   indeterminate 332
Gonadal stromal tumors 157
Gonadoblastoma 157, 331
Gonadotropin 49, 316
   dependent puberty 46
   ectopic 37
   exogenous 316
   independent puberty 46
   injection 315
   releasing hormone 17, 28, 47, 49, 51,
      61, 165, 307, 315, 316
      agonist 63, 89, 113, 156
      antagonist 156
      dependent precocious puberty 37
      independent precocious
puberty 37
      secretion 50, 56
      testing 62
      therapy 321
   secretion, control of 94
   treatment, complications of 316
Gonococcal
   complement fixation test 129
   infection, disseminated 123, 130
   pelvic inflammatory disease 130
Gonorrhea 121-123, 128, 129, 189, 338
   acute 129
   chronic 129
   incubation period 128
   organism 128
   pathology 128
   signs of 129
   symptoms of 129
Graafian follicle 158
Granuloma inguinale 140, 141
   clinical features 140
   investigations 140
   organism 140
   treatment 141
Granulosa cell 14*f*, 157, 312
   tumor 40, 69, 158, 248, 387, 396
Greasy hair 46
Green-Armytage's forceps 228, 228*f*
Griseofulvin 168
Groove sign 140
Growth hormone 37, 49, 52
Gummata 136
Gynandroblastoma 159
Gynatresia 7
Gynecologic
   endoscopy 298
   oncology 361
   problems 28
   surgery, part of 298
Gynecological
   cancer screening 363
   disorders 22

   malignancy 421
   operations 261
   pathology 22*b*

H

Haemophilus ducreyi 139
Haemophilus influenzae 35, 118
Hagar's dilators 277
Hair-an syndrome 324
Haloperidol 427, 435
Hashimotos thyroiditis 331
Haultain's technique 295
Headaches 44
Heart 348
   disease 23
      congenital 170
      coronary 347*t*, 348, 352
Heavy bleeding, acute 88
Heavy menstrual bleeding 84, 86, 88, 91
   surgical management of 90
Hegar's dilator 223, 223*f*
Hemangioma 151
Hematocolpos 9, 9*f*, 242*f*
Hematoma, acute perianal 281
Hematometra 9, 56, 332
Hematuria 417
Hemochromatosis, primary 94
Hemoglobin levels 423
Hemorrhage 102, 105, 107, 160, 264, 272, 413
   intraperitoneal 416
   postpartum 295
   primary 272
   reactionary 272
   secondary 267, 272
   subepithelial 34
Hemorrhoids 281
   signs 281*t*
   treatment 281*t*
Hemostasis 301
Hemostatic clamps 267
Heparin 85
   A 126
      virus immunoglobulin 147
   B 126
      virus 147
   C virus 147
Hermaphrodite 50, 332, 336
Hermaphroditism, true 329, 332
Hernias 279
Herpes
   genitalis 126, 133, 151
      lesions 135
   infection, recurrent 133, 135
   primary 133
   simplex 189
      virus 126, 134, 141
   zoster virus infection 36
Hidden menses 9

High peak systolic velocities 238f
Hilar cell hyperplasia 324
Hilus cell tumors 159
Hip joints 24
Hirsutism 57, 58, 58t, 61, 319, 323, 324, 326
   drug-induced 325
   idiopathic 60
   management of 325
   managing 322
   pathophysiology of 323
   severity of 324
   signs of 318
Hormonal contraceptives 163, 166, 322
   drug interactions 168
   major problems 168
   mechanism of action 167
   side effects 167
Hormonal method, male 179
Hormonal oral contraceptive pills 131
Hormonal stimuli 109
Hormonal theory 78
Hormonal therapy 55
   effect of 347
   oral 80
   primary 336
Hormone 324
   anterior pituitary 338
   containing devices 171
   excess 54
   exogenous 370
   monitoring 164
   releasing intrauterine devices 172
   replacement therapy 22, 355
   therapy 343, 346, 348, 350-354
      benefit or no effect 352
      delivery systems 351
      menopausal 356
      risk 352
      side effects of 352
   thermogenic 339
Hormonogenesis 14
Horseshoe kidney 334
Hourglass appearance 34
Hulka-Clemens spring clip 176, 177f
Human chorionic gonadotropin 15, 54, 69
Human immunodeficiency virus 106, 126, 129, 144, 179
   clinical progression of 145
   infection 144, 145, 146
      chronic 147
      long-term 144
      primary 147
   transmission 145
      sources of 145t
Human menopausal gonadotropin 87, 316, 321, 315
Human papillomavirus 35, 70, 71, 126, 366, 374
   diagnosis of 191
   infection 106, 146, 366
   vaccines 366

Human sexuality, Masters and Johnson model of 182f
Hydatidiform mole 411, 412, 412t
   complete 248
   incidence of 411t
   invasive 248
   partial 248, 414
Hydrosalpinx 118, 128, 129
Hydroxylase deficiencies 333
Hymen 45
   imperforate 9, 36, 49, 51, 67, 71
Hymenal obstruction 9
Hyoscine hydrobromide 432
Hyperandrogenemia 49, 313, 319
Hyperandrogenism 58, 322
   causes of 59
   diagnosis of 58
   initial biochemical evaluation of 61t
   intra-ovarian 59
   mild symptoms of 58
   signs of 324
   treatment of 61
Hypercalcemia 429, 430, 433
   severe 433
   symptomatic 433
Hypercortisolism, adrenal 38
Hyperemesis gravidarum 412
Hyperinsulinemia, role of 319, 320fc, 322
Hyperplasia 98
   adrenal 39
   cellular atypia 394
Hyperprolactinemia 60, 98, 313-315, 324, 325
   cause of 98
   pathological causes of 313b
   severe 98
Hyperreacto luteinalis 243
Hyperseborrhea 58
Hypertension 23
   pregnancy induced 413
Hypertensive disorders 107
Hyperthyroidism 413
Hypertrichosis 323
Hypertriglyceridemia 351
Hypnosis 68
Hypoactive sexual desire disorder 183
Hypogastric nerve, resection of 81
Hypogonadism
   hypergonadotropic 48, 52, 313
   hypogonadotropic 48, 52, 312, 315
   primary 56
Hypomenorrhea 93
Hyponatremic crisis 47
Hypoplasia 7, 51
Hypothalamic
   disorders 53
   dysfunction 94
      cause for 315
   lesions 50, 56, 97
   maturation 311
   pituitary

      axis 15, 315
      dysfunction 96, 313
      failure 312
      ovarian axis 36, 43, 94, 307, 318
Hypothalamohypophyseal axis 94
Hypothalamo-pituitary ovarian system, oscillation of 17
Hypothalamus 52, 312
   pituitary region 96
Hypothyroidism 49, 217, 323
Hypoxic cells 422
Hysterectomy 91, 116, 262, 377
   abdominal 261-263
   bilateral salpingo-oophorectomy 114
   complications of 264
   laparoscopic 273, 274b
   postoperative care after 264
   prophylactic 415
   specimens, examination of 114
   subtotal 261
   total abdominal 261
   vaginal 155, 202, 261, 269
Hysterosalpingogram 288
Hysterosalpingography 99
Hysteroscope 277f
Hysteroscopy 87, 99, 276, 277, 277b, 288, 302, 303, 303f
   complications of 277
   operative 277
   timing of 303

I

Iatrogenic ureteral injury, causes of 282
Ibuprofen 65, 67, 428
Iliac fossa pain 280
Iliac spine, anterior superior 283
Imidazole derivative 326
Imiquimod 141
In vitro fertilization 340, 341
Incision
   choice of 262
   over vaginal epithelium overlying cystocele 201f
Incisional hernia, evidence of 23
Incontinence, neurogenic 208
Infection 50, 81, 105, 146, 160, 268
   parasitic 70
   recurrent 134
Infertile couple
   assessment of 338
   investigation of 339
Infertility 114, 190, 292, 322, 326, 334, 337
   causes of 337, 337f
   female 312
   male 338
   prolonged 337
   technologies 105
   unexplained 338

Index

Infibulation 103
Inflammatory disease 139
Infundibulopelvic ligament 265f
Injectable contraceptives 169
    combined 170
Injuries
    childbirth 193, 206
    sphincter 212
Insulin 319
    action of 320
    like growth factor 319, 320
    sensitivity 320
Internal genitalia, anatomy of 56
International Collaborative Ovarian Neoplasm 390
International Federation of Gynecology and Obstetrics Staging for Cervical Carcinoma 378t
International Obesity Task Force 104
Intersex 328
    diagnosis of 335
    management of 335
    syndromes 334
Interstitial salpingitis, chronic 119
Intertrigo 151
Intestinal obstruction 431
Intra-abdominal
    disease 261, 262
    masses, large 274
    pressure 290
Intracytoplasmic sperm injection 341
Intraepithelial neoplasia, severe 262
Intraperitoneal disease, disseminated 389
Intraurethral prostaglandin pellets 189
Intrauterine
    adhesions 413
    contraceptive device 22, 118, 221, 240, 274
    devices 79, 80, 163, 171, 172f, 179
        beneficial effects of 175
        complications 174
        copper-containing 171
        delayed complications 174
        inert 171
        removal 175
        technique of insertion 173
        types of 171
        unmedicated 171
    fetal death 126
    insemination 341
    pregnancy 416
    systems 172
Inversion
    acute 293
    chronic 295, 296
Ipratropium 432
Iron therapy 90
Irritable bowel syndrome 68, 279, 280
Irving technique 175, 176f
Itch 34
Ito test 139

J

Jaundice 416
    severe 417f
Johnson's maneuver 294
Jones classification 8

K

Kallmann's gene 334
Kallmann's syndrome 48, 94, 96, 97, 334
Kaposi's sarcoma 145, 148
Kegel's excercises 200, 210
Keloid formation 103
Keratoacanthoma 152
Ketaconazole 132, 326
Ketoprofen 65
Keyhole surgery 273
Kidney, ectopic 249
Killer disease 98
KISS1R gene 311
Kisspeptin 311
    signalling 311
Klebsiella granulomatis 140
Klinefelter syndrome 329, 330, 331
Knee joints 24
Kocher's artery forceps 227, 228f
Koilocytosis 365
Kroener's technique 176
Kronos Early Estrogen Prevention Study 348

L

Labia majora 45, 402f, 408f
Labia minora 33, 45, 408f
Labial adhesions 33
    etiology 33
    incidence 33
    treatment 33
    vulvitis 33
Labium majus 402f
Lactate dehydrogenase 69, 288
Lactational amenorrhea method 164, 179
Lactulose 280
Lamineria tent 230
Lanugo-like hair 325
Laparoscope 300f
Laparoscopic surgery
    indications of 298
    over conventional surgery, advantages of 302
Laparoscopy 65, 110, 113, 273, 288
    basic instruments of 275f
    close 274
    complications of 276, 276b, 302
    contraindications of 274, 274t
    equipment of 275t
    indications of 274t
    operative 273, 274
    over laparotomy, advantages of 273b
    procedure 301
    role of 66
    techniques of 274, 301
Laparotomy 388
Laser excisional conization 376
Laurence-Moon-Biedl syndrome 96
Leech Wilkinson's cannula 226, 226f
LeFort operation 272
LeFort repair 203
Leiomyoma 85, 151, 237f, 239, 395
    benign 395
    classification of 85
    hybrid 86
Leiomyosarcoma 395, 397
Lesions
    benign 150
    cystic 151
    pituitary 50, 56
Letrozole 113, 316
Leukemia 53
Leukocytes 364
Leuprolide 68
Levator ani 207f
    muscles 197
    plication 271f
Levomepromazine 435
Levonorgestrel 324
    releasing intrauterine system 90
Leydig cell 4, 338
    aplasia 333
Libido, loss of 21
Lichen planus 151
Lichen sclerosus 34, 150
    diagnosis 34
    treatment 34
Lichen simplex chronicus 151
Lidocaine 134
Ligase chain reaction 127
Lignocaine 134
Lipid cell tumors 157
Lipschutz ulcers 151
Lithotomy position 301f, 303
Liver 167
    diseases 351
    function tests 149
LNG-IUS 20 172
Lowenstein-Jensen medium 287
Lower urinary tract 206, 207, 346
    and bowel, neural control of 207f
Lump, abdominal 20
Lung 416
    cancer 354
    metastases 417f
Luteal phase dysphoric disorder 62
Luteinizing hormone 28, 47, 49, 51, 54, 61, 165, 185, 313, 316, 318, 338
    monitoring 339
    receptor abnormality 333

Lymph node
  inguinal 139
  metastases 379, 403
Lymphadenectomy 405
  para-aortic 398
Lymphangioma 151
Lymphatic glands 139
Lymphedema 96, 379, 422, 434
  lower limb 398
  postoperative 403
  severe 379f
Lymphogranuloma venereum 126, 139, 141, 151
  clinical features 139
  investigations 140
  treatment 140
Lymphorrhea 434
Lynch syndrome 396, 397b

M

Mackenrodt's ligament 266f
Macroadenoma, pituitary 314f
Macular degeneration, age-related 355
Madlener technique 176
Malabsorption syndrome 56
Malaria 107
Malignant cells, absence of 288
Malignant disease 273, 372
Malmstrom cup 229, 229f
Malnutrition 52
Mammogram 217
Mammography 217
Manchester operation 269
Manchester repair 203
Mantoux test 286
Manual vacuum aspirator 224, 224f
Masculinized female 329, 332, 333
Mass
  abdominal 386
  hypoechoic 236f
  tubo-ovarian 118, 128, 129
Mastalgia 44, 216
Mastitis 217
  acute 220
  periductal 219
Maternal estrogen exposure 29
Mathew-Duncan dilator 223, 223f
  complications 223
  uses 223
Maturation, psychologic 310
Mayer-Rokitansky-Küster-Hauser syndrome 52, 334
McCall culdoplasty 202
McCune-Albright syndrome 37-40, 46
McIndoe operation 9
McIndoe procedure 9, 10
McIndoe technique 52
Mechanical bowel obstruction 430
Medroxyprogesterone 38, 395

Mefenamic acid 56, 67
Mefipristone 171
Meig's syndrome 247
Melanomas 401
Meloxicam 428
Menarche 97
  delayed 50t
  physiology of 94
Menopausal problems
  early 345
  late 347
Menopause 191, 212, 343, 344
  artificial 335
  genitourinary symptoms of 346
  premature 355
  signs of 345
  symptoms of 345
  transient 419
  transition 344
Menorrhagia 93, 94, 393
Menorrhea 77
Menstrual bleeding
  abnormal 20
  irregular 170
  normal 84
Menstrual cycle 16f, 17t, 343
  irregular 59, 104
  normal 338
  proliferative phase of 232
  several 157
Menstrual disorders 52
Menstrual function 94, 203
Menstrual history 21, 22b, 339
Menstrual irregularities, improving 322
Menstrual loss, normal 84
Menstrual periods, regular 15
Menstrual phase 16
Menstrual problems 13, 146
Menstruation 13, 16, 51, 52, 59, 72
  cessation of 13
  physiology of 93
Mesenchymal origin, nonspecific 385
Mesenchymal tumors, nonspecific 386, 386b
Mesenchymoma, virilizing 159
Mesonephric ducts 4
Mesonephroid tumor 158
Metabolic disorders 323
Metabolic syndrome 59, 60, 311
Metaplasia, squamous 373
Metastatic lesions, typical rounded 417f
Metformin 321, 322
  mechanism of action of 321
Methylnaltrexone 431
Metoclopramide 431
Metronidazole 122, 131
Metrorrhagia 67
Metyrapone 60
Meyer's coelomic epithelium transformation 109
Miconazole 132

Microadenomas, prolactin secreting 324
Midluteal serum progesterone 339
Migraines 179, 351
Mikulicz cells 140
Minilaparotomy 175
  complications of 176
Minoxidil 323
Mirena 172
Miscarriage 133, 337
  risk of 104
Mitomycin C 380
Mittelschmerz syndrome 64
Mixed gonadal dysgenesis 32, 329, 331
Molar pregnancy
  diagnosis of 413
  management of 413
Mole
  complete 412t
  invasive 411, 414
  partial 412t, 414f
Molluscum contagiosum 36
Moniliasis 131
Mood swings 44
Morbidity, cause of 347
Mother-to-child transmission 144
  prevention of 148
Motion sickness 430
Müllerian abnormalities 71
  diagnosis 71
Müllerian agenesis 95, 96, 97
Müllerian anomalies 8, 50, 51
  classification of 8t
Müllerian duct 4, 6, 8, 329, 331, 385
  anomalies 7, 11
  development of 7
  regress 329
  regression 5
  syndrome, persistent 334
Müllerian dysgenesis 49
Müllerian hormone 329
Müllerian hypoplasia, segmental 8
Müllerian inhibiting substance 69
Müllerian metaplasia theory 109
Müllerian structures 32, 333
  well-developed 331
Müllerian system, development of 7
Müllerian transformation 109
Multiple pituitary hormone deficiencies 49, 52
Mumps oophoritis 313
Mycobacterium
  bovis 285
  tuberculosis 285
Mycoplasma hominis 118
Myocardial infarction 351
Myoma, subserosal 237f
Myomectomy 155, 293
  laparoscopic 156f
  principle of 155
Myometrial calcification 236f, 239

Myometrial contractility 79
Myometrial invasion 414
Myometrial ischemia 79
Myometritis 239
Myometrium 87, 232, 238f, 239f, 285
    anterior 235f
    benign
        conditions 234
        tumors 234
    diseases of 234
    malignant tumor 234
    thickened
        anterior 115f
        posterior 115f

N

Nabothian cysts 241
Nafarelin 68
Nail clipping, regular 281
Naproxen 65, 428
    sodium 67
National AIDS Control Organization 144
Natural family planning method 163, 164
Nausea 66, 422, 429
    cause of 430, 430t
Necklace sign 244
Necrosis, postpartum pituitary 98, 99
Neisseria gonorrhoeae 66, 67, 117, 118, 121, 122, 128, 129
Neonatal death rates 107
Neonatal disease 126
Neoplasia 98
Neurofibroma 151
Neurological deficit, evidence of 134
Neurosyphilis 136, 138
    asymptomatic 137
Night's sleep 427
Nipple discharge 217
    physiological 217
Nocturnal pruritus 34
    diagnosis 34
    treatment 34
Nocturnal sperm emissions 308
Nodular echogenic lesion 238f
Nodule, endometriotic 299f, 416f
Nonclassic adrenal hyperplasia 58-61
    clinical aspects 60
    diagnosis 60
Non-hormonal therapy 346
Non-pigmented endometriotic lesion, laparoscopy view of 111f
Nonsexual terminal hair 323
Nonspecific antigen tests 137
Nonsteroidal anti-inflammatory drugs 67, 79, 88, 111, 217
Noradrenaline 429
Norepinephrine 429
Norethisterone 324

Normal menstruation 93
    clinical features of 18
Normal pubertal process, landmarks of 310f
Norplant rods 170f
Nortestosterone-derived progestins 60
Novel vaginoplasty techniques 10
Nucleic acid amplification
    techniques 129, 131, 140
    tests 127
Nystatin 132

O

Obesity 103, 318
    abdominal 311
    central 103
    maternal 104
    medical complications of 104f
Obturator fossa 211f
Obturator internus muscle 233f
Ofloxacin 128
Oligomenorrhagia 99
Oligomenorrhea 56, 59, 93, 99, 104, 318, 324
Omental cake 386f, 387f
Omental flap 214f
Omeprazole 432
Oocytes
    after expulsion of 15
    retrieved 341
Oophorectomy
    bilateral 185
    medical 63
    prophylactic 262, 385
    surgical 63
Oophoritis 117
Ophthalmia 126
Oral contraceptive 54, 55, 61, 79
    pill 18, 384, 385
        combined 18, 51, 56, 65, 89, 111, 166, 179, 326
Oral medications 427
Oral mucositis, severe 419f
Oral progestins 89
Organisms
    aerobic 35
    anaerobic 35
Orgasmic disorder 183
Oropharynx 432
Osmotic laxatives 431
Osteoarthritis 355
Osteopenia 72
Osteoporosis 343, 349, 349t, 350
    treatment 349
Ovarian agenesis 8
Ovarian cancer 353, 354, 368, 383-385, 390, 424
    advanced 387f
    anatomy 384
    diagnosis 386

    epidemiology 383
    etiological factors 384
    examination 387
    mode of spread 384
    preoperative evaluation 387
    prevention of 385
    risk of 353, 385
    screening, current status of 369
    signs 386
    stages of 387
    symptoms 386
    syndrome, hereditary 385
Ovarian carcinoma 23, 383, 389
    epithelial 388
    treatment of 388
Ovarian cycle 13, 14, 37, 39, 68, 338
Ovarian cyst
    clinical presentation 39
    diagnosis 40
    malignant 369
    massive 390, 390f
    rupture of 121, 160
    types 39
Ovarian cystectomy 161
Ovarian dermoid 247
    cysts 243
Ovarian drilling 317
    laparoscopic 317
Ovarian dysfunction, pathophysiology of 13
Ovarian edema, massive 246
Ovarian events 17
Ovarian failure 50, 313
    premature 47, 56, 61
    primary 48, 94
Ovarian fibroma 159
Ovarian follicle development 312
Ovarian fossa 282f
Ovarian function, preservation of 379
Ovarian germ cell tumors 389
Ovarian hormones, postovulatory secretions of 17
Ovarian hyperandrogenism, functional 61
Ovarian hyperstimulation 244f
    syndrome 244, 316, 340
        complications of 321
Ovarian insufficiency, primary 355
Ovarian lesions, additional 239
Ovarian ligament 269
Ovarian lymphoma 248
Ovarian mass 383
    evaluation of 248
Ovarian neoplasms 242, 246
    benign 157
    classification of 385
Ovarian parenchyma 244f, 245f
Ovarian remnant syndrome 244
Ovarian sonography 242
Ovarian stroma 385
Ovarian structure, benign cystic lesion of 243

Ovarian torsion 66, 245
Ovarian tumor 59, 60, 60, 69, 386f
    benign 157t
    complications of 160
    functional 325
    gross specimen of 159f, 160f
    infection of 160
    malignant 157t
    multilocular 246f
    solid 157t
    torsion of 160f
    twisted 121
Ovarian vascular lesions 242, 245
Ovarian venous thrombosis 246
Ovarian vessels 282
Ovary 8, 232, 285, 312
    benign tumors of 156
    bilateral papillary serous
        cystadenocarcinoma of 386f
    carcinoma of 401
    connective tissue of 159
    development of 4
    enlarged 244f, 246f
    fossa 232
    into pelvis, descent of 5f
    lesions of 243ff
    neoplastic enlargement of 69
    non-neoplastic enlargement of 68
Ovulation 13
    disorders of 54, 312
    induction 315, 320t, 340
        clinical correlation for 18
        methods 321
        surgical induction of 317, 321
        years of 384
Ovulatory cycle 93
Ovulatory disorders 312
Ovulatory dysfunction 85, 338, 340
Ovulatory free fluid in cul-de-sac, small amount of 234f
Ovulatory mechanism, regular 338
Oxytocin infusion 413

P

Paget's cells 408
    typical 409f
Paget's disease 409f
Pain 66
    abdomen, acute 118
    abdominal 130
    acute 64
    character of 63
    chronic 64
    control 427
        invasive techniques for 429
    cyclic 64
    hypogastric 280
    lower abdominal 279, 332
    midcycle 67
    neuropathic 428
    non-menstrual 113
    recurrent abdominal 63
    types of 64
PALM-COEIN classification 86
    salient features of 86
Panmural myomas 239
Pap smear
    screening 366
    test 370
Papanicolaou smear 364
Papillary erosion 152
Paramesonephric cord 4
Paramesonephric ducts 4
Parametritis 117
Parametrium 261
Paraovarian structure, benign cystic lesion of 243
Parkland technique 176
Partial androgen insensitivity syndrome 32
Pelvic abscess 105, 118, 128, 177
Pelvic adhesions 66, 68, 188, 293
Pelvic endometriosis 114, 121
Pelvic examination 45, 45t, 339, 369
    routine 369
Pelvic floor 197, 206
    anatomy of 196
    disorders, etiology of 194
    dysfunction 188, 206
    layer of 196
    muscle training 210
    relaxation 194
    repair 269
    support system, anatomy of 207f
Pelvic infections 129
Pelvic inflammation 129
Pelvic inflammatory disease 67, 103, 106, 107, 117, 117b, 117t, 119, 127, 165, 170, 245, 262, 267, 273, 291, 293, 298
    acute 23, 119, 121, 286
    chronic 120
    diagnosis of 119b, 121
    hydrosalpinx 118
    sequelae of 119fc
    treatment of 121, 122
Pelvic irradiation, adjuvant 379
Pelvic kidney 249, 334
Pelvic lymph nodes 261
Pelvic lymphadenectomy 379
    role of 398
Pelvic masses, assessment of 274
Pelvic operations posterior 282f
Pelvic organ 23
    prolapse 193, 196t, 206
        classification of 194t
        clinical features of 198t
        quantification system 195f
        treatment of 200, 201t
    support quantification 195f
Pelvic pain 20, 63, 110
    acute 66
    causes of 21b
Pelvic peritoneum 245
Pelvic peritonitis 117
Pelvic relaxation 194t
Pelvic splanchnic nerve 207f
Pelvic support defects 199
Pelvic surgery 188
Pelvic ultrasound 287, 376f
Penile implants 189
Per vaginal bleeding, abnormal 110
Perianal pain, acute 281, 281b
Pericardial effusion 341
Perifollicular flow 233f
Perimenopause 344
Perineal
    body 195f
    congestion 281
    dilation 52
Perineorrhaphy 202f, 204
Perineum 200, 207f
Peritoneal cavity 398
Peritoneal wash 284
Peritoneum 287f, 398
Peritonitis 105, 128
Pessary complications 227
Pessary test 293
Pessary treatment 292
Pfannenstiel transverse abdominal incision 262f
Phenytoin 168, 323
Phosphodiesterase inhibitors 189
Phyllodes tumor 218
    malignant 218
Pigmentation, disorders of 151
Pigmented endometriotic lesion, laparoscopy view of 111f
Piles 280
Pills
    high dose 167
    low dose 167
    mini 169
    missed 168
    monophasic 167
    multiphasic 167
Pinard's fetal stethoscope 230, 230f
Pituitary gonadotropin
    depression of 17
    orchestrate 17
    secretion 17
Placental site trophoblastic tumor 248, 411, 415
Plasma 145
Plasminogen activator 18
    inhibitor 89
Pnemocystitis carinii 144
    pneumonia 145
Pneumonia 145
    bacterial 145

Index

Pneumoperitoneum 300
Podophyllin 141
Podophyllotoxin 141
Polycystic ovarian syndrome 42, 47, 49, 54, 59, 61, 85, 244, 313, 318-320, 320t, 322, 393
    adolescent 46
    diagnosis of 313, 319
    etiology of 313
    mechanism of onset of 319, 319fc
    pathogenesis of 319, 320fc
    phenotypes 60
    transvaginal ultrasound of 314f
Polycystic ovaries 313, 318, 319
    evidence of 319
    transvaginal sonogram of 244f
    typical of 318
Polydimethylsiloxane 90
Polydioxanone 282, 283
Polyglactin 283
Polyglycolic acid 282, 283
    suture 9
Polyhydramnios 136
Polymenorrhea 93
Polymerase 423
    chain reaction 127, 137, 287
Polypropylene mesh 211f
Polyps 85, 302f
    pedicle 239f
Pomeroy technique 175, 175f
Porphyria cutanea tarda 323
Portahepatis 416
    region of 417f
Positive pelvic nodes, distribution of 379f
Postcoital douche 164
Posterior vaginal wall 193, 198
    defect, repair of 204
Postmenarchal cycles 44
Postnatal sexual problems, management of 190t
Post-tubal sterilization syndrome 178
Potassium sparing diuretic 433
Pouch of Douglas 26, 27, 119, 202f, 233, 246f, 270f
Povidone iodine 284
Powder burn 110
Prader-Willi syndrome 96
Precocious development, treatment of 38
Precocious puberty 36, 46
    central 46
    clinical forms of 46t
    diagnosis of 38
    dissociated 46
    forms of 39
    major classes of 37
    management of 38
    peripheral 46
    secondary central 37
    treatment of 38
Prednisolone 326

Pre-eclampsia 104, 412
Pregnancy 130, 138
    adolescent 72
    carries 281
    complications 53
    ectopic 23, 66, 120, 178, 273, 298, 337
    loss 321
    multiple 316
    termination of 72, 190
    with herpes 133
Premature pubarche 46
    decision tree for 47fc
Premature sexual maturation 332
    disorders of 37
Premature thelarche 46
    decision tree for 47fc
Premenstrual syndrome 62, 167
Primary amenorrhea 8, 9, 46, 49, 50fc, 56, 95, 95fc, 334
    causes of 48t
    management of 96, 97t
    treatment of 97
Primidone 168
Problematic uterine smooth muscle tumors, classification of 395t
Procedentia 296
Proctitis 129
Proctological diseases 280
Progesterone 15f, 339
    only pills 169
    receptor modulators 171
    treatment 88
Progestin 333, 351
    only pill 56, 179
    only protocols 65
Progestogen 156, 350, 351
    types of 352
Prokinetic agents 431
Prolactin 54, 324
Prolactinoma 98, 217
Prolapse 193
    degree of 204f
    uterus 198b
Prostaglandin 428
    intracavernous 189
    synthase inhibitors 65, 156
    theory 78
Protease inhibitor 148
    monotherapy 148
Pruritus 346
    vulvae 70
Pseudohermaphroditism 328
Pseudopuberty, precocious 37, 46
Psoas hitch 282
Psoriasis 151
Psychosexual element 182
Psychosexual medicine 187
Psychosexual problems 181
Psychosocial sex-deviations 334
Psychotherapy 68

Pubarche 309
Pubertal development 50t
    chart 310f
    stages of 43
Pubertal events, summary of 44
Pubertal phenotypic changes, sequence of 309
Puberty 42, 51, 307, 310, 319
    absent 46
    advanced 46
    changes during normal 42
    delayed 47, 48f, 97
    factors influencing 308b
    physical
        changes of 309
        landmarks of 309t
    physiological
        hyperandrogenism of 58
        landmarks of 309t
    physiology of 307
    psychologic changes of 310
Pubic hair 43, 97
    development 309
    growth of 36
    premature 61
Pudendal nerve 207, 207f
Puerperal inversion, prevention of 294
Puerperal ligation 175
Punch biopsy forceps 225, 225f
Purandare cervicopexy 272
Pure gonadal dysgenesis 48, 52, 329
Pyelogram, intravenous 267
Pyometra 242f
Pyosalpinx 118, 119, 128, 129

Q

Q-tip test 199f, 209
Quinolones 130

R

Radiation
    ionizing 421
    therapy, primary 380
Radical electrocoagulation diathermy 375
Radical hysterectomy 27, 261, 377f, 379
    complications of 379
    laparoscopic 273
Radical vulvectomy 405f, 406f, 408f
    specimen 405f
Radioactive isotopes 421
Radiotherapy 399, 421
    image-guided 422
Raised intracranial pressure 429, 430
Randomized controlled trials 398
Ranitidine 432
Rectal
    examination 26, 296
    treatments 431

Rectocele 201
Rectovaginal examination 27, 27f
Rectovaginal fistula 213f
Rectovaginal septum 245
Rectovaginal space 271
Rectum 200, 206, 207f
Rectus muscle 275f
Rectus sheath 262f
Red rubber catheter 225, 225f
Reinke crystals 159
Reiter's syndrome 123, 126, 127
Renal anomalies 9
Renal disease 56
Renal failure 103, 308, 430
Reproductive
   aging, basis of 345
   endocrinology 305
   function 203
   health 101, 107
   system, female 110
   tract, female 7
Respiratory disorders 22
Respiratory system 110
Respiratory thorax 110
Rete cysts 243
Retropubic approach 211f
Retropubic space 211f
Retroversion 291
   degrees of 291
   symptoms of 291
Richardson's tetractor 227
Rifampicin 168
Ring pessary 226, 226f
Rokitansky-Kuster-Hauser syndrome 49
Rotterdam consensus 60
Round ligament 263f, 269
   abdominal 203
Rudimentary left horn 11f

S

Saccharomyces cerevisiae 131
Salbutamol 432
Saliva 145
Salpingitis 117, 129
   chronic 127
   edema 128
   stage of 118
Salpingo-oopherectomy, bilateral 114, 261, 379, 388, 398
Salpingo-oophoritis 118
Salvage surgery, secondary 390
Sampson's retrograde menstruation 109
Sarcoma, undifferentiated 394
Scoliosis 96
Scratch 34
Screening test 145
Seborrheic keratosis 152

Secondary amenorrhea 46, 56, 57, 97, 99fc
   cause of 98
   evaluation of 57fc
   management of 98t
Secondary trocar 276
   insertion 301
Selective estrogen receptor modulators 350
Semen 145
Sensate focus program 187f
Sentinel node localization 407f
Septae, multiple 158f
Septate uterus 8, 11, 234
   surgical management of 11
Septic secondary infection 135
Septum 303f
   abnormalities, resorption of 8
Serological tests 127
Serosa 86
Sertoli-Leydig cell tumors 159, 248, 387
Sex assignment 33
Sex cord 3243, 247, 368
   stromal tumors 386, 386b
     benign 158
   tumors 157
Sex determination 30
Sex determining region 328
Sex differentiation 30, 329
Sex education 187b, 311
Sex genotype 329
Sex hormone 351
   binding globulin 61, 62, 313, 316, 320
Sex steroids, action of 39
Sexual abuse 35, 73, 191
Sexual activity 101
Sexual ambiguity 30
Sexual arousal disorder 183
Sexual behavior change, patterns of 189
Sexual characteristics, secondary 56, 57
Sexual contact 131
Sexual desire disorders 183
Sexual development
   delayed 46
   disorders of 329, 335
   secondary 97
Sexual differentiation 330f
   classification of 329
   disorders of 30, 33, 328, 329
Sexual difficulties 187b
   management of 185
   presentation of 182
Sexual disorders 183
   female 183
   primary 182
Sexual dysfunction 21, 181, 189, 189t
   aspects of 181
   female 182, 186
Sexual function 30, 190, 203
   female 186
Sexual health 181
Sexual history 22, 184

Sexual indifferent stage 329
Sexual intercourse 123, 145
Sexual medicine 186t
Sexual pain disorders 183
   noncoital 184
Sexual partners, treatment of 122
Sexual precocity, signs of 38
Sexual problems 188t
Sexual violence 102
Sexually transmitted diseases 45, 117, 125, 126, 165, 190, 366
Sexually transmitted infections 44, 66, 101, 106, 125, 126
   bacterial 126
   fungal 126
   protozoa 126
   types of 126fc
   viral 126
Sheehan's syndrome 94, 98, 99
Shigella flexneri 35
Shining radiotherapy beams 421
Shirodkar's abdominal sling operation 272
Shirodkar's hook 226, 226f
Shirodkar's modification of Manchester repair 203
Shirodkar's vaginal repair 268, 269
Shock, obstetric 295
Silastic ring 176
Sildenafil 189
Sim's anterior vaginal wall retractor 222
Sim's double ended uterine curette 223, 223f
Sim's vaginal speculum 25, 221, 221f
Sinovaginal bulbs 6
Sister Joseph's nodules 23
Skeinitis 129
Skene's glands 6
Skin
   bridge metastases 405
   changes 347
     treatment 347
   closure, primary 406f
   incision 405f
   necrosis 419f
   rash 136
   toxicity 423
Small serum-ascites albumin gradient 288
Smith-Hodge pessary 226
Smooth muscle tumor 395
Society of Gynecologic Oncologists Statement guidelines 397b
Solid ovarian lesion, cystic 248f
Somatic nervous system 206, 207
Sonohysterography 240, 241f
   saline infusion 87
Spasmodic dysmenorrhea 78
   types of 81
Specula, types of 25f
Sperm factor, investigation of 339
Spermatogenesis 332, 338

Index

Spermatozoa 338
    competent 338
Spermicidal preparations 166
    advantages 166
    disadvantages 166
Sperms decides genetic sex 329f
Spinal cord 428
    surgeries 209
Spironolactone 61, 326, 433
Sponge holding forceps 229, 230f
Squamous cell carcinoma 377, 401, 402, 402f
    large clitoral 402f
    superficial ulceration of 402f
Squamous cell hyperplasia 150, 151
Squamous intraepithelial lesion 375
    low grade 71, 365
Standard days method 164
Staphylococcus aureus 35
Stein-Leventhal syndrome 318
Stem cells 210
Sterilization 162
    interval 175
    laparoscopic 176
    male 178
    postabortal 175
    postpartum 175
    procedures 178
    reversal of 178
    surgical 175
    tubal 298
Steroids
    anabolic 60
    androgenic 156
    exogenous 54
    hormones 374f
    urinary excretion of 62
Stomach cancer 384
Stool, involuntary loss of 206
Strassman procedure 10
Streptococcus 220
    pneumoniae 35
Stress 54
    incontinence 21
    test 209
    urinary incontinence 199f, 208, 210
Stroke 351, 352
Stroma, echogenic 246f
Stromal tumor, mixed endometrial 395
Struma ovarii 247
Subdermal estrogen implants 351
Suction cannula 224, 224f
    uses 224
Sulbactam 122
Suprapubic mass, large 389f
Surface epithelial
    inclusion cysts 243
    stromal tumors 246
Surface-Wetting agents 431
Surgery, cytoreductive 390

Swelling, inguinal 140
Swyer syndrome 331
Symptothermal method 164
Synechiae 240
Syphilis 129, 135, 136, 138
    classification of 135, 136fc
    clinical presentation 135
    congenital 136
    early 137, 138
    gummatous 138
    incubating 138
    late 137t, 138
    management of 137
    organism 135
    primary 135, 137, 151
    secondary 137
    symptomatic late 136
    tertiary 136
    transmission 135
    treatment of 137
Syphilitic ulcer 135
Systemic diseases 54, 94, 95
Systemic lupus erythematosus 355

T

Tabes dorsalis 137
Tadalafil 189
Tamoxifen 22, 217, 396
Tanner's staging 43t
Tears 145
Teeth 355
Telescopes 300
Tenaculum 222, 223f
Tenesmus 110
Tenofovir plus emtricitabine 148
Tension free vaginal tape 211f
Teratoma
    immature 247, 386f, 387
    mature 158
Terminal hair 323
Testes
    ectopic 335
    unilateral 32
Testicular feminization 336
    syndrome 95, 97, 333, 335
Testicular hormones, absence of 5
Testosterone 69, 185, 313, 324, 330
    stimulates 329, 335
    exogenous 31
Thalassemia 56, 94
Thayer-Martin media 129
Theca cell 14, 14f
    tumors 159
Theca lutein cysts 243
Thecoma 247, 396
Thelarche 309
    isolated premature 46
Thermachoice III uterine balloon system 90

Thermal balloon ablation 90
Three swab test 214t
Thrombocytopenia 53
Thromboembolism 104
    venous 23, 343, 348, 349, 352
Thrombophilias 351
Thyroid
    dysfunction 87
    hormone 308
    replacement 39
    stimulating hormone 49, 51, 54, 314
Tibial nerve stimulator, posterior 211
Tibolone 356
Tinidazole 131
Tissue, ectopic 152
Torsion 23
Toxic shock syndrome 166
Toxoplasma 145
Tranexamic acid 55, 56, 89
Transabdominal scan 237f, 242
Transabdominal surgical repair 215
Transabdominal survey scan 87
Transdermal patch 169
Transformation zone 365
    large loop excision of 367, 376
Transitional cell
    carcinoma 407, 408f
    tumors 247
Transvaginal color Doppler 231
    scan 245f, 247f
    sonogram 239f
Transvaginal probe 19
Transvaginal scan 232f, 235f, 239f, 242f, 244f
Transvaginal sonogram 246f, 249f
Transvaginal sonography 87
    high resolution 231
Transvaginal ultrasound 110
Transverse vaginal septum 49, 51, 71
Trauma 38
Treponema pallidum 137
    infection 136, 139
Treponemal enzyme immunoassay 137
Treponemal pallidum 137
Treponemata 137
Trichloroacetic acid 141
Trichomonas 35
    vaginalis 70, 130, 131
    vaginitis
        clinical features 130
        investigations 131
        treatment 131
Triglycerides 147
Trocar 300f
Trophoblastic malignancy 413
Tropical azole group antifungal 132
Tubal factor 338
Tubal pregnancy, ectopic 412
Tubercle
    echogenic 247f
    presence of 288f

Tubercular bacillus 118
Tuberculin test 286
Tuberculosis 51, 145, 279, 285
    genitourinary 285
    vulval 286
Tubo-ovarian complex 245
Tuboplasty 123, 293
Tubule dysgenesis, seminiferous 330
Tumor 386f
    adrenal 59, 60
    adrenocortical 62
    benign 239
        mucinous 247f
    cystic 157t
    endometrioid 246
    epithelial 152, 394
        trophoblastic 411, 415
    infiltration 429
    markers, serum 69f, 368
    mass, large 417f
    maternal 333
    metastatic 243, 248
    mixed epithelial-nonepithelial 395
    mucinous 246
    nonepithelial 151, 394
    pituitary 52, 217
    serous 246
    sessile 295
    stromal 243, 247
    trophoblastic 425
Turner's syndrome 8, 32, 47, 52, 57, 94-97, 313, 329, 331
    stigmata of 48
Two cell, two gonadotropin system 14f
Twombley-Ulfelder technique, modified 405

U

Uchida technique 176, 176f
Ulceration, severe 433
Ulcerative granulomatous disease, chronic 140
Ulcers 140
    vulval 151
Ulipristal acetate 171
Ultrasonography, transabdominal 115
Ultrasound
    abdominal 287
    scan 217
Umbilical
    area, cross-section view of 275f
    cord cutting scissor 227, 227f
    trocar insertion 275, 276f
United Nations Population Fund 102
Upper vagina 95, 329
    examination of 30
Uremia 429
Ureteral reconstruction, surgical techniques of 282t

Ureteric colic 279, 280
Ureteric injury 268, 282
    causes of 282b
Ureteric reimplantation 282
Ureteroneocystostomy 283f
Ureteroureterostomy, end-to-end 283f
Urethra 199, 207, 207f, 211f, 405, 408f
Urethral catheter 211f
Urethral prolapse 36
Urethral sphincter, external 207f
Urethritis 129
Urethrocele 201
Urethrovesical angle, mobility of 199f
Urge incontinence 208, 211, 212
Urinary bladder 207, 207f, 211f
Urinary diseases 70
Urinary fistula 213, 379
Urinary incontinence 20, 207-208, 210, 355
    causes of 209
    classification 208
    pathophysiology 207
    prevalence 207
    types of 208, 208t, 210
Urinary infection 209
Urinary pregnancy test 414
Urinary problems 379
Urinary sphincter, artificial 210
Urinary symptoms 21, 130
Urinary system 110
Urinary tract 267
    anomalies, upper 334
    infection 121, 267, 279, 346
        recurrent 355
    injuries 267
Urine 145
    involuntary loss of 206
    microscopy 210
    protein 147
Urogenital ducts 4f, 5f
Urogenital membrane 6
Urogenital sinus 4, 6, 329
Uropathy, obstructive 433
Urorectal septum 4
    fusion of 5f
Uterine abnormalities 53, 81
Uterine adenosarcoma 395, 396
Uterine anomalies 9
Uterine artery ligation 265f
Uterine bleeding
    abnormal 20, 53, 84, 87, 377
        acute 86
        chronic 86
        classification of 84
        common complaint of 87
        evaluation of 86
        FIGO classification of 85
        management 88
Uterine cancer 394, 396
Uterine cavity 90, 412f, 413
    diseases of 236

Uterine choriocarcinoma, appearance of 416f
Uterine corpus carcinoma 248
Uterine curette 223
Uterine descent 193
    pull of 198
    Shaw's degrees of 194t
Uterine didelphys 8
Uterine displacements 290
Uterine fibroids 236f
Uterine inversion 290, 293
    degrees of 294f
Uterine ligaments 245
Uterine malignancy 393
    epidemiology 394
    histopathology 394
    risk factors 394
Uterine manipulator 300
Uterine masses, cavitated 82
Uterine myoma 338
Uterine perforation 105
Uterine polyps 156
Uterine prolapse 201
    complete 296
Uterine relaxants 294
Uterine sarcoma 296, 397
    high grade undifferentiated 394
Uterine segment, lower 267
Uterine shape 234
    abnormal 235f
Uterine sound 222, 222f, 303
    uses 222
Uterine tubes 329
Uterine vessel 269, 282f
    clamping of 265f
    ligation 270f
Uterine wall 94
Uterosacral ligaments 198
Uterosacral nerve ablation, laparoscopic 114
Uterovaginal prolapse 21, 202, 203t
Uterovesical fold 266f
Uterus 9, 26, 95, 109, 193, 206, 207f, 214f, 231f, 232, 232f, 234f, 239, 261, 266f, 287f, 290-293, 329
    anteverted 231f, 290f, 292f
    benign tumors 152
        classification 153
        expectant management 155
        hysterectomy 155
        intramural 153
        microscopic appearance 154
        pathophysiology 153
        signs 153
        subserosal 153
        symptoms 153
    development of 5
    didelphys 234
        nonobstructed 10
    double 10f
    evaluation of 234

fundus of 237f
heterogenous 239f
intact 353
investigation of 340
lateral displacement of 291
malignant disease of 393
measures 232
parts of 234
retroflexed 291f
retroverted 232f, 290f-292f
small 242f
subseptus 8f
T-shaped 234
ultrasound of 234
unicollis 234, 235f
unicornuate 7, 7f, 8
upward displacement of 290
wall of 4189f

V

Vacuum
  aspiration 106
  delivery 229
  devices 189
  extractor 229
Vagina 9, 207f, 242, 346
  absent 51
  benign lesions of 152
  carcinoma of 401
  development of 6
  distended 242f
  double 10f
  noncanalization of 9
  short 51
  single 10f
  upper third of 261
  visualization of 25
Vaginal abnormalities 53
Vaginal agenesis 9
  surgical management of 9
Vaginal angles 266f
Vaginal approach 177
Vaginal atresia 71
Vaginal bleeding 30, 396, 416
  intermittent 295
  irregular 295
Vaginal brachytherapy 399
Vaginal cancer 425
Vaginal candidiasis 146
Vaginal cuff 200
Vaginal cysts 152
Vaginal delivery 135
Vaginal diaphragms 165, 166
  advantages 165
  disadvantages 165
  side effects 166
Vaginal discharge 35, 70, 70t, 130, 377
  abnormal 21, 396
  causes of 35, 70t

persistent 30
  premenarchal 35
Vaginal dryness 21, 343, 346
Vaginal epithelium 202f
Vaginal estrogen therapy 346
Vaginal examination 45, 209
Vaginal flora 35
Vaginal hysterectomy, laparoscopically
  assisted 298
Vaginal irrigation 36
Vaginal irritation 35
Vaginal laceration 105
Vaginal length, total 195f
Vaginal lumen 408f
Vaginal mass pelvic organ prolapse 200t
Vaginal metastasis 416
  of choriocarcinoma, typical location
    of 416f
Vaginal mycoses, treatment of 281
Vaginal operations 268
Vaginal packing 271
Vaginal prolapse 193
Vaginal reconstruction operations 11
Vaginal repair 214
Vaginal retractor, anterior 222f
Vaginal ring 169
Vaginal secretions 130
Vaginal speculum examination 377
Vaginal support, Delancey's levels of 197f
Vaginal tablets 132
Vaginal tape 210
Vaginal tuberculosis 286
Vaginal vault 271f
  closure of 267f
  prolapse 201
Vaginismus 183
Vaginitis 38, 129
Vaginoplasty, sigmoid 10
Vague symptoms 21
Valaciclovir 134
Vardenafil 189
Varicose veins 282
Vas deferens, congenital absence of 338
Vascular injuries 284
Vasectomy 178
  reversible 178
Vasomotor symptoms 21
Vault prolapse 22, 193, 203
Vecchietti and Davydov procedures 10
Venereal disease 137
Venlafaxine 429
Veress needle 274, 300, 301,301f
  insertion of 275f
Vesicocervical plane 269f
Vesicouterine fistula 213f, 215
Vesicovaginal fistula 105, 209, 213f, 214
  clinical presentation 214
  diagnosis 214
  types 214
Viagra 189
Villus hair, conversion of 323

Vincristine 389
Viral infections 35
Virilization, presence of 325
Virus colonize 133
Viscero-fascial layer 196
Vital signs, monitoring of 264, 271
Vitamin
  D
    insufficiency 349
    supplementation 349
  D_2 349
  D_3 349
Vomiting 66, 429, 430
  causes of 430t
von Willebrand disease 85
Vulsellum forceps 222, 223f
  disadvantages 222
  uses 222
Vulva 45, 132
  benign lesions of 150
    classification 150
  benign tumors of 151
  cancer 403f
    varies, incidence of 401
  carcinoma of 21, 401, 407, 407f
  extensive squamous cell carcinoma
    of 403f
  extramammary Paget's disease of 408,
    408f, 409f
  lower 402f
  malignant melanoma of 407
  Paget's disease 409f
  squamous cell carcinoma of 402f
  tuberculosis of 286
Vulval diseases 70
Vulval lesion 409f
Vulvar cancer 401
  diagnosis 403
  etiology 401
  management of 404
  pattern of spread 403
  special situations 405
Vulvar hygiene 34
Vulvar irritation 408
Vulvar lesion 408
Vulvar malignancies 407
Vulvar pruritus 408
Vulvar sarcomas 407
Vulvitis 33, 129
Vulvovaginal candidiasis 131, 132
  chronic 132
    treatment 132
  clinical features 132
  investigations 132
  organism 131
  predisposing factors 131
  recurrent 133
  treatment 132
Vulvovaginal complaints 70
Vulvovaginal disorders 33
Vulvovaginal masses 21b

Vulvovaginitis 34, 35, 66
    infectious 35
    nonspecific 34

W

Wart 152
Waterfall sign 241f
Web neck 96
Weeping umbilicus 23
Weight loss 145
Wertheim's hysterectomy 261
WHO eligibility criteria, revised 163
WHO prognostic scoring system, modified 418t
William's vaginoplasty 52
William's vulvovaginoplasty 10
Wilson's disease 94
Wolffian ducts 4, 329
    degenerate 329
    structures 331
Women's Health Initiative Study 348
Wounds
    dehiscence 268
    malodorous 434

X

X-chromosome 328
    normal 28
    partial deletion of 48

X-linked testicular feminization syndrome 333
X-spermatozoa 328

Y

Yolk sac tumor 69, 247
Yoon ring 176

Z

Zidovudine 148
    plus lamivudine 148
Zolendronate 433